Handbook of Life Stress,
Cognition and Health

Handbook of Life Stress, Cognition and Health

SHIRLEY FISHER
Department of Psychology,
The University of Dundee,
Scotland

and

JAMES REASON
Department of Psychology,
The University of Manchester,
England

JOHN WILEY & SONS
Chichester · New York · Brisbane · Toronto · Singapore

Library of Congress Cataloging-in-Publication Data:

Handbook of life stress, cognition, and health.

  Includes bibliographies.
    1. Medicine, Psychosomatic. 2. Stress (Psychology)
3. Cognition. 4. Health. I. Fisher, S. (Shirley)
II. Reason, J. T. [DNLM: 1. Cognition. 2. Health.
3. Life Change Events. 4. Stress, Psychological.
WM 172 H2364]
RC49.H326 1988   616.08   87-34096
ISBN 0 471 91269 7

British Library Cataloguing in Publication Data:

Handbook of life stress, cognition and
  health.
  1. Stress (Psychology) 2. Stress
  (Physiology)
  I. Fisher, Shirley   II. Reason, James
  155.9   BF575.S75

  ISBN 0 471 91269 7

Typeset by Inforum Ltd, Portsmouth
Printed and bound in Great Britain by
Anchor Brendon Ltd, Colchester, Essex

To Reg Pittman

Contents

**Section V: Cognitive Developments with Implications for Coping
                   and Health**

List of Contributors

WOLFGANG BATTMANN: *Institute fur Psychologie der Freie Universitat, Berlin, West Germany.*

ADINA BIRNBAUM: *Department of Psychology, Temple University, Philadelphia, Pennsylvania, USA.*

BRUCE BOMAN: *Department of Veterans Affairs, Repatriation General Hospital, Concorde, New South Wales, Australia.*

CLARE BRADLEY: *Department of Psychology, The University of Sheffield, UK.*

CHRIS R. BREWIN: *MRC Social Psychiatry Unit, The Maudsley Hospital, London, UK.*

GEORGE W. BROWN: *Department of Social Policy and Social Science, Royal Holloway and Bedford College, The University of London, UK.*

JENNIFER BROWN: *Department of Psychology, The University of Surrey, UK.*

RACHEL BRYANT-WAUGH: *Department of Psychological Medicine, The Hospital for Sick Children, Great Ormond Street, London, UK.*

BRAM P. BUUNK: *Department of Psychology, The University of Nijmegen, The Netherlands.*

FRANCES CLEGG: *The National Hospital for Nervous Diseases, Maida Vale, London, UK.*

RAYMOND COCHRANE: *Department of Psychology, The University of Birmingham, UK.*

CARY L. COOPER: *Department of Management Sciences, The University of Manchester, UK.*

TOM COX *Department of Psychology, The University of Nottingham, UK.*

CLIFF C. CUNNINGHAM: *Hester Adrian Research Centre, The University of Manchester, UK.*

JOHN BOOTH DAVIES: *Department of Psychology, The University of Strathclyde, Glasgow, UK.*

D. DOWLATSHAHI: *Department of Psychiatry, St George's Hospital Medical School, London, UK.*

INEZ DOOTJES DUSSUYER: *Community Services Victoria, Melbourne, Australia.*

JOSEPH EYER, *Department of Anatomy, The University of Pennsylvania School of Medicine, Philadelphia, USA.*

MICHAEL W. EYSENCK: *Department of Psychology, Royal Holloway and Bedford New College, The University of London, London, UK.*

SHIRLEY FISHER: *Department of Psychology, The University of Dundee, Scotland, UK.*

ABE FOSSON: *Department of Pedriatrics, Albert Chandler Medical Center, The University of Kentucky, USA.*

DAVID FRYER: *Department of Psychology, The University of Stirling, Scotland, UK.*

PAUL GILBERT: *Pastures Hospital, Derby, UK.*

IAN GOODYER: *Department of Psychiatry, The University of Cambridge, UK.*

IAN HOWARTH: *Department of Psychology, The University of Nottingham, UK.*

RONNIE JANOFF-BULMAN: *Department of Psychology, The University of Massachusetts, Amherst, USA.*

MARIE JOHNSTON: *Psychology Unit, The Royal Free Hospital of Medicine, London, UK.*

CHRISTINA KNUSSEN: *Hester Adrian Research Centre, The University of Manchester, UK.*

MARSHA M. LINEHAN: *Department of Psychology, The University of Washington, Seattle, USA.*

JANET E. MALLEY: *Department of Psychology, The University of Boston, USA.*

FRANS H.G. MARCELISSEN: *TNO Institute of Preventive Health Care, Leiden, The Netherlands.*

SUZANNE M. MILLER: *Department of Psychology, Temple University, Philadelphia, Pennsylvania, USA.*

RUDOLF H. MOOS: *Social Ecology Laboratory, Department of Psychiatry and Behavioral Sciences, Stanford University and Veterans Administration Medical Centers, Palo Alto, California, USA.*

KEITH OATLEY: *Department of Psychology, The University of Glasgow, Scotland, UK.*

FIONA O'DOHERTY: *Department of Psychology, The University of Strathclyde, Glasgow, Scotland, UK.*

EUGENE PAYKEL: *Department of Psychiatry, The University of Cambridge, UK.*

JAMES W. PENNEBAKER: *Department of Psychology, The Southern Methodist University, Dallas, Texas, USA.*

RICHARD RAHE: *Department of Psychiatry, The University of Nevada School of Medicine, Reno, Nevada, USA.*

JAMES REASON: *Department of Psychology, The University of Manchester, UK.*

MICHAEL ROSENBAUM: *Department of Psychology, The University of Tel-Aviv, Israel.*

YONA TEICHMAN: *Department of Psychology, The University of Tel-Aviv, Israel.*

RICHARD TOTMAN: *Department of Experimental Psychology, The University of Sussex, UK.*

WOLFGANG SCHÖNPFLUG: *Institut fuř Psychologie der Freie Universität Berlin, West Germany.*

EWARD N. SHEARIN: *Department of Psychology, The University of Washington, Seattle, USA.*

PETER STERLING: *Department of Anatomy, The University of Pennsylvania School of Medicine, Philadelphia, USA.*

ABIGAIL J. STEWART, *Department of Psychology, The University of Boston, USA.*

DANIEL M. WEGNER: *Department of Psychology, Trinity University, San Antonio, Texas, USA.*

JACQUES A.M. WINNUBST: *Department of Clinical Psychology, State University of Utrecht, The Netherlands.*

Preface

BACKGROUND TO THE HANDBOOK

Within the last 25 years there has been increasing interest in the effects of stressful life events on human behaviour, efficiency, welfare and health. During the same period, research into the biological and clinical aspects of disease has resulted in an increased awareness of the importance of elusive factors such as morale and the determination to recover, or in some cases to die, as factors in the progress of disease. What used to be thought of as psychosomatic medicine is now fast becoming the domain of modern medical science.

Perhaps the most useful illustration of the role of psychological factors in health is the statistical data provided by Berkson (1962), some of which is reproduced in Chapter 32. The divorced are shown to be more at risk for a variety of physical illnesses as well as for accidents and suicide as compared with single or married individuals; the single fare worse than the married in this respect. The roles of marital status and social status in general have been confirmed as factors in the risk of ill-health by other studies (see, for example, Dodge and Martin, 1970). Data from UK records confirm the vulnerability of the widowed, especially immediately following the death of their spouse; men over 55 years of age have mortality rates which are 40% above the expected rate for age-matched married groups (Connolly, 1975). On first consideration, it is hard to escape the conclusion that not being married can damage your health, although as Cochrane (Chapter 8) shows, there are some contradictions in this respect.

There are, however, numerous difficulties in the interpretation of findings such as these. Firstly, statistical associations do not imply causation: more drivers wearing seat belts are involved in car accidents and yet no-one would want to argue that the wearing of seat belts causes car accidents. Even when causal links can be more reliably established in the context of prospective studies, the direction of causation cannot be easily anchored. The life event may be cause or consequence of a particular disorder or there may be some third, unknown, factor which influences both the event and the disorder. Self-selection factors may also operate; the established link between, for example, geographical mobility and health (see Chapter 3) could be explained in terms of self-selection factors—maybe the ambitious or the unhappy are more likely to migrate.

Investigation of relationships for specific cases of illness involves further problems relating to validity. Self-report of life history events may be subject to error. The bias towards making sense of a current illness in terms of the events which precede it is so well established in the literature on stress and coronary heart disease that the phrase 'effort after meaning' is commonly used to describe the tendency of patients to over-report stressful life events. There is evidence to suggest that depression, whether occurring as a primary condition or as a secondary factor accompanying illness, might bias recall in favour of unhappy life events (see, for example, Rappaport, 1961; Lloyd and Lishman, 1975).

Explaining a valid association between a stressful experience and ill-health is difficult. There may be behavioural links between certain experiences and ill-health (see Chapter 32). There may be differences in the attitude of others to the victim of adversity, and this might be especially likely following a divorce or bereavement. George Brown (Chapter 24) has indicated that a possible link between early parental loss and subsequent depression in adult life is the lack of care-giving from remaining relatives. There may be more direct effects on cognitive and biological state. Trait anxiety might, for example, change the parameters of the perceptions of threatening objects (see Eysenck, Chapter 25). Prolonged states of distress and anxiety caused by protracted stressful experiences might create biological memories which could trigger reminiscence of unhappy events (see the psychobiological model of depression proposed by Gilbert, Chapter 31). Moreover, continuous high levels of arousal could increase the risk of functional abuse of bodily systems, leading to structural changes, or create states of immunosuppression thus weakening the body's defence against antigens.

THE IMPORTANCE OF COGNITIVE FACTORS

This volume emphasizes the linking and moderating role played by a person's knowledge of himself, his efficiencies and skills, and the world around him, in understanding the impact and outcome of life stresses. In order to show how interest in this area has evolved, it is useful to consider the development and shortcomings of the main approaches in historical perspective.

The need to provide a valid measure for the assessment of the incidence and magnitude of life events was recognized in the mid-sixties in response to clinical observations concerning the prevalence of stressful events in the immediate life history of physically ill patients (see Holmes and Rahe, 1965). The resulting Social Readjustment Rating Scale consisted of 42 items, developed from the ratings of physically well populations, concerning the stressful nature of life events, relative to marriage, which was given a base value of 500. A weighting for each item on the scale based on the scores was then calculated (average score per item/10), and the resulting score in terms of Life Change Units could be used to compare individuals who were ill with matched counterparts, either prospectively or retrospectively, to predict illness. A great deal of research was devoted to the assessment of the predictive validity of the scale, which assumed that life events were additive in changing the risk of illness. The general conclusion was that there was some predictive validity, especially for illness in general, although the power to predict specific illnesses was often of marginal significance (see Birley and Connolly, 1976). Even in the case of cardiovascular disease, the predictive validity may be improved by the addition of key variables. Rahe (Chapter 17) identifies 'emotional' factors such as hostility, home problems, life dissatisfaction, as well as 'behavioural' factors such as overwork and time urgency as those which need consideration.

One of the reasons why the predictive validity of a preweighted, additive scale of stressful life events might be low is the failure to take into account the prevailing circumstance at the time of the event, as well as background factors in the life of the individual. The death of a pet bird may be as important to an old and lonely person as the death of a person, and may even convey the symbolic losses associated with earlier bereavements.

In response to the problem of including 'personal meanings', Brown (1974) developed an interview procedure which involved careful attempts to obtain details of contextual aspects of life events. Although time consuming, the approach, researched mainly with psychiatric groups, provided a more sensitive measure. In the case of the death of a pet bird, for example, the overall circumstance such as the life, age and loneliness of the person who looks after the bird could be taken into account in determining the impact. The greatest difficulty with contextual analysis is that much still depends on the intuitions of the investigators as to the overall weighting that should be given.

The introduction of the issue of 'personal meanings' now provides the challenge for the cognitive scientist and is compatible with existing cognitive and clinical research interests. Research into the response to a wide variety of life events indicates large differences in sensitivity and reaction. Some people seem to survive the most horrendous of life experiences and others seem to break down or become disturbed by apparently lesser threats. A probabilistic model developed by Schulberg and Sheldon (1968) assumes that the probability the event will occur, that the individual will be exposed to the event, and the existence of counterharm resources combine multiplicately to determine outcome. Fisher (1984) provided the grounds for distinguishing 'extrinsic' and 'intrinsic' risk factors in crisis and illness. Extrinsic risk represents vulnerability levels which evolve from the outcomes of previous experience: thus an orphaned child would be expected to have a higher extrinsic risk of adverse reaction to a stressful experience in later adult life. Intrinsic risk factors are dictated by the contextual and central elements of a particular stressful experience. The two forms of risk are multiplicative determinants of outcome and were argued to be manifest in bias in decision making concerned with personal and interpersonal control.

Research on the effects of specific life stresses (such as bereavement, divorce, work stress, unemployment, assault) on the individual increasingly provides identification of complex moderating variables which appear to be influential. In particular, perceived control or helplessness, level of self-esteem, attributional style and the tendency to accept or reject blame for negative outcomes, cognitive failure level, learned resourcefulness and hardiness, self-image, social disruption, rule breakdown, prevailing or state conditions such as anxiety, are forming the focus for intensive research programmes. Research into these concepts, although necessarily complex, offers great insight into the precise nature of the literature with environmental contingencies and may well influence the therapies of the future.

In compiling this volume, a particular focus has been, therefore, the role of the structure and utilization of personal knowledge as an essential part of the perception and response to stress. This includes knowledge of both reality and self. The approach provides the potential for insight into how 'personal meanings' arise, how contexts and situations are influential and why illness is an outcome on some occasions and not others.

There are obvious implications for preventative medicine. If we can understand the factors that affect the risk of illness, then it might well be possible to find ways to educate the victims of unfortunate experiences in terms of the skills for coping and avoiding later illness penalties. It is not at all obvious why some events in life are so devastating in impact and yet others have only minor effects. This alone raises a major problem for the understanding of the sorts of ways a person appraises the threat imposed by the world around him.

Jennifer Brown's account, in Chapter 7, of the impact of threats associated with the building of nuclear reactors and the occurrence of nuclear accidents, suggests that the level and prevalence of fear and worry in sampled populations are less than might be supposed given the magnitude of the effects of an error; the effect of stress created by, for example, personal relationships at work, or unemployment, is likely to be much greater.

How do we explain such differences? Perhaps it is necessary to take into account the perceived likelihood of a nuclear accident, the belief in the protection afforded by the state for its citizens, or the sense of uninvolvement that is created by implementation of an essentially new technology when there is lack of detailed information on its performance and the consequence of error. These are aspects of a person's knowledge which will determine the sorts of threats that are pertinent. It is possible that low frequency events, albeit of high consequence, are not pertinent in the thinking of most people. Thus car accidents, aircraft accidents etc., will not govern daily thinking unless they become high probability events. When the likelihood of a terrorist attack on trans-Atlantic flights increased because of the Libyan crisis, there was a reported boycot of American tourist flights to London. The probability of an air disaster had changed and the behaviour of the public reflected the perceived increased risk.

By contrast, personal catastrophies such as financial disasters, personal loss or illness and handicap may be perceived as more probable sources of threat given relevant circumstances. They are threats to security and existing lifestyle. The probability of an adult experiencing a significant bereavement is high; after all, one of every married couple will have to endure the death of the other. The potential for anticipating these threats and 'worrying in advance' could be much greater than for low probability albeit high cost environmental accidents.

Increasingly, research into the effects of specific stresses is beginning to emphasize the importance of ruminative activity which may occur in prospect or in retrospect. The powerful ideational components of depression were identified by Beck in his work in the 1970s with psychiatric groups; appropriate ideations could be easily triggered by specific remarks and relevant ideational content was found to feature in the dreams of these patients (see, for example, Beck, 1967; 1970). The triggering of the relevant thoughts was found to be capable of driving the appropriate affective states.

The importance of worrying and ruminative activity as factors in the risk of illness was explored by Fisher (1986). Persistent ruminative activity, whether externally or internally controlled, may have functional origins in allowing old plans to be gradually replaced as new situations arise, or in providing the anticipatory activity necessary for setting up the appropriate plans for dealing with contingencies relevant to threatening situations. Chapter 5, by Johnston, identifies some of the sources of worry for patients awaiting surgical operations. The sources may be expected to vary between individuals, but involve themes concerned with all aspects of the circumstances of impending surgery.

A number of chapters on specific stresses have noted the importance of mental preoccupations. 'Living with the dead' has long been recognized as a major feature of bereavement and may be attributed to a focus based on a primitive need to search for the lost person. This absorption with the cause of grief serves to propagate it, and yet internal control over the mental process itself may be difficult. Fisher (Chapter 3) identifies the strong compulsive, ruminative activity which is contingent on leaving home for between 50% and 70% of most school and student populations. Constantly thinking about home could drive physiological states of anxiety and depression which raise the risk of illness in the long term. Moreover, the existence of such states reduces the possibility of a commitment to the new environment because of preoccupation with irrelevant thoughts.

Although perhaps initially functional, states of ruminative activity serve to retain the problem (or rehearse its impact in advance) and may prolong the existence of adverse hormone states. Fisher (Chapter 32) argues that the risk of ill-health is increased as a function of the magnitude, duration and frequency of stress hormone levels. Thus, being able to control a stressful problem means that there is a constraint on the duration of the hormone states that accompany that problem. Conversely, loss of control implies protracted experience, with implications for the duration and frequency of elevated hormone levels; control, in effect, is determined externally.

One consequence of use of mental resources for ruminative activity is reduction of attentional capacity available for other aspects of life. States of absent-mindedness indexed by measures of cognitive failure have been found to be sensitive to exposure to stressful environments and may have 'state' properties in that those high in absent-mindedness are more likely to react adversely to stressful environments (see Reason, Chapter 22).

The role of inefficiency as a determinant of the feedback loops which potentiate further stress was identified by Fisher (1984); inefficiencies have a direct effect on the world outside and may be responsible for new problems. Equally, there may be changes in confidence and self-esteem as a function of perceived inefficiency, especially when a person does not make allowances for circumstances or accepts the blame for unfortunate consequences.

Pennebaker (Chapter 36) provides a sound case for the therapeutic reduction of ruminative activity. Those who are encouraged to talk or write about their problems may gain benefits (even if they lose friends in the process!). Wegner (Chapter 37) shows how difficult it might to be practise direct suppression of ruminative content. Merely trying not to think about a specified object by attempting to activate alternative thoughts may be self-defeating; the alternative thoughts then become linked to the undesirable thought content and can trigger it. Hence, the development of obsessive thinking may be a further consequence.

Schönpflug and Battmann (Chapter 38) provide some convincing arguments for the suggestion that coping with stress may have negative as much as beneficial consequences. Problems labelled by others as self-induced may be a consequence of an attempted coping strategy which has not been made explicit. It could well be argued that attempts to interfere with the persistence of ruminative activity might create some unfortunate side-effects. Perhaps when confronting stressful life events and stressful problems, thinking can damage your health, but trying not to think can make it worse! An alternative to direct attenuation of ruminative activity or exhaustion by continuous productions of the thoughts is to create competing demands which at least temporarily take up attentional resources and interrupt the adverse effects of ruminative activity (see Fisher, Chapter 3).

The effects of a violent assault such as rape have been shown by Janoff-Bulman (Chapter 6) to have a profound influence on cognitive activity. The victim must come to terms with a step function change in beliefs about the outside world in order to accommodate the fact of the existence of violence and cruelty. This deduction could of course be made from regular reading of the press, but it would appear that a personal experience is more profound and more radical in effect. The victim must also come to terms with personal esteem and the probability of the attack being repeated. Janoff-Bulman notes that attributional decisions may be a very important feature of subsequent adjustment; behavioural blame can lead to a sense of raised control over the occurrence of such an event in the future. She distinguishes this from characterological blame, which would have a more negative implication.

Thus it is useful to distinguish *behavioural* blame, which could be functional in some cases and actually increases control over future threats (thus reducing the probability of their occurrence), and *characterological* blame, which may be associated with depression and loss of control. Repeated episodes of behavioural blame might however eventually lead to characterological blame if there is a logical tendency to make the inductive generalization from behavioural blame to a more abstract concept of personal responsibility.

The role of attributional style as a major factor influencing the effects of adversity is presented by Brewin (Chapter 23) and underlines the importance of the way information might be utilized in these decisions. One suggestion of importance is that blame should be partitioned into feelings of causal responsibility (self-blame) as compared with culpability (avoidability). On this analysis, the tendency to generalize from particular incidents of behavioural blame to more global self-blame concepts often found prevalent as themes in the cognition of the depressed, could be prevented. In general, the perception of control may have either negative or positive consequences for the individual as a function of circumstances. Again, the role of situational factors and personal meanings is emphasized.

There are important causal implications of the widespread recognition of the significance of psychogenic explanations of illness. On first consideration, a consequence is that responsibility (and control) is given back to the patient.

Smokers may have become used to feeling guilty about the habit and feeling responsible for their own chest ailments; those with cardiovascular disease may be led to feel that they are behaviourally responsible (and this to a Type A personality means failure). Other groups may also be made to feel responsible for their own conditions. The attributional tendencies which arise when the protection of the medical model is reduced should be taken seriously by clinicians and therapists.

In emphasizing a psychogenic approach, there is no denial of the influence of other factors such as genetic dispositions, diet, or exercise. We are essentially considering a probabalistic model in which stress factors create risk. Thus it is perfectly possible for a person living an apparently high stress existence, who is isolated and lonely, to remain healthy, just as it is possible for some cigarette smokers to reach old age.

There is a need for caution in assuming that causal factors once identified can be utilized as part of the cure. The fact that smoking causes lung cancer does not mean that giving up smoking will reverse the condition. Just this assumption is sometimes made by those who adhere to psychogenic principles in explaining illness: thus, if loss of control is shown to be a major factor in a particular illness, restoring control cannot be assumed necessarily to benefit the illness. Causal and ameliorating roles of cognitive variables in illness need to be independently investigated. When once biological changes have taken place, reversibility may not be that easy.

There is, however, a major role for the development of the understanding of cognitive mediators of life stress and health in preventative medicine. On the assumption that most people experience major stresses in their lives from time to time, methods of coping with those stresses could be made explicit. Perhaps once, in more religious climates, ministers of religion accepted the role of confident and provided social support not available through family or friends. Perhaps more latterly, the role has fallen to busy general medical practitioners. Maybe trained professionals could occupy this role. It has to be remembered that both nationalized health services and insurance companies benefit from reduction in patient input. Trained professionals in stress management may ultimately be cost saving and should reduce the strain on the health-care professions.

THE PSYCHOBIOLOGICAL BASIS OF ILLNESS

No attempt to make sense of the relationship between life events and disease would be complete without exploring the relationship with existing biological 'markers' or vulnerabilities, in relation to the biological changes which result from human decision making. Ultimately, the preparations for infectious and chronic disease must be understood in terms of short- and long-term changes in biological and biochemical state. The way in which there is facilitation for, or attenuation of, incoming antigens must be understood in terms of the complex interplay of various aspects of the body's immunological defence mechanisms. The way in which functional abuse of cardiovascular systems may prepare the way for anatomical changes which raise the risk of cardiovascular illness must be understood. Ultimately, there is a need to link psychological concepts concerning decision making in life with accompanying biological states. The most obvious links to explore are those provided by hormone states which change metabolic function and which are themselves stress sensitive. The stress hormones may play this vital linking role.

The distinction between homeostasis and allostasis is made by Sterling and Hyer in Chapter 34. Biological activity (demand) is argued to rise to meet the essential demands imposed by a threatening situation rather than to reflect a homeostatic adjustment to it. A different perspective is taken through the complex dynamics of the total response to stress and leads to different predictions. One outcome is that harmonious biological states of equilibrium may be overridden during a stressful experience. Human decision becomes an important precursor of pathological arousal states and hence the risk of illness.

The key question of individual differences in susceptibility to different types of illness remains a mystery, but the approach through the impact of human decision might help to partition and thus unravel some of the complex biological changes which specify the risks selectively. Some biological patterns might trigger auto-immune reactions, raising the risk of a number of chronic states. Others may interact with existing biological markers to influence anatomical changes. Others may impair the immune response and increase the risk of an antigen becoming established, or may attenuate natural killer cell activity and increase the risk of the survival of cancerous divisions.

THE ORGANIZATION OF THE VOLUME

In Section I, some of the most well-established researchers who work with specific stress conditions such as bereavement, unemployment, divorce and stress at work have been invited to try to provide an indication of the psychological and physical impact of particular stresses and to locate the common denominators relevant to the causes of strain. Once thought to be the domain of social psychology and social psychiatry, this research is now of such relevance as to be of interest to medical and cognitive science.

In Section II, a number of leading researchers who have researched factors in specific illnesses and disorders such as cardiovascular disease, cancer, diabetic disorder, depression, anorexia nervosa as well as abnormal behaviours such as drug addiction, parasuicide and suicide, provide evidence of the role of stressful life events as causal or moderating variables in the progress and treatment of the condition.

In Section III, we have drawn from the talents of clinical, social, experimental psychologists, cognitive scientists and sociologists to try to develop a better understanding of the way in which different sociocognitive concepts are of importance in understanding the impact of threatening experiences.

In Section IV, there are some attempts to develop psychobiological models in which human decision is linked to biological response and ultimately to the risk of disorder. There are illustrations with respect to a variety of disease processes and to depression.

In Section V, some of the implications of the cognitive involvement in the stress–illness relationship are explored in terms of new issues in management and coping. We have selected researchers whose contributions are innovative and who make new points of relevance to the understanding of coping and stress management.

FINAL COMMENTS

It is intended that this book will be of interest to all those groups in teaching, research and clinical practice who have an interest in stress and mental or physical disorders. It has been impossible to comment on the innovative content of many of the chapters in the volume. Collectively they do present a story with recurring themes highlighted from different perspectives.

I am indebted to the authors who have been so cooperative in producing accounts which combine the skills needed to provide up-to-date accounts of modern research in ways that create readable text, accessible to a variety of professional groups. The demands of writing about broad issues and detailed research findings within relatively small space limitations became, for some, a form of 'author-stress' but was necessary if we were to produce all these contributions within the same volume.

In common with other editors, I too have learned that it is easier to write a book than act as editor. I am grateful to many of my colleagues in Dundee and at La Trobe University in Melbourne, where I spent a term during the preparation of the volume, for helpful encouragement and, most importantly, for tolerance of my absent-mindedness.

I am grateful to so many of the authors for helpful comments and much appreciated encouragements. I would especially like to thank Dr Chris Brewin, The Maudsley Hospital, London; Dr Paul Gilbert, Pastures Hospital, Derby; Professor Danny Wegner, The Department of Psychology, The University of San Antonio, Texas; Professor Abe Fosson, Department of Pediatrics, The Albert Chandler Medical Center, The University of Kentucky.

I owe a great debt to Mr Alan Wilkes, Department of Psychology, The University of Dundee, for constant support, helpful criticism and much encouragement. I am delighted that Dr Nicholas Wade, The Department of Psychology, The University of Dundee, was persuaded to design the cover for the volume.

Finally, I do not know how my husband put up with the constant intrusions into life at home, but I am very grateful that he did. His encouragement for the venture and tolerance of the side-effects were much appreciated. The fact that he now finds A4 paper threatening is something that we are learning to cope with!

Shirley Fisher
Dundee

REFERENCES

Beck, A.T. (1967). *Depression, clinical, experimental and theoretical aspects*. New York: Harper and Row.

Beck, A.T. (1970). The core problem in depression: the cognitive triad. *Science and Psychoanalysis, 17*, 45–55.

Berkson, J. (1962). Mortality and marital status. Reflections on the derivation of aetiology from statistics. *American Journal of Public Health, 52*, 1318.

Brown, G. (1974). Methodological research on stressful life events. In B.S. Dohrenwend & B.P. Dohrenwend (eds), *Stressful life events*. New York: Wiley.

Connolly, J. (1975). Circumstances, events and illness. *Medicine, 2*,10, 454–458.

Dodge, D.L., & Martin, W.T.(1970). *Social stress and chronic illness*. Indiana: Notre Dame Press.

Fisher, S. (1984). *Stress and the perception of control*. London: Lawrence Erlbaum Associates.

Fisher, S. (1986). *Stress and strategy*. London: Lawrence Erlbaum Associates.

Holmes, T.H., & Rahe, R. (1967). The social readjustment rating scale. *Journal of Psychosomatic Research, 11*, 213–218.

Lloyd, G.G., & Lishman, W.A. (1975). Effects of depression on the speed of recall of pleasant and unpleasant events. *Psychological Medicine, 5*, 173–180.

Rapaport, D. (1961). *Emotions and memory*. The Menninger Clinic Monograph Series No 2. New York: Science Editions.

Schulberg, H., & Sheldon, A. (1968). The probability of crisis and strategies to preventative intervention. *Archives of General Psychiatry, 18*, 553–558.

Acknowledgements

We would like to acknowledge the help given by the following in reading and commenting on specific chapters: Professor Keith Oatley, Dr Nick Emler, Dr David Fryer, Mr Alan Wilkes, Professor Marie Jahoda, Professor Ray Over, Dr Margaret Foddy.

We would like to thank Mrs Marilyn Laird for looking after the correspondence from the contributors during the period of the principal editor's leave in Australia, and Anna Shewan, Mair Rowans, Margaret Grubb, and Anne Anderson for occasional help with letters to contributors. Ms Sarah Griffiths helped compile the indexes.

We would like also to thank all the authors for their careful and thoughtful chapters and for their efforts to meet the deadlines.

We would like to acknowledge the help and encouragement provided by Dr Paul Gilbert, Dr Chris Brewin, Professor Dan Wegner, Professor Abe Fosson and Mr Alan Wilkes.

Finally, we would like to acknowledge the help given by the Publishers. In particular, we would like to thank Wendy Hudlass and Michael Coombs for the considerable help and attention given throughout the preparation of the volume. We would also like to pay tribute to the skill and expertise of Cliff Morgan and the copy editor, Mrs Jane Smith.

The Royal Bank of Scotland kindly helped with some of the production costs of the volume.

SHIRLEY FISHER
JAMES REASON

Section IA
Specific Life Stresses

Handbook of Life Stress, Cognition and Health
Edited by S. Fisher and J. Reason
© 1988 John Wiley & Sons Ltd.

1

Expectant Parenthood

Yona Teichman
Tel-Aviv University

INTRODUCTION

Expectant parenthood is a developmental stage experienced by most adults. In Western society, due to the availability of contraceptives and the liberalization of abortion, in most instances pregnancy is a planned and socially approved state. As such it is defined by the prospective parents and their social context as a positive event. According to common belief, folklore and artistic expression, transition to parenthood is considered as the greatest joy and a self-fulfilling experience. On the other hand, when theoretical propositions, clinical impressions and research findings are examined, pregnancy emerges as a stressful life event. A review of the literature on expectant parenthood reveals a concentration on the crisis aspects of this experience and almost an exclusive focus on the feminine point of view.

This chapter will examine physical, psychological and contextual factors which are involved in determining the experience of expectant parenthood from women's, men's and couple's perspectives. Within this frame of reference, topics such as differences in reactions to first and subsequent pregnancies, age and pregnancy, work and pregnancy, modern medical technology and its influence on pregnancy will be presented and discussed. Based on the consideration of these issues, the question of whether pregnancy is a crisis or a developmental progression will be readdressed, and a compromise which defines expectant parenthood as a period with crisis potentials will be offered.

BECOMING A MOTHER

The understanding of the psychological processes that unfold during the transition to motherhood was first attempted by Freud (1925). Freud suggested that the psychological experiences in pregnancy and childbirth are related to the frustration and anxiety experienced by the young girl upon becoming aware of her psychological inferiority in not possessing a penis. Pregnancy, which represents a man's love, and the prospect of having a male baby resolve these problems and

3

lead to the development of mature femininity. Other psychoanalytically oriented scholars (incidentally all of whom were women) continued to develop Freud's ideas, but introduced more elaborated views about pregnancy (Deutsch, 1945; Benedek, 1959; Bibring, 1959). They argued that pregnancy is a complex psychological experience which stimulates unconscious conflicts and anxieties about identity, relationship with significant others, dependency and regressive tendencies. In this respect pregnancy is a developmental crisis; however, the transformation to motherhood and mature womanhood resolves this crisis. Deutsch (1945), Benedek (1959) and Bibring (1959) illuminated important aspects of the properties of psychological experiences during pregnancy, but, as stated by Grossman *et al.* (1980), their thinking was primarily intrapsychic: they viewed the woman in isolation from any meaningful context.

According to Freud, the wish to have a child, especially a son, represents women's desire to compensate for their physiological inferiority. These ideas were investigated by examining actual preferences that women express regarding the gender of their child. Hammer (1970) asked single and married college students and married noncollege adults the question: 'If you knew for sure that you could have only one child, would you prefer that child to be a male or a female?' (p. 54). Results for both college samples lend some support to Freud's contention: 78% of the unmarried and 73% of the married female students expressed a preference for a boy. On the other hand, only 30% of the married noncollege women expressed a preference for a boy. Male subjects expressed an overwhelming preference for a boy (83%–90%) and they, according to Freud, do not have to resolve any physical inferiority complex. In another study, Rabinowici (1985) asked 197 married expectant mothers in Israel to indicate whether they would prefer a boy or a girl, but they were also allowed a third choice of 'don't care'. Twenty-nine percent of the respondents stated that they would prefer a boy, 33% a girl and 38% did not care. The conclusion that may be drawn from both studies is that married, more mature women express lower preference for a son, while younger women and men in general express a higher preference for sons. These findings may be interpreted as representing the sensitivity of younger women to men's expectations and the balanced attitude of more mature women regarding this issue. However, in Freudian terms these findings can be attributed to repression of the real needs. Thus, although these are interesting results, from the theoretical point of view their implications are not clear. Furthermore they point but the difficulties in examining theoretical ideas which are based on unconscious processes while in most instances data are collected on the conscious level.

Grossman *et al.* (1980) reviewed studies which investigated motivations for pregnancy without considering the Freudian hypothesis. They mention several reasons that people indicate for wanting children, such as liking children, seeking immortality through children, or anticipating feelings of pride. More pathological motivations which are mentioned, mainly in clinical literature, are the wish to save the marriage, to restore self-esteem, to be like other women or to demonstrate how to raise a child well (Blitzer and Murray, 1964; Wenner and Cohen, 1968).

Grossman *et al.* (1980) approached the study of motivations quantitatively.

They investigated women's attitudes towards their pregnancy on conscious and unconscious levels and correlated them with adaptation to pregnancy. Women who described themselves as unambivalently positive about having the child, on the conscious level, were judged as better adapted to pregnancy. On the other hand, when unconscious motivations were considered, women who revealed ambivalence were judged as better adapted. It seems that motivations expressed on different levels may differ, and that ambivalence may have positive outcomes. According to Grossman *et al.* (1980), ambivalence represents psychological investment in the process of becoming a mother which has a positive effect on the general adjustment to pregnancy.

Emotional Experience During Pregnancy

Before looking at the emotional experiences women report during pregnancy, it has to be mentioned that the data concerning these experiences were obtained mainly from first-time expectant mothers. The findings of most studies indicate that pregnancy is an emotionally strenuous time. Pregnant women describe themselves as experiencing emotional stress, fatigue, depression, emotional lability, loneliness, fears and concerns (see, for example, Leifer, 1980; Osofsky and Osofsky, 1984; Shereshefsky and Yarrow, 1973; Wenner and Cohen, 1968; Zajicek and Wolkind, 1978). Considering these findings, Lips (1985) argues that in describing pregnancy, the negative tone prevails, but little information is available 'about the actual extent to which such symptoms occur differentially among pregnant women as opposed to other adults'. Using discriminant analysis and trend analysis, Lips (1985) compared pregnant women's self-descriptions in three stages of pregnancy and postpartum. In all stages, the scores of pregnant women were compared with those of two other groups of adults (husbands and nonpregnant women). Lips' findings show that indeed, in contrast to other adults, the scores of pregnant women on 'negative emotional state' and depression increased over time. However, it is important to note that the significant increase in the 'negative emotional state' occurred mainly during the end of pregnancy and postpartum, and the largest elevation in depression occurred between the middle and end of pregnancy. Despite this elevation, pregnant women's scores did not exceed the level of normal depression. According to Lips (1985), the emotional changes reflect reactions of pregnant women to increased bodily stresses in the last trimester of pregnancy and the feeling 'that the pregnancy has gone on for ever'.

Another in-depth look at women's emotional experience during pregnancy is described by Hees-Stauthamer (1985), who evaluated the subjective experiences of four women during their first pregnancy. The methodology which was applied was a longitudinal case study. Although not quantitative, this intensive inquiry into the psychological processes during expectant motherhood reveals that emotional experiences in pregnancy are much more complex than the negative stereotypes which emerged from popular beliefs, clinical descriptions and early research. Hees-Stauthamer's findings also confirm Lips' (1985) conclusion that emotional experiences change during pregnancy.

Despite the fact that the women in Hees-Stauthamer's study became pregnant under very favourable personal, marital and economical conditions, their initial reactions to their pregnancies were mixed. On the one hand they experienced excitement, an enhanced sense of feminity and commitment to the marital relationship, yet on the other hand they felt distress, emotional sensitivity, lability, disorientation and turmoil. In the second trimester, after experiencing the quickening, reactions were great excitement, intensified internal imagery of the child and an increased sense of the baby's 'aliveness'. These experiences increased the awareness of 'motherliness' and the identification with the newly developing mother role. However, the women also reported instances of sudden increase in emotional lability, preoccupation with pregnancy, concerns and conflicts, and reduced interest in sex. In the third trimester, the women described themselves as impatient with the pregnancy, irritable and still emotionally labile. They also resented being alone and expressed feelings of vulnerability and dependency. A characteristic feeling in the last part of pregnancy was ambivalence. Women expressed great concern, anxiety and empathy for the child, yet on the other hand they also experienced feelings of detachment from the baby, occasional rejection, and frustration with having to subordinate their own well-being to that of the baby.

Beyond the description of emotional reactions during pregnancy it is interesting to examine what determines them. Findings from studies which addressed this question indicate that physical, psychological and contextual variables influence women's emotional adjustment to pregnancy.

Physical Factors and Emotional Well-being

Pregnancy is a long physical process accompanied by hormonal and bodily changes. In most cases, all through the pregnancy regular contact with medical services or medical personnel is maintained. The interrelationship between these physiological aspects and psychological reactions during and post pregnancy has been explained by two points of view. The medical point of view considers physiological factors as independent variables which influence emotional adjustment to pregnancy and postpartum. Studies which represent this perspective investigated the influence of hormonal activity on mood (Dalton, 1971; Hamburg *et al.*, 1968; Melges, 1968; Nott, 1976), influence of biological causes on nausea and vomiting (Fitzgerald, 1984), and the influence of illness during pregnancy on psychological adjustment (Gordon and Gordon, 1959). As noted by Grossman *et al.* (1980) and by Sherman (1971), the findings of most of these studies are inconclusive and often contradictory.

The alternative point of view considers physiological symptoms as dependent variables, caused by the pregnant women's intraphchic state. Studies which represent this perspective investigated the effect of negative attitudes towards pregnancy, neuroticism and anxiety on pregnancy-related symptoms such as nausea, vomiting, backache, dizziness, fatigue, gastrointestinal discomfort and pregnancy complications. Results usually indicated a positive relationship between the personality variables and physical symptoms or complications (Brown,

1964; Davids and DeVault, 1962; Fitzgerald, 1984; Gorusch and Key, 1974; Shereshefsky and Yarrow, 1973; Zemlick and Watson, 1953).

Psychological Factors and Emotional Well-being

In addition to the interest in the influence of intrapsychic variables on physiological well-being, and vice versa, very extensive interest has been directed to the study of the effects of these variables on the psychological well-being of mothers to be. Variables which were considered were ego strength, nurturance, the capacity to visualize oneself as a mother, feminine identification, and previous level of emotional adjustment (Shereshefsky and Yarrow, 1973; Wenner *et al.*, 1969; Grossman *et al.*, 1980). Two intrapsychic variables attracted more interest than others: these are the pregnant woman's perceived relationship with her own mother, and anxiety.

The idea that the expectant mother's perception of her own mother affects her psychological well-being was influenced by the ideas expressed by Bibring (1959), Chertok (1969), Deutsch (1945) and other psychoanalytically oriented theorists. Findings of studies which investigated this proposition prove that positive attitudes of pregnant women toward their mothers or their ability to use them as positive models determine their psychological adjustment to pregnancy and help them to reconcile themselves to the transition to motherhood (Breen, 1975; Osofsky and Osofsky, 1984; Shereshefsky and Yarrow, 1973; Weigert *et al.*, 1968).

Another variable which attracted a good deal of attention is anxiety. Anxiety has been investigated as an antecedent which influences emotional adaptation or as a consequence which represents it. Grossman *et al.* (1980) were interested in anxiety as an antecedent. They differentiated between two kinds of anxiety, expressed anxiety and anxiety inferred from clinical data. The first type had a negative influence on women's adaptation to pregnancy, while the second type was a predictor of positive adjustment. Grossman *et al.* suggested that some anxiety during pregnancy is inevitable. The psychological changes that occur during pregnancy, especially the first one, evoke anxiety, and coming to terms with this anxiety is one of the tasks confronting expectant mothers. Thus, signs which indicate that anxiety exists represent positive adjustment, while its denial represents difficulties in integrating the psychological processes which unfold during this period in the woman's life. Grossman *et al.*'s (1980) differentiation between expressed and suppressed anxiety demonstrates an important methodological problem in its study. It appears that anxiety is a multidimensional construct, different kinds of which, in the same situation, may have different meanings and influences. The need to differentiate 'anxieties' has been discussed extensively in the literature (Endler, 1982; Spielberger, 1966; Teichman, 1978). The findings of Grossman *et al.* (1980), show that in the study of pregnancy, generalizations regarding anxiety may be misleading, and a clear specification of the aspects of anxiety which have been investigated is necessary.

A study which took into account different types of anxiety and investigated it as a consequence during pregnancy was reported by Rabinowici (1985). Based on

Spielberger's (1966) theory which differentiates between situational anxiety (A-state) and predisposition to experience anxiety (A-trait), Rabinowici (1985) hypothesized that expectant mothers with high trait anxiety will experience a higher level of state anxiety. She also hypothesized that a discrepancy between the expected and actual gender of the fetus will elevate the level of state anxiety, while congruency will reduce it. Elevation in anxiety was particularly expected in pregnant women who already had children of the currently unpreferred gender (mothers who had two daughters and preferred a son, or mothers who had two sons and preferred a daughter). Rabinowici's (1985) results support her hypothesis regarding the relationship between trait and state anxiety during pregnancy and yield only partial support for her second hypothesis. Women with high trait anxiety had significantly higher scores in state anxiety than women with low trait anxiety, but in the first pregnancy, irrespective of whether the preference was for a boy or a girl, incongruency between the preferred gender of the fetus and the actual gender did not cause a significant elevation in state anxiety. On the other hand, in the third pregnancy, incongruency caused a very significant elevation in the level of state anxiety. This was especially evident in women who had two sons and preferred a daughter.

These findings demonstrate the need to investigate the contribution of individual differences in determining the level of experienced anxiety during pregnancy. They also contribute to the body of research relevant to the Freudian hypothesis regarding women's motivations for childbirth. Contrary to Freud's proposition, Rabinowici's (1985) findings indicate that, in the first pregnancy, the gender of the fetus, or even a discrepancy between preferred and actual gender, did not influence anxiety level. The findings regarding women in the third pregnancy who already had two sons and preferred a daughter indicate that having a daughter is emotionally very meaningful for women.

In any stress-related research, anxiety is a frequently used concept. The review of studies which investigated anxiety during pregnancy demonstrates that attention has to be paid to the differentiation between anxiety as antecedent or as a consequence, expressed or suppressed anxiety, state or trait anxiety. Last, but not least, the level of anxiety has to be considered. Despite the fact that it is assumed that during pregnancy women experience elevation in anxiety, there has been no study that the author is aware of showing, that anxiety changes during pregnancy or that pregnant women experience higher level's than comparable nonpregnant women.

It may be summarized that expectant mothers experience emotional upheavals, but their feelings are differentiated, and change during the pregnancy. Their experiences are influenced by physiological and psychological factors and influence them in return. However, pregnancy occurs in context, and contextual variables also affect an expectant mother's emotional experiences and well-being. Contextual variables will be discussed in the next section.

Contextual Variables and Emotional Well-being

Contextual variables which influence emotional well-being during pregnancy may be divided into the following factors: sociocultural and socioeconomic factors, age, previous life stress, marital relationship, support system, work situation, and contact with medical services. The interest in most of these factors is relatively new, but even the sporadic data that are available indicate their importance in contributing to the emotional well-being of expectant mothers.

Anthropologists have devoted attention to the sociocultural dimension of pregnancy. According to anthropological reports, sociocultural norms and values determine concrete behavior during pregnancy and reactions to it (Mead, 1948; Newman, 1978). In Western society the isolation of the nuclear family and its mobility are often mentioned as factors that add to the strains of pregnancy. So is the changing role and status of women in family and society which may create conflicts regarding the choice between the demands of career and motherhood as well as tensions with the husband (Cowan and Cowan, 1987; Hees-Stauthamer, 1985; Osofsky and Osofsky, 1984).

Socioeconomic factors influence emotional reaction during pregnancy as well. These factors have direct implications on the financial resources available to families to deal with pregnancy-related expenses. They also contribute to family stability (Cutright, 1971). In this respect it is interesting to note that most of the longitudinal studies which are the main source of information about the processes that occur during pregnancy, investigated married, economically well-to-do expectant mothers (Grossman *et al.*, 1980; Hees-Stauthamer, 1985; Shereshefsky and Yarrow, 1973).

A variable closely related to the issue of women's status in society and to socioeconomic factors is the age of expectant mothers. As previously mentioned, most of the literature on pregnancy is based on the first pregnancies of women in their twenties. In recent years a significant number of women are postponing pregnancy and motherhood and adjusting it to academic or career needs. This changes the personal and environmental context of pregnancy and most probably has an influence on some of the processes that occur during it. An attempt to understand experiences during the first pregnancy of women in their thirties is described by Hees-Stauthamer (1985), but a comparative study of women of different ages has not yet been attempted.

Previous life stress is another contextual factor. It gained more empirical attention than the previously mentioned ones, but investigators were concerned mainly with its impact on birth and postpartum complications. The findings which are available regarding pregnancy indicate that previous life stresses are related to adaptation to pregnancy (Shereshefsky and Yarrow, 1973) and, more specifically, that women with few psychological assets are especially vulnerable to prepregnancy stresses (Nuckolls *et al.*, 1972).

The influence of the perceived quality of marital relationship on emotional experiences during pregnancy has been the most investigated of the contextual factors. Marital relationship at this point will be examined from the women's point of view. As can be expected, studies that investigated the effect of marital relationship on pregnancy report that the support that the pregnant woman receives from her husband is an important factor in determining her emotional well-being. According to Grossman *et al.* (1980), the expectant mother's perception of the quality of her marital relationship was one of the two most important predictors of the optimal adaptation to pregnancy. (The second predictor was the woman's general level of psychological adaptation.) Grossman *et al*, maintain that the main components in the marriage of expectant couples which determine whether the pregnant woman will feel isolated or supported, vulnerable or secure are the woman's ability to express dependency and to ask for help, and the husband's ability to respond appropriately. The need to deal with dependency and renegotiate with the husband patterns of dominance and submission was mentioned also by Weigert *et al*. (1968). On the other hand, Shereshefsky and Yarrow (1973) mention that marital disharmony before and during pregnancy increases the pregnant woman's experience of stress. Another dimension of marital relationship is communication. Osofsky and Osofsky (1984) report that women who were able to share their concerns with their husbands had better adjustment to their pregnancy.

In exploring the marital dimension during pregnancy, it is interesting to look at Hees-Stauthamer's (1985) detailed description of changes in expectant mothers' attitudes towards marital relationship during pregnancy and following childbirth. She points out the following sequence: 'The first trimester was experienced as a confirmation of the couple relationship, although new concerns about the husband as a potential father also emerged. These new concerns, together with increased awareness of gender differences, led to greater differentiation within the couples' relationship during the second trimester. Women felt more in tune with universal aspects of female experience and were generally closer to their women friends. Feelings of anger or distance in the marital relationship were especially common at the end of the fifth and the beginning of the sixth month of pregnancy. The differentiation experienced as a result of these events was resolved as the couple worked together to prepare for labor and delivery. After the birth of the child, both confirmation of the couple in terms of deepened commitment and differentiation in terms of the distance introduced by the child's presence into the marital dynamic were consolidated into a richer, more complex relationship' (p. 112).

In the reality of modern society, in which young people often form families away from their family of origin, spouses depend on support from each other. However, the husband is not the only source of support; two other kinds may be differentiated: informal support by friends and relatives, and formal, professional support. As suggested by Grossman *et al*. (1980), it is logical to assume that the amount and the availability of interpersonal support to the expectant mother will determine her well-being during her pregnancy. The function of the informal support is to give the expectant mother an opportunity to share experiences and gain information from other pregnant women and young mothers. According to Hees-Stauthamer (1985), in the second trimester of pregnancy expectant mothers very much appreciate this kind of support; they also increase contact with their own mothers. Due to the special strains in the first pregnancy, it may be assumed that first-time expectant mothers would manifest a greater need for this kind of support than mothers in second or subsequent pregnancies. These ideas, however, are based on intuition and they await empirical examination.

The fact that expectant parenthood is associated with high stress potentials led to the development of many preventative programs for expectant mothers. In contrast to the informal support, this type of support is often empirically evaluated, and results indicate that it is effective in reducing postpartum depression, maternal anxiety, and need for medication. It also contributes to awareness during birth and satisfaction with the childbirth experience (Enkin *et al.*, 1971; Davenport-Slack and Boylan, 1974; Klusman, 1975; Zax *et al.*, 1975). A question still remains regarding the influence of these programs on emotional well-being and adjustment during pregnancy and their long-term efficacy.

The last two contextual variables to be discussed are work and contact with medical services. The systematic evaluation of the impact of employment on pregnancy complications and outcomes was conducted mainly by the medical profession. In a recent review of this literature Saurel-Cubizolles and Kaminski (1986) showed that the interest in the influences of work on the medical aspects of pregnancy can be traced to the end of the 19th century, and that untill the middle of the current century all studies reported that employment has very adverse effects on pregnancy.

On the other hand, research published during the 1970–1980 decade shows that employment ceased to be a risk factor for perinatal outcome and that the incidence of premature delivery is lower among working women. The authors attribute these changes to the following reasons. Early findings are based on hospital records, which mainly represent poor women; the proportions and difference in social characteristics of working women changed; working conditions improved; and medical services became much more readily available. Female employment, which nowadays is a widespread phenomenon in western society, is regarded as the norm, and from the medical point of view does not have any negative implications for pregnancy.

In contrast to the medical literature, psychological knowledge of the impact of work during pregnancy is very limited. Hees-Stauthamer (1985) provides interesting information about changing attitudes to work during pregnancy. Based on interviews with four women who were highly committed to their careers before pregnancy, she states that 'only one woman was able to integrate her personal and professional worlds fully'. The others went through a process which started in the first trimester and lasted untill the end of pregnancy, a process which reoriented them from work to motherhood. This does not mean that they gave up long-term professional goals, but towards the end of pregnancy they had different priorities. Owing to the centrality of work in the lives of modern women, Hees-Stauthamer's (1985) findings have to be reexamined with larger samples and quantitative methodology.

Dealing with contextual variables, it is impossible not to mention contact with medical services. In modern society most pregnant women are, one way or another, in regular contact with the medical profession. This contact increases their awareness of the medical aspects of pregnancy. It is obvious that regular medical supervision has a substantial preventative role in reducing physical complications for the mother and infant, but the psychological implications of the close association with medical services were only rarely investigated. Oakley

(1980) maintains that technological intervention at birth is associated with post-partum depression. She argues against the 'colonization of birth by medicine' and for more control to be given to women over the normal processes occurring in their bodies. Oakley (1980) directed attention to the postpartum emotional consequences of medical interventions at birth, but since modern technology is widely used also during pregnancy, it is logical to assume that this has consequences as well. A technological procedure which is almost a routine is that of ultrasound scanning which is performed in the first trimester of pregnancy. Several studies have evaluated women's attitudes and emotional reactions of this procedure. Pregnant women usually accept ultrasound scanning enthusiastically. They describe it as enhancing 'bonding' with the baby and reducing anxiety (Hyde, 1986; Kohn et al., 1980; Milne and Rich, 1981; Rabinowici, 1985; Reading and Cox, 1982). A very important aspect related to ultrasound scanning is the feedback it provides regarding the fetal image. Hyde (1986) mentions that insensitively provided feedback may have negative or even harmful psychological effects.

Routine medical examinations and ultrasound scanning are experienced by most pregnant women. However, women who have difficulties in conceiving or who experience complications during pregnancy are subject to medical treatments which employ medical technology as well; the psychological aspects of such procedures are unknown. The appropriate evaluation of the effects of these interventions may serve as a guideline for the development of support programs for expectant parents who are exposed to these stressful situations.

BECOMING A FATHER

Expectant fatherhood has been much less explored than expectant motherhood, but changing sociocultural norms regarding gender-related roles in family and society stimulated interest in the processes experienced by men during the transition to parenthood. As in the case of motherhood, the first attempt to explain the emotional experiences and psychological motivations of expectant fathers has to be traced to Freudian thinking. Freud's (1925) theory of fatherhood is related to the resolution of the Oedipal conflict by repression of the sexual desire for the mother and identification with the father. The identification with the father orients the boy toward assuming the male's functions in family and society, one of which is fatherhood. Contrary to women, men express overwhelming preference for a male child. Mead's (1949) explanation of this preference as representing men's desire for immortality is still accepted today.

The experiences of men during their wives' pregnancies were often associated with the revival of Oedipal and other childhood conflicts. Thus for men as well, expecting a child, especially the first one, was generally seen as a stressful period, with strong potentials for crisis or even pathology. However, the interest in factors that determine the expectant father's well-being is relatively limited. The most prevailing interest regarding expectant fathers was and still is in their physical and emotional reactions.

Physical Reactions

While expecting a child, men do not undergo biological or hormonal changes, yet many of them experience physical symptoms. The timing, amount, intensity and frequency of these symptoms may change. When they appear at the beginning of pregnancy and disappear after birth they are referred to as the couvade syndrome (Trethowan and Conlon, 1965). The couvade syndrome is explained as identification with the wife or as a displacement of feelings or conflicts. Despite the many clinical examples of this syndrome, only a few studies have investigated it empirically. There are studies which report that expectant fathers complain of more physical symptoms than control, non-expecting men (Liebenberg, 1967; Lipkin and Lamb, 1982; Teichman and Lahav, 1987; Trethowan and Conlon, 1965; Wolkind, 1981). Yet another study (Quill et al., 1984) found that expectant fathers did not ask for medical help more than controls (who were non-expectant fathers) and had a significantly lower visit rate during their partner's pregnancy than before conception or after delivery. The authors attribute this finding to the fact that they utilized a behavioral measure of symptoms-related behavior, which caused men to refrain from admitting acting weak or sick.

An additional finding regarding the physical symptoms of expectant fathers was reported by Teichman and Lahav (1987). They found that first-time expectant fathers reported experiencing more physical symptoms than control, non-expecting men and than men expecting a second or a subsequent child. This finding suggests that for expectant fathers as well, the first pregnancy is more stressful than subsequent pregnancies. The relationship between physical and emotional reactions will be discussed in the following section.

Emotional Reactions

The interest in the emotional reactions of expectant fathers may be traced to Zilboorg's (1931) work. He identified pregnancy as a potential precipitating event for mental illness in men. Since then, research into men's reactions to pregnancy has been dominated by an orientation towards psychopathology (Curtis, 1955; Fishbein, 1981; Freeman, 1951; Ginath, 1974; LaCoursiere, 1972; Wainwright, 1966). Beail (1982), Einzig (1980), Lewis (1982), Parke, (1981) and Scott-Heyes (1982) criticized this orientation as too psychoanalytic and therefore unrepresentative. The emotional reactions of normal men, who constitute the majority of expectant fathers, were seldom investigated. Recently, however, four studies have attempted to elucidate different aspects of emotional reactions, mainly anxiety, of normal expectant fathers (Trethowan and Conlon, 1965; Gerzi and Berman, 1981; Scott-Heyes, 1982; Teichman and Lahav, 1987). Trethowan and Conlon (1965) focused mainly on physical reactions, but also investigated the relationship between anxiety and symptoms. They found the two to be negatively correlated, i.e. men who denied feeling anxious reported more physical symptoms, while men who admitted being anxious reported fewer symptoms. A replication of this finding was reported by Teichman and Lahav (1987).

Gerzi and Berman (1981) compared the anxiety scores of expectant fathers who were expecting their first child with those of married childless men. They found that expectant fathers were significantly more anxious. Scott-Heyes (1982) criticized Gerzi and Berman's methodology of comparing expectant fathers with childless men. She suggested that their results regarding anxiety may be attributed to parenthood generally rather than specifically to pregnancy. As an alternative, Scott-Heyes (1982) evaluated the emotional reactions of expectant fathers longitudinally. She measured anxiety, depression and hostility in two stages during pregnancy and twice postpartum. Her findings indicate emotional stability; analysis of variance showed no significant differences among the four different measures of the three emotions. However, Scott-Heyes' study did not compare expectant fathers with any control group, and thus nothing can be concluded regarding the level of the emotions of these men. An additional finding reported by Scott-Heyes is that late in pregnancy, men expecting their first child were more depressed than other expectant fathers. This finding corresponds to Lips' (1985) finding regarding the time in pregnancy when expectant mothers report an elevation in depression. The implications of these two findings will be discussed later.

Teichman and Lahav (1987) took into account Scott-Heyes' criticism of Gerzi and Berman's (1981) study. They compared two groups of expectant fathers (first child and second or subsequent child) with a group of men who were fathers but not in the expectant phase of fatherhood. Viewing pregnancy as a clearly defined state, they used a direct measure of state anxiety (Spielberger et al., 1970). Contrary to their prediction, expectant fathers, particularly those who were expecting their first child, reported lower levels of anxiety.

Similarly to Quill et al. (1984), Teichman and Lahav (1987) attributed their findings to the direct measure of anxiety which they used. They suggest that at a time when personal and social expectations increase, men tend to manifest responsibility, dependability, and maturity, rather than admitting emotional strain and vulnerability. The idea is that direct confrontation with anxiety activates defensiveness, and anxiety is denied. It is interesting to note that Grossman et al. (1980) who investigated anxiety in expectant fathers and used the same measure of anxiety, also reported that expectant fathers had low anxiety scores.

Dealing with the problem of denial of anxiety by expectant mothers, Grossman et al. (1980) suggested that this is a positive indication which represents the working through and emotional adjustment to the new role. In the case of expectant fathers, however, the denial is less positive. It is most probably caused by conformity to stereotypical social expectations and as such creates additional strain. This strain is expressed in physical symptoms. Younger men expecting their first child are more vulnerable in this respect, and it may be recommended that preventative programs that are planned for expectant fathers will address this issue.

Two additional topics regarding expectant fathers' anxiety have to be addressed: what determines their anxiety level and how they cope with anxiety. According to Grossman et al. (1980), the best predictor of expectant fathers' anxiety towards the end of pregnancy (eighth month) is their state anxiety level in the beginning of pregnancy (first trimester). Grossman *et al.*, also investigated the effect of sex role identification as assessed by the scale developed by Bem (1974) on the anxiety level of expectant fathers. Contrary to Bem's theory, 'masculine' men felt more comfortable with their wives' pregnancies. Lahav (1984) reinvestigated this issue and he reported findings more in line with Bem's theory. In his study, expectant fathers who described themselves as more androgynous, and thus better capable of relating to both feminine and masculine aspects of their personality, had the lowest state anxiety scores. The highest scores were obtained by men who described themselves as masculine. The contradiction between the findings of Grossman *et al.* (1980) and those of Lahav (1984) may be attributed to the different cultural contexts in which the two studies were conducted (in the USA and Israel). This line of thinking suggests the need for further cross-cultural research regarding expectant parenthood.

The last question is whether the stress and anxiety experienced by expectant fathers can be reduced, and which coping strategies are more effective. Wolkind (1981) and Scott-Heyes (1982) suggested that expectant fathers' emotional involvement in their wives' pregnancies affects their well-being. However, while Wolkind found that husbands who were highly involved with their wives' pregnancies had pregnancy type symptoms, Scott-Heyes' findings indicate that men who expressed more willingness to be involved in pregnancy-related activities had significantly lower levels of depression and hostility during the pregnancy and lower anxiety scores in the beginnings of pregnancy. These opposing findings can be attributed to the fact that in the two studies, different types of involvement were investigated. Whereas Wolkind (1981) investigated the husbands' emotional involvement as perceived by their wives, Scott-Heyes (1982) investigated more active involvement such as accompanying wives to antenatal checkups and preparing for the baby. Based on this differentiation, Teichman and Lahav (1987) hypothesized that expectant fathers who have high levels of emotional involvement with their wives' pregnancies will report a high level of anxiety and a high frequency of experiencing physical symptoms, while expectant fathers who are actively involved will report low levels of anxiety and a low frequency of experiencing physical symptoms.

Teichman and Lahav's results support their hypothesis regarding physical symptoms. They found that emotional involvement was associated with increase in physical symptoms, while active involvement was not. These results help to interpret the contradictory findings of Wolkind (1981) and Scott-Heyes (1982) as actually complementing each other because they investigated different types of involvement. The differentiation between types of involvement of expectant fathers in their wives' pregnancies seems to be an important predictor of their psychological well-being and deserves future investigation.

Departing from the direct consideration of anxiety and looking at other variables which affect psychological adjustment of expectant fathers, it is interesting to note variables such as satisfaction with sexual life and the men's feelings about their relationships with their own mothers. Grossman *et al.* (1980) report that in their study, men who felt satisfaction with their sexual relationship with their wives and men who felt that they were loved, nurtured and had a sense of their wives being like their own mothers were judged as better adapted to expectant fatherhood. It is interesting to remember that the emotional reactions of expectant mothers were also affected by their relationship with their own mothers. The repeated findings regarding the importance of the relationship between both expectant parents and their own mothers have relevance to the psychoanalytic conceptualization of pregnancy in men and women.

Contextual Factors

The interest in the effect that contextual factors have on expectant fathers has been very sporadic. One of the few variables that was looked at is socioeconomic status. Grossman *et al.* (1980), Duvall (1971) and Kohn (1963) report that socioeconomic status, especially of first-time expectant fathers, determines their attitudes and general adjustment to pregnancy. Men of lower socioeconomic status were less pleased with the pregnancy and the coming birth than men of higher socioeconomic status and had lower general adjustment to pregnancy.

It is striking to note how rarely the quality of marital relationship and social support, as perceived by expectant fathers, were investigated as affecting their well-being. Osofsky and Osofsky (1984), who interviewed expectant couples, mention the importance of the strength of the marital relationship as perceived by the father in determining his ability to grow during the experience of expectant fatherhood. Grossman *et al.* (1980) point out the importance of a satisfactory sexual relationship, and Parke (1981) mentions the need of expectant fathers for informal support of friends, relatives and especially their own mothers. Providers of formal support started to offer programs for expectant fathers and expectant couples (Bittman and Zalk, 1978; Clulow, 1982; Osofsky & Osofsky, 1984; Cowan and Cowan, 1987). These developments are very encouraging, but, as stated by Cowan and Cowan (1987), the evaluation of the processes that take place in most of these interventions and their short- and long-term results are mainly descriptive. When expectant fathers are considered, contextual factors such as age, work situation and contact with medical services, are still ignored. It is logical to assume that these factors affect expectant fathers as well, and they also await systematic investigation.

THE EXPECTANT COUPLE

Expectant parenthood, or even the phase when pregnancy and becoming parents is planned, start the process of transition to parenthood. During expectant parenthood both partners undergo many meaningful changes, overt and covert experiences. Some of these changes and experiences occur in both spouses simultaneously, others according to an individual timetable. As a couple, they have to reorganize patterns of behavior and communication, to redefine roles and reschedule hierarchies of needs. It is inevitable that these processes will fail to be reflected in the couple's relationship. Despite this fact, most of the research which has investigated the effect of a couple's relationship on the transition to parenthood, or the effect of the transition to parenthood on the couple's relationship, has focused on the phase when couples actually become parents, namely, on early parenthood (Cherlin, 1977; Cowan *et al.*, 1985; Cowan *et al.*, 1986; Dyer, 1963; Feldman, 1971; Grossman *et al.*, 1980; Hobbs and Cole, 1976; LeMasters, 1957; Rossi, 1968; Russell, 1974; Shereshefsky and Yarrow, 1973). Issues related to the couple during the first phase of transition to parenthood in the pregnancy were only seldom investigated.

Considering the individual perspectives of expectant parents, it is evident that the experiences of each spouse during the pregnancy have the potential for stress in the marital relationship. Women have to deal with unpleasant physical symptoms and physical discomfort, they become concerned with bodily, identity and lifestyle changes. They become preoccupied and introverted. They experience worries, concerns, anxiety and depression. They become dependent, vulnerable, emotional, ambivalent and at times they experience reduced interest in sex. Men also have occasionally to cope with physical symptoms which resemble those of their wives (couvade syndrome). They, as well, face identity problems, ambivalence, worries, concerns, anxieties and depression, the expression of which is unacceptable. Social expectations from expectant fathers are for maturity, strength, dependability and the ability to act supportively towards their wives. Although these difficulties are accompanied by pride, satisfaction, positive feelings as well as individual and marital confirmation, they put great strain on the marital relationship. The strain is increased by the fact that at times husband and wife have the same reactions and at other times they may experience competing needs. Some similarities were empirically confirmed. In comparing reactions to different pregnancies, it was demonstrated that both men and women experience the first pregnancy as more difficult and emotionally demanding (Grossman *et al.*, 1980; Osofsky and Osofsky, 1984; Teichman and Lahav, 1987). Physical symptoms are most prevalent in the beginning of pregnancy (Trethowen and Conlon, 1965), and elevation in depression is reported for both spouses towards the end of pregnancy (Lips, 1985; Scott-Heyes, 1982). Differences in needs were reported as well. Grossman *et al.* (1980) maintain that men's adjustment to pregnancy depends very much on sexual satisfaction. On the other hand, Hees-Stauthamer (1985) reports that in the second part of pregnancy women feel a reduced need for sex, and in the last part of pregnancy sex is often avoided.

It can be suggested that couples capable of handling the similarities and differences while expecting a child are those who eventually reach the mutual goal of becoming a family and grow with the experience, while those who have difficulties in resolving the problems caused by pregnancy become frustrated and alienated. If things continue to deteriorate, eventually the marriage is terminated. Indeed there are reports that many marriages are dissolved shortly after children are born (Bumpass and Rindfuss, 1979).

Borrowing Bernard's (1974) concept of 'his and hers marriage', Cowen *et al.* (1986) introduced the concept of 'his, her and their transition to parenthood'. Based on the preceding discussion, there is no doubt that there is also 'his, her and their pregnancy'. Keeping in mind the fact that many divorces occur when couples enter parenthood, it is recommended that the expectant phase of the transition to parenthood be systematically investigated, and interventions which take into account his, her and their pregnancy be offered.

A very impressive example of preventative intervention for couples becoming parents which focused mainly on couple issues was described by Cowan and Cowan (1987). Expectant couples who participated in Cowan and Cowan's program, when compared with expectant couples who did not participate in it, had higher self-esteem, were more satisfied with their role arrangement, and maintained stability in marital satisfaction. Considering Cowan and Cowan's results, it is logical to suggest that professional interventions shall be organized to offer support to both expectant parents and be provided during the pregnancy. Intervention has to address physical, emotional and relationship issues and focus both on pregnancy-related stress and preparation for childbirth and parenthood.

IS EXPECTANT PARENTHOOD A CRISIS?

Integrating the findings about her, his and their pregnancy, it is interesting to readdress the question, whether expectant parenthood is a crisis. The theoretical thinking about pregnancy, which was influenced by psychoanalysis, led to the conceptualization of pregnancy as a crisis. This trend of thinking triggered protest. Beail (1982), Einzig (1980), Lewis (1982), Parke (1981) and Scott-Heyes (1982) claim that the crisis orientation to pregnancy is unrepresentative and that normal adults on the verge of parenthood do not necessarily experience it is as a debilitating experience. Osofsky and Osofsky (1984) argued that 'conceptualizing pregnancy and new parenthood as a crisis does not appear to convey adequately the developmental adjustments and potential growth that may characterize this period' (p. 373).

The research reviewed in this chapter points to the conclusion that the fact that an event is positive, anticipated and has growth components does not mean that it is free from crisis potentials. Throughout the pregnancy, men, women and couples have to face new, intensive and at times unpleasant experiences which demand reorganization of old adjustment patterns. This in itself corresponds to Parad and Caplan's (1965) definitions of crisis. According to them, crisis is caused by confrontation with a situation of basic importance to the individual combined with difficulty of solution by familiar methods or available resources.

Despite the strenuous tasks which confront men, women and couples while expecting a child, and despite the correspondence of the situation to the most widely accepted definition of crisis (Parad and Caplan, 1965), it is proposed not to label this period as a crisis but rather as a period with crisis potentials. This slight differentiation takes into account the fact that an event becomes a crisis depending on the definitions and meanings attributed to it (Hill, 1965), and allows for individual differences. On the other hand, the acknowledgement of crisis potentials during this period legitimizes the need for support experienced at this time and motivates further exploration of variables which may contribute to the crisis or diminish it. Future research on expectant parenthood has to continue to focus on men, women and couples, describe and understand the processes that they undergo, relate them to their past experiences, to their present context and to adaption during and post pregnancy.

SUMMARY AND CONCLUSIONS

Assuming a parent's role has meaningful personal, marital and social implications. Recently the interest in these implications was intensified and their empirical investigation expended. This chapter has focused on the first phase of transition to parenthood—on the pregnancy—and examined it from men's, women's and couples' points of view. This examination leads to the conclusion that experiences during pregnancy are determined by physical, emotional and contextual factors, and influence them in return. Additionally it can be concluded that for men, women and couples, pregnancy is a strenuous time, a period with crisis potentials.

Based on this conclusion, it is suggested that interventions during pregnancy be planned to include both spouses and to relate to physical, emotional and couple issues.

REFERENCES

Beail, N. (1982). The role of the father during pregnancy and childbirth. In N. Beail & J. McGuire (eds.), Fathers' psychological perspectives. London: Junction Books.

Bem, S.L. (1974). The measurement of psychological androgyny. *Journal of Consulting and Clinical Psychology, 42*, 155–162.

Benedek, T. (1959). Parenthood as a development phase. *Journal of American Psychoanalytic Association, 7*, 389–417.

Bernard, J. (1974). The Future of Marriage. New York: World.

Bibring, G.L. (1959). Some considerations of the psychological processes in pregnancy. In *Psychoanalytic study of the child*, Vol. 14, New York: International University Press.

Bittman, S., & Zalk, S.R. (1978). *Expectant Fathers*. New York: Hawthorn Books.

Blitzer, J.R., & Murray, J.M. (1964). On the transformation of early narcissism during pregnancy. *International Journal of Psychoanalysis, 45*, 89–97.

Breen, D. (1975). The birth of the first child: Towards an understanding of femininity. London: Tavistock.

Brown, J. (1964). Anxiety in pregnancy. *British Journal of Medical Psychology, 37*, 27–57.

Bumpass, L., & Rindfuss, R.R. (1979). Children's experience of marital disruption. *American Journal of Sociology, 85*, 49–65.

Cherlin, A. (1977). The effect of childen on marital dissolution. *Demography, 14*, 264–272.

Chertok, L. (1969). *Motherhood and personality*. London: Tavistock.

Clulow, C.F. (1982). *To have and to hold*. London: Aberdeen University Press.

Cowan, C.P., & Cowan, P. (1987). In C.F.Z. Boukydis (ed.), *Research on support for parents and infants in the postnatal period*. New Jersey: Ablex.

Cowan, C.P., Cowan, P., Heming, G. (1986). Risks to the marriage when partners become parents: Implications for family development. Paper presented at the American Psychiatric Association Meeting. Washington, DC.

Cowan, P.C., Cowan, A.P., Heming, G., Garrett, E., Coysh, W.S., Curtis-Boles, H., & Boles, A.J. (1985). Transition to parenthood: His, hers and theirs. *Journal of Family Issues, 6*, 451–481.

Curtis, T.L. (1955). A psychiatric study of 55 expectant fathers. *US Armed Forces Medical Journal, 5*, 937–950.

Cutright, P. (1971). Income and family stability. *Journal of Marriage and the Family, 33*, 294–306.

Dalton, K. (1971). Perspective study of puerperol depression. *British Journal of Psychology, 118*. 689–692.

Davenport-Slack, B., & Boylan, C. (1974). Psychological correlates of childbirth pain. *Psychosomatic Medicine, 24*, 215–233.

Davids, A., & DeVault, S. (1962). Maternal anxiety during pregnancy and childbirth abnormality. *Psychosomatic Medicine, 5*, 464–470.

Deutsch, H. (1945). *Psychology of women. A psychoanalytic interpretation.* Vol. II, *Motherhood.* New York: Grune and Straton.

Duvall, E.M. (1971). *Family development.* Philadelphia: Lippincott.

Dyer, E.D. (1963). Parenthood as crisis: A restudy. *Marriage and Family Living, 25*, 196–201.

Einzig, J.E. (1980). The child within: A study of expectant fatherhood. *Smith College Studies in Social Work, 50*, 117–164.

Endler, N.S. (1982). Interactionism: A personality model, but not yet a theory. *Nebraska Symposium on Motivation*, 155–200.

Enkin, M., Smith, S.L., Dermer, S.W., & Emmet, J.O. (1971). An adequately controlled study of effectiveness of PPM training. In N. Morris (ed.), *Psychosomatic medicine in obstetrics and gynecology.* New York: S. Karger.

Feldman, H. (1971). The effects of children on the family. In A. Mitchael (ed.), *Family issues of employed women in Europe and America.* Leiden: Brill.

Fishbein, E.G. (1981). Fatherhood and disturbances of mental health: A review. *Journal of Psychiatric Nursing and Mental Health Services, 19*, 24–27.

Fitzgerald, C.M. (1984). Nausea and vomiting in pregnancy, *British Journal of Medical Psychology, 57*, 159–165.

Freeman, T. (1951). Pregnancy as a precipitant of mental illness in men. *British Journal of Medical Psychology, 24*, 49–54.

Freud, S. (1925). Some psychological consequences of the anatomical distinction between the sexes. In *Collected Papers*, Vol. 5. New York: Basic Books (Reprinted 1959).

Gerzi, S., & Berman, E. (1981). Emotional reactions of expectant fathers to their wives first pregnancy. *British Journal of Medical Psychology, 54*, 259–265.

Ginath, Y.V. (1974). Psychoses in males in relation to their wives pregnancy and childbirth. *Israel Annals of Psychiatry, 12*, 227–237.

Gordon, R.E., & Gordon, K.K. (1959). Social factors in the prediction and treatment of emotional disorders of pregnancy. *American Journal of Obstetrics and Gynecology, 77*, 1074–1083.

Gorsuch, R., & Key, M. (1974). Abnormalities of pregnancy as a function of anxiety and life stress. *Psychosomatic Medicine, 36*, 352– 362.

Grossman, F., Eichler, L., & Winickoff, S. (1980). *Pregnancy, birth, and parenthood.* San Francisco: Jossey-Bass.

Hamburg, D.A., Moos, R.H., & Yalom, I.D. (1968). Studies of distress in the menstrual cycle and the postpartum period. In R.P. Micheal (ed.), *Eneocrinology and human behavior.* London: Oxford University Press.

Hammer, J. (1970). Preference for gender of child as a function of sex of adult respondents. *Journal of Individual Psychology, 31*, 54–56.

Hees–Stauthamer, J.C. (1985). *The first pregnancy. An integrating principle of female psychology.* Ann Arbor, Michigan: Umi Research Press.

Hill, R. (1965). Genetic features of families under stress. In H.J. Parad (ed.), *Crisis intervention: Selected readings.* Family Service Assocation of America.

Hobbs, D.F., & Cole, S.P. (1976). Transition to parenthood: A decade replication. *Journal of Marriage and the Family, 38*, 723–731.

Hyde, B. (1986). An interview of pregnant women's attitudes to ultrasound scanning. *Social Sciences and Medicine, 22*, 587–592.

Klusman, L.E. (1975). Reduction of pain in childbirth by the alleviation of anxiety during pregnancy. *Journal of Consulting and Clinical Psychology, 43*, 162–165.

Kohn, M.L. (1963). Social class and parent–child relationships: An interpretation. *American Journal of Sociology, 68*, 471–480.

Kohn, C.L., Nelson, A., & Weiner, S. (1980). Gravidas' responses to real-time ultrasound fetal image. *Journal of Obstetrics, Gynecology and Nursing*, March/April, 77–80.

LaCoursiere, R. (1972). Fatherhood and mental illness. *Psychiatric Quarterly*, *46*, 109–124.

Lahav, Y. (1984). Psychological aspects of men during their wives' pregnancy. Unpublished MA Theses, Tel-Aviv University.

Leifer, M. (1980). *Psychological effects of motherhood: A study of first pregnancy*. New York: Praeger.

LeMasters, E.E. (1957). Parenthood as crisis. *Marriage and Family Living*, *19*, 352–355.

Lewis, C.V. (1982). A feeling you can't scratch?: The effect of pregnancy and birth on married men. In N. Beail & J. McGuire (eds.), *Fathers psychological perspectives*. London: Junction Books.

Liebenberg, B. (1967). Expectant fathers. *American Journal of Orthopsychiatry*, *37*, 358–359.

Lipkin, M., & Lamb, G.S. (1982). The couvade syndrome: An epidemiologic study. *Annals of Internal Medicine*, *96*, 509–511.

Lips, H.M. (1985). A longitudinal study of the reporting of emotional and somatic symptoms during and after pregnancy. *Social Science and Medicine*, *21*, 631–640.

Mead, M. (1949). *Male and female*. London: Victor Gollancz.

Melges, F.T. (1968). Postpartum psychotic syndrome. *Psychosomatic Medicine*, *30*, 95–108.

Milne, L.S., & Rich, O.J. (1981). Cognitive and affective aspects of the responses of pregnant women to sonography. *Maternal–Child Nursing Journal*, *10*, 15–39.

Newman, L.F. (1978). Symbolism and status change: Fertility and the first child in India and the United States. In W. Miller & L.F. Newman (eds), *The first child and family formation*. North Carolina: University of North Carolina.

Nott, P.N. (1976). Hormonal changes and mood in the peurperium. *British Journal of Psychiatry*, *128*, 379–383.

Nuckolls, K., Cassel, J., & Kaplan, B. (1972). Psychological assets, life crisis and the prognosis of pregnancy. *American Journal of Epidemiology*, *95*, 431–441.

Oakley, A. (1980). *Women confined: Towards a sociology of childbirth*. Oxford: Martin Robertson.

Osofsky, J.D., & Osofsky, H.J. (1984). Psychological and developmental perspectives on expectant and new parenthood. In R.D. Parke, R.N. Emde, H.P. McAdoo, & G.P. Sackett (eds), *Review of child development research*, Vol. 7: *The Family*. Chicago, Ill.: The University of Chicago Press.

Parad, H.J., & Caplan, G. (1965). A Framework for studying families in crisis. In H.J. Parad (ed.), *Crisis intervention: Selected readings*. New York: Family Services Association of America.

Parke, R.D. (1981). Fathers. Harvard University Press, Cambridge.

Quill, T.M., Lipkin, M., & Lamb, G.S. (1984). Health-care seeking by men in their spouse's pregnancy. *Psychosomatic Medicine*, *46*, 277–283.

Rabinowici, D. (1985). Psychological adaptation during pregnancy and postpartum as related to knowledge of fetal sex and personality traits. Unpublished MA Thesis. Tel-Aviv University.

Reading, A.F., & Cox, D.N. (1982). The effects of ultrasound examination on material anxiety levels. *Journal of Behavioural Medicine*, *5*, 237–247.

Rossi, A.S. (1968). Transition to parenthood. *Journal of Marriage and the Family*, *30*, 26–39.

Russell, C.S. (1974). Transition to parenthood: Problems and gratifications. *Journal of Marriage and the Family*, *36*, 294–301.

Saurel-Cubizolles, M.J., & Kaminski, M. (1986). Work in pregnancy: Its evolving relationship with perinatal outcome. (A review). *Social Science and Medicine*, *22*, 431–442.

Scott-Heyes, G. (1982). The experience of prenatal paternity and its relation to attitudes to pregnancy and childbirth. In N. Beail & J. McGuire (eds), *Fathers psychological perspectives*. London: Junction Books.

Shereshefsky, P.M., & Yarrow, L.J. (1973). *Psychological aspects of a first pregnancy.* New York: Raven.

Sherman, J.A. (1971). *On the psychology of women: A survey of empirical studies.* Springfield, Ill.: Charles C Thomas.

Spielberger, C.D. (1966). Theory and research on anxiety. In C.D. Spielberger (ed.), *Anxiety and behavior.* New York: Academic Press.

Spielberger, C.D., Gorsuch, R.L., & Lushene, R.L. (1970). *State–trait anxiety manual.* Palo Alto: Consulting Psychologist Press.

Teichman, Y. (1978). Affiliative reaction in different kinds of threat situations. In C.D. Spielberger and I.G. Sarason (eds), *Stress and anxiety*, Vol. 5. Washington: Halsted Press.

Teichman, Y., & Lahav, Y. (1987). Expectant fathers, emotional reactions, physical symptoms and coping. *The British Journal of Medical Psychology, 60*, 225–232.

Trethowan, W.H., & Conlon, M.H. (1965). The couvade syndrome. *British Journal of Psychiatry, 3*, 57–66.

Wainwright, N.H. (1966). Fatherhood as a precipitant of mental illness. *American Journal of Psychiatry, 123*, 40–44.

Weigert, E.V., Wenner, N.K., Cohen, M.B., Fearing, J.M., Kavarnes, R.G., & Ohaneson, E.M. (1968). Emotional aspects of pregnancy. Final Report of Washington School of Psychiatry Project. Clinical Study of the Emotional Challenge of Pregnancy. Washington, DC: Washington School of Psychiatry.

Wenner, N., & Cohen, M.B. (1968). Emotional Aspects of Pregnancy. First report of the Washington School of Psychiatry Project. Washington, DC: Washington School of Psychiatry.

Wenner, N.K., Cohen, M.B., Weigert, E.V., Kavarnes, R.G., Obaneson, E.M., & Fearing, J.M. (1969). Emotional problems in pregnancy. *Psychiatry, 32*, 389–410.

Wolkind, S. (1981). Fathers. In S. Wolind & E. Zajicek (eds), *Pregnancy a psychological and social study.* London: Academic Press.

Zajicek, E., & Wolkind, S. (1978). Emotional difficulties in married women during and after the first pregnancy. *British Journal of Medical Psychology, 59*, 379–385.

Zax, M., Sameroff, A., & Farnum, J. (1975). Childbirth education, maternal attitudes and delivery. *American Journal of Obstetrics and Gynecology, 123*, 185–190.

Zemlick, M.J., & Watson, R. (1953). Maternal attitudes of acceptance and rejection during and after pregnancy. *American Journal of Orthopsychiatry, 23*, 570–584.

Zilboorg, G. (1931). Depressive reactions related to parenthood. *American Journal of Psychiatry, 87*, 927–962.

KEY WORDS

Expectant parenthood, transition to parenthood, expectant mothers, expectant fathers, expectant couples, pregnancy, physical factors, emotional factors, contextual factors, emotional well-being, anxiety, crisis, crisis potentials, couvade syndrome, age, work, medical technology, formal support, informal support, prevention, intervention.

Handbook of Life Stress, Cognition and Health
Edited by S. Fisher and J. Reason
© 1988 John Wiley & Sons Ltd.

2

Stress in Childhood and Adolescence

I.M. GOODYER
University of Cambridge

INTRODUCTION

Children are developing organisms whose optimal physical and mental growth is a result of complex and interrelated processes of biological, psychological and social factors. This chapter considers the contribution of recent stressful life events and ongoing family and social difficulties to the development of distress and mental disorder in childhood and adolescence.

The early environment, the family, social experiences and the effects of disasters will be discussed. The potential differences in children's appraisal of stressors, and subsequent behavioural responses at different stages of development are outlined. Understanding the mechanisms by which social stressors exert their effects will not be achieved without further clarification of the psychological and physiological processes involved.

The present state of knowledge does not allow for a clear development theory of stress to be proposed. It is suggested that progress in the area of stress research will require closer multidisciplinary collaboration from biological, psychological, social developmental and clinical scientists.

INFANCY AND THE PRESCHOOL CHILD

From conception, the human organism is subjected to stressful life 'events': it is self-evident that birth is stressful and eventful, as are other biological innate developmental milestones such as crawling and walking. However, there are many external concomitants of these innate characteristics which are critical in negotiating necessary developmental stages. For example, starvation may lead to a failure of normal development or render a child vulnerable to chronic illness resulting in significant delays in physical development. Similarly, the presence of well-being in the young child provides the platform for later normative and necessary tasks and events (i.e. those we expect to occur as a result of

23

development) that are potentially stressful, such as the attainment of friendship and school entry.

By and large, the state of stress of normal infants is defensive, with a great deal of diversive behaviour. Lipsitt (1983) indicates that in infancy there are many risks and hazards to be negotiated in order to continue with normal development. Defensive responses such as crying occur most in the first months of life and decrease in quantity from thereon throughout childhood. Social withdrawal characterized by listlessness and a poverty of interaction with caretakers can be seen (in the abscence of physical disease) as pathological defensive reactions as described, for example, in extreme forms of child abuse (MacCarthy, 1974; Mrazek and Mrazek, 1985).

It becomes apparent therefore that human beings are subject to stresses from early infancy that may be independent of their own actions and to which aversive and defensive coping behaviours (such as crying) are likely results. To determine what antecedents influence these behavioural repertoires and whether or not these early styles reflect a rehearsal for later coping styles is, as Lipsitt argues, a task for developmental research.

Kagan (1983) asserts that, for developmentalists, stress must be viewed as an interaction between 'want and response' and will not be adequately understood if either of these factors is studied in isolation from the other. Thus stress reflects reciprocal activity between an infant and its environment. Stress may arise because of deficits in the infant, the environment or their interactions.

Evidence to date suggests that both continuities and discontinuities in development are likely to occur (Emde and Harmon, 1984). At present there is little research to tell us if stressful events of a discrete nature cause undesirable pathologic effects in infancy in the medium to long term. There is, however, a substantial literature to show that more enduring long-term difficulties do exert unwanted effects on infants (Rutter, 1983). In particular, mothers who are unable to nurture as a result of pyschiatric disorder, personality difficulties or lack of intimate confiding relationships in their own lives seem unable to provide an environment for optimal normal development. Their children show increased rates of psychiatric disorder in early childhood (Ghodsian et al., 1984; Richman, 1977; Pound et al., 1985).

As Rutter (1983, 1984) has indicated, a striking feature of these early identity difficulties is that the infant is continually exposed to the effects of maternal stresses. These findings suggest that in infancy and during the preschool years, stress exerts effects through deficits in both nurturing and protection. Quinton and Rutter's (1985a) studies of children raised in care demonstrate, however, that the outcome is far from gloomy in all cases and that, for some children, removal from continuous undesirable stress to a better caretaking environment can result in good later adjustment.

Present evidence indicates that if caretaking deficits are to exert stressful effects they must be ongoing long-term difficulties. The resilience of infants and young children is also apparent when such difficulties are neutralized by improving the environmental conditions.

STRESS AND MIDDLE CHILDHOOD

For the infant and preschool child, present evidence indicates a powerful role of the environment in the influence of stressful experiences on development and psychiatric disorder, but it also suggests that there are intrinsic factors of young children which promote resilience and may be important precursors for coping responses in the presence of social adversity.

In middle childhood the effects of the environment, especially the family, continue to play a major role in protecting children from stress or being a cause of stress. By this stage of development the child has an increased repertoire of responses and coping strategies to stressful experiences.

In broad terms there are three factors of normal development for which middle childhood can be considered to be different to early childhood:

    a)   peer relations
    b)   cognitive development
    c)   behavioural response to stress.

It is likely that these three factors are mutually interdependent, although to what degree and under what conditions are not yet understood.

Increasing the number of peer relations brings greater opportunities for specific and discrete life events to impact on the child directly, both within school and in social and leisure pursuits.

Cognitive development brings a greater sense of enquiry and exploration of the world, with resulting desire for the mastery of tasks and the accompanying risk of potential failure and personal danger.

By middle childhood the child's responses to stress may be more subtle and less direct than the care-elicting or seeking responses that predominate in infancy and preschool children. The increased repertoire of behavioural responses to social experiences broadens the opportunity for clinicians and researchers to identify patterns of abnormal signs and symptoms as a result of stressful events and difficulties. Thus in this age group affective expression (sadness, misery, anger) and behavioural expression (disruptiveness, school refusal, obsssional phenomena) became apparent. Consequently, psychopathological states in middle childhood may assume a different form of expression as a result of stress.

Whether or not some stresses result in different forms of behavioural response at different levels of development is not yet clear. There is some evidence that such an effect does exist. For example, Ferguson (1979) has shown that previous experience of hospitalization may reduce fears of hospitals in school-age children but not in preschoolers.

There is also some evidence to indicate a lack of specificity between the type of recent stressful life event and the form of disorder (Goodyer *et al.*, 1985). This research demonstrated, for example, that recent stressful life events such as family disharmony, illness or accident can occur with equal frequency in cases of both conduct disorders with predominant symptoms of disturbed behaviour, and emotional disorders with predominant symptoms of mood disturbance.

In contrast to the occurrence of recent stresses, Rutter (1983, 1985) has shown that chronic family and marital difficulties and continuous exposure to psychiatric disturbance in parents are significantly more common in conduct than in emotional disorder, indicating that there is some evidence for greater specificity between ongoing long-term difficulties and presenting with behavioural symptoms rather than with mood disturbance.

The relative contribution, however, of recent stressful events, ongoing difficulties and social disadvantage as causal factors in conduct and emotional disorders in this age group has yet to be evaluted. At present, therefore, the mechanisms by which social factors exert their effects in distress reactions and different psychiatric disorders remain unclear.

STRESS AND ADOLESCENCE

For the adolescent, increasing social development continues to alter the balance of the individual's orientation between family and peer group. Thus, there is further privacy and personal responsibility associated with a widening social network, with further decreases in the amount of time spent in the family home. Whether these shifts reflect qualitative changes in orientation, from parents and siblings to friends, for example, with less intimacy and personal support is not clear. However, adolescents are just as likely as those in middle childhood to be exposed to stressful life events (Goodyer et al., 1986). What is different is that the type of event is increasingly more likely to be personal and not necessarily to involve family members. In particular, sexual events become important. Furthermore adolescents may consider the personal meaning and potential impact of events differently from their parents. Indeed, recent research suggests that stressful experiences occurring in the lives of children and young adolescents (less than 15 years of age) may be reliably reported by their mothers but for older adolescents mothers can be unaware of personal stressful events and those adolescents are more reliable with their own reports (Moncke and Dobbs, 1985).

Thus, the social experience of adolescence is broader, wider and qualitatively different, from that of middle childhood. With increasing personal autonomy comes a potentially increasing risk of experiencing events that may not be ameliorated by family factors previously seen as protective against stressful events and difficulties. There is a shift of emphasis towards peer identification and a greater use of personal coping away from family protection.

The developmental issues briefly referred to indicate that social experiences can be considered in three ways when evaluating their effects. Firstly, their form may change with development, for example mothers' protective and nurturing function in infancy is substantial. By adolescence, mothers are less instrumentally protective, may be more advisory and consultative and make less of a relative contribution to the quantity of time spent with their child. If mothers maintain their protective functions as in infancy at adolescence, this may reflect a non-normative process which is now undesirable.

Secondly, the content of social experiences alters. Thus the relative contribution of family and peer group relations and the quality of such relationships change with age. For example, by late adolescence increasing confiding relationships with peers contrasts with decreasing intimacy with mothers.

Thirdly, the process of experiences changes. The want and response relationship between infant and mother may become more complex and multivariate. A wakeful crying infant may invariably require feeding, but a wakeful crying adolescent requires enquiry before response can be made.

Clearly the context of events and difficulties must be understood if their impact is to be measured. The relative contributions of discrete stressful life events and ongoing difficulties must be evaluated in relation to a child's stage of development and the successes and failures of social development that have occurred during his lifetime.

Finally, there may be hidden advantages to certain stressful experiences in the course of development. For example, the development of individual competence may be enhanced by stresses that are necessary but overcome (e.g. school entry) or occur in a qualitatively acceptable way (e.g. minor physical illness). Garmezy (1985) and others (e.g. Parmalee, 1986) have referred to the positive consequences of these adversities as steeling effects, and postulate that they contribute to the development of self-esteem and resilience in the face of other perhaps similar adversities at other points in time, possibly by influencing cognitive–emotional perceptions of social circumstances.

THE PERCEPTION OF STRESS

To consider children in isolation from family and peers is clearly unhelpful and misleading. We can see that stressful experiences may exert different effects at different ages and, furthermore, what may be desirable at one age may clearly be undesirable at another. The relationship between factors that protect against stressful events as well as the importance of understanding the relative contribution of recent events in the presence of ongoing difficulties and disadvantage have been highlighted. Finally it is clear that the impact of life events may not always be detrimental, and the quality of events, rather than the number alone, may determine effects at different ages.

Identifying stressful family and social events and difficulties that are potentially causal factors in distress and psychiatric disorder is a continuing task for the researcher in developmental psychopathology. It is equally as important, however, to understand the cognitive and emotional processes that are involved in the appraisal of these phenomena.

For example, the psychological mechanism of denial has advantages in protecting against stress in adults (Lazarus, 1981). In childhood the value of denial is less clear. Firstly, it becomes less apparent as children get older and, secondly, its utility may depend on the situation—i.e. state related—rather then the child's capacity for denial—i.e. trait related—(Smith and Rossman, 1986). Secondly, there is some evidence to indicate a development shift in children's concept of emotion between 6 and 11 years of age, but little change thereafter. Thus younger children focus on the publicly observable components of emotion whilst older children consider the hidden mental aspect (Harris et al., 1981). The elucidation of relationships between emotions, cognitions and behaviours in normal and disturbed children is important to the understanding of intrinsic mechanisms for perceiving and responding to stressful experiences (Izard *et al.*, 1984).

LIFE EVENTS AND PSYCHIATRIC DISORDER

The use of semi-structured interviews to discriminate between events as potential causes rather than consequences of psychiatric disorder has resulted in a much greater understanding of the role of acute stress in psychiatric disorder, particularly depression in young adults (Brown, 1974; Brown and Harris, 1978; Paykel, 1983).

The role of recent stressful life events as potentially causal factors in psychiatric disorders of childhood and adolescence has been examined in few studies, only one of which evaluates events on a prospective sample of children using a semi-structured interview approach (Goodyer *et al.*, 1985). Results from this study suggest that moderate to severely undesirable life events occurring in the 12 months before disorder are potentially causal factors in about 60% of new cases attending psychiatric clinics. This study also showed that mildly undesirable events are potentially causal factors for conduct but not emotional disorders.

These findings suggest that for conduct disorders the quality of stressful events is relatively unimportant and they exert a rather non-specific mechanical effect on the onset of behavioural symptoms. By comparison, the quality of events is important for emotional disorders as only events considered likely to be substantially undesirable cause mood disorder. Furthermore, the results highlight the fact that recent stresses are only one causal factor, even in emotional disorders, as 40% of cases in the study had no recent stresses. Overall, the findings from this study suggest that:

    a)   in some two thirds of cases, moderate to severely undesirable recent life events may provoke new episodes of psychiatric disorder;

    b)   some well children experience severe events but do not develop psychiatric disorder, suggesting they are protected in some way (either by other social experiences or different appraisal).

Classifying Events

Events may be classified in ways other than by their degree of undesirability. For example, events may be classified according to their general characteristics (such as marital, family, illness or accident) and as to whether or not they consitute permanent separations (termed exit events) or additions (entrance events) to the child's social field.

Although exit events appear less commonly, they may be more important for severe anxious and depressive emotional disorders and children presenting with somatic complaints (Goodyer *et al.*, 1985). These latter findings are made on the basis of rather small sample size but are of interest as they are analogous to the associations between this class of life events and the onset of depression in adults.

An understanding of the associations between psychiatric disorder and events may be improved by considering certain other psychological qualities which events may carry. For example, a single event may be undesirable, out of the child's control, impact directly on the child or indirectly via a parent, and have consequences that inevitably alter the child's environment (e.g. divorce) or return it to the previous state (e.g. serious but successfully treated illness). As yet, such multidimensional measures of life events have not been examined in children, although the evidence from adult studies suggests exploration would be worthwhile (Finlay-Jones and Brown, 1981; Miller and Ingham, 1983).

The Number and Timing of Events

The causal relationship between events and disorder may also be strengthened if there is an association between event occurrence and the time of onset of signs and symptoms. For example, in school-age children, whilst events occur throughout the 12 months prior to the onset of disorder, they tend to cluster in the 16 weeks closest to onset of symptoms, supporting the inference that events cause disorder (Goodyer et al., 1987). Furthermore, children who have experienced two or more events in the preceding 12 months are more likely to report an event in the 16 weeks before onset. This suggests that in some cases a degree of additivity between events occurs over time to produce a stressful effect.

The type of mechanism involved in this additivity effect of stressors may be different for different types of disorder. For conduct disorders there appears to be a non-specific quantitative addition dependent mainly on the number of events. Under these circumstances, therefore, symptoms may occur independent of any meaning inherent in the events, implying a threshold of stress above which psychiatric disorder is likely.

The association for emotional disorders is less clear, and more qualitative factors may also influence additivity as well as impact. These may be the presence of particular links or connections between the events or perhaps through the personal significance unrelated to the events but reflecting intrinsic psychological associations made by the child. Under these circumstances the meaning of events is important and symptoms are more likely to occur as a consequence.

In contrast there is no association between the number of reported events and disorder in cases where onset of disorder occurs within four weeks of an event. This suggests that there are rapid and perhaps direct effects of a single stressful event in some cases. Whether rapid effects are a result of qualities in the event itself or a particular type of appraisal by the child has not been examined.

It may be that there are differential effects of both the timing and number of events at different ages. The study described above was carried out in school-age children, and similar systematic research has not been carried out for children of other ages. There are suggestions in the literature, however, that age is important in determining the effect of events. For example, studies on hospitalization in childhood suggests that it is multiple not single admissions that are likely to result in long-term distress (Douglas, 1975; Quinton and Rutter, 1976).

The Influence of Sex Differences on Recent Life Events

The influence of sex differences on the impact of stressful social experiences is an important factor in developmental research. There is some evidence that there are sex differences in the appraisal of stressful events but not necessarily in the occurrence of such events. Thus Burke and Weir (1978) have suggested that girls perceive more stress in their lives than boys, and Dweck and colleagues (Dweck and Bush, 1976; Dweck et al., 1978) have reported observational data in a classroom setting indicating that boys respond with greater efforts following criticism of performance from adults, whereas girls tend to give up and blame their own lack of ability. Perhaps girls are more likely to attribute external stressors to their own personal shortcomings, insurmountable through personal effort alone. Adverse social experiences that adults bring to bear on children may be important in this regard: for example the popular view that girls are emotionally more labile or more suggestible than boys is not supported by research findings (Maccoby and Jacklin, 1978).

These appraisal differences are important, but it is not clear if they are a result of the events per se or the consequence of adults' responses to events, as seems the case with classroom experience.

The evidence, at least for school-age children, is that there is surprisingly little difference in the number and type of stressful life events occurring in the lives of boys and girls (Goodyer et al., 1986). The present evidence suggests that girls may be more likely to experience severe mood disturbances than boys, but overall it is the lack of sex differences that is striking.

Measuring Events

An important issue is how and by whom events should be rated. We do not know if adults' concepts and perceptions of threat, undesirability and other dimensions of events are necessarily the same as those of young people themselves. This issue needs addressing and investigating, perhaps using well children at different ages to rate how threatening events might be perceived. Furthermore, what of subjective ratings of the child patients themselves? Whilst patients with acute disorder may overrate the undesirable qualities of events, this may not be true for more quiescent phases of illness or during recovery.

Some preliminary evidence suggests that events rated by adults and adolescents show substantial concordance when severely undesirable but low concordance when only mildly undesirable. In particular, adolescents with psychiatric disorders are significantly more likely to rate mild events as severe compared with well adolescents or adults (Gannon et al., 1987). This suggests that adolescents with recent disturbance may overestimate the impact of events and this may be a function of disorder. This work is in a preliminary phase, but tentatively suggests that young people's ratings of events may be prone to the same sorts of invalidity as ratings for adults, in particular there are similar errors due to overestimating the degree of undesirability and therefore confounding the association between events and disorder.

Methodologically there will be developmental limitations in obtaining children's ratings of events and it is unlikely that children under 7 or 8 years old would be able to evaluate the impact of life events over time.

A further measurement issue concerns the conditions in which an event occurs. Children and adolescents may not be in a position to (a) take independent action or (b) guard against being adversely influenced by events happening to other family members. In some events, the impact may be filtered by parents or others dealing with the practical issues required, e.g. nursing a sick family member of home, or providing direct support to the child by explanation and reassurance of their sibling's condition. In other circumstances the effects of events may be amplified, e.g. the failure to nurse a sick sibling adequately may indirectly increase the effects of this event on a child.

These issues illustrate some of the methodological complexities required if reliable and valid measurement of life events is to be achieved for young people.

The Relative Contribution of Events to Psychiatric Disorder

The complexities of theory, measurement, statistical models and data interpretation applied in many adult studies in an effort to elucidate the social and psychological mechanisms of anxiety and depression in adults have not yet been applied fully to studies of psychiatric disorder in children. From what little we can surmise, recent events will be of interest both in terms of their aetiological significance and as models for examining individual and family coping responses to stressful social experiences.

At present the meaning and mechanisms of stressful events in young people are probably best further illustrated by the studies which have concentrated on a particular type of stressor. Three of these, divorce, birth of a sibling and bereavement, are used to illustrate how stressful events may exert their effects.

Divorce

Divorce is an outcome event of ongoing difficulties in marital relationships and constitutes a major adverse stress in the lives of children (Wallerstein and Kelly, 1980). The stressful effects that divorce brings to bear on children depends on:
a) antecedent relationships between parents
b) antecedent child/parent interaction
c) post divorce relationships between biological parents
d) post divorce child/parent interaction
e) post divorce social experiences (i.e. access arrangements, social migration resulting in school and peer relationship changes and new adult relations).

Conceptually, one difference between divorce and other stressful events is that divorce is arrived at intentionally in an effort to end unwanted and intolerable marital disharmony. From the child's point of view, marital disharmony, particularly involving physical violence between parents, is associated with psychiatric disorder in children (Wallerstein, 1983; Quinton and Rutter, 1976). In these circumstances, divorce may have a beneficial effect on a child as a result of separation from unwanted experiences.

However, as other researchers have shown, this is only likely in cases where divorce has the required effect, i.e. stops or significantly diminishes parental discord. When discord continues, children remain in ongoing stressful circumstances and the risk of maladjustment remains (Wallerstein, 1983).

The process of divorce may exert unwanted stressful effects even when it succeeds in relieving marital disharmony. This may be because separation from either parent is unwanted, even in the presence of disharmony, and because, unlike other stressors (e.g. acute illness or burglary), there is no return to a previously desirable steady state. Furthermore, for the child there is no predicting how the environment will be in the future. Divorce as a disrupter is therefore largely uncontrollable, with negative as well as positive outcome options.

Differential effects of divorce at different ages. The form of expression of children's response to the stresses of divorce changes with development (Wallerstein and Kelly, 1980; Hetherington *et al.*, 1978, 1979). The preschool child's responses are dominated by sleep disturbance, irritability, aggression and inhibited play. In middle childhood, signs of depression, with fearfulness of a parental replacement, social withdrawal and increased risk of educational underachievement are more characteristic. In late childhood and adolescence, overt anger may accompany depression, continuing difficulties with education and peer relations may be reported, and a parent's own social behaviour can be stimulating but distracting from normal adolescent pursuits.

Furthermore, the evidence suggests that girls are more disrupted in the acute phase, although late adjustment seems unrelated to sex and more to the quality of life in the post-divorce family (Hetherington *et al.*, 1979).

The importance of understanding cognitive mechanisms related to stressful events is demonstrated by the different attributions and possible coping strategies of children of different ages that may occur as a result of divorce. Thus Hetherington and her colleagues (1979) have shown, for example, that in younger children marital disharmony and subsequent divorce may be attributed to their personal failures, whereas the older child is more likely to blame one or other parent. How social and cognitive factors interact to influence children's emotional responses, such as feelings of loss, disappointment, anger, depression and personal blame, is less well understood.

Birth of Sibling

An example of the transactional effects of stress within families has been examined from a different point of view with regard to the birth of a sibling (Dunn and Kendrick, 1980a,b). This important research highlights how for many families a normative event (i.e. the birth of a child) is stressful. For some first-born children the development of behaviour problems with the arrival of a sibling was found to be linked to individual differences in the children's temperament and to marked changes in interaction between the first-born child and mother. Thus mothers tended to engage in less playful interaction with their first-born children and also showed more prohibitions, confrontations and negative verbal inter-actions. Furthermore, depressed mothers were more likely to exhibit signs of withdrawal from the first-born. Dunn and her colleagues conclude that the normal relationship between a 2–3 year old and its mother is often stressful, and the complex changes that occur around the birth of a sibling heighten these difficul-ties, even when the second child is born at home so that there is no separation of the mother and first-born.

The transactional effects of the birth of a sibling and the consequences for ongoing relationships suggest that an adequate analysis of stressful events and difficulties requires an analysis not merely of marital effects, but of the patterns of interactions within a family (Dunn, 1986; Emde and Harmon, 1984).

Bereavement

There are surprisingly few studies on the effects of bereavement as a stressor in childhood (Garmezy, 1983). In the only prospective controlled report to date, Van Eerdewegh and colleagues (1982) compared a cohort of children, randomly selected and aged 2 to 11 years, 1 and 13 months after the death of one of their parents, with age- and sex-matched controls with no such loss. At 1 month there were signs of depressive mood in over three-quarters of the bereaved children compared with a third of the non-bereaved controls. By 13 months, however, the reactions in the bereaved group were considerably diminished, and depressive symptoms were rare, although disinterest in school persisted in some adolescents. The results suggest that, in comparison with earlier clinical descriptive studies (Furman, 1974), for many children the immediate consequences of bereavement may be severe but of a relatively short duration.

There is a suggestion that in adolescence the loss of the same sex parent is more likely to result in prolonged and more depressive type symptoms (Lifschitz *et al.*, 1977; Raphael, 1982; Rutter, 1966). At present, however, it has to be said that we know little of either the short or medium term effects of bereavement on children. The long-term effects of bereavement in childhood have received greater atten-tion in the adult literature as researchers have examined the relative contribution of bereavement to adult depression. A review of this literature is beyond the scope of this chapter; however, the present evidence suggests that where bereavement exerts a long-term effect into adulthood, it may do so because of its consequences for the child's subsequent care rather than because of the impact of loss per se (Brown *et al.*, 1986).

Retrospective studies of separation and loss effects at different times in childhood have indicated that it is children of middle childhood who may be the most vulnerable to later difficulties as adults, perhaps because it is children of this age group who respond with greatest difficulty to institutionalization, either in a children's home or with foster parents (Tennant *et al.*, 1982). The research to date, however, has not considered in any systematic way the develop-mental effects that may influence the impact of bereavement. For example, the relationship between cognitive understanding of death, coping responses used by children and their subsequent adjustment merits systematic study.

Overall, the immediate impact of bereavement carries an understandable degree of stress. The duration of bereavement, however, may depend on the quality of relationships antedating the loss and the subsequent relationships in the child's life.

THE STRESS OF EVERYDAY LIFE

The subsequent and possibly coercive patterns of behaviour between family members as a result of a stressful event and circumstances represent a process that can change patterns of behaviour over time. Patterson (1982, 1983) points out that by concentrating on the major patterns of life events in the search for causal factors of stress-related disorders, the minor everyday hassles may be overlooked although they may have profound effects on adjustment. Rather than attempting to develop a general theory of stress, it may be more productive to identify critical parameters that characterize specific stress situations. Patterson's detailed studies of the relationship between boys and their parents using direct observation show that aggression between mother and child is a consequence of mutually coercive interdependent behaviour. Families with both coercive interactions and everyday hassles are significantly more likely to produce conduct disorder than families with everyday hassles but no coercive interactions.

BUFFERING AND PROTECTIVE FACTORS AGAINST STRESS

Social and Family Supports

The effects of stresses may be attenuated by other factors in the child's life. Children who develop and maintain good relationships with one or both parents, have a previous record of scholastic achievement, and maintain or develop social supports with their peers are significantly less likely to develop psychiatric disorder (Rutter, 1979, 1983). These findings suggest that the availability of adequate and intimate relationships with others (siblings, friends, extended family) protects against the effects of ongoing stressful difficulties in general. There have been no published studies to date examining the success of these protective or buffering factors in the presence of recent stressful life events. Furthermore, we have yet to examine the importance of supportive factors under different conditions. For example, we do not know if support at a time of crisis is the same as everyday support.

There are differences in the way children's friendships and confidants develop over time that are part of normal social development (Hartup, 1983). A closer examination of these friendship processes in disturbed children will provide clues as to how social relationships interrelate with stressful events and difficulties.

The appraisal of social relations by children requires closer examination as there is some evidence to suggest that certain individual characteristics such as the development of self-esteem and personal resilience, are a result of successful interpersonal experiences (Hartup, 1983; Rutter and Garmezy, 1983; Harre, 1984; Hunter, 1983). These personal qualities may be important factors in determining children's coping abilities in the presence of stressful experiences.

Intrinsic Mechanisms of Stress

There is considerable evidence that children vary greatly in their individual temperamental styles (Porter and Collins, 1982). Various studies have shown the importance of these temperamental differences in determining the risk of developing conduct or emotional disorder (Rutter, 1983).

The work of Dunn and Kendrick (1980a) suggests that temperamental differences in the children in their study were predictive of behaviour problems following the birth of a sibling. Other research has also hinted at the importance of temperament in stressful circumstances as a consequence of increasing children's vulnerability to stress and/or as producing stressful events and circumstances by inducing more negative responses from others (Rutter, 1983; Quinton and Rutter, 1985b). At present, however, the processes and mechanisms involved in the associations between temperament and stress are not well understood.

The associations between other internal markers of stress such as physiological changes in the autonomic nervous system of endocrine responses (such as cortisol growth hormone, prolactin and β-endorphins) have also received relatively little attention and their role in the development of psychiatric disorders is unclear. Understanding the maturation of these biological systems may be important in understanding transactions between physiochemical change and stressful experiences (Levine, 1983; Price *et al.*, 1983). In animal models, correlates between brain opioids and social emotions, endocrine and immune responses to stress and the effect of neurophysiological and chemical lesions on affiliative behaviour suggest potential integration of psychobiological models of human development (Reite and Field, 1985). It has to be said, however, that so far there is little evidence in children that there are specific psychophysiological or neurochemical models of response to stressful events (Rutter, 1983).

ONGOING STRESSFUL DIFFICULTIES

Rutter and colleagues (1979, 1983) have identified a number of social and family adversities that increase the risk of psychiatric disorder and reflect ongoing chronic difficulties. Unemployment, paternal criminality and being taken into care by the social services can all increase the risk of psychiatric disorder in children. The presence of psychiatric disorder in parents (especially, mother and, in particular, personality difficulties) is an important chronic stress in children's lives (Quinton and Rutter, 1985a). These results suggest that it is the persistence of adverse effects in the child's life that increases the risk of disorder.

PATTERNING AND MULTIPLE STRESSES

The work of Rutter and colleagues (Rutter, 1985) indicates that there are important interactions between chronic persistent stresses that potentiate their adverse effects and increase risk of distress and disorder, especially for disorders of conduct. There is also some evidence that the presence of chronic stresses makes it more likely that children will suffer effects from acute stresses (Rutter, 1979). The finding that those with conduct disorders have experienced greater numbers of stressful life events than those with emotional disorders further suggests that chronic adversities may increase the rate of occurrence of acute stressful events (Goodyer et al., 1985). The importance of investigating interactions between stresses in well children as well as of improving the specificity of the association with psychiatric disorder is an important ongoing task for stress research.

DISASTER, COPING AND ADJUSTMENT

Studies of extreme circumstances can allow some important observations to be made on children's coping reactions and subsequent adjustment. Disasters such as war, massive trauma, personal assault or evacuation to another country without parents or family members, have highlighted how children's psychological responses operate as a result of profound experiences of loss, deprivation and personal intrusion (Kinzie et al., 1986; Sack et al., 1986; Blom, 1986; Anthony, 1986; Garmezy, 1983). The finding and maintaining of a social and family support system after the disaster are predictive of good social adjustment. This suggests that the permanent loss of all previously significant relationships does not result in irrevocable disturbance providing subsequent social relations can be obtained that are adequate and sufficiently intimate.

This is not the case for all children who experience this degree of trauma, and individual differences reflecting the effects of temperament, genetic or other biological factors influence adjustment.

Therapeutic intervention for child victims of disaster has often been aimed at alleviating the immediate distress of traumatic experiences with counselling techniques. In some cases, however, adjustment may be facilitated through a more guided cognitive as well emotional re-experiencing, restructuring and re-enacting of the disaster event under controlled circumstances (Galante and Foa, 1986; Pynoos and Eth, 1986).

There has been little systematic research into treatment interventions for different types of stress-related disorders, and the implication that attention to cognitive as well as emotional factors in the children may be important for well-being in some cases merits further study.

SUMMARY AND CONCLUSIONS

There is clearly no satisfactory definition of 'stress' which will encompass the social, psychological and biological issues as they pertain to children.

Long-term exposure to ongoing family and social disadvantages can have profound adverse effects on subsequent development and increase the risk of psychiatric disorder throughout childhood. Acute stresses, too, substantially increase the risk of psychiatric disorder. There is a need to build on these important findings to improve our knowledge of the different effects that stresses may bring to bear at different stages of development.

Factors that provoke, facilitate and maintain exposure to undesirable social experiences must be considered concurrently with factors that protect, buffer and neutralize such experiences. The relevance of personal appraisal cannot be ignored as it has implications for treatment strategies. Also, research into the way children think about emotions and social experiences will help us clarify the mechanisms by which stressful experiences exert their effects.

We need to improve our understanding of the differential effects of stressful events on family process at different stages in the family life cycle. How, for example, would children in middle childhood or adolescence respond to the birth of a new sibling? What effects do prior experiences of divorce and their differential consequences have on children whose parents remarry? What effect does cognitive development exert on individual competence in the presence of stressful events and differential degrees of parental protection? Are there different physicochemical factors involved with different types of stressful experience?

It is apparent that clinical, epidemiological and experimental methods all have their place in the domain of stress research and will clearly require the skills of many. Greater exphasis must be placed on closer multidisciplinary research collaboration between neuroscientists, developmental psychologists and clinical researchers with an interest in, and a commitment to, children's mental health.

REFERENCES

Anthony, E.J. (1986). Terrorizing attacks on children by psychotic parents. *Journal of the American Academy of Child Psychiatry, 25*, 3, 226–235.

Blom, G.E. (1986). A school disaster—intervention and research aspects. *Journal of the American Academy of Child Psychiatry, 25*, 3, 336–345.

Brown, G.W. (1974). Meaning, measurement and stress of life events. In B.S. Dohrenwend & B.P. Dohrenwent (eds.), *Stressful life events, their nature and effects*. New York: John Wiley.

Brown, G., & Harris, T. (1978). *The social origins of depression*. London: Tavistock Press.

Brown, G., Harris, T., & Bifulco, A. (1986). Long term effects of loss of parent. In M. Rutter, C. Izard & P. Reed (eds.), *Depression in young people, developmental and clinical perspectives*. New York, London: Guilford Press.

Burke, R., & Weir, T. (1978). Sex differences in adolescent life stress, social support. *Journal of Psychology, 98*, 277–288.

Douglas, J.W.B. (1975). Early hospital admissions and later disturbances of behaviour and learning. *Development Medicine and Child Neurology, 17*, 456–480.

Dunn, J. (1986). Stress, development and family interaction. In M. Rutter, C. Izard & P. Reed (eds.), *Depressions in young people*. New York, London: Guilford Press.

Dunn, J., & Kendrick, C. (1980a). Studying temperament and parent–child interaction: comparison of interview and direct observation. *Development Medicine and Child Neurology, 4*, 484–496.

Dunn, J., & Kendrick, C. (1980b). The arrival of a sibling: Changes in patterns of interaction between mother and first born child. *Journal of Child Psychology and Psychiatry, 22*, 1–18.

Dweck, C.S., & Bush, E.S. (1976). Sex differences in learned helplessness. I. Differential deliberation with peer and adult evaluations. *Developmental Psychology, 12*, 147–156.

Dweck, C.S., Davidson, W., Nelson, S., & Emde, B. (1978). Sex differences in learned helplessness. II. The contingency of evaluative feedback in the classroom, and II. An experimental analysis. *Developmental Psychology, 14*, 268–276.

Emde, R., & Harmon, R. (1984). *Continuities and discontinuities in development*. New York, London: Plenum Press.

Ferguson, B.F. (1979). Preparing young children for hospitalisation: A comparison of two methods. *Pediatrics, 64*, 656–664.

Finlay-Jones, R., & Brown, G. (1981). Types of stressful life events and the onset of anxiety and depressive disorders. *Psychological Medicine, 11*, 803–815.

Furman, E. (1974). *A child's parent dies: studies in childhood bereavement*. New Haven: Yale University Press.

Galante, R., & Foa, D. (1986). An epidemiogological study of psychic trauma and treatment effectiveness for children after a natural disaster. *Journal of the American Academy of Child Psychiatry, 25*, 3, 357–363.

Gannon, B., Goodyer, I., & Rivlin, E. (1987). The appraisal of life events by adolescents. Unpublished manuscript.

Garmezy, N. (1983). Stresses of childhood. In N. Garmezy & M. Rutter (eds.), *Stress, coping and development in children*. New York: McGraw-Hill.

Garmezy, N. (1985). Stress-resistant children: the search for protective factors. In J. Stevenson (ed.), *Recent research in developmental psychopathology*. Oxford: Pergamon Press.

Ghodsian, M., Zajicek, E., & Wolkind, S. (1984). A longitudinal study of maternal depression and childhood behaviour problems. *Journal of Child Psychology and Psychiatry, 25*, 97–109.

Goodyer, I.M., Gatzanis, S., & Kolvin, I. (1987). The impact of recent stressful life events in psychiatric disorders of childhood and adolescence. *British Journal of Psychiatry*. (In Press).

Goodyer, I.M., Kolvin, I., & Gatzanis, S. (1985). Recent undesirable life events and psychiatric disorders of childhood and adolescence. *British Journal of Psychiatry, 47*, 517–523.

Goodyer, I.M., Kolvin, I., & Gatzanis, S. (1986). Do age and sex influence the association between recent life events and psychiatric disorders in children and adolescents—A controlled enquiry. *Journal of Child Psychology and Psychiatry, 27*, 5, 681–687.

Harre, R. (1984). Social elements as mind. *British Journal of Medical Psychology, 57*, 127–135.

Harris, P.L., Olthof, T., & Meerum Terwogt, M. (1981). Children's knowledge of emotion. *Journal of Child Psychology and Psychiatry, 22*, 247–261.

Hartup, W. (1983). Peer relations. In P. Mussen, (ed.). *Handbook of child psychology*, Vol. IV: *Socialisation, personality and social development*. New York, Chichester: John Wiley & Sons.

Hetherington, E.M., Cox, M., & Cox, R. (1978). The aftermath of divorce. In *Mother–child relations*. Washington, DC: National Association for the Education of Young Children.

Hetherington, E.M., Cox, M., & Cox, R. (1979). Family interaction and the social, emotional and cognitive development of children following divorce. In V. Vaughan & T. Brazelton (eds), *The Family: setting priorities*. New York: Science and Medicine.

Hunter, W. (1983). Developmental perspectives on the self-system. In P. Mussen (ed.), *Handbook of child psychology*, Vol. IV: *Socialisation, personality and social development*. New York, Chichester: John Wiley & Sons.

Izard, C., Kagan, J., & Zajonc, R. (1984). *Emotions, cognition and behaviour*. Cambridge: Cambridge University Press.

Kagan, J. (1983). Stress and coping in early development. In N. Garmezy & M. Rutter (eds.), *Stress, coping and development in children*. New York: McGraw-Hill.

Kinzie, J.D., Sack, W.H., Angell, R.H., Manson, S., & Rath, B. (1986). The psychiatric effects of massive trauma on Cambodian children: I. The children. *Journal of the American Academy of Child Psychiatry, 25*, 3, 370–376.

Lazarus, R. (1981). The costs and benefits of denial. In B.S. Dohrenwend & B.P. Dohrenwend (eds.), *Stressful life events and their contexts*. Monographs in Psychosocial Epidemiology: 2. New York: Neale Watson.

Levine, S. (1983). A psychological approach to the ontogeny of coping. In: N. Garmezy & M. Rutter (eds.), *Stress, Coping and Development*. New York: McGraw-Hill.

Lifschtiz, M., Berman, D., Gallili, A., Gilad, D. (1977). Bereaved children: the effects of mother's perception and social system organisation on their short term adjustment. *Journal of the American Academy of Child Psychiatry, 16*, 3, 272–284.

Lipsitt, L. (1983). Stress in infancy: Toward understanding the origins of coping behaviour. In N. Garmezy, & M. Rutter (eds.), *Stress, coping and development in children*. New York: McGraw-Hill.

MacCarthy, O. (1974). Effects of emotional disturbance and deprivation (maternal rejection) on somatic growth. In J. Dobbing & J. Davis (eds.), *Scientific foundations of paediatrics*. London: Heinemann Medical; Philadelphia: W.B. Saunders.

Maccoby, R., & Jacklin, E. (1978). *The psychology of sex differences*. Stanford, California: Stanford University Press.

Miller, M., & Ingham, J.E. (1983). Dimensions of experience. *Psychological Medicine, 13*, 417–429.

Moncke, E., & Dobbs, R. (1985). Measuring life events in an adolescent population: Methodological issues and related findings. *Psychological Medicine, 15*, 841–850.

Mrazek, D., & Mrazek, P. (1985). Child maltreatment. In M. Rutter & L. Hersov (eds.), *Child and adolescent psychiatry: Modern approaches*. Oxford: Blackwell.

Parmalee, A.H. Jr. (1986). Children's illnesses: Their beneficial effect on behavioural development. *Child Development, 57*, 1–10.

Patterson, G.R. (1982). *Coercive family process: A social learning approach*, Vol. 3. Eugen, Oregon: Castalia Publishing Company.

Patterson, G.R. (1983). Stress: A change agent for family process. In N. Garmezy & M. Rutter (eds.), *Stress, coping and development*. New York: McGraw-Hill.

Paykel, E. (1983). Methodological aspects of life events research. *Journal of Psychosomatic Research, 5*, 27, 341–352.

Porter, R., & Collins, G.M. (1982). *Temperamental differences in infants and young children*. CIBA Foundation Symposium 89. London: Pitman Medical.

Pound, A., Cox, A.D., Puckering, C., & Mills, M. (1985). The impact of meternal depression on young children. In J.E. Stevenson (ed.), *Recent research in developmental psychopathology*. Oxford: Pergamon.

Price, D., Close, G., & Fielding, B. (1983). Age of appearance of circadian rhythm in salivary cortisol values in infancy. *Archives of Disease in Childhood, 58*, 454–456.

Pynoos, R.S., & Eth, S. (1986). Witness to violence: The child interview. *Journal of the American Academy of Child Psychiatry, 25*, 3, 306–319.

Quinton, D., & Rutter, M. (1976). Early hospital admissions and later disturbances of behaviour: Attempted replication of Daglos's findings. *Developmental Medicine & Child Neurology, 18*, 447–459.

Quinton, D., & Rutter, M. (1985a). Parenting behaviour of mothers raised in care. In Nicol, A.R. (ed.), *Longitudinal studies in child psychology and psychiatry*. Chichester: John Wiley & Sons.

Quinton, D., & Rutter, M. (1985b). Family pathology and child psychiatric disorder: A 4 year prospective study. In Nicol, A.R. (ed.), *Longitudinal studies in child psychology and psychiatry*. Chichester: John Wiley & Sons.

Raphael, B. (1982). The young child and the death of a parent. In C.M. Parkes & J. Stevenson-Hinde (eds.), *The place of attachment in human behaviour*, 131–150.

Reite, M., & Field, T. (eds.) (1985). *The psychobiology of attachment and separation*. New York, London: Academic Press.

Richman, N. (1977). Behaviour problems in preschool children: Family and social factors. *British Journal of Psychiatry, 131*, 523–527.

Rutter, M. (1966). *The children of sick parents: an environmental and psychiatric study.* Institute of Psychiatry Maudsley Monographs 16. London: Oxford University Press.

Rutter, M. (1979). Protective factors in children's responses to stress and disadvantage. In M.W. Kent & E.J. Rolfe (eds.), *Primary prevention of psychopathology*, Vol. 3: *Social competence in children.* Idernacen: University Press of New England.

Rutter, M. (1983). Stress, coping and development: Some issues and some questions. In N. Gormezy & M. Rutter (eds.), *Stress, coping and development in children.* New York: McGraw-Hill.

Rutter, M. (1984). Continuities and discontinuities in socioemotional development: Empirical and conceptual perspectives. In R. Emde & R. Harmon (eds.), *Continuities and discontinuities in development.* New York: Plenum Press.

Rutter, M. (1985). Psychological therapies in child psychiatry: Issues and prospects. In M. Rutter & L. Hersov (eds.), *Child and adolescent psychiatry.* Oxford: Blackwell.

Rutter, M., & Garmezy, N. (1983). Developmental psychopathology. In P. Mussen (ed.), *Handbook of child psychology*, Vol. IV: *Socialisation, personality and social development.* New York, Chichester: John Wiley & Sons.

Sack, W.H., Angell, R.H., Kinzie, J.D. & Rath, B. (1986). The psychiatric effects of massive trauma on Cambodian children. II. The family, the home and the school. *Journal of the American Academy of Child Psychiatry, 25*, 377–383.

Smith, W., & Rossman, B. (1986), Developmental changes in trait and situational denial under stress during childhood. *Journal of Child Psychology and Psychiatry, 27*, 227–237.

Tennant, C., Hurry, J., & Bebbington, P. (1982). The relation of childhood separation experiences to adult depressive and anxiety states. *British Journal of Psychiatry, 141*, 5, 475–582.

Van Eerdewegh, M., Bieri, M., Parilla, R., Clayton, P. (1982). The bereaved child. *British Journal of Psychiatry, 140*, 1, 23–29.

Wallerstein, J. (1983). Children of divorce—Stress and developmental tasks. In N. Garmezy & M. Rutter (eds.), *Stress, coping and development.* New York: McGraw-Hill.

Wallerstein, J., & Kelly, J. (1980). *Surviving the breakup: How children and parents cope with divorce.* New York: Basic Books.

KEY WORDS

Infancy/pre-school, middle childhood, adolescence, perception of stress, life events — meaning/measurement, protective factors, intrinsic mechanisms, ongoing/multiple stresses, disasters, coping/adjustment.

3

Leaving Home: Homesickness and the Psychological Effects of Change and Transition

SHIRLEY FISHER
The University of Dundee

INTRODUCTION

The Common Denominators of Transition and Change

Transition and change are recurring features of life history, but may be associated with stressful experiences resulting in adverse effects on psychological and physical health. The form of transition and change varies greatly, but a common denominator is discontinuity in life pattern—existing forms of lifestyle and human relationships are replaced. This is characteristic of major losses and exits (bereavement, family break-up, divorce) and of more positive experiences (marriage, new jobs, geographical relocations).

The psychological effects of discontinuity are not necessarily uniform across the differing forms of change and transition; it is necessary to look more closely at the kind of change and transition that is being experienced. Research evidence increasingly suggests the importance of circumstantial and life history factors as determinants of reaction. Thus, a particular transitional experience might be positive for one individual and largely negative for another. Moreover, the way in which a person responds to a particular situation may be an important determinant of subsequent mental and physical health (Fisher, 1986).

Geographical Relocations as Aspects of Change

In the case of relocation, the individual experiences simultaneously loss of close experience of the familiar psychosocial environment and exposure to a new

The research on homesickness and the stress of the transition to university was supported by The Economic and Social Science Research Council, London, UK.

environment with new people and places, as well as perhaps cultural and linguistic differences. Since the individual generally moves for some reason, there may be contexts involving economic or social change. Additionally, the type of move may determine other features of context. In the case of 'moving home', the move may entail a shift of the complete home unit, involving family and sometimes close relatives. In other cases, the individual may leave home to reside elsewhere for a period of time. In the former case, close family support is continued although there may be breaks with close friends and neighbours. In the latter case, part of the context is the separation from close family at home.

THEORETICAL EXPLANATIONS OF THE EFFECTS OF TRANSITION

Separation-anxiety and Loss

Bowlby (1969, 1973, 1980) showed that maintenance of a close bond between child and parent creates a sense of security and is particularly sought at times of stress. Threat to the immediate availability of the attachment figure will result in protest and searching, accompanied by distress. Weiss (1975, 1978, 1982) has identified evidence of similar attachment behaviour in adults, within marriages, relationships between close friends or between parent and offspring in adult life. However, although attachment in adults has some characteristics in common with infant attachment, it differs in that the bond involves peer relationships rather than a caretaker relationship. The peer may be fostering the individual's capacity for mastering challenge. Attachment in adults does not appear to overwhelm other activities in the same way that it does in infants, and the focus of attachment together with the capacity to represent attachment and loss symbolically are age related. Weiss (1982) argues that as adolescents move on in their development, there are increasing intervals during which the accessibility of parents is not necessary for feelings of security, although they may require evidence of parental support. However, Weiss notes the similarity of the response to loss across all age levels, and this suggests the operation of a single perceptual emotional system which changes only in the object of focus.

Interruption of Lifestyle

Discontinuity is also inextricably linked with interruption. Laboratory studies of interruption have indicated the profound effects that interruption may have on cognitive systems. Zeigarnik (1927) reported enhanced recall of interrupted tasks. Although not all experimental evidence has shown this effect (see Van Bergen, 1968), there is some support for the notion of persistence in cognition of interrupted material.

Laboratory studies by Mandler (1975) have suggested that interrupted tasks create the conditions for raised tension, and when no response is available the consequence is anxiety, distress or fear. Mandler and Watson (1966) state that there is, in addition, (1) persistence toward completion of the interrupted sequence; (2) increased vigour with which the sequence is pursued; (3) substitution of alternative elements or sequences.

There is little direct evidence concerning how the interruption enforced by change and transition in life affects the individual. A possibility is that interruption has a powerful effect because plans which supervise daily routine behavior remain active, dominating cognition and driving inappropriate activity for the new environment. This might provide a basis for understanding the effects of moves. The domination of inappropriate plans reduces the resources available for coping with the new environment. It is also conceivable that the sense of separation and loss is triggered and maintained by the dominance of old plans. Thus, perhaps, the separation and interruption mechanisms have mutually reinforcing properties.

Reduced Control

Transition and change have been argued by Fisher (1986) to result in a period of reduced control, defined as power or mastery of the psychosocial environment. A person must learn about new places, people, routines and procedures. Separation from support offered by family and friends may additionally increase loss of control over a number of immediate problems. Because the post-transition environment is high in novelty, there may also be high demands on the individual. Karasek (1979) reported that in groups of Swedish and American workers, job strain is reported when demand (work load) is high and discretion (control) is low. The person who experiences loss, including separation from home, could be argued to encounter just this sort of job strain environment.

Fisher (1984) developed a cognitive model of the perception of control in terms of the resolution of the discrepancy between a desired goal and perceived reality. Failure for selected action to be successful implies an unmodified discrepancy in memory. After a series of unsuccessful trials, the unmodified discrepancy would be interpreted as evidence of 'no control' and would trigger the arousal system. In terms of this model the effects of separation might be to create reduced perceived control and an activated arousal system.

Role Change and Self-consciousness

A different conceptualization is that transition produces a change in perceived-role: one set of commitments ends and a new set is initiated. The necessity of taking on new roles has implications for self-concept. The focus of attention shifts from the environment to the self. The amount of perceived self-focus increases with the strangeness of a new environment (Wickland, 1982). Hormuth (1984) argues that lack of discrepancy between achieved and desired state of self will have a stabilizing function but if the transition involves the end of a commitment, then the self-concept is not stable. Following a relocation, a person is assumed to be motivated to avoid this aversive state by becoming familiar with the new environment. On this analysis, self-consciousness and striving would be expected psychological effects.

STUDIES OF THE EFFECTS OF RELOCATION

In this section some of the background of research on the effects of relocation is considered. Early studies, largely based on statistical evidence on the health of migrants and high mobility individuals, unavoidably confound mobility with the context of moves (social and educational mobility, previous life history) and leave open the possibility that those who move are self-selected.

Moving Home

A number of early studies, concerned with the relationship between moving and mental disorder, focused on the mental health of migrant communities as compared with the indigenous population. For example, Odegaard (1932) reported greater hospital admission rates for mental disorder amongst Norwegian immigrants to Minnesota than for either the native born of Minnesota or for the native born in Norway. Malzberg and Lee (1940) reported similar findings for the migrant and non-migrant populations of New York, even when age, sex, colour and time of immigration were controlled for.

Faris and Dunham (1939) attempted to focus on the psychological changes produced as a result of mobility by using 'home ownership' as compared with 'rental status' as indices of stability. They reported a negative association between rate of home ownership and incidence of schizophrenia and depression in different parts of the city of Chicago. The mobile, socially disorganized areas of the city were most likely to be associated with high rates of mental disorder, particularly schizophrenia. Their main conclusion was that social location may be the cause of psychopathology.

Research results that suggest that migration has no adverse effects are less frequent, but Kleiner and Parker (1959) showed that there were lower rates of mental disorder for southern migrants than for native-born Pennsylvanians, whereas northern migrants had higher rates than the native born. Kleiner and Parker (1963) further demonstrated the relative vulnerability of the native-born migrant in terms of: higher rates of mental illness, and greater prevalence of psychoneurotic and psychosomatic symptoms. There were no differences between the migrant or native born groups in terms of status inconsistency, but some indication that the variance in the discrepancy between educational aspiration and achievement was greater for the native born group. This underlines the importance of consideration of personal and circumstantial factors.

Research evidence across the last 60 years has demonstrated the vulnerability of migrant populations to physical ill-health. In particular, cardiovascular disorders, gastric disorders and infectious illness have been found to be more likely in migrant populations than in the initial or 'receiving' communities (see Medalie and Kahn, 1973; Cruze Coke *et al.*, 1964; Wolff, 1953; Holmes, 1956; Christenson and Hinkle, 1961). The problem of confounding mobility with circumstantial factors remains and in addition there may be self-selection factors operating. Migration may also create intermediate conditions which do not favour healthy living (crowding, diet, sanitation etc.), and it remains possible that moving provides a focus for the attribution of negative experiences.

In order to identify the effects of relocations on the mental and physical health of the individual, more detailed examination of psychological state and reaction pattern is needed. One of the first to meet this need was a longitudinal study of the effects of slum clearance by Fried (1963). Pre- and post-relocation interviews showed that psychological reactions were intense, overwhelming, prolonged and characterized by grief-like responses for the old home: 'I felt as if the heart was taken out of me'. Depressive mood and a sense of helplessness were major features. The results of Fried's study are particularly interesting because there was no separation from family as a result of the move. The findings emphasize the importance of loss of *objects* such as building surrounds and features of the old home. Perhaps these are symbols of aspects of security and familiarity, or perhaps they become associated with happy memories of the previous existence. The finding challenges the assumption that it is separation from close human relationships that is a determinant of unhappiness following a relocation.

Fried's studies also emphasized the importance of a number of factors associated with successful adjustment and coping. First, the status of the individual (defined by occupational, educational and income factors) was positively associated with successful coping: 72% from the high education—high occupation group adjusted successfully to the move, but only 20% from the low education—low occupation group adjusted successfully. Groups with one or both foreign born parents had greater adjustment difficulties. Equally, there were predictors of adaptation success in terms of whether or not the move was originally planned for: 52% of those who had planned to move were more well adjusted, but 24% of those who had initially planned to resist moving were well adjusted. Fried argued in favour of 'preparedness for transition' as a critical determinant of the success of adaptation; 'mastery', defined in terms of the determination to struggle and persist against all opposition, was seen as a sign of 'inner preparedness'.

In more recent research on relocations, an emerging optimistic view is that residential mobility is an adaptive response to a modern fast-moving society and that rapid communication systems mean that the individual is not bound by the immediacy of social relationships. (Butler *et al.*, 1973). Demographic trends within the USA indicate that about 20% of the population are mobile and that many people do change residence voluntarily and positively, perceiving the process to be part of upward social mobility. Only those individuals affected by poverty, racial discrimination or physical infirmity are likely to be at risk (Fischer and Stueve, 1977). Thus it would follow that relocation need not be a stressful life event but may be part of upward mobility and success.

Stokols *et al.* (1983) attempted some reconciliation of these two possibilities by advocating emphasis on the contextual analysis of a particular relocation in terms of life history and future aspirations. One interesting outcome of a longitudinal study of the effects of relocation by Stokols *et al.* (1983) was an indication that moving may create or reflect poor health status. A study of 242 adult employees, 121 of whom completed a follow-up study of emotional and physical well-being 3 months after a move, showed that frequent relocation was associated with a greater number of illness-related symptoms. The effect was greater amongst those with low tendency to explore and establish themselves in the new environment. Additionally, raised symptom levels also characterized those low in relocation frequency who perceived low choice of residence and low congruence with expectations.

Leaving Home and Homesickness

A form of relocation involving a temporary move from home might be expected to increase the sense of grief and loss because family and friends as well as objects and life routines are left behind. The effect of the break with contact with supporting relationships may be balanced against the fact that the move is less likely to be permanent and home still remains to be visited in the holidays. Children as young as 7 years old may endure such a break when sent away to boarding school for primary education. Students and those needing vocational training or seeking employment are likely to be the predominant groups encountering the experience.

The Psychological State of Homesickness

The term 'homesickness' is commonly used to describe any condition of unhappiness or malaise following the transition to a new environment. Dictionary definitions include 'pining for home' (*Chambers Dictionary*, 1972); 'depressed by absence from home' (*Concise Oxford Dictionary*, 1964). In spite of the lack of modern research, there was early attention to the importance of 'homesickness' in medical texts of the 17th and 18th centuries where the association with protracted grief and somatic symptoms such as giddiness, weakness and insomnia were noted (Corp, 1791; Harder, 1678). The term homesickness was introduced in a dissertation by Harder (1678), who referred to 'Heimweh' or 'maladie du pays' to describe the patterns of behaviour and health following leaving home to take up residence elsewhere. Early medical texts provide descriptions of the nature of the adverse mental and physical reactions to leaving home. Corp (1791) observed the response of young men forced to leave home to take up active service, reporting that they often became dejected, had poor health and even died. Symptoms such as weakness, giddiness, noise in the ears, bad dreams, insomnia, dietary change, and melancholy were reported by Corp as characteristic.

The issue of whether homesickness is determined by personality or environmental factors was discussed by Harder, who favoured the view that the determinants were external and likely to involve differences in climate, customs, habits and food as well as insults and injuries. By contrast, Zuckert (1768) gave greater emphasis to personality factors; the homesick person was seen as unstable and disposed to feeling insecure.

The semantics of homesickness.   One of the problems with investigations of self-reported psychological states following loss is that there are semantic factors involved. A person may not understand a particular concept appropriately or may fail to use the label as a description of perceived symptoms. These are problems for the self-assessment of all forms of mental disorder. At least one reason why mental disorders such as depression are diagnosed by experts, is that patients may not categorize personal states appropriately. Early studies of homesickness revealed a 'labelling' problem: when the term 'homesickness' was omitted, only 16% of pupils spontaneously mentioned it (Fisher *et al.*, 1984). When the term was provided, incidence levels were about 60–70% (Fisher *et al.*, 1986, 1988). Thus, the majority will not spontaneously label their adverse experiences in this way, but recognize the label as appropriate when it is available.

Written, personal definitions obtained across a number of studies (Fisher *et al.*, 1985, 1986; Fisher and Hood, 1986a,b,c) showed that the cognitive elements were given paramount importance and centred on ruminations concerned with home. Symptoms included dizziness, anxiety, feeling overwhelmed, unhappiness, depression, loneliness, and somatic complaints. There were no differences between homesick and non-homesick subjects in this respect. Thus in terms of reported phenomenology, 'homesickness' is a complex cognitive–motivational–emotional state with much in common with bereavement. It involves cognitive elements focused on all aspects of home, people, objects, places and routines, together with varying motivational and emotional symptoms. One way of envisaging the state might be as an agitated depression with a cognitive profile flavoured by antecedents concerned with loss of home. The cognitive profile thus differentiates it from other forms of depressed and anxious mood. As a result of these considerations, Fisher (1988) has proposed a descriptive model of depression based on hierarchical order in which cognitive features retain superordinate positions and drive common groups of symptoms (loss of volition, crying, agitation).

The phenomenology of homesickness. Diary studies conducted with boarding school children (Fisher *et al.*, 1986) have provided further information on the phenomenology of homesickness. The pupils endorsed a column headed 'homesickness' to indicate periods during the day when homesickness was experienced. Results showed that homesickness is reported as occurring in episodes, usually during the early morning or late evening. The reporting pattern was different for males and females in that the former were more likely to report homesickness in the morning and the latter were more likely to report it in the evening. For the majority of individuals the episodic nature of reporting suggests that the day's activity might help to keep homesickness at bay. However, this was not the case for about 10–15% of subjects who characteristically used all the cells of the column and reported themselves as highly distressed and continuously homesick. It would appear that for these individuals, activity does not prevent the homesickness experience from dominating mental resources.

A diary study in which the pupils only reported on homesickness and its surrounding circumstance (Fisher *et al.*, 1986) indicated that for the episodic reporters homesickness was strongly associated with periods of passive mental activity. The evidence also suggested that about 20% of episodes can be triggered during the day by reminders (familiar music, a letter from home).

A model is needed in which the day's events have the potential to compete with the signals generated by the separation and interruption mechanisms in gaining access to a limited capacity attentional resource. The model must allow for cases where the strength of the competing signals is so strong that the day's events do not provide effective competition.

The cognition of the homesick. A central aspect of cognition in the homesick is attentional focusing on the immediate past. Whereas this may occur because of separation or because of interruption of previous well-established plans (see Section II), it remains possible that the tendency to continue to be dominated by the plans of the immediate past following a transition may be an organizational feature of planned activity. Dominant plans continue to exist, have access to memory and action systems, and provide a pertinent source of attentional demand. The individual might literally lapse and forget his new location.

If so, then non-homesick and homesick individuals should show similar focusing. The difference between the two populations would be assumed to be quantitative rather than qualitative: the homesick are more frequently possessed by home-focused thoughts. Some support for this was provided by the results of our early diaries completed by boarding school pupils of daily problems and associated periods of worrying for the first 2 weeks of the new school term (Fisher *et al.*, 1984). From the content of descriptions provided, problems were classified by the investigators into *school related* (e.g. 'losing my books'; 'whether the history teacher likes me'; 'mathematics test') and *home related* (e.g. 'my mother's health'; 'whether my dog gets his walks'; 'missing my bedroom'). Periods when a pupil remembered worrying about each problem were indicated by endorsements in cells marked out in 1-hour units against a time scale on a column relating to each reported problem. The resulting data were expressed as a ratio of worries against problems for each major problem category. The lower the value of the ratio, the greater the mental preoccupation with the problem and hence, by operational definition, the greater its intensity. It was found that the number of reported school problems exceeded the number of home problems but that the latter were associated with significantly lower problem–worry ratios, indicating more ruminative activity.

On first analysis, any cognitive system which allows domination of the plans of the immediate past should not be biologically adaptive because efficiency and ultimately survival depend on adaptive focusing on the present and future. However, Fisher (1984) argued that one benefit of reflective ruminative activity might be as an aid to revising and adapting existing plans or consolidating previously acquired resources. Bridge and chess players often have 'regurgitation' sessions where the previous moves and counter-moves of a game are analysed. These reflective analyses have the potential for improving and up-dating strategies. On this analysis, the homesick may be assumed to overindulge in reflective ruminative activity, and symptoms of distress could be argued to result from overly prolonged regurgitations. This might imply that the homesick were carrying out planning procedures more likely to benefit them in the long term, although an immediate penalty would be failure to become committed and to engage tasks in the new environment.

On the 'regurgitation model', the content of home thoughts should not differentiate homesick and non-homesick subjects. However, Fisher (to be published) showed that when asked to estimate the proportion of home-oriented thoughts concerned either 'problems created because of leaving home', 'on-going problems' or 'uncontrollable home imagery', it was found that uncontrollable imagery predominated for the homesick (average percentage 73%), whereas problems created by leaving home predominated for the non-homesick (63%). Thus, there was no support for the regurgitation theory as outlined above; the homesick appear to have qualitative differences in the content of reported home-related thoughts.

One possible explanation of the above finding of a qualitative difference in the features of home thoughts is that homesick people cannot prevent themselves thinking about home because of potence of home thoughts in memory. The potence model would predict that the homesick have an organization in memory in which home-related events predominate. This would suggest a cognitive organization in which immediacy effects are strong determinants of memory structure.

A study by Fisher (to be published) compared a group of homesick students, non-homesick students and depressed (non-homesick) students (between group design) on the time required to produce the first verbal utterance when asked to recall, as quickly as possible, a list of either positive or negative experiences associated with home. The homesick were significantly slower than either the control or the depressed group to have negative thoughts of home, but faster than the other two groups to have positive thoughts of home. When asked to report positive or negative experiences concerning university, the homesick were similar to the depressed (non-homesick) students in that they were faster to produce negative experiences and slower to report positive experiences compared with the control group.

The memory of the homesick thus seems to be organized with respect to a system based on valence. It seems that dominant structures are positive-home and negative-university memories. Perhaps, therefore the homesick are dominated by thoughts of home because they enjoy reliving these memories. They might seek escape from perceived current unpleasantness by thinking about the pleasantries of the past. The short-term gain of reliving pleasant past experiences might then carry the penalty of reactivating distress due to separation. The homesick person might be likened to an addict who tries to give up the psychological dependence on the source of addiction but the existing schema continue to drive memory of the source of the addictive habit.

Homesickness, psychological disturbance and health.   Reports from university students experiencing homesickness (Fisher *et al.*, 1985) indicated that about a third experienced loss of concentration, had poor attendance at lectures, or handed in work late. There were also positive correlations between the perceived frequency of episodes and (a) the degree to which work was reported as affected ($r = 0.46$); (b) lack of concentration ($r = 0.47$); (c) work handed in late ($r = 0.42$). There was evidence to suggest raised levels of absent-mindedness (as assessed by the Cognitive Failures Questionnaire; Broadbent *et al.*, 1982). Additionally, laboratory comparisons between homesick and non-homesick subjects on a task requiring the repeated typing of a single, overlearned word in the absence of visual feedback (see Fisher, 1988) showed the homesick to be more error prone and less likely to report self-produced typing errors. They were also more likely to give a pessimistic, discrepant global estimate of total errors than non-homesick subjects.

Fisher and Hood (1987) have shown in the context of a longitudinal study that homesick students have raised levels of psychological disturbance after the transition to university (The Middlesex Hospital Questionnaire; Crown and Crisp, 1966). Symptoms most likely to be elevated are depression, obsessionality, somatic symptoms, phobias and anxiety. There was also evidence of lower adaptation to university. (The College Adaptation Questionnaire; Crombag, 1968), indicating perhaps lack of commitment to the new environment or high levels of inefficient behaviour.

There is also evidence to support the view that homesickness is associated with poor physical health; Fisher et al., (1986) reported that homesick boarding school pupils reported more non-traumatic ailments (colds, influenza, mild infections) but not traumatic ailments, which argues against a response bias hypothesis. Homesick pupils also had more days off school and more visits to a doctor. Kane (1986) reported that the general health of homesick university students was lower than that of non-homesick students. Fisher and Hood (1987a) found that somatic symptom reporting was greater in the homesick as compared with the non-homesick. Thus there is an accumulation of evidence to suggest that there is a relationship, whether by cause or consequence, between homesickness reporting and ill-health.

Moderating and Controlling Factors in Homesickness Reporting

Given the above considerations, the interesting question is why only about 60–70% of any sample report homesickness. It remains possible that some people might more readily label post-transition experiences in this way, but it is also possible that there are other important differences between the groups. Results have indicated that factors such as distance from home, decisional control over the move, satisfaction with the new environment, and initial state of mental health, combine in very complex ways with the circumstances of the new environment to determine reaction.

Fisher et al. (1985) found that the geographical distance of the move was greater for homesick students and although they desired more home visits than they had had by the sixth week of term, the number of visits home did not differ. This indicates the importance of perceived distancing. The first possible explanation is that culture shock varies as a function of distance from home. An alternative explanation is that control over visits home has a moderating influence: increased distance means increased travel costs and therefore decreased potential for home visits.

There was also greater decisional involvement in the transition to university for the non-homesick group. Again, there is the possibility that decisional involvement reflects self-selection, or that it represents a form of control over the move.

This underlines the point made by Fried (above) that planning for a move might be an important determinant of adjustment.

When these same factors were examined in the context of a boarding school environment, they did not differentiate the homesick and non-homesick groups. One possible reason is that circumstances make geographical distance less critical for school children because they are restricted in home visits. Also, financial factors may be less influential because boarding schools in the UK are part of private sector education and attract a high socioeconomic catchment. Equally, children may expect less decisional involvement about whether to go to a particular school or not.

Fisher (1984, 1986) proposed a hierarchical model of decision making concerning control. If control is perceived as possible initially, then subsequent tests of whether control facilities are available at a lower level of the hierarchy are possible. For students there is the *potential* for control, but those who are homesick perceived reduced facility for exercising it because of, for example, parental dominance or, in the case of home visits, financial cost. School children do not perceive the potential for control in the first place and therefore the remainder of the tests is irrelevant. On this argument, children are assumed to have less control overall and so there should be higher incidence of homesickness compared with students. However, the results indicate that incidence levels do not distinguish children and student groups.

The longitudinal study of Fisher and Hood (1987a) also showed that homesick students were distinguished from nonhomesick counterparts, in terms of raised levels of psychological disturbance *prior to leaving home*. In particular, there were raised MHQ subscale scores of obsessionality, somatic symptoms and depression. Covariate analysis (MANOVA) showed that the homesick group had greater gains in overall psychological disturbance, anxiety, somatic symptoms and obsessionality following the transition. Fisher and Hood hypothesized that raised symptom levels in those who later become homesick might reflect *anticipatory stress*. Equally the effect might represent an existing state of *vulnerability*— perhaps those with high symptom levels are less likely to become involved in challenge (see Fisher, 1988).

Cognitive Models of Homesickness

The competing demands model of homesickness.   One model which makes sense of many of the above findings is the competing demands model represented in Figure 3.1. It is assumed that, due to the effects of separation from home and the interruption of familiar routines, there are potent sources of information which compete with information from the new (university) environment for access to a limited capacity attentional resource. First, the effects of separation and loss may have the potential to create anxious searching behaviour, the focus of which is dominant in memory. Secondly, there may be problems arising because of leaving home which create demands on attentional resource. Finally, it remains possible that plans and routines once interrupted continue to exert a dominant influence on thinking.

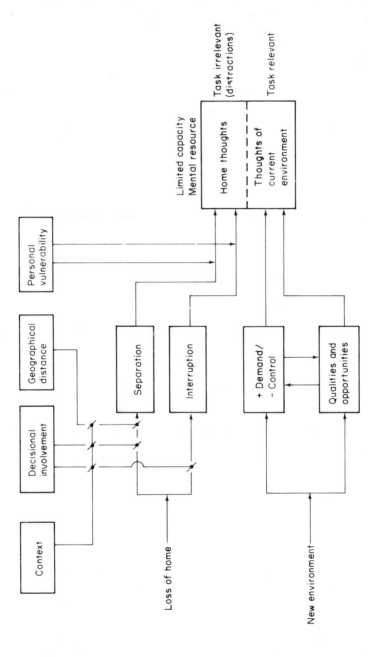

FIG. 3.1 The competing demands models of homesickness: homesickness imagery competes with environmental demand in mental resource.

It is assumed that signals concerned with the features of the new environment (new locations, rules, routines, friends, institutional and academic aspects) compete for attention. On the assumption that the attentional resource is of limited capacity, the two streams of information may need to compete for the resource. If the demands of the new environment are stronger because the individual is committed and motivated towards challenge, it is possible that homesickness thoughts are suppressed. Conversely, very strong 'home-orientated' ideations could force out the possibility of commitment to the new environment: the homesick person may be absent-minded, distressed and 'home-focused' to the extent that the challenges of the new environment cannot be taken up.

Thus the individual may be caught in a loop whereby the failure to engage the challenge of the new environment because of strong past-oriented ideations effectively blocks an important step in the adaptation process, namely the accepting of commitment and challenge and the replacement of home-ideations by content relevant to the new environment. The homesick person may be the one for whom separation and interruption are so compelling that the attentional resource remains dominated; or the one who fails to become committed and therefore fails to gain the benefits from competition provided by the challenge of the new environment. Evidence from the longitudinal study described previously, suggesting that homesick students show signs of greater disturbance prior to leaving home, might be interpreted in terms of the failure of depressed individuals to take on the challenge of a new place and to become committed. As illustrated in Figure 3.1, vulnerability factors might be envisaged either as amplifying systems which strengthen the output of the separation and interruption mechanisms, or as determinants of commitment to the new environment and hence as determinants of the strength of competing information.

The results of the diary studies lend some support to the competing demands model in that, for the majority of homesick school children who are episodic reporters, reporting of homesickness is more likely at night or first thing in the morning, suggesting that the days' events offer effective competition for attention. The small proportion of strongly homesick individuals show reporting patterns which suggest that home-thoughts remain dominant all day and that daily activities do not provide effective competition. The model gives weight to the importance of the new environment in all its aspects and to the ability of the individual to become actively involved and committed.

The model also illustrates the possibility that factors such as decisional control over the move and control over visits home determine the degree to which the separation and interruption mechanisms become active in producing trains of competing signals. The model further allows for contexts and personal situations to act as gate devices which determine whether these moderating factors operate. This takes account of the comparative finding that university students and boarding school children appear to differ in the extent to which factors such as geographical distance and decisional control are influential.

The job strain model of homesickness. More recent research has suggested that an additional model is needed which provides for the possibility that the properties of the new environment might directly precipitate the homesickness experience. In other words, the new environment may not merely have the potential for attenuating the homesickness experience, it may in some cases actively create it. This is especially likely when the new environment provides a source of strain.

The first clue arose as a result of the longitudinal study by Fisher and Hood (1987a) which showed that *all students* showed a rise in overall level of psychological disturbance; symptoms included increased depression, somatic symptoms, obsessionality and absent-mindedness. Exposure to the university environment was, by operational definition, more stressful. Since residential and home-based students were not distinguished in this respect, the results emphasize that the new university environment constitutes a main source of stress.

Analysis of data on reported problems suggested that over 60% of both the residents and the home-based students were concerned with academic pressures: 'worried about standards'; 'not coping with lectures'; 'failing'; 'work load'; 'finding time for study'. There were also problems specific for each group. Residents reported problems due to sharing life in an institution and managing financial affairs (lack of privacy; financial management; loneliness; being overwhelmed by people etc.). Home-based students reported problems based on the need to integrate university and home life. Collectively, the results are consistent with the idea that students experience job strain when they attend university.

A second clue is provided by homesickness reporting patterns observed by Fisher and Hood (1987a): whilst the majority of homesick university students assessed in the sixth week of their first term reported being homesick in the first week and the sixth week, or being homesick in the first week and not the sixth week, 35% reported not being homesick initially but *becoming homesick as the term progressed*. Thus, it could be that for some individuals homesickness develops as a reaction to the experience of a new environment.

A third clue is provided by the finding that certain mobility experiences in previous life history might immunize a person against the experience of homesickness. Fisher *et al.* (1986) reported that boarding school children who had been to a boarding school in primary education were less likely to be homesick. A study of self-reported mobility history in relation to homesickness reporting in university students by Fisher and Hood (1987b) confirmed the immunizing effect of previous school experiences and holidays away from home. Leaving home for other reasons did not appear to be influential. One conclusion is that it is not leaving home per se that is important, it is experience of exposure to comparable environments. This again emphasizes the importance of the features of the new environment as a possible factor in determining homesickness. Perhaps the individual grieves for the past when the new environment is a source of strain and unhappiness. Fisher *et al.* (1985) reported that satisfaction with aspects of the university environment is lower for homesick students. Thus the idea of hedonizing (see above) or turning away from challenge to the security of the immediate past might provide an alternative account of homesickness.

On the competing demands model (see Figure 3.1), the failure to become committed to the new environment implies lack of an effective source of signals to attenuate the effects of separation and interruption. By contrast, analysis in terms

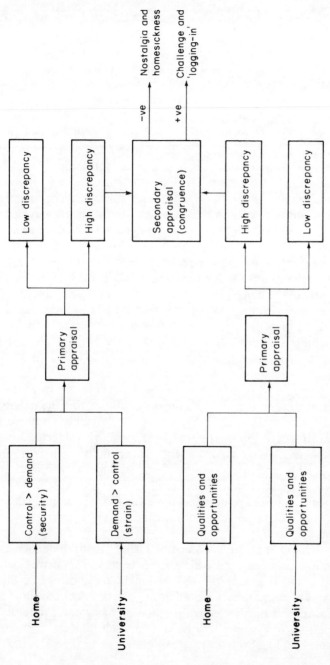

FIG. 3.2 Computational job strain model of homesickness.

of a job strain model assumes that dissatisfaction and unhappiness can create the conditions for homesickness. Karasek (1979) showed that job strain is more likely when demand (work load) is high and discretion (control) is low. When demand is high but discretion is high the result is more likely to be one of challenge. It should follow therefore that homesick students would be more likely to report high demand and low control over the new environment than non-homesick students.

Fisher and Hood (1987c) designed a study in which control and demand were independently rated on 5-point scales. Results showed that homesick students assessed demand as greater than control, whereas the reverse was the case for non-homesick students. Comparison of level of demand showed that it was significantly greater for homesick as compared with non-homesick groups. Level of control did not distinguish the groups. On the job strain model these co-ordinates suggest the environment involves challenge and effort. Students do typically have a great deal of jurisdiction over how they spend their day as compared with those who work in structured environments for payment. Therefore perhaps a more sensitive set of questions might be needed in order to answer this question.

Figure 3.2 represents a job strain model of homesickness. It is a computational model which assumes that the individual weighs the features of the new environment against those of the home environment. If the new environment is characterized by high demand relative to control, but the home environment has the reverse properties, then perhaps memories of home will be actively selected. There are self-confirming properties, in that failure to become committed to the new environment will reduce the potential for control and will increase the feeling of being lost and overwhelmed.

On this model, the individual is not dominated mechanically by past events but is actively engaging in ruminations as a means of attenuating the unhappiness of the current environment. In other words, ruminating might be strategic 'hedonizing': the pleasantries of the home environments are actively selected as a means of blocking out the unpleasant environment. The penalty is that the individual revitalizes separation and interruption effects, as when a reformed addict imagines the source of his addiction. Vulnerability effects are explained by assuming that those who are depressed prior to leaving home fail to respond to the challenge of the new environment and engage in ruminative activity concerned with home as a consequence.

The risk of physical ill-health is argued by Fisher (1986) to be increased when prolonged rumination associated with distress occurs. This drives pathological states of arousal and increases the risk of functional abuse of bodily systems (cardiovascular, gastrointestinal) as well as the risk of infectious illnesses due to raised immunosuppression. Reflective rumination has greater potential for sustaining long periods of distress because it is less self-limiting than anticipatory stress. It provides an ideal way of increasing the risk of illness.

SUMMARY AND CONCLUSIONS

Moves are associated with adverse mental and physical health, but research has frequently confounded mobility with circumstantial factors such as social and educational mobility or housing. Detailed investigation of the psychological effects suggests that homesickness affects 60% of populations who leave home. The *competing demands* model assumes that separation-anxiety and interruption create sources of information which dominate a limited capacity attentional resource. The demands of the new environment provide signals which can attenuate the effect. The vulnerable individual is the one who fails to engage the challenge offered by the new environment. The *computational job strain* model assumes that the individual fails to be committed to the new environment and perceives the security of home as more attractive. Thus, home-related thoughts begin to dominate cognition. Reflective ruminative activity is not self-limiting and provides an ideal basis for perpetuation of high arousal and distress, thus raising the risk of illness because of the effect of hormones such as cortisol on the immune response system (see Fisher, 1986, Chapter 12).

REFERENCES

Bowlby, J. (1969). *Attachment and Loss*, Vol. 1: *Attachment*. New York: Basic Books.

Bowlby, J. (1973). *Attachment and Loss*, Vol. 2: *Separation, anxiety and anger*. New York: Basic Books.

Bowlby, J. (1980). *Attachment and Loss*, Vol. 3: *Loss: sadness and depression*. New York: Basic Books.

Broadbent, D.E., Cooper, P.F., Fitzgerald, P., & Parkes, K.R. (1982). The Cognitive Failures Questionnaire (CFQ) and its correlates. *British Journal of Clinical Psychology, 21*, 1–16.

Butler, E.W., McAllister, R.J., & Kaiser, E.J. (1973). The effects of voluntary and involuntary residential mobility on females and males, *Journal of Marriage and the Family, 35*, 219–227.

Christenson, W.W., & Hinkle, L.E. (1961). Differences in illnes and prognostic signs in two groups of young men. *Journal of the American Medical Association, 177*, 247–253.

Corp, R. (1791), An essay on the changes produced in the body by operations of the mind by the late Dr. Corp of Bath, Cited in Rather (1965).

Crombag, H.F.M. (1968). *Studie motivatie en studie attitude*. Groningen: Walters.

Crown, S., & Crisp, A.M. (1966). A short clinical diagnostic self-rating scale for psychoneurotic patients: The Middlesex Hospital Questionnaire (MHQ). *British Journal of Psychiatry, 112*, 917–23.

Cruze-Coke, R., Etcheverry, R., & Nagel, R. (1964). Influences of migration on blood pressure of Easter Islanders, *Lancet*, 28 March, 697–699.

Faris, R.E.L., & Dunham, H.W. (1939), *Mental disorders in urban areas*, Chicago: University of Chicago Press.

Fischer, C.S., & Stueve, C.A. (1977). Authentic community: The role of place in modern life. In C.S. Fischer, R.M. Jackson, C.A. Stueve, K. Grierson, L.M. Jones & M. Baldassare (eds). *Networks and places: Social relations in an urban setting*. New York: The Free Press.

Fisher, S. (1984). *Stress and the perception of control*. London: Lawrence Erlbaum Associates.

Fisher, S. (1986). *Stress and strategy*. London: Lawrence Erlbaum Associates.

Fisher, S. (1988). *Homesickness and the psychological effects of transition and change*. London: Lawrence Erlbaum Associates.

Fisher, S., Frazer, N., & Murray, K. (1984). The transition from home to boarding school: A diary style analysis of the problems and worries of boarding school pupils. *Journal of Environmental Psychology, 4*, 211–221.

Fisher, S., Murray, K., & Frazer, N. (1985). Homesickness, health and efficiency in first year students. *Journal of Environmental Psychology, 5*, 181–195.

Fisher, S., Frazer, N., & Murray, K. (1986). Homesickness and health in boarding school children. *Journal of Environmental Psychology, 6*, 35–47.

Fisher, S., & Hood, B. (1987). The stress of the transition to university: A longitudinal study of vulnerability to psychological disturbance and homesickness. (Submitted for publication).

Fisher, S., & Hood, B. (1987). Mobility history and psychological disturbance following the transition to university. (Submitted for publication).

Fisher, S., & Hood, B. (1987). Job strain and psychological disturbance in university students. (Submitted for publication).

Fried, M. (1963). Transitional functions of working class communities: implications for forced relocation. In M.B. Kantor, (ed.) *Mobility and mental health*. Springfield, Illinois: Charles C. Thomas.

Harder, J.J. (1678). *Dissertation medico de nostalgia order heimweh praeside*. Basle: Johannes Heferno. Cited in Rather (1965).

Holmes, T.H. (1956). Multidiscipline studies of tuberculosis. In P.G. Spooner (ed.). *Personality, Stress and Tuberculosis*.

Hormuth, S. (1984). Transitions in commitments to roles and self concept change: relocation as a paradigm. In V.L. Allen and E. van de Vliert (eds.), *Role transitions: explorations and explanations*. New York: Plenum Press.

Kane, G. (1986). Unpublished doctoral thesis.

Karasek, R.A. (1979). Job demands, job decision latitude and mental strain: implicated for job redesign. *Administrative Science Quarterly, 24*, 43–48.

Kleiner, R.J., & Parker, S. (1959). Migration and mental illness: a new look. *American Sociological Review, 24*, 687–690.

Kleiner R.J., & Parker, S. (1963). Goal striving and psychosomatic symptoms in a migrant and non-migrant population. In M.B. Kantor (ed.). *Mobility and Mental Health*. Springfield, Illinois: Charles C. Thomas.

Leff, M.J., Roatch, J.F., & Bunney, W.E. (1970). Environmental factors preceding the onset of severe depressions. *British Journal of Psychiatry, 33*, 293–311.

Malzberg, B., & Lee, E.S. (1940). *Migration and mental disease: a study of first admissions to hospital for mental disease*. New York: Social Science Research Council (1956).

Mandler, G. (1975). *Mind and emotion*. New York: John Wiley & Sons.

Mandler, G., & Watson, D.L. (1966). Anxiety and interruption of behaviour. In C.D. Spielberger (ed.). *Anxiety and behaviour*. New York: Academic Press.

Medalie, J.H., & Kahn, H.R. (1973). Myocardial infarction over a five year period. 1. Prevalence, incidence and mortality experience. *Journal of Chronic Diseases, 26*, 63–84.

Murphy, H.B.M. (1965). Migration and the disorders: a reappraisal. In M.B. Kantor (ed.), *Mobility and mental health*. Springfield, Illinois: Charles C. Thomas.

Odegaard, O. (1932). Emigration and insanity: a study of mental disease among the Norwegian born population of Minnesota. *Acta Psychiatrica et Neurologica*, Supplement 1–4.

Odegaard, O. (1945). The distribution of mental disease in Norway: A contribution to the ecology of mental disorder. *Acta Psychiatrica et Neurologica, 20*, 247–284.

Rather, D.J. (1958). *Mind and body in eighteen medicine: A study based on Jerome Gamb's Regimine Mentis*. London: Wellcome Historical Library.

Stokols, D., Schumaker, S.A., & Martinez, J. (1983). Residential mobility and personal well being. *Journal of Environmental Psychology, 3*, 5–19.

Totman, R. (1979). *Social Causes of Illness*. Souvenir Press.

Van Bergen, A. (1968). *Task interruption*. Amsterdam: North Holland.

Weiss, R.S. (1975). *Marital separation*. New York: Basic Books.

Weiss, R.S. (1978). Couples' relationships. In M. Corbin (ed.), *The couple*. New York: Penguin.

Weiss, R.S. (1982). Attachment in adult life. In C.M. Parkes & J. Stevenson-Hinde (eds), *The place of attachment and loss in human behaviour*. London: Tavistock Press.

Wickland, R.A. (1982). Self-focused attention and the validity of self-reports. In M.P. Zanna, E.T. Higgins and C.P. Herman (eds.), *Consistency in social behaviour: the Ontario Symposium*, Vol. 2. Hillsdale, N.J.: Lawrence Erlbaum Associates.

Wolff, H.G. (1953). *Stress and disease*. Springfield, Illinois: Charles C. Thomas.

Zeigarnik, B. (1927). Das behalten erledigter und unerledigiter, handlungen. *Psychologisches Forschung, 9*, 1–85.

Zuckert (1768). *Von den Leidenschaften*. Berlin. (Cited in Rather, 1958).

KEY WORDS

Relocation, geographical moves, moving, mobility, homesickness, life events and mental health, life events and physical health, transition and change, loss, attachment, interruption, bereavement, grief, control, demand, job strain, migration, depression, schizophrenia, anxiety, obsessionality, personal vulnerability, transition to university, university stresses, academic pressures, problems, worries, vulnerability.

Handbook of Life Stress, Cognition and Health
Edited by S. Fisher and J. Reason
© 1988 John Wiley & Sons Ltd.

4

Bereavement

FRANCES CLEGG
*The London Hospital**

DEFINITIONS AND CONCEPTUAL APPROACHES

Bereavement may be defined as the state which follows an actual or perceived loss. It may involve changes in any or all of the psychological, behavioural and physical dimensions, changes which may be seen following the loss of, or threat to, any valued object, state or relationship. To date, most research has been carried out on the state of bereavement following the loss of a person through death, although there is a growing body of knowledge on the sequelae to loss of employment (Warr, 1978, 1982; Burgoyne, 1985), loss of a pet (Keddie, 1977; Stewart *et al.*, 1985), loss of home (Fried, 1963; Parkes, 1972; Angrist, 1974), loss of a limb (Parkes, 1972; Shukla *et al.*, 1982), loss of health or faculties (Raphael, 1984), and loss through divorce rather than death (Jewett, 1982; Mitchell, 1985).

The state of bereavement is multifaceted, with many factors helping to shape its various social, cognitive, behavioural, physical and emotional manifestations. Cultural traditions and norms, the personality, circumstances and previous losses of the bereaved, the nature and quality of the lost or transformed relationship, and the existence and nature of support for the bereaved are perhaps the most crucial factors which work together to shape an individual's responses during bereavement.

Grief is almost synonymous with sorrow, but may be more technically defined as a series of reactions to the perception of loss. Parkes (1986) emphasizes the word *process*, and describes grief as a succession of clinical pictures which occur following loss, rather than a single symptom state which simply fades away after its most intense phase. It is perhaps this appreciation of grief as a succession of states that has led to the several stage theories of grief, the most important of which will be considered below.

Mourning is described by Parkes as an outward expression of loss, and a phenomenon which contrasts with grief, which is the experience of sorrow. It may

*Now at the National Hospital for Nervous Diseases.

be regarded as the aspect of bereavement which is most influenced by cultural norms (for instance see Stannard (1977), Danforth (1982) and Spencer (1982) for details of very different mourning rites), although in psychoanalytic theory, mourning is used to refer to conscious and unconscious psychological processes. When used this way, the term is close in meaning to grief, as it is in everyday language.

Although the pain of bereavement, and the perplexity which it often provokes in the bereaved, have been addressed by writers and poets from time immemorial, in recent years it seems to have attracted the interest of investigators with a medical background rather than psychologists, although, as we shall see, many psychologists will consider bereavement as subsumed within a wider area of interest. Freud (1917, 1926) had much to say about bereavement, and offered the first theoretical explanation of why it should be such a painful process. Mourning 'occurs under the influence of reality-testing'; successful mourning severs the ties that held the mourner to the lost object. However, every relationship provokes negative as well as positive feelings (e.g. sadistic impulses), and after bereavement the mourner attempts to deny these negative feelings by identifying with the lost love object. This impedes the process of detachment, and can lead to melancholic or hysteric symptoms. Bowlby (1969, 1980) subsequently challenged the central importance of identification, and developed a different conceptual approach, that of attachment theory. In his view, attachment is the instinctive development of bonds of affection, first appearing in the mother–child relationship. After childhood, adult–adult attachments are formed, unless disruption of childhood bonds has resulted in an inability to form new attachments. The threat of loss results in the activation of 'attachment behaviours', such as anxiety, clinging, crying and anger, together with a state of physiological arousal. After an experience of loss in early life, later losses (or even reminders of the loss) may reactivate attachment behaviours—either in an acute or a chronic episode of emotional upheaval.

Parkes, who was much influenced by Bowlby, has developed another conceptual framework, that of psychosocial transitions (Parkes, 1971). Essentially, an individual gets through life on sets of assumptions, but assumptions which can be completely overturned following a major loss. Parkes sees grief as the relinquishing of one set of assumptions and the adoption of a new and more appropriate set during the transitional period which almost inevitably follows a major loss. Three distinct 'tasks of grieving' must be successfully accomplished before a bereaved person may be considered to have fully come to terms with his or her loss (Parkes and Weiss, 1983). These tasks are:

a)   intellectual recognition and explanation of loss
b)   emotional acceptance
c)   adoption of a new identity.

Similarly, Worden (1982) identifies essential 'tasks of mourning' and suggests that they are:

a)   acceptance of the reality
b)   experiencing the pain of grief

c)   adjusting to the new environment

d)   withdrawing emotional energy and reinvesting it in new relationships.

In defining grief as a psychosocial transition, Parkes (1971, 1975) was departing from the medical model of grief. This latter approach can perhaps best be seen
in the classic paper written by Lindemann, a psychiatrist who was involved in
helping bereaved families after a fire in a night-club killed many youngsters
(Lindemann, 1944). The various emotional, physical and behavioural changes
exhibited by the grief-stricken survivors were labelled 'symptoms', and the whole
constellation of changes, the grief 'syndrome'. Lindemann distinguishes normal
from abnormal grief, and makes suggestions for the prognosis and management of
both forms of the disorder. It is of some interest, however, that in contrast to his
analysis of grief, his management programme is largely couched in psychological
or counselling terms, and does not necessarily call for the expertise of medically
trained staff or psychiatrists.

Many psychologists address bereavement within the context of stress research
or management. This approach has also been encouraged by the creation of a
category of disorder which has been specifically precipitated by trauma, the
post-traumatic stress disorder (PTSD; American Psychiatric Association, 1980).
PTSD covers loss-induced stress, whether caused by natural or man-made disasters, and in military or civilian contexts. Acute stress may be defined in psychological terms as the stage at which the events experienced by a person are
sufficiently overwhelming to cause a breakdown of his or her coping strategies.
Concurrently, homeostatic physiological changes take place which in the short
term activate the sympathetic nervous system, and give rise to the well known
'fight or flight' responses, but over a longer period of time may maintain changed
patterns of glandular secretion and immune response functioning. Worden (1982)
lists hollowness of stomach, tightness of throat or chest, oversensitivity to noise,
depersonalization, breathlessness, muscle weakness, lack of energy and dryness of
mouth as common physical sensations reported during the period of acute grief.
To this list may be added panic attacks, restlessness and increased muscle tension
(Parkes, 1970). It is hardly surprising that a newly bereaved person suffering from
some of these sympathetic nervous system sensations will frequently describe
himself or herself as feeling excessively anxious. Some sensations and physical
disturbances become so severe that they may be labelled as symptoms, or else are
so prolonged that they give rise to secondary problems. Maddison and Viola
(1968) list headache, dizziness, fainting spells, nightmares, insomnia, blurred
vision, skin rashes, sweating, appetite disturbance, indigestion, difficulty in
swallowing, vomiting, palpitations, chest pain, menstrual disturbance and general
aching as features which are sufficiently commonly experienced by newly bereaved people to be regarded as 'normal' grief reactions. Needless to say, the
sufferers do not usually label them as 'normal', and may fear for their sanity,
particularly if they 'hear' or 'see' the dead person. Rees (1975) states that 47% of
bereaved people report hallucinations following the death of their spouses. These
problems are perhaps even more serious when they result in prolonged changes in
physiological functioning, which may play a part in the subsequent illness or even

death of the newly bereaved person (see below). A stress approach to bereavement thus ties in with the life events theory, developed by Holmes and Rahe (1967); the death of a spouse is the event earning the most points on their Social Readjustment Rating Scale. Since it was first produced, the rating scale has been subject to various criticisms and modification, e.g. by Dohrenwend and Dohrenwend (1974), who suggest that some items on the scale are not independent. A distinction has been made between controllable and uncontrollable events, with the latter (which may include bereavement) being more stressful than events which are the result of deliberate decision making (Dohrenwend and Martin, 1978). Seligman considers lack of control and helplessness to be a major cause of depression (Seligman, 1975; Abramson *et al.*, 1978), but systematic work on attribution, labelling, and helplessness with specific reference to bereavement has yet to be developed.

Finally, a purely cognitive approach to bereavement has recently been developed. Neimeyer *et al.* (1984) are critical of the approaches to thanatalogical research, stating that they show 'a chaotic mosaic cluttered with duplication of effort, unconfirmed opinion, questionable research methodologies and paradigms, and a striking absence of anything approaching a coherent unifying base of psychological theory'. Reflecting upon the many disciplines which have an interest in thanatology, the same authors suggest that the unique contribution which psychologists can offer is the unified framework of Kelly's personal construct theory (Kelly, 1955) as a vehicle for future research. Kelly proposed that all people are scientists, and that they continually engage in an attempt to predict and control behaviour. With experience of life, individuals develop unique systems of constructs, a construct being a way in which objects, situations, people, concepts etc. can be construed as similar, yet differing. Constructs are, in fact, very similar to Parkes' assumptions as described above. Rowe (1984) uses clinical examples which illustrate how construct theory can be used with bereaved people; she also believes that the way people construe death is central to the whole structure of their cognitive system. A fuller account of a construct approach to bereavement is offered by Viney (1985), Woodfield and Viney (1985), and Hoagland (1984). Construct theorists have also done a considerable amount of work on measurement of death anxiety and, again, are critical of the more traditional approaches such as the Templer Death Anxiety Scale (Templer, 1970) and the Collett–Lester Fear of Death Scale (Collett and Lester, 1969). As an alternative, they have developed the Threat Index (Rigdon *et al.*, 1979; Neimeyer *et al.*, 1984) and, following criticisms of its unidimensional approach (Chambers, 1986), the Death Attitude Repertory Test (DART) (Neimeyer *et al.*, 1986). Neimeyer *et al.* believe that the DART may be useful in studying developmental constructions of life and death, and also suggest that this approach may provide a link with Beck's cognitive model of depression (Beck *et al.*, 1979).

STAGE MODELS OF LOSS

Possibly the most famous stage conception in bereavement is Kübler-Ross's five-stage sequence for the dying person: denial, anger, bargaining, depression, acceptance (Kübler-Ross, 1969). Since this work, stage models have proliferated. For example, Engel outlines the stages as shock and disbelief, developing awareness, restitution, resolving the loss, idealization and outcome (Engel, 1964); Kavanaugh's seven stages comprise shock, disorganization, volatile emotions, guilt, loss and loneliness, relief and re-establishment (Kavanaugh, 1972). Schneider (1984) compares the different observations of thirteen theorists in an extremely useful table.

Stage models of grief and loss are, however, two-edged swords. Although they offer an account of the changing picture of adjustment which may be predicted over the course of time in a bereaved person, and their descriptive elements can easily be grasped by the novice (Swain and Cowles, 1982), they can have serious drawbacks. The first problem arises from the incorrect usage of the stage conception itself. This has been taken from developmental psychology, and is meant to imply far more than a simple description of changing patterns of behaviour which occur in an invariant order. Stages are generally postulated when development proceeds by means of striking changes in complex patterns of behaviour, and, furthermore, the various segments of behaviour are meant to be grouped on the basis of an underlying theory (Mussen *et al.*, 1969). According to this definition, bereavement reactions cannot be appropriately accommodated within a stage model. Human beings do not move through invariant and discrete stages of grief, as is obvious to experienced clinicians. Both Kübler-Ross (1969) and Kavanaugh (1972) state quite explicitly that they expect to see patients or clients moving backwards and forwards between the stages, and this has been emphasized as a weakness by Bugen (1977) in his critique of stage models. However, less experienced workers can overlook this caveat, and adhere to a rigid stage conception (Leviton, 1977; Worden, 1982). The result is that moving backwards by the patient or client may be seen as 'regression', and an individual who fails to show the defined stages may be labelled as showing abnormal or pathological grief. In addition, the care-giver might feel a failure if he or she has not managed to move the client along the circumscribed path to an appropriate resolution of grief (Leviton, 1977). Finally, the correspondence between the proposed stages and human behaviour has been questioned by several clinicians, such as Schulz and Aderman (1974), Bugen (1977), and even Kübler-Ross herself (1969)!

Rando (1984) proposes that instead of stages, three broad phases of reactions to grief can be seen. These are the phase of avoidance, which encompasses shock, denial and disbelief; confrontation, the highly emotional state during which various aspects of loss are most keenly experienced; and re-establishment, when grief reactions dwindle and there is re-entry into the everyday world. However, even this conception does not do justice to the complexity of bereavement reactions. Shneidman (1976), whose experience with dying patients leads him to disagree with Kübler-Ross's conception, summarizes the limitations of any stage theory when he comments, 'What I do see is a complicated clustering of intellectual and affective states, some fleeting, lasting for a moment or a day or a week, set, not unexpectedly, against the backdrop of that person's total personality, his "philosophy of life" (whether an essential optimism or gratitude to life, or a pervasive pessimism and dour or suspicious orientation to life)'. This statement highlights an important limitation of stage models, namely that they cannot accommodate such variables as personality, previous experiences, current situational variables and cultural norms. A final criticism is that stage descriptions do not tend to stay consistently at the same level of analysis. That is, a single stage model may move through cognitive, emotional and behavioural dimensions, according to a principle of apparent domination. Ramsay (1977) suggests a solution whereby the sequential nature of grieving processes is recognized, but the term 'predominant component' offers a less confusing label than the word 'stage'.

THE NORMAL/ABNORMAL CONTINUUM

Throughout the literature on bereavement there are attempts to classify grief as either normal or abnormal. Perhaps because the word 'normal' has several meanings (e.g. statistically common, healthy or functioning), some writers have sought other labels, and so 'morbid' (Lieberman, 1978), 'atypical' (Parkes, 1986), 'complicated' (Engel, 1961), and 'pathological' (Raphael, 1975; Lynn and Racy, 1969) have been used as substitutes. Although the *Diagnostic and statistical manual of mental disorders* (DSM-III, American Psychiatric Association, 1980) has classified bereavement as a 'normal' (meaning common or healthy?) reaction rather than a form of mental disorder, some writers disagree with this and argue that even a straightforward reaction to loss causes derangement of sufficient magnitude to be classified as a mental disorder. Engel (1961), who may have been the first person to have used the labels 'complicated' and 'uncomplicated' to refer to bereavement reactions, clearly regards bereavement as similar to a disease; it involves suffering and causes impairment of functioning, it has a known cause and predictable symptomatology, and will generally tend to resolve itself in the same way that many wounds or infections do. Parkes (1965, 1986) also liked this analogy, although it was Parkes (1971, 1975) who subsequently moved away from the medical model when he looked at grief as a psychosocial transition. Those writers who see grief as a form of mental disorder do not all feel that the sufferers should be treated by medical personnel, however, and so the disease analogy is not taken to an extreme position. Kamm (1985) has likened grief to pregnancy: it is a normal process with a known starting point which progresses inexorably and with suffering, but which is benign, time limited and with an excellent prognosis.

DSM-III distinguishes uncomplicated bereavement (which may include guilt or depressive feelings) from bereavement which is complicated by the development of a separately identifiable mental disorder, such as major depression. Unfortunately though, as Hoagland (1984) and Melges and DeMaso (1980) observe, it is often quite hard to distinguish depression, the 'mental disorder', from depression which is the natural result of a severe loss. A possible link between these two conceptions of depression is the cognitive approach which has already been mentioned.

On the whole, clinicians regard 'abnormal' or 'complicated' grief as a pattern of responses which does not fit in with the general picture of progression, e.g. as outlined by Rando (1984) or Ramsay (1979). In an early paper, Parkes (1965) classified bereavement reactions, and although some of the psychiatric language used seems rather dated now, the broad conceptual framework has not been challenged as untenable. He has always been very sensitive to the fact that in order to classify something as statistically 'abnormal', there must be some knowledge of 'norms', and has been very energetic in collecting data which describe the typical progression of grief (Parkes, 1965, 1970). The inadequate conceptual basis for stage models of grief means that departure from the so-called norms they outline is not a sound basis for classifying a person's responses as either normal or abnormal.

However, there is some agreement about the general ways in which bereavement can cause problems for an individual. An absence of grief following a serious loss is considered to be unhealthy, in that inevitably, at some future point, the grief will be released. Grief which results in physical, psychosomatic or mental illness is considered to be unhealthy, and is often referred to as 'distorted' grief, whilst prolonged, (or 'chronic') grieving is yet another form of unhealthy response, sometimes postulated to be the result of secondary gain.

A somewhat different, and more complex, approach is taken to complicated grief by the psychoanalysts. Volkan (1983) states that complicated grief results in either depression or a syndrome termed 'established pathological mourning'. The latter is not simply chronic grief, but rather a strange state of ambivalence, in which the bereaved person wishes to complete his or her mourning, but at the same time persistently attempts to undo the reality of the death.

The confusion over defining grief as normal or abnormal is not merely academic, but has far-reaching practical results. Worden (1982) uses these terms as a basis for distinguishing grief therapy (identifying and resolving conflicts which preclude the completion of grief work) from grief counselling (the facilitation of mourning tasks with recently bereaved clients), and so uses the continuum to differentiate service provision. This distinction (although using different terminology, as bereavement counselling was then unknown) was also seen by Lindemann (1944), who said, 'Since it is obvious that not all bereaved persons, especially those suffering because of war casualties, can have the benefit of expert psychiatric help, much of this knowledge will have to be passed on to auxilliary workers. Social workers and ministers will have to be on the look-out for the more ominous pictures, referring these to the psychiatrist while assisting the more normal reactions themselves.' Thus the practical implications of assessing grief as typical or atypical are extremely important where help and support for bereaved people are available. The assessment and subsequent classification of grief by primary care-givers may be the most important factor in determining which bereaved people are offered help, by whom, and in which setting.

UNDESIRABLE OUTCOMES FOLLOWING BEREAVEMENT

Mortality Rates

Several studies have looked at the 'broken heart' phenomenon, which Parkes (1972) addresses in some detail, after citing the mortality statistics of 1657, in which a small proportion of people were noted to have died simply from 'griefe'. Jacobs and Ostfeld (1977) review thirteen reports published between 1940 and 1975, and conclude that excess mortality rates are found particularly in males and the younger widowed. The period of high risk can be up to 2 years, with the peak for men during the first 6 months, but the risk of suicide is elevated for several years. Apart from suicide, the causes of death include tuberculosis, influenza, pneumonia, cirrhosis, alcoholism, heart disease, cancer, diabetes and accidents.

An extremely thorough overview of the literature on mortality and illness risks following bereavement, in which sex differences are considered, is provided by Stroebe and Stroebe (1983). Despite different and often flawed methodologies, elevated mortality rates following loss are consistently reported, with men being more at risk than women.

Physical Disorders

Ill-health seems to be a more likely outcome of bereavement than actual demise. Some studies document the increased incidence of visits to a physician following bereavement (e.g. Maddison and Viola, 1968; Parkes, 1964, 1970; Weiner *et al.*, 1975), although the 'illnesses' may comprise a mix of physical, psychosomatic and psychological complaints, together with a need for some form of support (Raphael, 1984). One factor is probably people's unfamiliarity with the overwhelming physiological changes which occur during bereavement, and which lead them to label their state as illness. However, a state of intense or prolonged stress may result in a diagnosable illness, and Parkes and Brown (1972) found that the hospitalization rate was three times higher among the recently bereaved than in a control group. Both Raphael (1984) and Rando (1984) cite several further studies linking specific physical illnesses with loss. Lundin (1984) used registered sickness as a measure of ill-health, and found in his Swedish study that sudden bereavement in particular was associated with increased sickness during the 2 years following the loss.

With elderly people, an existing state of confusion which has an organic basis may be uncovered for the first time when a competent companion or spouse dies, or it may be greatly exacerbated by bereavement, as if the trauma is too much for an already impaired mind to cope with. A correlation between brain atrophy and bereavement was found in a study on healthy elderly people by Bird *et al.* (1986), who describe the finding as inexplicable. It has been suggested that elderly people seem prone to somatize their grief (Parkes, 1965; Stern *et al.*, 1951); although Stroebe and Stroebe (1983) disagree in the light of all findings to date. In the few studies in which sex differences are comparable, bereaved men are more at risk than bereaved women. In considering explanations for the greater vulnerability of men, these authors feel that the evidence supports the life events and stress model, but that the interpersonal protection theory (i.e. the beneficial effect of a good social support network) also offers a good explanatory model.

Finally, illness may be brought on directly by self-neglect or drug abuse. Clayton *et al.* (1968) found that non-drinkers or social drinkers did not take more alcohol when bereaved, but that heavy drinkers were more likely to cope by drinking more. The same pattern may occur with cigarette smokers, although there are no studies on this topic in the literature.

Psychosomatic Disorders

Since Lindemann (1944) suggested that psychosomatic illness could be considered a 'distorted' grief reaction, and named ulcerative colitis in particular, there have been several studies which link psychosomatic disorders with grief, or document physiological changes which may have a causative role in their development. Raphael (1984) gives an account of recent work in this area, and cites that of Bartrop *et al.* (1977) on changes in immune response and altered patterns of corticosteroid secretion (Chodoff *et al.* 1964). McDermott and Cobb (1939) suggested a link between loss and asthma, and Stamm and Drapkin (1966) describe how they treated a man who suffered from bronchial asthma after accidentally killing his own son. Leaverton *et al.* (1980) and Stein and Charles (1971) have linked loss to diabetes mellitus; Henoch *et al.* (1978) worked on juvenile rheumatoid arthritis, whilst Binger *et al.* (1969) noted general symptoms of malaise, such as enuresis, headaches, anxieties and abdominal pain, in children whose siblings died with leukaemia.

Psychiatric Disorders

There are several explanations as to why bereavement might be followed by an onset of mental disorder sufficiently severe to need psychiatric intervention. In itself, a severe loss is an understandable cause of sadness or depression, and particularly so if the cognitions of the bereaved person reinforce a hopeless, helpless view of the world. The difficulty of classifying depression when it occurs during bereavement has already been mentioned, but there is also some disagreement in the literature about when, if at all, active pharmacological or physical treatment for a depressive illness should be instituted. Several clinicians indicate that very severe depression should be treated medically (e.g. Lindemann, 1944; Melges and DeMaso, 1980), and Lynn and Racy (1969) describe successful resolution of grief following ECT. When depression is present but less extreme, Raphael (1984) suggests that antidepressants are not useful, but in an uncontrolled study, Bleich *et al.* (1986) report a generally successful strategy of combining psychotherapy with pharmacotherapy in helping Israeli soldiers recover from PTSD. Although depression is a reasonably common sequel to loss (Parkes, 1965; Stein and Susser, 1969; Parkes and Brown, 1972; Clayton *et al.*, 1972; Clegg, 1988), it need not always occur; it will often improve during the first year of the loss (Bornstein *et al.*, 1973; Crisp and Priest, 1972), and preventive work may be carried out beforehand by reducing ambivalence and increasing self-esteem (Raphael 1978, 1984). Stroebe and Stroebe (1983) found that when the general tendency for a greater incidence of depression in females is taken into consideration, males have a somewhat higher chance of becoming depressed during bereavement.

Although Lindemann (1944) mentioned overactivity combined with a feeling of zest and well-bring as a distorted grief reaction, mania is a relatively rare sequel to bereavement. However, Parkes (1965) found thirteen cases in the literature, Ambelas (1979) documented five cases, and Rosenman and Taylor (1986) provide a single case report.

The 'diathesis-stress' model (Rosenhan and Seligman, 1984) states that when there is a constitutional tendency towards a particular pathology, the experience of a severe stress may trigger off the first episode of the disorder or else bring about a relapse. This model may be applied to psychosomatic disorders, depression, or, perhaps more commonly, to schizophrenic disorders (Davison and Neale, 1986). Recently, Chung *et al.* (1986) found that threatening life events (including loss through death) were more strongly associated with the onset of briefer schizophreniform psychoses (DSM-III), and even with hypomania, than with schizophrenia.

INTERVENTION WITH BEREAVED PEOPLE

Bereavement Counselling

In the past a healthy bereaved person might expect considerable support from relatives and neighbours, who were likely to have experienced bereavement themselves. If a person became either physically or mentally ill, then aid would be sought (if available) from the appropriate sources of professional help. However, Gorer (1965) and Fulton and Fulton (1971) describe how sociocultural forces in the Western world have reduced public mourning rites to the barest minimum. This 'privatization' means that all too often nowadays the burden of grief is placed squarely upon an individual's shoulders, and that there are few opportunities to recount events and talk about the loss with supportive listeners. It is perhaps in recognition of the severe isolation experienced by bereaved people that there has recently been an enormous increase in the growth of professional, semi-professional and 'lay' bereavement counselling or suport services. For example, Cruse, a nationwide organization for bereaved people in Britain, has grown from having one small branch in 1959 to having over 14 000 members in 1986. There are now numerous branches of specialist bereavement organizations such as the Stillbirth and Neonatal Death Society (SANDS), the Foundation for the Study of Infant Deaths, and the Compassionate Friends (for parents who have lost a child). These organizations use their members' own experiences of loss and grief, sometimes supplemented by training in befriending and counselling skills, and in conjunction with professionals who can advise when needed. Besides offering counselling, many of the organizations just mentioned actively campaign to increase public awareness of the issues and promote improved conditions for terminal patients or bereaved people. For instance, following reports on the inadequacies of maternity care after stillbirth (e.g. Lovell, 1983), SANDS has encouraged local groups to campaign for better facilities and treatment during the hosptial stay, and for improved forms of memorialization for the life that never was.

Several books now give information about counselling approaches. Both

Rando (1984) and Raphael (1984) give comprehensive overviews of the psycho-logical literature on bereavement, with Raphael focusing on the bereaved client, and Rando on working with terminally ill people. Worden (1982), as mentioned above, offers a task-oriented framework in which therapy is differentiated from counselling.

A model of intervention which does not involve a distinction between 'abnor-mal' and 'normal' grieving has been developed by Le Poidevin (in prep.). In her multidimensional approach to understanding the many changes which a loss brings, she takes into consideration the acceptance of events, their practical consequences, social–cultural and family role changes, personal identity and sexual need, emotional expression and physical health. This system can serve as a basis for a counselling service, as well as giving good scope for evaluation of intervention (Le Poidevin, 1988). Finally, in an attempt to sort out the muddle which has arisen from stage conceptions of grief, Schneider (1984) outlines a holistic counselling approach in which physical, cognitive, emotional, spiritual and behavioural aspects are consistently used for purposes of assessment and intervention throughout the grieving process.

During the last decade many hospices financed by charitable donations have opened in Britain. They rely heavily on input from volunteers, and often offer a local bereavement counselling service. Parkes (1980) feels that when trained, such counsellors develop considerable expertise by working solely with the bereaved, and that they may come to rival professionals in the standard of care they are able to offer.

Professional Intervention

Compared with the literature on grief processes, there are few good publications on specific psychotherapeutic intervention strategies, and many of these are weak in their assessment of outcome.

Ramsay (1977, 1979) describes a behavioural approach in which flooding and prolonged exposure are used to help people whose avoidance of painful stimuli resembles the avoidance found in phobic conditions. Mawson et al. (1981) used a behavioural technique of 'guided mourning' on patients with chronic grief, and demonstrated some improvement compared with a control group whose members were actively encouraged to avoid painful reminders of the deceased. Hypothesiz-ing that incubation of distresss, social reinforcement of grief inhibition and lack of reinforcement of grieving underlie some patients' chronic grief, Gauthier and Marshall (1977) report rapid and good results from rearrangement of social contingencies together with flooding. Ramsay (1977) argues that interpretation is not necessary for successful treatment of complicated grief, although Volkan (1983) regards it as essential in his 're-grief' approach to established pathological mourning. Lieberman (1978) obtained successful results, as assessed with the morbid grief scale, using a semi-behavioural forced mourning procedure. He claims that it is beneficial if family members can be incorporated into the treatment procedure, but that forced mourning is not indicated when a patient lacks social support or has concurrent financial or social problems. Hodgkinson

(1982) reports on three cases in which a cathartic eclectic approach was used; Melges and DeMaso (1980) used imagery to restructure the memory of emotional events, and to reconstruct identity; and Horowitz *et al.* (1980) combined a cognitive and analytic approach to alter their patients' self-images.

Several studies attest to the efficacy of psychotherapeutic intervention following trauma or disasters, and Raphael (1984) gives a good overview of the work with disaster victims and workers. Hostages are faced with imminent death, and may witness it, and so are extremely likely to develop PTSD. In an effort to prevent full-blown development of PTSD, Sank (1979) used a treatment format based on Lazarus's multimodal behaviour therapy (Lazarus, 1976), with some success. A somewhat similar approach, based on rational–emotive, cognitive and problem-solving therapies, was adopted by Duckworth (1986), who reported beneficial changes in General Health Questionnaire status for police officers who had been involved in work at the Bradford fire disaster.

Who Needs Intervention?

A few studies to date have attempted to identify bereaved people whose special circumstances or characteristics suggest a high risk of undesirable sequelae.

Following the study in which they found several variables associated with poor outcome at 13 months, Parkes and Weiss (1983) put the information into a Bereavement Risk Index, which was later used with some success at St Christopher's Hospice. A controlled study subsequently showed that counselling by volunteers had beneficial effects upon general health as assessed during a 3-year follow-up period, and that the greatest benefit was shown by individuals previously assessed as high risk. Raphael (1977), in one of the few studies to evaluate the outcome of a counselling service, concluded that intervention had been beneficial; furthermore, the existence of a concurrent life crisis and the lack of a supportive social network were shown to be predictors of poor outcome, a conclusion corroborated by Stroebe and Stroebe (1983), La Greca (1985) and Berardo (1985).

Raphael (1984) suggests that the greatest value of intervention is with bereaved people who can be identified as high risk, and that there may be little value in offering support to bereaved people in general.

At the time of writing, the following variables should be considered as potential high risk indicators:

a) *Disposition of the bereaved person*: inadequate or potentially harmful coping strategies; earlier unresolved loss or losses; recent loss or losses; concurrent life crisis or crises; previous stress-related mental or physical illness; ambivalent relationship with the deceased; negative construed philosophy of life and death; feelings of helplessness or hopelessness; high dependence on the dead person.

b) *Social factors*: perceived lack of social support network; lack of warm environment in which emotional expression is accepted; over-protective atmosphere, in which painful reality is disguised.

c) *Circumstances of the death*: unexpected death; unpleasant death circumstances (e.g. following assault or mutilating accident).

Future Trends

It is likely that future research will focus on aspects of service provision, rather than on descriptive and theoretical approaches to bereavement. Issues to be addressed are the appropriateness of particular types of intervention for various client or patient groups, the style of service from which intervention is offered, the qualities sought in counsellors or therapists, and methods of service evaluation. We will probably see more research on the identification and predictive value of risk factors, comparative investigations of different therapeutic approaches, and further work related to the needs of specialist client groups, for instance mentally handicapped people (Strachan, 1981; McLoughlin, 1986), AIDS victims, the elderly (Lund *et al.*, 1985) and confused elderly, families, disaster victims and workers—military (Parson, 1986; Ørner, 1987) and civilian (Raphael, 1984; Eth and Pynoos, 1985). Finally, it is to be hoped that death education in Britain will start to grow in the same way that it has in the United States (Benoliel, 1982).

SUMMARY AND CONCLUSIONS

This chapter has looked at the processes of bereavement, grief and mourning, which typically follow an important loss. Psychoanalytic, attachment, medical, psychosocial, stress, and cognitive approaches have been outlined, followed by a critique of stage models of loss. The conceptualization of grief as normal or abnormal was discussed, before a review of studies indicating the various undesirable outcomes of bereavement: mortality, physical, psychosomatic or psychiatric illness, in which men generally fare worse than women. In the section on intervention, the growth of bereavement counselling was described, and preceded an account of some approaches offered by professional care-givers. Future research seems to lie in the direction of specialist input to clients with clearly defined needs, and aspects of service provision and evaluation, rather than in further work on the description of grief.

REFERENCES

Abramson, L.Y., Seligman, M.E.P., & Teasdale, J. (1978). Learned helplessness in humans, *Journal of Abnormal Psychology, 87*, 32–48.
Ambelas, A. (1979). Psychologically stressful events in the precipitation of manic episodes, *British Journal of Psychiatry, 135*, 15–21.
American Psychiatric Association (1980). *Diagnostic and statistical manual of mental disorders*, 3rd edn. Washington: American Psychiatric Association.
Angrist, S.S. (1974). Dimensions of well-being in public housing families. *Environment and Behaviour, 6*, 495–516.
Bartrop, R., Luckhurst, E., Lazarus, L., Kiloh, L.G., & Perry, R. (1977). Depressed lymphocyte function after bereavement. *Lancet* i, 834–836.
Beck, A.T., Rush, A.J., Shaw, B.F., and Emery, G. (1979). *Cognitive therapy of depression*. New York: Guilford.
Benoliel, J.Q. (1982). *Death education for the professional*. Washington: Hemisphere.
Berardo, F.M. (1985). Social networks and life preservation. *Death Studies, 9*, 37–50.
Binger, C.M., Ablin, A.R., Feuerstein, R.C., Kushner, J.H., Zoger, S., & Mikkelsen, C. (1969). Childhood leukemia: emotional impact on patient and family. *New England Journal of Medicine, 280*, 414–418.

Bird, J.M., Levy, R., & Jacoby, R.J. (1986). Computerised tomography in the elderly: changes over time in a normal population. *British Journal of Psychiatry, 148*, 80–85.

Bleich, A., Siegel, B., Garb, R., & Lerer, B. (1986). Post-traumatic stress disorder following combat exposure. *British Journal of Psychiatry, 149*, 365–369.

Bornstein, P.E., Clayton, P.J., Halikas, J.A., Maurice, W.L., & Robins, E. (1973). The depression of widowhood at thirteen months. *British Journal of Psychiatry, 122*, 561–566.

Bowlby, J. (1969). *Attachment and loss*, Vol. I: *Attachment*. London: Hogarth Press.

Bowlby, J. (1980). *Attachment and loss*, Vol. III: *Loss, sadness and depression*. London: Hogarth Press.

Bugen, L.A. (1977). Human grief: a model for prediction and intervention. *American Journal of Orthopsychiatry, 47*, 196–206.

Burgoyne, J. (1985). Marriage on the dole. *The Listener*, 13 June, 12–13.

Chambers, W.V. (1986). Inconsistencies in the theory of death threat. *Death Studies, 10*, 165–175.

Chodoff, P., Friedman, S.B., & Hamburg, D. (1964). Stress, defenses and coping behaviour: observations in parents of children with malignant disease. *American Journal of Psychiatry, 120*, 743–749.

Chung, R.K., Langeluddecke, P., & Tennant, C. (1986). Threatening life events in the onset of schizophrenia, schizophreniform psychosis and hypomania. *British Journal of Psychiatry, 148*, 680–685.

Clayton, P., Desmarais, L., & Winokur, G. (1968). A study of normal bereavement. *American Journal of Psychiatry, 125*, 168–178.

Clayton, P., Halikas, J.A., & Maurice, W.L. (1972). The depression of widowhood. *British Journal of Psychiatry, 120*, 71–78.

Clegg, F. (1988). Grief and loss in elderly people in a psychiatric setting. In E. Chigier (ed.), *First international symposium on grief and bereavement*, Vol. I: *Psychodynamics of grief and bereavement*. Tel Aviv: Freund.

Collett, L., & Lester, D. (1969). The fear of death and the fear of dying. *Journal of Psychology, 72*, 179–181.

Crisp, A.H., & Priest, R.G. (1972). Psychoneurotic status during the year following bereavement. *Journal of Psychosomatic Research, 16*, 351–355.

Danforth, L.M. (1982). *The death rituals of rural greece*. Princeton, NJ: Princeton University Press.

Davison, G.C., & Neale, J.M. (1986). *Abnormal psychology*, 4th ed. New York: Wiley.

Dohrenwend, B.S., & Dohrenwend, B.P. (eds.) (1974). *Stressful life events: Their nature and effects*. New York: Wiley.

Dohrenwend, B.S., & Martin, J.L. (1978). Personal vs. situational determination of anticipation and control of the occurrence of stressful life events. Paper presented at the annual meeting of the AAAS, Washington, DC.

Duckworth, D.H. (1986). Psychological problems arising from disaster work. *Stress Medicine, 2*, 315–323.

Engel, G.L. (1961). Is grief a disease? *Psychosomatic Medicine, 23*, 18–22.

Engel, G.L. (1964). Grief and grieving. *American Journal of Nursing, 64*, 93–98.

Eth, S., & Pynoos, R.S. (1985). *Post-traumatic stress disorder in children*. Washington: American Psychiatric Press.

Freud, S. (1917). Mourning and melancholia. In *Standard edition*, Vol. 14. London: Hogarth Press.

Freud, S. (1926). *Inhibitions, symptoms, and anxiety*. In *Standard edition*, Vol. 20. London: Hogarth Press.

Fried, M. (1963). Grieving for a lost home. In *The environment of the metropolis*. L.J. Dahl (ed.), New York: Basic Books.

Fulton, R., & Fulton, J. (1971). A psychosocial aspect of terminal care: anticipatory grief. *Omega, 2*, 91–99.

Gauthier, Y., & Marshall, W.L. (1977). Grief: a cognitive–behavioural analysis. *Cognitive Therapy and Research, 1*, 39–44.

Gorer, G, (1965). *Death, grief and mourning in contemporary Britain*. London: Cresset Press.

Henoch, M.J., Batson, J.W., & Baum, J. (1978). Psychosocial factors in juvenile rheumatoid arthritis. *Arthritis and Rheumatism, 21*, 229–233.

Hoagland, A.C. (1984). Bereavement and personal constructs: old theories and new concepts. In F.R. Epting & R.A. Neimeyer (eds.), *Personal meanings of death*. New York: Hemisphere.

Hodgkinson, P. (1982). Abnormal grief—the problem of therapy. *British Journal of Medical Psychology, 55*, 29–34.

Holmes, T.H., & Rahe, R.H. (1967). The social readjustment rating scale. *Journal of Psychosomatic Research, 11*, 213–218.

Horowitz, M.J., Wilner, N., Marmer, C., & Krupnick, J. (1980). Pathological grief and the activation of latent self-images. *American Journal of Psychiatry, 137*, 1157–1162.

Jacobs, S., & Ostfeld, A. (1977). An epidemiological review of the mortality of bereavement. *Psychosomatic Medicine, 39*, 344–357.

Jewett, C.L. (1982). *Helping children cope with separation and loss*. Harvard: Harvard Common Press.

Kamm, J.A. (1985). Grief and therapy: two processes in interaction. In E.M. Stern (ed.), *Psychotherapy and the grieving patient*. New York: Harrington Park Press.

Kavanaugh, R. (1972). *Facing death*. Harmondsworth: Penguin.

Keddie, K.M.G. (1977). Pathological mourning after the death of a domestic pet. *British Journal of Psychiatry, 131*, 21–35.

Kelly, G.A. (1955). *The psychology of personal consructs*. New York: Norton.

Kübler-Ross, E. (1969). *On death and dying*. New York: Macmillan.

La Greca, A.J. (1985). The psycho-social factors in surviving stress. *Death Studies, 9*, 23–36.

Lazarus, A.A. (1976). *Multimodal behavior therapy*. New York: Springer.

Leaverton, D.R., White, C.A., McCormick, C.R., Smith, P., & Sheikholislam, B. (1980). Parental loss antecedent to childhood diabetes mellitus. *Journal of the American Academy of Child Psychiatry, 19*, 678–679.

Le Poidevin, S. (1988). An organisational and training model for counselling the dying and bereaved. In E. Chigier (ed.), *First International Symposium on Grief and Bereavement*, Vol III: *Support systems*. Tel Aviv: Freund.

Le Poidevin, S. (In preparation). *Counselling for adjustment to stress, loss and change*. London: Croom Helm.

Leviton, D. (1977). Death Education. In H. Feifel (ed.), *New meanings of death*. New York: McGraw-Hill.

Lieberman, S. (1978). Nineteen cases of morbid grief. *British Journal of Psychiatry, 132*, 159–163.

Lindemann, E. (1944). The symptomatology and management of acute grief. *American Journal of Psychiatry, 101*, 141–148.

Lovell, A. (1983). Some questions of identity: late miscarriage, stillbirth and perinatal loss. *Social Science and Medicine, 17*, 755–761.

Lund, D.A., Dimond, M., & Juretich, M. (1985). Bereavement support groups for the elderly. *Death Studies, 9*, 309–321.

Lundin, T. (1984). Morbidity following sudden and unexpected bereavement. *British Journal of Psychiatry, 144*, 84–88.

Lynn, E.J., & Racy, J. (1969). The resolution of pathological grief after electroconvulsive therapy. *Journal of Nervous and Mental Disease, 148*, 165–169.

McDermott, N., & Cobb, S. (1939). A psychiatric survey of 50 cases of bronchial asthma. *Psychosomatic Medicine, 1*, 201– 204.

McLoughlin, I.J. (1986). Bereavement in the mentally handicapped. *British Journal of Hospital Medicine, 36,* October, 256–260.

Maddison, D.C., & Viola, A. (1968). The health of widows in the year following bereavement. *Journal of Psychosomatic Research, 12,* 297–306.

Mawson, D., Marks, I.M., Ramm, L., & Stern, R.S. (1981). Guided mourning for morbid grief. *British Journal of Psychiatry, 138,* 185–193.

Melges, F.T., & DeMaso, D.R. (1980). Grief-resolution therapy: reliving, revising and revisiting. *American Journal of Psychotherapy, 34,* 51–61.

Mitchell, A. (1985). *Children in the middle.* London: Tavistock.

Mussen, P.H., Conger, J.J., & Kagan, J. (1969). *Child development and personality.* New York: Harper and Row.

Neimeyer, R.A., Bagley, K.J., & Moore, M.K. (1986). Cognitive structure and death anxiety. *Death Studies, 10,* 273–288.

Neimeyer, R.A., Epting, F.R., & Krieger, S.R. (1984). Personal constructs in thanatology: an introduction and research bibliography. In F.R. Epting & R.A. Neimeyer (eds.), *Personal meanings of death.* Washington: Hemisphere.

Ørner, R. (1987). Survey of post-traumatic stress disorder. *Bulletin of the British Psychological Society, 40,* 27.

Parkes, C.M. (1964). The effects of bereavement on physical and mental health. *British Medical Journal, 2,* 274–279.

Parkes, C.M. (1965). Bereavement and mental illness. Part 1: A clinical study of the grief of bereaved psychiatric patients; Part 2: A classification of bereavement reactions. *British Journal of Medical Psychology, 38,* 1–26.

Parkes, C.M. (1970). The first year of bereavement: a longitudinal study of the reaction of London widows to the death of their husbands. *Psychiatry, 33,* 444–467.

Parkes, C.M. (1971). Psychosocial transitions: a field for study. *Social Science and Medicine, 5,* 101–115.

Parkes, C.M. (1972). The components of reaction to loss of a limb, spouse or home. *Journal of Psychosomatic Research, 16,* 343–349.

Parkes, C.M. (1975). What becomes of redundant world models? A contribution to the study of adaptation to change. *British Journal of Medical Psychology, 48,* 131–137.

Parkes, C.M. (1980). Bereavement counselling: does it work? *British Medical Journal, 281,* 5 July, 3–6.

Parkes, C.M. (1986). *Bereavement: Studies in grief in adult life,* 2nd edn. London: Tavistock.

Parkes, C.M., & Brown, R. (1972). Health after bereavement: a controlled study of young Boston widows and widowers. *Psychosomatic Medicine, 34,* 449–461.

Parkes, C.M., & Weiss, R.S. (1983). *Recovery from bereavement.* New York: Basic Books.

Parson, E.R. (1986). Life after death: Vietnam veteran's struggle for meaning and recovery. *Death Studies, 10,* 11–26.

Ramsay, R.W. (1977). Behavioural approaches to bereavement. *Behaviour Research and Therapy, 15,* 131–135.

Ramsay, R.W. (1979). Bereavement: A behavioural treatment for pathological grief. In P.O. Sjoden, S. Bates, & W.S. Dockens III (eds.), *Trends in behavioural therapy.* New York: Academic Press.

Rando, T.A. (1984). *Grief, dying and death: Clinical interventions for caregivers.* Champaign: Research Press.

Raphael, B. (1975). The management of pathological grief. *Australian and New Zealand Journal of Psychiatry, 9,* 173–180.

Raphael, B. (1977). Preventive intervention with the recently bereaved. *Archives of General Psychiatry, 34,* 1450–1454.

Raphael, B. (1978). Mourning and the prevention of melancholia. *British Journal of Medical Psychology, 51,* 303–310.

Raphael, B. (1984). *The anatomy of bereavement*. London: Hutchinson.

Rees, W.D. (1975). The bereaved and their hallucinations. In E. Schoenberg *et al.* (eds.), *Bereavement: Its psychological aspects*. New York: Columbia University Press.

Rigdon, M., Epting, F.R., Neimeyer, R.A., & Krieger, S.R. (1979). The threat index. *Death Education, 3*, 245–281.

Rosenhan, D.L., & Seligman, M.E.P. (1984). *Abnormal psychology*. New York: Norton.

Rosenman, S.J., & Taylor, H. (1986). Mania following bereavement. *British Journal of Psychiatry, 148*, 468–470.

Rowe, D. (1984). Constructing life and death. In F.R. Epting, & R.A. Neimeyer (eds), *Personal meanings of death*. Washington: Hemisphere.

Sank, L.I. (1979). Community disasters: primary prevention and treatment. *American Psychologist, 34*, 334–338.

Schneider, J. (1984). *Stress, loss, grief*. Baltimore: University Park Press.

Schulz, R., & Aderman, D. (1974). Clinical research and the stages of dying. *Omega, 5*, 137–143.

Seligman, M.E.P. (1975). *Helplessness: On depression, development, and death*. San Francisco: Freeman.

Shneidman, E.A. (1976). *Death: Current perspectives*, 3rd edn. Palo Alto: Mayfield.

Shukla, G.D., Sahu, S.C., Tripathi, R.P., & Gupta, D.K. (1982). A psychiatric study of amputees. *British Journal of Psychiatry, 141*, 50–53.

Spencer, A.J. (1982). *Death in Ancient Egypt*. Harmondsworth: Penguin.

Stamm, J., & Drapkin, A. (1966). The successful treatment of a severe case of bronchial asthma. *Journal of Nervous and Mental Disease, 142*, 180–189.

Stannard, D.E. (1977). *The puritan way of death*. Oxford: Oxford University Press.

Stein, S.P., & Charles, E. (1971). Emotional factors in juvenile diabetes mellitus. *American Journal of Psychiatry, 128*, 700–704.

Stein, Z., & Susser, M.W. (1969). Widowhood and mental illness. *British Journal of Preventive and Social Medicine, 23*, 106–110.

Stern, K., Williams, G.M., & Prados, M. (1951). Grief reactions in later life. *American Journal of Psychiatry, 108*, 289–294.

Stewart, C.S., Thrush, J.C., Paulus, G.S., & Hafner, P. (1985). The elderly's adjustment to the loss of a companion animal: people-pet dependency. *Death Studies, 9*, 383–393.

Strachan, J.G. (1981). Reactions to bereavement. *Apex, 9*, 20–21.

Stoebe, M.S., & Stroebe, W. (1983). Who suffers more? Sex differences in health risks of the widowed. *Psychological Bulletin, 93*, 279–301.

Swain H.L., & Cowles, K.V. (1982). Interdisciplinary death education in a nursing school. In J.Q. Benoliel (ed.), *Death education for the health professional*. Washington: Hemisphere.

Templer, D. (1970). The construction and validation of a death anxiety scale. *Journal of General Psychology, 82*, 165–177.

Viney, L.L. (1985). The bereavement process: a new approach. *Bereavement Care, 4*, 27 & 32.

Volkan, V.D. (1983). Complicated mourning and the syndrome of established pathological mourning. In S. Akhtar (ed.), *New psychiatric syndromes*. New York: Jason Aronson.

Warr, P. (1978). A study of psychological well-being. *British Journal of Psychology, 69*, 111–121.

Warr, P. (1982). Psychological aspects of employment and unemployment. *Psychological Medicine, 12*, 7–11.

Weiner, A., Gerber, I., Battin, D., & Arkin, A.M. (1975). The process and phenomenology of bereavement. In E. Schoenberg *et al.* (eds), *Bereavement: its psychosocial aspects*. New York: Columbia University Press.

Woodfield, R., & Viney, L.L. (1985). A personal construct approach to bereavement. *Omega, 16*, 1–13.
Worden, J.W. (1982). *Grief counselling and grief therapy*. London: Tavistock.

KEY WORDS

Definitions of bereavement, grief, mourning, psychoanalytic, attachment, psychosocial, task oriented, medical, stress, life events, cognitive, personal construct, death anxiety, stage models, normal/abnormal grief, outcome, mortality, physical, psychosomatic, psychiatric disorders, intervention, counselling, therapeutic approaches, risk factors.

5

Impending Surgery

MARIE JOHNSTON
Royal Free Hospital School of Medicine, London

INTRODUCTION

Surgery is a threatening event with many unpredictable and uncontrollable features. It is likely to tax the resources of most people and can therefore be seen as a stressful event. In the Schedule of Recent Experiences (Holmes and Rahe, 1967), 'major personal injury or illness' and 'major change in health of family' were seen to require considerable adjustment, warranting 53 and 44 life change units, compared with 50 for marriage. Surgery involves not just a significant illness, but also a significant treatment procedure.

Unlike most other traumatic events, surgery can usually be anticipated, as by far the majority of operations are planned or, elective, rather than emergency procedures. As a result, it offers an attractive natural stress paradigm within which models developed in laboratory work with humans and animals can be tested.

This chapter examines the features of the surgical experience which are stressful, before examining the response of patients at emotional, cognitive, and physiological levels. Factors which moderate the stressfulness of the experience have been conceptualized as features of the surgical situation, the clinical parameters, the predictability and the controllability of events or of the surgical patients, their demographic characteristics, their coping styles and strategies, and the social support available to them. The final two sections of the chapter briefly consider two areas that have been widely reviewed elsewhere: the implications of preoperative stress for the clinical outcomes of care (reviewed by Johnston, 1986), and the effects of psychological preparation for surgery in reducing stress and promoting recovery (reviewed by Mathews and Ridgeway, 1984, and Weinman and Johnston, in press).

WHAT IS STRESSFUL ABOUT SURGERY?

There are obvious potential threats for the surgical patient: anaesthesia, pain, physical restriction, life-threatening procedures, being away from home, meeting new people. Murphy *et al.* (1977) have suggested that sleep deprivation may be a significant stressor, and showed that patients on surgical wards get substantially less sleep than at home, principally due to early awakening.

Volicer and Bohannon (1975) have developed a scale, the Hospital Stress Rating Scale (HSRS), which ranks 49 events related to the experience of hospitalization. 'Knowing you have to have an operation' ranked 18th most stressful. Among the more stressful items were several which might be experienced by surgical patients including: being hospitalized far away from home (17); not having your questions answered by the staff (13); missing your spouse (12); not getting relief from pain medications (10); not being told what your diagnosis is (6); knowing you have a serious illness (4); thinking you might lose your sight (1).

Subsequent factor analysis identified nine factors, five of which showed differences between surgical and medical patients. Surgical patients showed more evidence of stress on unfamiliarity of surroundings, loss of independence, threat of severe illness, and medical patients showed more stress on financial problems, and lack of information.

These differences remained when age and seriousness of illness were allowed for. Overall, surgical patients reported higher levels of stress (Volicer *et al.*, 1977). This evidence confirms that there are features of the situation which are identified as potentially stressful.

EVIDENCE OF STRESS IN SURGICAL PATIENTS

Emotional

A number of scales have been developed which measure patients' anxiety about various aspects of hospitalization (e.g. Lucente and Fleck. 1972; Wilson-Barnett, 1976). In the latter study, 'anticipating a treatment or procedure which is likely to be painful' elicited a negative response (indicating apprehension, discomfort or embarrassment) in 109 out of 200 patients.

Numerous studies have shown elevated anxiety scores and stress ratings for presurgical patients. For example, on the State scale of the STAI (The State–Trait–Anxiety–Inventory) (Spielberger *et al.*, 1970), a twenty-item scale with scores ranging from 20 to 80, designed to measure transitory changes in anxiety, the typical patient scores in the low 40s on the day before surgery, whereas normal scores, when there are no identified threats, are in the low 30s (Johnston, 1980; Knight *et al.* 1983).

However, the scores after surgery continue to be high (Chapman and Cox. 1977; Johnston, 1980) and are higher than before surgery for some groups of patients. Previous results suggesting that anxiety was high before but not after surgery (Spielberger *et al.* 1973; Auerbach, 1973) are misleading, as the postoperative measures were not taken until each patient was 'relatively free from postoperative discomfort' and had been told that they were 'recovering from surgery without complications'. When the full course of anxiety over the total period is assessed, high levels of anxiety are seen both before and after surgery (Figure 5.1).

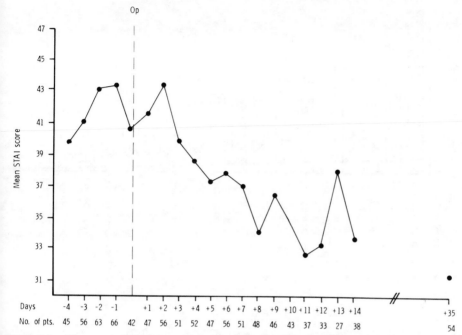

FIG. 5.1   Changes in STAI state anxiety levels over the course of surgery (from Johnston, 1980; reproduced by permission of the British Medical Association).

Compared with anxiety 5 weeks after surgery, scores are high on all 4 days before surgery, well before admission to hospital. There are no data to indicate how early the anticipatory anxiety begins.

Cognitive

Several studies have examined surgical patients' worries (Lucente and Fleck, 1972; DeWolfe *et al.*, 1966; Johnston, 1976, 1982a, 1987). The earlier studies observed significant worries that were not directly related to the procedures associated with surgery. Johnston (1987) found that patients' main worries were about the success of the operation and the subsequent return to normal, followed by concerns about home and family. Preoperative patients responded to a checklist of thoughts, identifying those which had worried them in the previous 24 hours, and selected their three main worries. The number of patients including each worry as a main worry is indicated in Figure 5.2. Concern about the lead up to the operation and about the operation itself was less frequently selected than worries about the outcome of the operation.

Weinman and Johnston (in press) have argued that the focus of research on patients' concerns about surgical procedures has distracted researchers from the study of potentially greater concerns about the *outcome* of the procedure. It is also of note that the patients worry significantly about normal everyday matters, perhaps exacerbated by hospitalization and the impending surgery, and that their worrying is not restricted to aspects of their illness and treatment.

As in the study of depression, the cognitive elements of surgical patients' stress

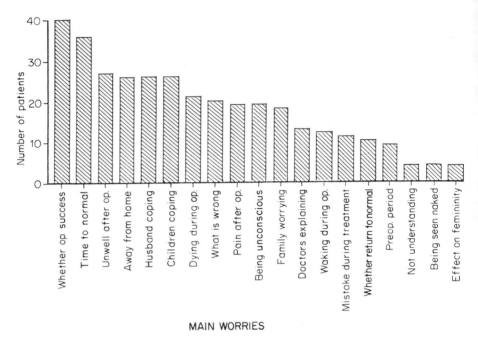

MAIN WORRIES

FIG. 5.2 Surgical patients' main worries (from Johnston, 1987).

response may be critical in indicating the most promising interventions to alleviate distress. Many approaches focus on giving information about surgical procedures, which, in terms of subjective reports obtained, are less important than those concerned with the outcome of the operation and with home and family worries. This might explain both the variable success of information interventions and the greater success of techniques that teach the patient strategies applicable to any worry that arises (e.g. the cognitive device taught by Langer *et al.*, 1975). Weinman and Johnston (in press), reviewing well-controlled intervention studies, noted that information interventions had reduced anxiety in only one out of nine studies, whereas cognitive approaches had been successful in the two studies in which they had been tried (see Table 5.1).

Physiological

It is particularly important to separate psychologically and physically induced physiological stress responses when mechanisms are being postulated and when interventions aimed at alleviating some of the undesirable consequences are being planned. Current evidence is severely limited by the lack of studies which combine sufficiently sophisticated models of stress (including the possibility of both physical and psychological stressors) and sufficiently sophisticated measurement techniques in both psychological and physiological domains. To date, very little work has been designed to investigate both psychological and physiological aspects equally.

The two commonly identified physiological stress axes, the sympathetic/

adrenomedullary and the pituitary/adrenocortical (Henry and Stephens, 1977; Feuerstein *et al.*, 1986), reveal rather different stress profiles in surgical patients. The most thorough research has been carried out on indices of *sympathetic–adrenomedullary* activity, both because they are readily measurable in surgical patients without complex, cumbersome and invasive techniques, and because this highly responsive physiological axis has been widely used in well-controlled laboratory studies of psychological stress.

Early work by Harrison *et al.* (1962) on the sympathetic–adrenomedullary axis, found a reduction in palmar sweating prior to surgery followed by recovery to normal levels postoperatively. Comparison with medical patient controls and careful monitoring of the sequence of events demonstrated that these results were not due to changes associated with hospitalization, altered diet or the administration of drugs. The patients' psychological states were not assessed, but the authors assumed that the palmar sweating changes were due to subjective stress.

Subsequent studies (Johnston, 1975; Johnson *et al.*, 1970; Vogele and Steptoe, 1986) have found the same pattern of palmar sweating over time in surgical patients as did Harrison *et al.* Figure 5.3 shows two of these data sets superimposed, and demonstrates the reliability of the finding that palmar sweating decreases prior to surgery and gradually returns to normal levels after surgery.

These later studies also measured psychological indices of stress. Using the STAI as a measure of psychological response, Johnston (1975) found no relationship between changes in palmar sweating and anxiety within individuals, although there tended to be a negative relationship between the two variables over days. Johnson *et al.* (1970) used a mood adjective checklist and found differences between subjects in palmar sweating related to self-reported fear and negative moods on the first day after surgery but to positive moods on the second day. Figure 5.4 illustrates the pattern of palmar sweating and self-reported moods over successive days. Palmar sweating does not correlate with the pattern of 'fear' ($r = 0.06$), but is more closely associated with 'arousal' ($r = 0.58$), and negatively associated with 'lethargy' ($r = -0.58$), replicating an earlier finding by the same group.

Taking these findings as a whole, a clear picture begins to emerge. Palmar sweating is not related to self-reported anxiety or fear in surgical patients, but is related to subjective feelings of energy and activity. The tendency for a negative correlation of anxiety and palmar sweating over time is probably spurious and may arise because both anxiety and energy levels relate to the time dimension, but by different mechanisms. It seems likely that changes in anxiety over time are due to changing patterns of threat, whereas changes in energy and palmar sweating over days are due to changes in activity levels associated initially with being confined to bed and subsequently with postoperative recovery.

Thus the palmar sweating pattern of surgical patients is related to the *effort* rather than distress aspect of stress (Frankenhauser, 1983). A similar interpretation of increases in sympathetic output postoperatively has been proposed by Wilson (1981). He found increases in postoperative excretion of epinephrine (adrenaline) in patients given relaxation training compared with controls; he suggests that the experimental group's increased sympathetic output may be due

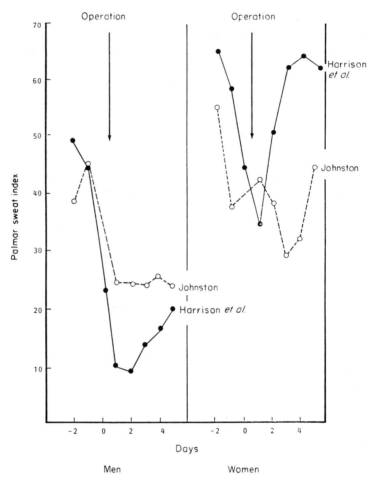

FIG. 5.3   Changes in palmar sweating over the course of surgery (adapted from Harrison *et al.*, 1962; and Johnston, 1975).

to an 'increased sense of energy and activity'. Others have related similar results of relaxation training to a hypothesized decrease in the sensitivity of adrenergic receptors following relaxation (Hoffman *et al.*, 1982).

Indices of cardiovascular activity may be even more difficult to interpret. Fleischman *et al.* (1976) showed reductions in platelet aggregation time and increases in blood pressure between admission and surgery. However, Goldstein *et al.* (1982) suggested that the cardiovascular responses to the stress of surgery are very complexly determined and may not be mediated by sympathetic influences. They found preoperative increases in heart rate, systolic blood pressure and cardiac output, but these persisted when noradrenaline (norepinephrine) responses were eliminated by diazepam sedation.

Turning to the second physiological stress axis, measures of *pituitary/ adrenocortical* activity show in increase with surgery (e.g. Murray, 1967; Bridges and Jones, 1966; Czeisler *et al.*, 1976; Cohen *et al.*, 1982). While this is readily

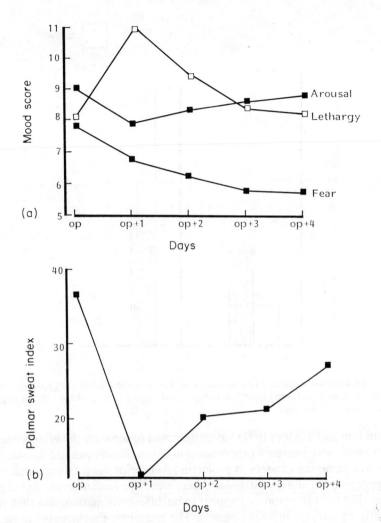

FIG. 5.4   Changes in (a) mood and (b) palmar sweating over the course of surgery (adapted from Johnson *et al.*, 1970. © 1970 American Journal of Nursing Company. Reprinted with permission from *Nursing Research*, Jan/Feb 1970, Vol. 19, No. 1.).

interpreted as a 'stress' response, it has been more difficult to separate the effects of psychological and physical stressors, as psychological states, if considered at all, have typically been inferred rather than measured.

Czeisler *et al.* (1976) have explored the time course of the cortisol response by means of frequent blood samples obtained using an indwelling catheter, and find no evidence of *chronic* activation of the pituitary/adrenocortical axis in preoperative patients. Instead, in the four patients studied, they found raised levels between 9 p.m. and 11 p.m. on the evening before surgery, the time when preoperative preparations such as shaving and enema were scheduled. As the authors point out, it is not clear whether the critical stimulus is the physical manipulation or the psychological implications of these procedures.

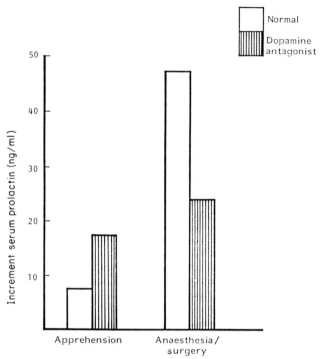

FIG. 5.5   Prolactin release due to apprehension and anaesthesia/surgery with and without dopamine antagonist (adapted from Corenblum and Taylor, 1981). Reproduced by permission of *Fertility and Sterility*.

Corenblum and Taylor (1981) have attempted to separate the effects due to the stress of anticipating surgery (apprehension) from the stresses of anaesthesia and surgery by examining changes in prolactin levels prior to and during procedures. Both apprehension and anaesthesia/surgery were shown to increase serum prolactin levels, but the two responses appear to be differently mediated as they reacted differently to various blocking agents. For example, the increase in prolactin preoperatively was enhanced by a dopamine antagonist, whereas the anaesthesia/surgery increase was diminished (see Fig. 5.5). The authors concluded that the preoperative apprehension effect is due to release of a prolactin-releasing factor, and the anaesthesia/surgery effect to inhibition of a prolactin-inhibiting factor. While the role of prolactin release is unclear and the complexity of neuroendocrine factors make such results difficult to interpret fully, the implication that psychologically and physically induced effects can have a similar result (increased serum prolactin) via different mechanisms is important.

Further information on the relationship between changes in the patient's psychological state and adrenocortical activity is presented by Boore (1978), who found that patients given psychological preparation for surgery had lower rates of secretion of urinary corticosteroids postoperatively than a control group. There is clearly enough evidence to suggest that the psychological threat of surgery may influence pituitary/adrenocortical activity independently of the physical threats, but the mechanisms are still open to speculation.

Other studies examine other physiological pathways, e.g. suppression of immune functioning (Linn and Jenson, 1983; Slade *et al.*, 1975), or increases in serum lipids (Sane and Kukreti, 1978; Sane *et al.*, 1981), but do not report on psychological states. The results presented here are only a small sample of the many studies which present data only on physiological changes associated with stress in surgical patients. As the above studies illustrate, it is difficult to separate the psychological effects of the threatening features of surgery from the direct physical effects unless one can obtain frequent measures of the physiological parameter, as with palmar sweating. Apart from the anaesthesia and surgery itself, changes may be caused by alterations in diet and by medications, especially starvation before surgery and premedication or sedation on the night prior to surgery. While these problems have at least been partly dealt with in the studies of the sympathetic/adrenomedullary axis, studies of other pathways are still at a very early stage and cannot support any firm conclusions.

MODERATORS OF SURGICAL STRESS

Demographic and Clinical

While women appear to be more distressed about the prospect of surgery and hospitalization than men (Lucente and Fleck, 1972; Wilson-Barnett, 1976), this may simply reflect their generally higher trait and state levels of anxiety (Knight *et al.*, 1983). Evidence of a sex difference in the pattern of change in anxiety over time in orthopaedic patients (Johnston, 1980) may be confounded with the different types of injury or disorder and resulting variations in their operations. Similarly, it is difficult to interpret age differences (e.g. showing reduced anxiety with age; Lucente and Fleck, 1972) as they may relate both to anxiety and surgical procedure differences.

One might expect simple differences between major and minor operations, but even this is not consistently found. For example, Johnston (1987) found no difference in STAI scores of women awaiting major and minor gynaecological procedures, and B.A. Johnson *et al*, (1970) found no difference in the anxiety on admission of patients having major and minor vaginal surgery. In terms of the anticipated physical trauma, these results make very little sense, but consideration of the psychological event offers a possible explanation. Typically, minor gynaecological procedures are diagnostic or investigative, or as in in-vitro fertilization, associated with uncertain procedures (Johnston *et al.*, 1987). Major procedures such as hysterectomy are typically therapeutic, following full assessment, and with relatively little ambiguity about the course of events. Thus the psychological threat may balance the anticipated physical threat, resulting in similar anxiety levels for those having major and minor surgery.

Lucente and Fleck (1972) found gynaecological and orthopaedic patients to be more anxious than general surgical patients, and cancer patients to be more anxious than those with other conditions. In each case, the more anxious patients are facing procedures which carry threats beyond the immediate threat of surgery.

The best predictors of the stressfulness of surgery are likely to be those which take account of the patients' appraisal of the event rather than simply the physical trauma.

Predictability and Control

An important theory in the field has been that accurate expectations reduce the stress of surgery, especially postoperatively (Johnson and Leventhal, 1974). Studies using this approach have involved giving patients additional information about procedures and expected sensations, and have had some success in reducing pain, analgesic use and length of hospital stay (Hayward, 1975; Johnson et al., 1978a, 1978b; Wallace, 1984)—and some failures. For example, Staite (1978) and Visser (1982) found no benefits in their informed patients compared with controls. Staite's experimental group showed increased accuracy in their expectations without the accompanying reductions in stress levels either pre- or postoperatively.

Others predict that such information, while having the potential to reduce postoperative stress, is likely to increase preoperative anxiety. Janis (1958) proposed that preoperative information would *increase* the preoperative anxiety of the non-anxious patients and thus alert them to engage in the 'work of worrying' which he predicted would be beneficial in terms of reducing postoperative distress and hostility levels. However, controlled studies of information giving have not resulted in increases in preoperative anxiety (Vernon and Bigelow, 1974); on the contrary, Wallace (1984) found *reduced* anxiety levels in the experimental group.

Johnston (1981) found that the accuracy of the patients' expectations about pain was not a predictor of the postoperative anxiety experienced, as Johnson and Leventhal (see above) hypothesized, but that an expectation in excess of the level of pain actually experienced was associated with lower anxiety. It is unlikely that predictability per se is the critical variable as patients cope well when pain turns out to be less than expected. On the other hand, predictability may reduce stress when it increases the likelihood of control.

Patients may attempt to control emotions or the environment (Leventhal, 1970; Johnson et al., 1971). Most events on the surgical ward are controlled by ward staff or by hospital organizational policies and very little is left in the control of patients. Even when they appear to be able to choose their meal from a menu, they frequently find that they have chosen for the patient who will occupy the bed tomorrow and that they will have been moved to another position where another patient has chosen the meal. Johnson et al., chose to assess the patients' success in influencing management decisions regarding analgesic administration and discharge from hospital. Greater analgesic use and longer hospital stay were taken as indications of greater environmental control. In other studies (see Weinman and Johnston, in press), these same two indices have been used as indices of failure, showing poor recovery by the patients with high scores.

Interventions with surgical patients have attempted to increase control over both emotions and the dangers in the situation and have shown improved coping with emotions and with recovery in the postoperative period. Mathews and

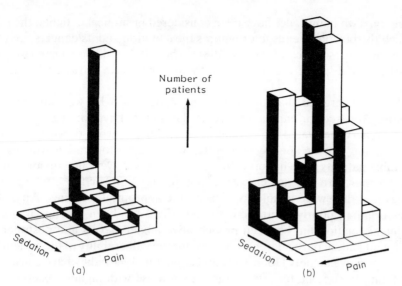

FIG. 5.6   Pain and sedation levels in postoperative patients (a) with and (b) without control over anasthesia (adapted from Atwell *et al.*, 1984). Reproduced by permission of *Journal of Urology*.

Ridgeway (1984) concluded that the evidence from adequately controlled studies shows cognitive coping approaches to be superior, and speculate that this is due to promoting the patients' sense of control.

However, it may be possible to minimize the emotional response without achieving reductions in length of hospital stay, and vice versa (Johnson, 1984; Johnston, 1984). Weinman and Johnston (in press) have argued that interventions may have specific effects, and that different interventions may give control of different outcomes.

Thus two problems arise in studies of control in surgical patients. On the one hand, it may be unproductive to think of patients gaining control of the dangers or of the ward environment. On the other, a general non-specific increase in control or perceived control may not be predictive of reduced stress as indicated by improved mood or successful recovery. Instead, patients may gain control or be able to cope with particular aspects of the situation and therefore show quite specific benefits.

An illustration of this more specific approach is given by Atwell *et al.* (1984) who compared postoperative patients given standard analgesia with patients who controlled their own anaesthetic administration by triggering a modified infusion pump. The latter group showed less pain, lighter sedation and greater activity as rated by observers than did those on the standard regimen (Fig. 5.6). The authors did not investigate other outcomes, but, for example, reduced pain and sedation levels might, by enabling faster mobilization, facilitate faster recovery.

Coping Styles and Strategies

It has been suggested that the individual's coping style may alter the stressfulness of surgery. Two main styles have been considered in surgical patients: the extent to which the person attends to or ignores the situation and its dangers, and their perception of personal control (Ray, 1981). These styles will be referred to here as 'sensitizing' and 'perceived control', although they have attracted a variety of labels.

It has been argued that the sensitizing patient will be well informed and therefore prepared for unpleasant events. Janis (1959) hypothesized that preoperative anxiety motivated the patient to carry out the 'work of worrying' which would enable him or her to cope better with the postoperative stresses. The vulnerable patients were hypothesized to be those who were not anxious enough and who therefore did not engage in this preparation, or those who were so anxious that they were unable to focus on the appropriate worries. Apart from Janis's original, poorly controlled, studies, there has been no support for this curvilinear relationship between preoperative anxiety levels and postoperative adjustment and, in particular, no evidence for the vulnerability of the patient with low preoperative anxiety (Johnston and Carpenter, 1980); they have consistently been found to cope better after surgery than those with higher anxiety.

It is still possible that the cognitive rather than emotional aspects of the hypothesis are valid, i.e. that the sensitizing strategy, thinking about the operation and the postoperative situation, whether or not motivated by anxiety, is helpful. Sensitizing has been investigated as vigilance, information seeking and denial. Cohen and Lazarus (1973) found that patients who adopted a 'vigilant' coping disposition fared worse postoperatively (longer length of stay and more minor complications) than patients using an 'avoidant' strategy. Similarly, Wilson (1981) found patients scoring high on 'denial' made better postoperative progress in terms of length of stay and medications for pain. Sime's (1976) 'information seekers' did not show any benefits or harmful effects. It would appear that those who actively think about the situation do not benefit and, in two of these studies showed worse outcomes than those who avoid thinking about it. Thus there is no support for the notion that being sensitized to the threats is helpful.

It is of interest that these above coping strategies relate to length of stay, complications and pain outcomes and not to the patients' emotional state. One possible explanation is that the avoidant or denying patient continues to suffer as much as the sensitizers but fails to communicate this suffering to ward staff, and as a result receives less medical and nursing attention and is more readily perceived as ready for discharge.

The measures discussed so far index coping strategies specifically in the surgical situation; it is also possible to examine a more general coping style as measured by scales such as repression–sensitization (R–S) and its variants. Cohen and Lazarus (1973) found R–S unrelated to any index of postoperative adjustment.

Sensitizing coping styles may interact with psychological interventions with surgical patients. For example, Andrew (1970) found that avoiders required more postoperative medication when given preoperative information; sensitizers were unchanged; and neutrals showed faster recovery and required fewer medications. It would appear that the coping of the repressor or avoider can be disrupted by information giving; Shipley *et al.* (1978), in work with endoscopy rather than surgical patients, also found that repressors could be disrupted by information. Using a different form of preoperative teaching involving instruction by nurses, Kinney (1977) found little difference between patients with different coping styles apart from a suggestion of immediate heart rate increases in sensitizers but not in repressors.

Mathews and Ridgeway (1981) have concluded that the evidence of positive correlations between measures of sensitizing and measures of neuroticism or trait anxiety indicates that they are measuring the same dimension, and that sensitizing might be reinterpreted as high neuroticism. It is well demonstrated that pre-operative anxiety is predictive of postoperative distress, and this relationship may be due to the persistent mediation of trait anxiety (Johnston, 1981). Preoperative anxiety is also related to postoperative pain and may be related to poorer re-covery, although results are not consistent over studies (Johnston, 1986). It is plausible that trait anxiety reflects a coping style, and recent results suggest that trait-anxious surgical patients worry in a different manner from the less anxious: Johnston (1987) found that high trait anxiety was associated with *number* of worries rather than the *duration* of time spent thinking about having surgery. In a laboratory study of anxious psychiatric patients by Macleod *et al.* (1986), patients were found to attend more to threatening cues. Sensitizers and high trait-anxious individuals may share a coping style which results in additional attention being paid to the dangers of the hospital and surgical situation.

Attention to the threatening cues may prove unhelpful if there is nothing that the surgical patient can do to protect him or herself from the perceived dangers. If one examines the worries that are most commonly experienced by these patients, it can be seen that few are within the patient's current control; the outcome of the operation and the course of recovery are unpredictable and it is even more difficult than usual to control events at home. Some patients will perceive greater control than others, but perceived control has largely been studied as an enduring style of the patient rather than as a strategy or specific belief in this situation.

Early work by Johnson *et al.* (1971) proposed that locus of control would predict patients' attempts to control the dangers and that this would be inde-pendent of emotional control in their parallel processing model. They found that the internal–external control dimension was indeed related to the patient's ability to influence care; internals received more needed analgesics than externals. Levesque and Charlebois (1977) did not replicate this finding, and showed no differences between internals and externals. There is some suggestion that inter-nals may benefit more from information (Auerbach *et al.*, 1976; Pickett and Clum, 1982), but this has not been found in other studies (e.g. Wallace, 1983). As in other areas where locus of control or some other construct of perceived control is used, a clear pattern of results is unlikely to emerge until more situation-specific measures are developed. Given the confusion in studies of surgical patients about what can be controlled (see section on controllability and coping) and what constitutes successful control, is it hardly surprising that trait measures of locus of control are producing inconsistent results.

Social Support

Social support is frequently cited as a moderator of the effects of stress, and while this may be true for surgical patients, it has not yet been clearly demonstrated. Patients are very positive about the social support they receive (Wilson-Barnett, 1976); of sixteen items eliciting predominantly positive responses in hospital patients, eight referred to some kind of social support from other patients, relatives, the junior doctor, the consultant, sister, visitors, student nurses and the staff nurse, in ascending order, with talking to the staff nurse second only to early-morning tea. Surgical patients perceive different kinds of support coming from different individuals (Ray and Fitzgibbon, 1979). 'Information' and 'reassurance' were sought primarily from the surgeon and the nurse, 'direction' from spouse and nurse, 'distraction' and 'ego-enchancement' from spouse and fellow patients. Using a different questioning approach, Richards and McDonald (1985) found the house surgeon to be the most important source of information and the one to whom patients directed most of their questions.

While nurses and surgeons are likely to be well informed about hospital and surgical procedures, they are unlikely to be well informed about patients' concerns (Lucente and Fleck, 1972; Johnston, 1976, 1982b; Richards and McDonald, 1985). It would appear that nurses tend to underestimate patients' pain (Johnston, 1976; Cohen, 1980) and overestimate the number of worries which patients have, and while they achieve some accuracy in identifying the most common worries, they are poor at assessing an individual patient's worries, being less accurate than other patients (Johnston, 1982b), although Ray and Fitzgibbon's (1979) study suggests the latter are not a potent source of reassurance. It is clear that patients who arrive on the surgical ward concerned about the common worries are likely to receive optimal reassurance as they will not only find others who share their concerns, but their worries are the ones that the nurses are most likely to deal with.

Even where the doctors are agreed to be an important source of information, their perception of patients' needs may render them ineffective. Richards and McDonald (1985) found that the house surgeons underestimated patients' knowledge, and that the four subjects they claimed to avoid included two major causes of concern, to the patients: 'postoperative pain and discomfort', and 'risks of surgery'. The other two subjects were 'outcome without surgery' and 'alternatives to surgery'.

Most interventions to alleviate the stress of surgery involve some social interaction, and this may contribute to the effectiveness of the procedures, although this has not been specifically evaluated. It is clear that their effects go beyond simple social support, as benefits are obtained using booklets (Wallace, 1984) with a relatively limited social input and also in studies where appropriate control groups have been used (see Mathews and Ridgeway, 1984).

IMPLICATIONS OF PREOPERATIVE STRESS

While the emotional, cognitive and physiological experiences of the preoperative patient may be unpleasant in themselves, much of the research has focussed on the implications of these experiences for the outcomes of the patient's clinical care. There is now a considerable body of evidence showing that patients who are most anxious before surgery are likely to fare worse on a variety of indices in the postoperative period than the less anxious patients (see review by Johnston, 1986). In addition, they may require more anaesthesia for adequate sedation, and anaesthetists tend to take account of the patient's anxiety level in calculating required amounts; Williams *et al.* (1975) have suggested that this may make the preoperatively anxious patient more vulnerable to the risks of anaesthesia, including that of death. As suggested earlier, this group of patients is likely to meet nurses and other patients who have less understanding of their concerns. They may even derive less benefit from preoperative psychological interventions than the less anxious patient (Wilson, 1981; Wallace, 1983).

One possibility is that these are the people who fare worst in all of life's situations and that there is nothing special about surgery. However, in the surgical situation, their anxiety may be associated with physiological changes which may make them more vulnerable to physical problems. Mathews and Ridgeway (1981) concluded that patients scoring high on neuroticism scales were likely to have slower postoperative recovery.

Models of Stress and Surgery

Three quite different types of hypothesis have already been alluded to which might explain a link between preoperative anxiety and postoperative recovery: cognitive–behavioural, psychophysiological, and communication hypotheses.

The *cognitive–behavioural* hypotheses suggests that the way in which the patient thinks about the operation or the care received might alter what he or she does and thereby affect their recovery. For example, believing that there is personal responsibility for postoperative mobilization might promote earlier ambulation and thus faster recovery. Many forms of this hypothesis have been proposed, as indicated earlier, including Janis's emotional drive hypothesis which asserts that the emotional state motivates the adaptive cognitive preparation. An alternative, simpler notion relies more parsimoniously on amount of cognitive preparation preoperatively as the predictor of postoperative adaption. As the evidence stands, it is possible that a particular style rather than quantity of thinking about the operation may facilitate optimal behaviours and that the non-anxious patient is more likely to adopt this style. Wilson's (1981) finding that patients trained in relaxation techniques had raised epinephrine (adrenaline) levels and faster recovery patterns was interpreted as due to greater activity levels in the more relaxed patients, who had an increased sense of their own energy and control. This greater activity may have been the critical component in achieving faster recovery. However, these speculations are largely untested.

Similarly, there are *psychophysiological* hypotheses. Increased physiological arousal in the anxious patients may result in increased doses of anaesthetics or analgesics (Williams *et al.*, 1975) which limit patients' postoperative alertness and therefore recovery; or the increased cortisol secretion may suppress immune function and leave the anxious patient more susceptible to infection (Bradley, 1982); or increased cortisol secretion may be associated with increased postoperative morphine requirements (Cohen *et al.*, 1982) and therefore to slower postoperative progress; or increased platelet aggregation time (Fleischman *et al.*, 1976) may lead to postoperative deep vein thrombosis (DVT), resulting in increased duration of bed rest and slower recovery. All of these hypotheses are plausible, but unproven and largely untested.

Two forms of *communication* hypothesis are possible. The first suggests that the anxious patient's behaviour communicates a different level of recovery to the nurses and doctors who decide on medication and discharge; since these parameters are usually taken as indices of recovery, the patient's measured progress will appear retarded if he or she describes or acts as if in greater pain, and the anxious patient may therefore be seen to be making a slower recovery. Alternatively, anxious patients may get less reassurance on the surgical ward because the nurses are unaware of, and most other patients do not share their concerns (Johnston, 1982b). It is noteworthy (see above) that these patients do not benefit as much from preoperative communications, perhaps because their concerns are not addressed or because they find it difficult to attend to the messages. Again, these hypotheses are largely untested.

Clearly the three types of hypothesis have very different implications, especially for the care of surgical patients and for the type of intervention which might be beneficial.

PSYCHOLOGICAL PREPARATION FOR SURGERY

Since Egbert *et al.*'s (1964) original work on preparing patients for surgery, there have been many investigations of numerous techniques of potential benefit to patients. The researchers have been primarily psychologists and nurses, with the psychologists focusing on theoretical issues and the mechanisms of stress reduction, and the nurses on the more practical issues of improving patient care (Wilson-Barnett, 1984). The studies vary in the extent to which they use adequate research designs with appropriate, randomly allocated control groups and sufficient numbers of patients, in the type of intervention being used, and in the type of outcome studied. Nevertheless, Mathews and Ridgeway (1984) found 22 studies which allowed them to consider which interventions had been shown to be most effective, and Mumford *et al.* (1982) concluded that, on the basis of meta-analysis, there was evidence for the effectiveness of such interventions.

Interventions have included the giving of procedural or sensation information, instructions, group discussions, psychotherapy, relaxation instruction, teaching of cognitive coping techniques, and stress inoculation. The outcomes have been diverse, and have included effects on mood (mainly anxiety and depression), pain, medications (mainly analgesics and sedatives), behaviour on the ward, length of hospital stay, patient complaints, return to normal activities and to work, and various clinical (e.g. postoperative vomiting, complications) and physiological indices (e.g. heart rate, catecholamine excretion).

There has been a primary focus on the inputs, psychological techniques developed in other spheres being adapted and applied to the surgical patients. In this context, it is worth noting that the cognitive methods which are currently proving successful are direct translations of techniques used for patients with other types of stress or anxiety complaint. There has been rather poor conceptualization of the output, perhaps with the unstated assumption that all outputs were tapping the same dimension. However, this is clearly not the case. Measures of outcome are frequently poorly correlated, and different studies produce benefits on different outcome variables. Both pain and analgesic use are taken as measures of recovery, whereas, on the basis of other information about these factors, one might expect them to be negatively correlated. The lack of definition of recovery has inhibited the development of measures with construct validity, and when a full analysis, with appropriate conceptual and statistical basis, is performed, there is evidence of more than one dimension accounting for the hotch-potch of measures of convenience (Johnston, 1984).

As Wilson-Barnett (1984) notes, even when success has been demonstrated, the procedures have not been incorporated as part of normal clinical practice. One can understand the reticence about introducing a technique which would require an additional member of staff, as would appear to be implied by the psychologists' studies. On the other hand, the nursing studies have not been adopted by their own profession as a part of nursing routine. Again the fault may lie in the lack of attention to the output and the general impression that any benefit is equally valuable.

The concentration on inputs has resulted in very little information being available on the specificity of the techniques. Thus one now has evidence that techniques are effective without knowing what they affect. Weinman and Johnston (in press) reconsidered the twenty-two well-controlled investigations reviewed by Mathews and Ridgeway (1984) to give a cross-tabulation of the inputs and outputs (Table 5.1). The table presents the number of times a particular outcome has been assessed for a particular type of intervention and the number of times it has been effective, i.e. better than a placebo or other treatment; starred cells indicate inputs which have been effective on at least 50% of the occasions on which they have been tested.

Clearly, even treatments which have been effective have not been equally so for all outcomes, and all outcomes which have been achieved have not been achieved equally readily with any input. Of particular note is the surprising failure rate on 'mood' and 'pain', success being achieved for mood on only 6 out of 21 studies and then mainly when emotion-focused or cognitive interventions were used, and for pain on 5 out of 15, mainly when relaxation and cognitive approaches were adopted. By contrast, psychological interventions are quite likely to be effective in reducing drug intake and length of hospital stay, and most approaches that have been tried have been beneficial. This analysis suggests that mood and pain are altered by specific inputs but that the clinical indices may be influenced by a variety of interventions, the shared effect perhaps being mediated by a final common pathway of how ward staff perceive the patient to be progressing.

It is suggested that targeting outcomes as well as tailoring inputs may serve to make interventions more effective, but may also lead to their wider adoption. A

Table 5.1 Psychological interventions and their effects on different outcome measures

Intervention	Effect							
						Recovery		
	No. of studies	Drugs	Mood	Length of stay	Pain	Behaviour	Physical	Rating
Information (I)	6	2* / 3	0 / 3	1* / 2	0 / 1	0 / 2	–	0 / 1
Behavioural instructions (BI)	1	1* / 1	1* / 1	0 / 1	–	–	–	1* / 1
Combination of I & BI	8	3* / 6	1 / 6	3* / 4	1 / 6	1 / 5	1 / 5	1 / 3
Emotion focused	5	2* / 3	2* / 4	2* / 4	–	1* / 1	2* / 4	0 / 1
Relaxation	5	2* / 4	0 / 3	1* / 2	2* / 4	1* / 1	2* / 2	0 / 2
Sensation information	2	1* / 2	0 / 2	1* / 2	0 / 2	0 / 2	–	–
Cognitive	3	2* / 3	2* / 2	0 / 1	2* / 2	0 / 1	0 / 1	1* / 2
Total	22	13* / 22	6 / 21	8* / 16	5 / 15	3 / 12	5* / 10	3 / 10

Each cell indicates total number of studies (bottom right), total with significant effect of the intervention (top left), and * where at least half of the interventions had a significant effect

closer collaboration between the investigations of mechanism and of alleviation of stress could contribute to the development of each, as the mechanism analysis suggests new, and potentially more effective, interventions with specific targets and the interventions offer the best test of hypothesized mechanisms.

SUMMARY AND CONCLUSIONS

Evidence that surgical patients experience stress exists at emotional, cognitive and physiological levels. The emotional and cognitive data have been limited by prior assumptions about when and what the patients worry about. The failure to include subjective measures in studies with physiological indices has resulted in difficulty in separating changes due to the perceived stress and to the physical traumas.

It is not clear that any demographic, clinical or coping variables are reliably related to the stress experienced, although they may moderate the effectiveness of therapeutic interventions. Similarly, the importance of perceived control and social support has not been elaborated.

Preoperative stress does predict some important outcomes, and many successful psychological interventions have shown that benefits can be obtained. The links between the interventions and the specific benefits has hardly been addressed, and to do so may provide insights into stress mechanisms as well as immediate alleviation of patients' distress.

REFERENCES

Atwell, J.R., Flanigan, R.C., Bennett, R.L., Allen, D.C., Lucas, B.A., & McRoberts, J.W. (1984). The efficacy of patient-controlled analgesia in patients recovering from flank incisions. *Journal of Urology, 132,* 701–703.

Andrew, J.M. (1970). Recovery from surgery with and without preparatory instruction for three coping styles. *Journal of Personality and Social Psychology, 15,* 233–226.

Auerbach, S.M. (1973). Trait–state anxiety and adjustment to surgery. *Journal of Consulting and Clinical Psychology, 34,* 264–271.

Auerbach, S.M., Kendall, P.C., Cuttler, H.F., & Levitt, N.R. (1976). Anxiety, locus of control, type of preparatory information, and adjustment to dental surgery. *Journal of Consulting and Clinical Psychology, 44,* 809–818.

Boore, J.R.P. (1978). *Prescription for recovery.* London: Royal College of Nursing.

Bradley, C. (1982). The contribution of psychological factors. In J. Watkins & M. Salo (Eds.), *Trauma, stress and immunity in anaesthesia and surgery* (pp. 334–361). London: Butterworth.

Bridges, P.K., & Jones, M.T. (1966). Diurnal rhythm of plasma cortisol concentration in depression. *British Journal of Psychiatry, 112,* 1257–1261.

Chapman, C.R., & Cox, G.B. (1977). Determinants of anxiety in dental surgery patients. In C.D. Spielberger & I. Sarason (Eds.), *Stress and anxiety,* Vol. 4, pp. 269–290. New York: Wiley.

Cohen, F.L. (1980). Postsurgical pain relief: patients' status and nurses' medication choices. *Pain, 9,* 265–274.

Cohen, F., & Lazarus, R.S. (1973). Active coping processes, coping dispositions and recovery from surgery. *Psychosomatic Medicine, 35,* 375–389.

Cohen, M.R., Pickar, D., Dubois, M. *et al.* (1982). Clinical and experimental studies of stress and the endogenous opioid system. *Annals of the New York Academy of Science, 398,* 424–432.

Corenblum, B., & Taylor, P.J. (1981). Mechanisms of control of prolactin release in response to apprehension stress and anaesthesia. *Fertility & Sterility, 365,* 712–715.

Czeisler, C.A., Ede, M.C., Regestein, Q.R. *et al.* (1976). Episodic 24-hour cortisol secretory patterns in patients awaiting elective cardiac surgery. *Journal of Clinical Endocrinology and Metabolism, 42,* 273–283.

Egbert, L.B., Battit, G.E., Welch, C.E., & Bartlett, M.K. (1964). Reduction of postoperative pain by encouragement and instruction of patients, *New England Journal of Medicine, 270,* 825–827.

Feuerstein, M., Labbe, E.E., & Kuczmierczyk, A.R. (1986). *Health psychology: A psychobiological perspective.* New York: Plenum Press.

Fleischman, A.I., Bierenbaum, M.L., & Stier, A. (1976). Effect of stress due to anticipated minor surgery upon in vivo platetet aggregation in humans. *Journal of Human Stress, 2,* 33–37.

Frankenhauser, M. (1983). The sympathetic–adrenal and pituitary-adrenal response to challenge: comparison between the sexes. In T.M. Dembroski, T. Schmidt & G. Blumchen (Eds.) *Biobehavioural bases of coronary heart disease* (pp. 91–105). Basel: Karger.

Goldstein, D.S., Dionne, R., Sweet, J. *et al.* (1982). Circulatory, plasma catecholamine, cortisol, lipid, and psychological responses to a real-life stress (third molar extractions): effects of diazepam sedation and of inclusion of epinephrene with the local anaesthetic. *Psychosomatic Medicine, 44,* 259–271.

Harrison, J., Mackinnon, P., & Monk-Jones, M.E. (1962). Behaviour of the palmar sweat glands before and after operation. *Clinical Science, 23,* 371–377.

Hayward, J. (1975). *Information: a prescription against pain.* London: RCN.

Henry, J.P. & Stephens, P.H. (1977). *Stress, health and the social environment.* New York: Springer-Verlag.

Hoffman, J.W., Benson, H., Arna, P.A., Stainbrook, G.L., Landsberg, L., Young, J.B., & Gill, A. (1982). Reduced sympathetic nervous system responsivity associated with the relaxation response. *Science, 215,* 190–192.

Holmes, T.H., & Rahe, R.H. (1967). The social re-adjustment rating scale. *Journal of Psychosomatic Research, 11,* 213–218.

Janis, I.L. (1958). *Psychological stress.* New York: John Wiley & Sons.

Johnson, B.A., Johnson, J.E., & Dumas, R.G. (1970). Research in nursing practice: the problem of uncontrolled situational variables. *Nursing Research, 19,* 337–342.

Johnson, J.E. (1984). Psychological interventions and coping with surgery. In A. Baum, S.E. Taylor & J.E. Singer (Eds.), *Handbook of health psychology,* Vol 4, (pp. 167–188). Hillsdale, NJ: Erlbaum.

Johnson, J.E., Dabbs, J.M., & Leventhal, H. (1970). Psychological factors in the welfare of surgical patients. *Nursing Research, 19,* 182–188.

Johnson, J.E., & Leventhal, H. (1974). Effects of accurate expectations and behavioural instructions on reactions during a noxious medical examination. *Journal of Personality and Social Psychology, 29,* 710–718.

Johnson, J.E., Leventhal, H., & Dabbs, J.M. (1971). Contributions of emotional and instrumental response processes in adaptation to surgery. *Journal of Personality and Social Psychology, 20,* 55–64.

Johnson, J.E., Fuller, S.S., Endress, M.P., & Rice, V.H. (1978a). Altering patients' responses to surgery: an extension and replication. *Research in Nursing and Health, 1,* 111–121.

Johnson, J.E., Rice, V.H., Fuller, S.S., & Endress, M.P. (1978b). Sensory information, instruction in a coping strategy, and recovery from surgery. *Research in Nursing Health, 1,* 4–17.

Johnston, M. (1975). STAI and PSI in surgical patients. Unpublished paper.

Johnston, M. (1976). Communications of patients' feelings in hospital. In A.E. Bennett (Ed.). Oxford: Oxford University Press. (pp. 30–43).

Johnston, M. (1980). Anxiety in surgical patients. *Psychological Medicine, 10,* 145–152.

Johnston, M. (1981). Emotional distress immediately following surgery. In J.W.G. Tiller & P.R. Martin (Eds.), (pp. 35–42). Melbourne: Geigy.

Johnston, M. (1982a). Anxiety and worries in surgical patients. In H. van der Ploeg & P. Defaresz (Eds.), *Stress en Angst in de Medische Situatie,* Alphen aan den Rijn: Stafleu.

Johnston, M. (1982b). Recognition of Patients' worries by nurses and by other patients. Recognition of Patients' worries by nurses and by other patients. *21,* 255–261. *British Journal of Clinical Psychology.*

Johnston, M. (1984). Dimensions of recovery from surgery. *International Review of Applied Psychology, 33,* 505–520.

Johnston, M. (1986). Pre-operative emotional states and post-operative recovery. *Advances in Psychosomatic Medicine, 15,* 1–22.

Johnston, M. (1987). Emotional and cognitive aspects of anxiety in surgical patients. *Communication & Cognition, 20,* 261–276.

Johnston, M., & Carpenter, L. (1980). Relationship between pre-operative anxiety and post-operative state. *Psychology and Medicine, 10,* 361–367.

Johnston, M., Shaw, R.W., & Bird, D. (1987). 'Test-tube baby' procedures: stress and judgements under uncertainty. *Psychology and Health, 1,* 25–38.

Kinney, M.R. (1977). Effects of pre-operative teaching upon patients with differing modes of response to treatment stimuli. *International Journal of Nursing Studies, 14,* 49–59.

Knight, R.G., Waal-Manning, H.J., & Spears, G.F. (1983). Some norms and rehability data for one state-trait anxiety inventory and the Zung self-rating depression scale. *British Journal of Clinical Psychology, 22,* 245–250.

Langer, E., Janis, I1J., & Wolfer, J.A. (1975). Reduction of psychological stress in surgical patients. *Journal of Experimental Social Psychology, 11,* 155–165.

Leventhal, H. 1970. Findings and theory in the study of fear communications. *Advances in Experimental Social Psychology, 5,* 119–186.

Levesque, L., & Charlebois, M. (1977). Anxiety, locus of control, and the effect of pre-operative teaching on patients' physical and emotional state. *Nursing Papers 8,* 11–26

Linn, B.S., & Jenson, J. (1983). Age and immune response to a surgical stress. *Archives of Surgery, 118,* 405–409.

Lucente, F.E., & Fleck, S. (1972). A study of hospitalization anxiety in 408 medical and surgical patients. *Psychosomatic Medicine, 34,* 304–312.

Macleod, C., Mathews, A., & Tata, P. (1986). Perceptual bias with emotional stimuli in normal and abnormal populations. *Journal of Abnormal Psychology, 95,* 15–20.

Mathews, A., & Ridgeway, V. (1981). Personality and surgical recovery: a review. *British Journal of Clinical Psychology, 2,* 243–260.

Mathews, A., & Ridgeway, V. (1984). Psychological preparation for surgery. In A. Steptoe & A. Mathews (Eds), *Health care and human behaviour* (pp. 231–259). London: Academic Press.

Mumford, E., Schlesinger, H.J., & Glass, G.V. (1982). The effects of psychological intervention on recovery from surgery and heart attacks: an analysis of the literature. *American Journal of Public Health, 72,* 141–151.

Murphy, F., Bentley, S., Ellis, B.W., & Dudley, H. (1977). Sleep deprivation in patients undergoing operation: a factor in the stress of surgery. *British Medical Journal, 2,* 1521–1522.

Murray, D. (1967). Cortisol binding to plasma proteins in man in health, stress and at death. *Journal of Endocrinology, 39,* 571–591.

Pickett, C., & Clum, G.A. (1982). Comparative treatment strategies and their interaction with locus of control in the reduction of post-surgical pain and anxiety. *Journal of Consulting and Clinical Psychology, 50,* 439–441.

Ray, C.J. (1981). The surgical patient: psychological stress and coping resources In. J.R. Eiser (Ed.) *Social psychology and behavioral medicine* (pp. 483–507). Chichester: John Wiley & Sons.

Ray, C.J., & Fitzgibbon, G. (1979). Socially mediated reduction of stress in surgical patients. In D.J. Osborne, M.M. Gruneberg & J.R. Eiser (Eds.), *Research in psychology and medicine,* Vol. 2 (pp. 321–327). London: Academic Press.

Ray, C.J., & Fitzgibbon, G. (1981). Stress arousal and coping with surgery. *Psychology and Medicine, 11,* 741–746.

Richards, J., & McDonald, P. (1985). Doctor–patient communication in surgery. *Journal of the Royal Society of Medicine, 78,* 922–924.

Sane, A.S., Chary, T.M., Kukreti, S.C., & Multani, S. (1981). Effect of surgical stress on serum lipid levels. *Panminerva Medica, 23,* 207–209.

Sané, A.S., & Kukreti, S.C. (1978). Effect of pre-operative stress on serum cholesterol levels in humans. *Experientia, 34,* 213–214.

Shipley, R.H., Butt, J.H., Horowitz, B., & Farby, J.E. (1978). Preparation for a stressful medical procedure: effect of stimulus pre-exposure and coping style. *Journal of Consulting and Clinical Psychology, 46,* 499–507.

Sime, M. (1976). Relationship of pre-operative fear, type of coping, and information received about surgery to recovery from surgery. *Journal of Psychology, Personality and Social Psychology, 40,* 33–38.

Slade, M.S. Simmons, R.L., Yunis, E., & Greenberg, L.R. (1975). Immunodepression after major surgery in normal patients. *Surgery, 78,* 363–372.

Spielberger, C.D., Auerbach, S.M., Wadsworth, A.P., Dunn, T.M., & Taulbee, E.S. (1973). Emotional reactions to surgery. *Journal of Consulting and Clinical Psychology, 40,* 33–38.

Spielberger, C.D., Gorsuch, R.L., & Lushene, R.E. (1970). *State trait anxiety inventory manual.* Palo Alto: Consulting Psychologists Press.

Staite, S.A. (1978). The effect of giving information about post-operative sensations on mood and pain in patients and undergoing gynaecological surgery. Unpublished MPhil. thesis, University of London.

Vernon, D.T., & Bigelow, D.A. (1974). Effects of information about a potentially stressful situation on responses to stress impact. *Journal of Personality and Social Psychology, 29,* 50–59.

Visser, A. (1982), Situational and individual determinants of state anxiety of Situational and individual determinants of state anxiety of surgical patients. In C.D. Spielberger, P. Defares & I.G. Sarason (Eds.) *Stress and anxiety.* Academic, New York: Academic Press.

Vogele, C., & Steptoe, A. (1986). Physiological and subjective stress responses in surgical patients. *Journal of Psychosomatic Research, 30,* 205–215.

Volicer, B.J., & Bohannon, M.W. (1975). A hospital stress rating scale. *Nursing Research, 24,* 352–359.

Volicer, B.J., Isenberg, M.A., & Burns, M.W. (1977). Medical–surgical differences in hospital stress factors. *Journal of Human Stress, 3,* 62–77.

Wallace, L.M. (1983). Psychological studies of the development and evaluation of preparatory procedures for women undergoing minor gynaecological surgery. Unpublished PhD thesis, University of Birmingham.

Wallace, L.M. (1984). Psychological preparation as a method of reducing the stress of surgery. *Journal of Human Stress, 10,* 62–77.

Weinman, J., & Johnston, M. (in press). Stressful medical procedures: an analysis of the stressfulness of the procedures. In S. Maes, P. Defares, I.G. Sarason & C. Spielberg (Eds.) *Proceedings of the First International Expert Conference on Health Psychology* Chichester: John Wiley & Sons.

Williams, J.G.J., Jones, J.R., Workhoven, M.N., & Williams, B. (1975). The psychological control of pre-operative anxiety. *Psychophysiology, 12,* 50–54.

Wilson, J.F. (1981). Behavioural preparation for surgery: benefit or harm? *Behavioural Medicine, Journal of 4,* 79–102.

Wilson-Barnett, J. (1976). Patients' emotional reactions to hospitalization: an explanatory study. *Journal of Advances in Nursing, 1,* 351–358.

Wilson-Barnet, J. (1984). Interventions to alleviate patients' stress: a review. *Journal of Psychosomatic Research, 28,* 63–72.

KEY WORDS

Accuracy of expectations, anaesthesia, analgesia, anxiety, catecholamine, cognitive, cognitive–behavioural, communication, coping, emotion, hospital stay, Hospital Stress Rating scale (HSRS), life threatening, pain, palmar sweating, physiological, pituitary-adrenocortical, postoperative, predictability and control, preoperative, preparation for surgery, procedural information, recovery, relaxation, sensory information, social support, surgery, sympathetic–adrenomedullary, work of worrying, worries.

Handbook of Life Stress, Cognition and Health
Edited by S. Fisher and J. Reason
© 1988 John Wiley & Sons Ltd.

6

Victims of Violence

RONNIE JANOFF-BULMAN
University of Massachusetts

INTRODUCTION

Violence is an all too common feature of modern life. Media presentations are filled with images of people hurting one another, and although much attention is given to scenes depicting violence and even to perpetrators of violence, little is given to victims (Bard and Sangrey, 1979). Violence involves physical force with the intent to harm another, and from an observer's perspective, victims' injuries seem best measured in terms of physical harm. The plight of the victim, in other words, is generally understood in terms of physical violation. Yet injury to victims of violence involves not only physical violation, but psychological violation as well. The aftermath of violence for victims must be understood by considering threats not only to their bodily integrity, but to their psychological integrity. Victims are forced to confront directly the possible loss of physical functioning and even death. They are also forced to confront directly the possible breakdown of the cognitive structures that had been so instrumental in providing psychological stability.

The suffering of victims of violence varies from person to person, but is generally far more intense than might be predicted from a simple examination of physical injury. Victims of rape, robbery, assault, sexual abuse, and physical abuse often have similar responses to their victimization (Janoff-Bulman and Frieze, 1983; Krupnick and Horowitz, 1980); victims frequently feel helpless, out of control, depressed, ashamed, anxious, frightened, and disorganized. Behavioural reactions include sleep disturbances (e.g. insomnia, nightmares), uncontrollable crying, restlessness, deterioration of personal relationships, and increased use of drugs (Frieze *et al.*, 1984). For many victims, the trauma of violent victimization is resolved within 6 months to a year (Horowitz, 1976); for others, the stress of victimization persists. Research with rape victims, for example, has found that psychological symptoms often last beyond a year. Rape victims have been found to be more depressed a year after their victimization than a control sample of women (Ellis *et al.*, 1981), and many feel they have not recovered as much as 4 to 6 years after the rape (Burgess and Holmstrom, 1976, 1979; also see Sales *et al.*, 1984).

Persistent, severe, yet not uncommon responses of victims of violence are best described by post-traumatic stress disorder (PTSD), a new diagnostic category of the *Diagnostic and Statistical Manual* (DSM III) of the American Psychiatric Association (1980). In addition to a recognizable stressor, diagnostic criteria for PTSD include: (a) re-experiencing the trauma via intrusive thoughts, dreams or memories; (b) numbing of responsiveness, demonstrated by constricted affect, feelings of detachment from others, or diminished interest in important activities; and (c) the presence of at least two other symptoms, including sleep disturbance, exaggerated startle response, guilt, memory impairment, trouble concentrating, and phobias about activities triggering recollection of the event. In its discussion of PTSD, the American Psychiatric Association (1980) does not make distinctions between different stressor events; rather, the stressor is simply presented as 'a traumatic event that is generally outside the range of usual experience'. Thus, PTSD is intended to describe intense psychological responses of many types of victims, including not only victims of violence, but also victims of natural disasters, accidents, and diseases. The only mention of any distinction to be drawn between these types of victimization is in a single sentence that reads, 'The disorder is apparently more severe and longer lasting when the stressor is of human design' (American Psychiatric Association, 1980, p.236). Victims of violence, unlike victims of natural disasters, accidents, or diseases, are victims of a stressor that is human induced and intended (i.e. designed) by a perpetrator. Such victims are particularly apt to experience severe psychological distress.

FEAR AND ANXIETY

One way to begin to understand the reactions of victims, and of victims of violence in particular, is to recognize that PTSD is classified as an anxiety disorder (American Psychiatric Association, 1980). Anxiety and fear are clearly predominant emotional responses of victims of violence (Frederick, 1980; Krupnick and Horowitz, 1980). Among rape victims, for example, the most prominent, persistent reactions include general diffused anxiety and intense fears of rape-related situations (Calhoun *et al.*, 1982; Nadelson *et al.*, 1982). In their study of rape victims 3–6 months post rape, Kilpatrick *et al.* (1979) found that the victims differed from non-victims only on measures of fear and anxiety, and not on other distress measures.

Anxiety and fear are frequently presented as common reactions of victims, and the two emotional reactions often are not distinguished. This is understandable in light of the fact that fear and anxiety are generally indistinguishable from an observer's perspective. The manifestations of both include autonomic hyperactivity, apprehensive expectation, motor tension, and vigilance (American Psychiatric Association, 1980). Nevertheless, they represent two distinct psychological responses by an individual.

Generally, the distinction drawn between fear and anxiety relates to the identifiability of the source of stimulation; that is, in the case of fear, the source is readily identified, whereas in the case of anxiety it cannot be (see, for example, Freud, 1926; cf. Rachman, 1978). In other words, victims can tell someone else what they fear, and it appears that victims of violence frequently report fears, particularly those of being alone, a recurrence of the victimization, and death (Frieze *et al.*, 1984). In the case of fear, the threat of danger is consciously recognized and generally external (American Psychiatric Association, 1980), and generally the fears of victims are strongly related to physical violation. In contrast, anxiety is more closely associated with psychological violation and does not involve a consciously recognized danger nor an external threat. Yet, a better understanding of anxiety can provide important clues to the psychological trauma often experienced by victims of violence.

Unlike fear, the primary threat in the case of anxiety is internal, for the cardinal feature of anxiety is cognitive disintegration (Averill, 1976). 'Many of the features commonly ascribed to anxiety can be traced directly or indirectly to the disintegration of cognitive systems. For example, a disruption of cognitive systems leaves the person feeling uncertain and helpless' (Averill, 1976, p.120). Threats that produce anxiety are related to our symbolic systems of ideas, values, and concepts. Anxiety results when these symbols, or cognitions, no longer fit reality, when they no longer enable individuals to relate meaningfully to the world around them (Lazarus and Averill, 1972). Cognitive disintegration may arise in a number of ways; it could be a result of excessive stimulation that may tax the ability to process information, or of intrapsychic conflict when two cognitions are incompatible, or of unusual information that is impossible to interpret (Averill, 1976; Lazarus and Averill, 1972). Violent victimization produces considerable anxiety in victims, suggesting that victims of violence experience cognitive disintegration. Understanding the reactions of victims of violence, then, involves better understanding the cognitive, or symbolic, systems that are affected by violent victimization.

ASSUMPTIVE WORLDS

Recent work in social psychology has stressed the importance of cognitive schemas for understanding people's perceptions, memories, and inferences (e.g. Abelson, 1981; Cantor, 1980; Fiske and Taylor, 1984; Markus, 1977). A schema is 'a cognitive structure that represents organized knowledge about a given concept or type of stimulus' (Fiske & Taylor, 1984, p.140). Our interactions in the world are primarily defined by top-down processing; that is, we start with schemas and understand phenomena through these cognitive structures. In processing information, we rely upon schemas without necessarily being aware of their content. Further, these schemas are generally resistant to major changes, for ordinarily we alter our perceptions and memories so as to render them schema consistent; we persevere in maintaining our schemas (see discussions in Nisbett and Ross, 1980, and Fiske and Taylor, 1984).

Although work on schemas has generally dealt with our 'theories' of particular categories of people or events, the psychological perspective represented by this work is consistent with the orientations of psychologists who have been interested in more global theories or assumptions people hold about themselves and their world. Parkes (1971, 1975), for example, maintains that people strongly hold a set of assumptions, their 'assumptive world', that represents their view of reality and is built and confirmed by years of experience. Bowlby's (1969) 'world models', Marris' (1975) 'structures of meaning', and Epstein's (1973, 1979, 1980) 'theory of reality' all represent this same conceptual system that guides our perceptions and actions. As Epstein (1980) and Parkes (1971) maintain, we operate on the basis of these theories or assumptions, and yet we are generally unaware of their content. Further, because we perceive the world through these assumptive lenses, it is very difficult to invalidate them. They generally persist and are resistant to change. Our assumptive world provides us with a stable conceptual system that affords us psychological equilibrium in a constantly changing world.

Although our basic assumptions about the world and ourselves are generally not questioned or challenged, occasionally particular events force us to objectify and confront them. In the realm of science, paradigms provide the basis for all work during 'normal science' (Kuhn, 1962), just as our basic assumptions underlie 'normal' (i.e. day-to-day) living. Yet, there are occasions in science when crises arise. When anomalies call into question fundamental aspects of the paradigm and the old paradigm is 'pushed too far', the result is a scientific revolution (Kuhn, 1962). Similarly, there are occasions in people's lives when their assumptive worlds are seriously challenged. Violent victimization represents one such experience. Victims of violence can no longer automatically rely upon their assumptive worlds to account for the data of their experience, and the stability of their conceptual system is threatened. The psychological trauma experienced by victims of violence can be understood in terms of the potential breakdown of their assumptive worlds. There is disorganization within their conceptual systems, and the individuals are thrown into a state of psychological crisis.

CORE ASSUMPTIONS

The threat to the victim's assumptive world occurs because victimization cannot readily be assimilated into his or her conceptual system. A cluster of assumptions, all of which relate to the general perception of relative invulnerability, are challenged by victimization, particularly by violent victimization. A very common reaction following victimization is an intense feeling of vulnerability. Most people, prior to any serious victimization, feel relatively invulnerable to negative events (Janoff-Bulman and Lang-Gunn, in press; Perloff, 1983; Weinstein, 1980; Weinstein and Lachendro, 1982). Victims can no longer say, 'It can't happen to me.' Rather, they experience a lost sense of safety and security, whether they are victims of crime (e.g. Bard and Sangrey, 1979; Fischer, 1984; Krupnick, 1980; Notman and Nadelson, 1976), disease (e.g. Taylor, 1983; Weisman, 1979; Wortman and Dunkel-Schetter, 1979), or disasters (e.g. Lifton and Olson, 1976; Titchener et al., 1976; Wolfenstein, 1957). In his work with individuals exhibiting post-traumatic stress, including people who had been assaulted, had undergone a near-fatal experience, and had lost a loved one, Horowitz (1982) found that the most common theme expressed by these victims was discomfort over their own vulnerability.

This sense of vulnerability appears to be tied to the disruption of certain core assumptions about the self and the world. In particular, people generally seem to operate on the basis of three fundamental assumptions related to invulnerability: (a) the world is benevolent; (b) events in the world are meaningful; and (c) the self is positive and worthy. A benevolent world is not only one in which good things happen, but one in which people are good. A meaningful world is one in which events 'make sense' because they predictably follow certain accepted 'social laws' (Janoff-Bulman and Frieze, 1983; Silver and Wortman, 1980). In Western cultures, events are meaningful if they follow principles of justice (i.e. people get what they deserve; Lerner, 1980) or controllability (i.e. people's actions determine their outcomes; Seligman, 1975). A positive view of the self involves seeing oneself as decent and worthy, and thereby deserving of good outcomes.

These three vulnerability-related assumptions may form a central core of our assumptive world. Work on the child's earliest experiences suggests that the groundwork for these assumptions is laid in the child's early interactions. Essentially, the development of the child during the first year involves learning to trust the world, learning that he or she is not vulnerable, but rather is protected and secure (Erikson, 1950, 1968, 1980). The establishment of a sense of relative invulnerability seems grounded in early relationships with caregivers (Bowlby, 1969; Fairbairn, 1952; Sullivan, 1940, 1953). Typically, the child comes to perceive the world as benevolent through predictable interactions with a responsible caregiver. Through positive interactions in which the child's needs (physical and emotional) are met, the child learns that his or her world is controllable, dependable, and just. Simultaneously, the child begins to develop a sense of self-worth, in that he or she is the recipient of positive caregiving. The process is one of mutual regulation, in which the child perceives 'friendly otherness' and 'personal trustworthiness' through sensitive, dependable care. During the first year, as children learn that others are good, they also learn that they are good and that the world is orderly and predictable. Generally, they come to believe that they are not helpless in a hostile environment (Horney, 1937, 1939), but capable and cared for in a benevolent world.

The assumptions of benevolence of the world, meaningfulness of events, and self-worth are grounded in the early preverbal experiences of the child and are therefore apt to be core assumptions in our conceptual system. Though certainly not the only assumptions an individual holds, these three vulnerability-related assumptions are no doubt very 'high-order postulates' (Epstein, 1980) or, in Lakatos' (1974) terms, components of our 'metaphysical hard-core'. As such, their maintenance is essential to our psychological stability; threats to these core assumptions result in a great deal of psychological distress. Victimization threatens these assumptions, and the psychological responses of victims indicate their decreased sense of self-worth coupled with a perception of the world that is malevolent and arbitrary.

Although these three basic assumptions are threatened by the experience of non-violent victimization (e.g. disease, accidents, natural disasters), violent victimization seems to provide even greater threats and challenges to the assumptive worlds of victims (Janoff-Bulman, 1985). For victims of violence, the world is not only a place in which negative events occur (i.e. unfortunate outcomes become salient; Kahneman and Tversky, 1973), but people can no longer be trusted. Both the impersonal world and the personal world appear hostile. As Bard and Sangrey (1979) write. 'Because crime is an interpersonal event, the victim's feeling of security in the world of other people is seriously upset' (p. 14). For those victimized by an individual they know well (e.g. date, spouse, parent, friend), the breakdown in the assumption of a benign world is particularly acute. Considerable emotional trauma follows the experience of rape by a partner or friend (Burgess and Holmstrom, 1974; Medea and Thompson, 1974). Victims of rape and sexual abuse often have a great deal of difficulty establishing a sense of trust in subsequent close relationships (Miller *et al.*, 1982; Nadelson & Notman, 1984). The individual who is victimized by a stranger often suffers a loss of trust in people as well, for the experience forces a direct confrontation with the realization that people can be malevolent; the world of people becomes suspect (Fischer, 1984).

Victims of violence, as well as victims of accidents, disease and natural disasters, experience serious threats to their assumption of meaningfulness. They have been brought face to face with arbitrariness or randomness, and it is difficult to make sense of their victimization. Once again, however, the intent to harm by another human being suggests the possibility of unique difficulties for victims of violence. They must confront the existence of 'evil' and the breakdown of a moral universe (see Lifton, 1967). Diseases, accidents, and natural disasters do not raise the question of evil; it is as if to be evil, something has to be intended, as is the case in violent victimizations (Janoff-Bulman, 1985).

There is considerable evidence that victims in general experience a marked decrease in their sense of self-worth (Horowitz *et al.*, 1980; Krupnick, 1980). They perceive themselves as having been singled out for misfortune, and this leads to self-questioning, a perception of deviance and self-stigma (Coates and Winston, 1983). Victims of violence are apt to experience the greatest threats to their self-worth, for being victimized by another who has intended harm is likely to exaggerate one's sense of powerlessness and helplessness, as well as one's sense of 'losing' to another human being. One has been overpowered by another person and has thereby experienced a direct 'violation of the self' (Bard and Sangrey, 1979). This sense of weakness and helplessness in contrast to the dominance of an evil other is apt to be experienced as humiliation, shame, and a loss of self-respect.

COPING AND 'INAPPROPRIATE' REACTIONS

Coping with violent victimization involves coming to terms with the cognitive disorganization precipitated by the experience. Assumptions and personal theories that had provided psychological stability over the years are seriously challenged and often shattered. For victims of violence, intense anxiety—with all of its emotional, physiological, and behavioral manifestations—reflects the disruption in their cognitive systems, and the road to adjustment and decreased anxiety entails reorganizing and rebuilding their assumptive world.

The work of Horowitz (1976, 1980, 1982) is instructive in understanding the process of coping with victimization. According to Horowitz, people's 'inner models' change as a result of serious life events, and he calls the tendency to integrate one's inner models and reality the 'completion tendency'. Prior to this integration, or completion, information from and reactions to the traumatic experience are stored in active memory and account for the intrusive thoughts experienced by victims. These intrusions cease when the information has been integrated and thereby is no longer stored in active memory.

From a cognitive perspective, the key to the victim's recovery process is the reestablishment of an integrated, organized set of basic assumptions or schemas. The traumatic event must be assimilated into the victim's assumptive world, or the assumptive world must accommodate to the new data (Piaget, 1971). In either case, anxiety will dissipate as the victim's cognitive system becomes integrated and viable as a means for understanding and responding to his or her world.

This focus on the victim's assumptive world renders the internal reality of the victim paramount in the process of understanding victims' reactions to traumatic events. Once the significance of this internal reality is recognized, certain reactions of victims that ordinarily appear inappropriate or maladaptive from an outsider's perspective begin to be comprehensible. Thus, Janoff-Bulman and Timko (1987) maintain that the often-maligned process of denial is natural and often necessary and can, in fact, facilitate adaptation to traumatic experiences by modulating the attack on a victim's assumptive world. Denial allows the victim slowly and gradually to face the realities of the victimization and incorporate them into his or her internal world. Certainly, it can be argued that it is easier to use denial in the case of victimization by disease than violent victimization, for the latter involves another person and a discrete event. Nevertheless, other apparently 'odd' reactions of victims, particularly victims of violence, can better be understood by recognizing their role in the process of building and rebuilding a stable, integrated assumptive world for the victim.

The 'Stockholm syndrome', sometimes found among hostages, is a case in point. The name derives from the case of a Stockholm bank robbery, in which several of the hostages captured during the hold-up defended their captors when released. This syndrome is now used to describe this alignment of positive affections by hostages towards their captors (Eitinger, 1982; Ochberg, 1986; Strentz, 1982; Symonds, 1982). Although typically explained via the psychoanalytic concept of identification with the aggressor, it seems possible that the victims' needs for a stable conceptual system may play a role in this phenomenon as well. By regarding their captors positively, hostages are able to maintain a belief in a benevolent environment in which their own safety and security are maximized. Their situation appears relatively benign, thereby minimizing the terror associated with their predicament.

Perhaps the best example of a victim response that may be better understood by noting the internal reality and cognitive needs of victims is that of self-blame. Self-blame is a common response by victims of violence (Bard and Sangrey, 1979; Frieze et al., 1984; Geis, 1981). Victims often seem unnecessarily willing to blame themselves for their victimization. The apparent inappropriateness of such a response is illustrated by Burgess and Holmstrom (1974) in their discussion of a woman who was assaulted outside her apartment one afternoon, while searching through her purse for her keys. Although the woman fought back, even managing to take her assailant's knife, the man forced his way into her apartment, beat and raped her. Surprisingly, the woman later engaged in self-blame and said she should have acted differently when she first saw the man; then neither she nor the rapist 'would be in trouble'. This tendency to accept blame is frequently found among victims of rape (Burgess and Holmstrom, 1974; Medea and Thompson, 1974; Weis & Weis, 1975). In a survey of rape crisis centers across the country, center workers reported that fully 74% of the women they see blame themselves at least in part for the rape (Janoff-Bulman, 1979). Battered women, too, often seem to engage in self-blame (Frieze, 1979; Hilberman and Munson, 1978; Walker, 1979). Geis (1981), based on his work with crime victims, writes, 'It must be particularly appreciated that the crime victim rarely is able to see himself as an entirely guiltless person . . . If nothing else, he must satisfactorily resolve questions relating to the lottery of human existence that resulted in injury being visited upon him rather than another' (p. 63). Geis (1981) goes on to note that too many alternative ways of behaving usually had been available to the crime victim (e.g. more care in choosing one's route, a better lock, staying aware from certain people), and 'almost inevitably, then, some blame attaches to the self' (p. 61).

This focus on behavior as a basis for self-blaming is important in understanding the role of self-blame in the coping process of victims. There are (at least) two distinct types of self-blame, one of which has been labelled 'behavioral self-blame', the other 'characterological self-blame' (Janoff-Bulman, 1979). The former involves blaming one's behaviors for a negative outcome such as victimization, whereas the latter involves blaming one's character or enduring qualities. Thus, a rape victim can blame herself by saying she should not have hitchhiked or should not have walked alone at night (behavioral self-blame), or she can say that she is too trusting, a bad person, or the type of person who attracts rapists (characterological self-blame). An important distinction between the two types of attributions concerns the perceived controllability (i.e. modifiability through one's own efforts) of the factor(s) blamed. This difference in perceived controllability has led Janoff-Bulman (1979; also see Wortman, 1976) to posit that behavioral self-blame may be an adaptive response to victimization, for it enables victims to minimize their perception of vulnerability by allowing them to believe that altering their behaviors in the future can minimize the likelihood of a recurrence. Behavioral self-blame may not involve only the avoidability of the particular negative outcome in question, but may promote a general belief in one's ability to avoid or control future negative outcomes in general (Janoff-Bulman, 1979; Janoff-Bulman and Lang-Gunn, in press). Characterological self-blame, on the other hand, involves self-esteem deficits, and is the type of self-blame generally associated with depression (Beck, 1967; Janoff-Bulman, 1979). Empirical support has been found for the adaptive value of behavioral self-blame (e.g. Affleck et al., 1985a, 1985b; Baum et al., 1983; Bulman and Wortman, 1977; Fischer, 1984; Peterson et al., 1981; Tennen et al., 1986; Tennen et al., 1984; Timko and Janoff-Bulman, 1985), although not consistently (e.g.

Kiecolt-Glaser and Williams, in press; Meyer and Taylor, 1986; Taylor *et al.*, 1984; Witenberg *et al.*, 1983).

Behavioral self-blame often seems to be psychologically adaptive; further, it is frequently manifested following victimization, perhaps especially by victims of violence who have been singled out for harm by another human being. Certainly, any self-blame attribution provides a meaningful response to the question of selective incidence: 'Why me?' A full understanding of why behavioral self-blame is so common and why it can be psychologically adaptive following victimization involves going beyond its control implications and considering, once again, the internal reality of victims and their need for a stable, integrated cognitive system. By engaging in behavioral self-blame, victims are able to minimize the threats and challenges to their assumptive worlds. They are essentially able to re-establish their conceptual systems such that cognitive disintegration can largely be avoided. Prior assumptions about the benevolence of the world, meaningfulness, and self-worth are not severely threatened when victims engage in behavioral self-blame. By maintaining that the event was due to their own behaviors (or behavioral omissions), victims need not change their view of how benign their environment is. Further, the victimization 'makes sense', in that it was controllable via their own actions, and can thus be avoided in the future; the event was not simply random and arbitrary. And behavioral self-blame generally does not result in decreased self-esteem, in that it is an attribution to a specific behavior and does not involve generalizations to one's overall evaluation of the self, as does characterological self-blame. Engaging in behavioral self-blame, then, may be protective for the victim, who seeks to maintain cognitive stability in the face of an unexpected, negative, extreme event.

SUMMARY AND CONCLUSIONS

Reactions of victims of violence can be understood within a framework that emphasizes the significance of the victim's conceptual system following victimization. The intense anxiety experienced by victims of violence reflects their cognitive disintegration in the face of a traumatic external event. Basic unquestioned assumptions, built over years of experience, are suddenly challenged. In particular, assumptions about the benevolence of the world, the meaningfulness of events in the world, and self-worth are seriously threatened. Although these assumptions are no doubt threatened by the experience of any victimization, they are more severely challenged when an individual is the victim of harm by another person. The process of coping for victims involves reestablishing an integrated, stable system of basic assumptions that are viable in the face of their traumatic experience. Common victim reactions such as self-blame may appear inappropriate from the perspective of an observer; yet these responses become readily comprehensible when considered from the perspective of the victim's need to rebuild his or her assumptive world.

REFERENCES

Abelson, R.P. (1981). The psychological status of the script concept. *American Psychologist*, *36*, 715–729.

Affleck, G., Allen, D.A., Tennen, H., McGrade, B.J., & Ratzan, S. (1985a). Causal and control cognitions in parent coping with a chronically ill child. *Journal of Social and Clinical Psychology*, *3*, 369–379.

Affleck, G., McGrade, B.J., Allen, D.A., & McQueeney, M. (1985b). Mothers' beliefs about behavioral causes for their developmentally disabled infant's condition: What do they signify? *Journal of Pediatric Psychology*, *10*, 193–303.

American Psychiatric Association (1980). *Diagnostic and statistical manual of mental disorders* (DSM III), 3rd edn. Washington, DC: American Psychiatric Association.

Averill, J. (1976). Emotion and anxiety: Sociocultural, biological, and psychological determinants. In M. Zuckerman and C.D. Spielberger (eds), *Emotion and anxiety: New concepts, methods and applications*. New York: Erlbaum-Wiley.

Bard, M., & Sangrey, D. (1979). *The crime victim's book*. New York: Basic Books.

Baum, A., Flemming, R., & Singer, J.E. (1983). Coping with victimization by technological disaster. *Journal of Social Issues*, *39*, 119–140.

Beck, A.T. (1967). *Depression: Clinical, experimental, and theoretical aspects*. New York: Harper & Row.

Bowlby, J. (1969). *Attachment and loss*, Vol. 1: *Attachment*. London: Hogarth.

Bulman, R.J., & Wortman, C.B. (1977). Attributions of blame and coping in the 'real world': Severe accident victims react to their lot. *Journal of Personality and Social Psychology*, *35*, 351–363.

Burgess, A., & Holmstrom, L. (1974). Rape trauma syndrome. *American Journal of Psychiatry*, *131*, 981–985.

Burgess, A., & Holmstrom, L. (1976). Coping behvior of the rape victim. *American Journal of Psychiatry*, *13*, 413–417.

Burgess, A., & Holmstrom, L. (1979). Adaptive strategies and recovery from rape. *American Journal of Psychiatry*, *136*, 1278–1282.

Calhoun, K.S., Atkeson, B.M., & Resick, P.A. (1982). A longitudinal examination of fear reactions in victims of rape. *Journal of Counseling Psychology*, *29*, 665–661.

Cantor, N. (1980). Perceptions of situations: Situation prototypes and person–situation prototypes. In D. Magnusson (ed.), *The situation: An interactional perspective*. Hillsdale, NJ: Erlbaum.

Coates, D., & Winston, T. (1983). Counteracting the deviance of depression: Peer support groups for victims. *Journal of Social Issues*, *39*, 171–196.

Eitinger, L. (1982). The effects of captivity. In F.M. Ochberg and D.A. Soskis (eds), *Victims of terrorism*. Boulder, Colorado: Westview Press.

Ellis, E., Atkeson, B., & Calhoun, K. (1981). An assessment of long-term reaction to rape. *Journal of Abnormal Psychology*, *90*, 263–266.

Epstein, S. (1973). The self-concept revisited, or a theory of a theory. *American Psychologist*, *28*, 404–416.

Epstein, S. (1979). The ecological study of emotions in humans. In P. Pilner, K.R. Blanstein & I.M. Spigel (eds), *Advances in the study of communication and affect*, Vol. 5: *Perception of emotions in self and others*. New York: Plenum Press.

Epstein, S. (1980). The self-concept: A review and the proposal of an integrated theory of personality. In E. Staub (ed.), *Personality: Basic Issues and current research*. Englewood Cliffs, NJ: Prentice-Hall.

Erikson, E. (1950). *Childhood and society*. New York: Norton.

Erikson, E. (1968). *Identity: Youth and crisis*. New York: Norton.

Erikson, E. (1980). *Identity and the life cycle*. New York: Norton.

Fairbairn, W.R.D. (1952). *An object-relations theory of the personality*. New York: Basic Books.

Fischer, C.T. (1984). A phenomenological study of being criminally victimized: Contributions and constraints of qualitative research. *Journal of Social Issues*, 40, 161–178.

Fiske, S.T., & Taylor, S.E. (1984). *Social cognition*. Reading, Ma: Addison-Wesley.

Frederick, C. (1980). Effects of natural vs. human-induced violence. *Evaluation and change*. Special issue: Services for survivors, 71–75.

Freud, S. (1926). Inhibitions, symptoms, and anxiety. *Standard edition*, Vol. 20. London: Hogarth, 1959.

Frieze, I.H. (1979). Perceptions of battered wives. In I.H. Frieze, D. Bar-Tal & J.S. Carroll (eds), *New approaches to social problems: Applications of attribution theory*. San Francisco, CA: Jossey-Bass.

Frieze, I.H., Hymer, S., & Greenberg, M.S. (1984). Describing the victims of crime and violence. In S.S. Kahn (ed.), *Victims of crime and violence*. Final report of the APA task force on the victims of crime and violence. Washington, DC: American Psychological Association.

Geis, G. (1981). Victims of crimes of violence and the criminal justice system. In B. Galway & J. Hudson (eds), *Perspectives on crime victims*. St. Louis, Miss.: Mosby.

Hilberman, E., & Munson, K. (1978). Sixty battered women. *Victimology*, 2, 460–471.

Horney, K. (1937). *The neurotic personality of our time*. New York: Norton.

Horney, K. (1939). *New ways in psychoanalysis*. New York: Norton.

Horowitz, M. (1976). *Stress response syndromes*. New York: Aronson.

Horowitz, M. (1980). Psychological response to serious life events. In V. Hamilton & D. Warburton (eds), *Human stress and cognition*. New York: Wiley.

Horowitz, M.J. (1982). Stress response syndromes and their treatment. In L. Goldberger & S. Breznitz (eds), *Handbook of stress*. New York: Free Press.

Horowitz, M.J., Wilner, N., Marmar, C., & Krupnick, J. (1980). Pathological grief and the activation of latent self-images. *American Journal of Psychiatry*, 137, 1137–1162.

Janoff-Bulman, R. (1979). Characterologial versus behavioral self-blame: Inquiries into depression and rape. *Journal of Personality and Social Psychology*, 37(10), 1798–1809.

Janoff-Bulman, R. (1985). Criminal vs. non-criminal victimization: Victims' reactions. *Victimology*, 10, 498–511.

Janoff-Bulman, R., & Frieze, I.H. (1983). A theoretical perspective for understanding reactions to victimization. *Journal of Social Issues*, 39, 1–17.

Janoff-Bulman, R., & Lang-Gunn, L. (in press). Coping with disease and accidents: The role of self-blame attributions. In L.Y. Abramson (ed.), *Social cognition and clinical psychology*. New York: Guilford.

Janoff-Bulman, R., & Timko, C. (1987). Coping with traumatic life events: The role of denial in light of people's assumptive worlds. In C.R. Snyder & C. Ford (eds), *Coping with negative life events: Clinical and social psychological perspectives*. New York: Plenum.

Kahneman, D., & Tversky, A. (1973). On the psychology of prediction. *Psychological Review*, 80, 237–251.

Kiecolt-Glaser, J.K., & Williams, D. (in press). Self-blame, compliance, and distress among burn patients. *Journal of Personality and Social Psychology*.

Kilpatrick, D.G., Veronen, L.J., & Resick, P.A. (1979). The aftermath of rape: Recent empirical findings. *American Journal of Orthopsychiatry*, 49, 658–669.

Krupnick, J. (1980). Brief psychotherapy with victims of violent crime. *Victimology*, 5, 347–354.

Krupnick, J., & Horowitz, M. (1980). Victims of violence: Psychological responses, treatment implications. *Evaluation and change*. Special issue: Services for survivors, 42–46.

Kuhn, T.S. (1962). *The structure of scientific revolutions*. Chicago: The University of Chicago Press.

Lakatos, I. (1974). Falsification and the methodology of scientific research programs. In I. Lakatos and A. Musgrave (eds), *Criticism and the growth of knowledge*. London: Cambridge University Press.

Lazarus, R.S., & Averill, J.R. (1972). Emotion and cognition: With special reference to anxiety. In C.D. Spielberger (ed.), *Anxiety: Current trends in theory and research*. New York: Academic Press.

Lerner, M.J. (1980). *The belief in a just world*. New York: Plenum.

Lifton, R.J. (1967). *Death in life: Survivors of Hiroshima*. New York: Simon and Schuster.

Lifton, R.J., & Olson, E. (1976). Death imprint in Buffalo Creek syndrome: Symptoms and character change after a major disaster. In H.J. Parad, H.L.P. Resnik & L.G. Parad (eds), *Emergency and disaster management*. Bowie, MD: Charles Press.

Markus, H. (1977). Self-schemata and processing information about the self. *Journal of Personality and Social Psychology*, *35*, 63–78.

Marris, P. (1975). *Loss and change*. Garden City, NY: Anchor/Doubleday.

Medea, A., & Thompson, K. (1974). *Against rape*. New York: Farrar, Straus, & Giroux.

Meyer, C.B., & Taylor, S.E. (1986). Adjustment to rape. *Journal of Personality and Social Psychology*, *50*, 1226–1234.

Miller, W.R., Williams, M., & Bernstein, M.H. (1982). The effects of rape on marital and sexual adjustment. *American Journal of Family Therapy*, *10*, 51–58.

Nadelson, C.C., & Notman, M.T. (1984). Psychodynamics of sexual assault experiences. In I.R. Stuart and J.G. Greer (eds), *Victims of sexual aggression: Treatment of children, women, and men*. New York: Van Nostrand Reinhold.

Nadelson, C.C., Notman, M.T., Jackson, H., & Garnick, J. (1982). A follow-up study of rape victims. *American Journal of Psychiatry*, *139*, 1266–1270.

Nisbett, R.E., & Ross, L. (1980). *Human inference: Strategies and shortcomings of social judgment*. Englewood Cliffs, NJ: Prentice-Hall.

Notman, M.T. & Nadelson, C.C. (1976). The rape victim: Psychodynamic considerations. *American Journal of Psychiatry*, *133*, 408–413.

Ochberg, F. (1986). The victim of terrorism. In R.H. Moos (ed.), *Coping with life crises*. New York: Plenum Press.

Parkes, C.M. (1971). Psycho-social transitions: A field of study. *Social Science and Medicine*, *5*, 101–115.

Parkes, C.M. (1975). What becomes of redundant world models? A contribution to the study of adaptation to change. *British Journal of Medical Psychology*, *48*, 131–137.

Perloff, L.S. (1983). Perceptions of vulnerability to victimization. *Journal of Social Issues*, *39(2)*, 41–62.

Peterson, C., Schwartz, S.M., & Seligman, M.E.P. (1981). Self-blame and depressive symptoms. *Journal of Personality and Social Psychology*, *41*, 253–259.

Piaget, J. (1971). *The construction of reality in the child*. New York: Basic Books.

Rachman, S.J. (1978). *Fear and courage*. San Francisco: W.H. Freeman.

Sales, E., Baum, M., & Shore, B. (1984). Victim readjustment following assault. *Journal of Social Issues*, *40*, 117–136.

Seligman, M.E.P. (1975). *Helplessness: On depression, development, and death*. San Francisco: W.H. Freeman.

Silver, R.L., & Wortman, C.B. (1980). Coping with undesirable life events. In J. Garber & M.E.P. Seligman (eds), *Human helplessness: Theory and application*. New York: Academic Press.

Strentz, T. (1982). The Stockholm syndrome: Law enforcement policy and hostage behavior. In F.M. Ochberg and D.A. Soskis (eds), *Victims of terrorism*. Boulder, Colorado: Westview Press.

Sullivan, H.S. (1940). *Conceptions of modern psychiatry*. New York: Norton.

Sullivan, H.S. (1953). *The interpersonal theory of psychiatry*. New York: Norton.

Symonds, M. (1982). Victim responses to terror: Understanding and treatment. In F.M. Ochberg and D.A. Soskis (eds), *Victims of terrorism*. Boulder, Colorado: Westview Press.

Taylor, S.E. (1983). Adjustment to threatening events: A theory of cognitive adaptation. *American Psychologist*, *38*, 1161–1173.

Taylor, S.E., Wood, J.V., & Lichtman, R.R. (1983). It could be worse: Selective evaluation as a response to victimization. *Journal of Social issues*, *39(2)*, 19–40.

Tennen, H., Affleck, G., & Gerschman, K. (1986). Self-blame among parents of infants with perinatal complications: The role of self-protective motives. *Journal of Personality and Social Psychology*, *50*, 690–696.

Tennen, H., Affleck, G., Allen, D.A., McGrade, B.J., & Ratzan, S. (1984). Causal attributions and coping with insulin-dependent diabetes. *Basic and Applied Social Psychology*, *5*, 131–142.

Timko, C., & Janoff-Bulman, R. (1985). Attributions, vulnerability, and psychological adjustment: The case of breast cancer. *Health Psychology*, *4*, 521–544.

Titchener, J.L., Kapp, F.T., & Winget, C. (1976). The Buffalo Creek syndrome: Symptoms and character change after a major disaster. In H.J. Parad, H.L.P. Resnik & L.G. Parad (eds), *Emergency and disaster management*. Bowie, MD: Charles Press.

Walker, L.E. (1979). *The battered woman*. New York: Harper & Row.

Weinstein, N.D. (1980). Unrealistic optimism about future life events. *Journal of Personality and Social Psychology*, *39*, 806–820.

Weinstein, N.D., & Lachendro, E. (1982). Egocentrism as a source of unrealistic optimism. *Personality and Social Psychology Bulletin*, *8*, 195–200.

Weis, K., & Weis, S. (1975). Victimology and the justification of rape. In I. Drapkin and E. Viano (eds), *Victimology: A new focus*. Vol. 3. Lexington, Mass.: Lexington Books.

Weisman, A.D. (1979). *Coping with cancer*. New York: McGraw-Hill.

Witenberg, S.H., Blanchard, E.B., Suls, J., Tennen, H. McCoy, G., & McGoldrick, M.D. (1983). Perceptions of control and causality as predictors of compliance and coping in hemodialysis. *Basic and Applied Social Psychology*, *40*, 650–663.

Wolfenstein, M. (1957). *Disaster: A psychological essay*. Glencoe, Ill.: The Free Press.

Wortman, C.B. (1976). Causal attributions and personal control. In J.H. Harvey, W.J. Ickes & R.F. Kidd (eds), *New directions in attributions research*, Vol. 1. Hillsdale, NJ: Lawrence.

Wortman, C.B., & Dunkel-Schetter, C. (1979). Interpersonal relationships and cancer: A theoretical analysis. *Journal of Social Issues*, *3(5)*, 120–155.

KEY WORDS

Victim, victimization, violence, psychological reactions, post-traumatic stress disorder, fear, anxiety, cognitive disorganization, assumptive world, schema, conceptual system, core assumptions, vulnerability/invulnerability, benevolence of the world, meaningfulness of event, self-worth, early childhood interactions, trust, coping, inappropriate victim reactions, psychological stability, internal reality, denial, Stockholm syndrome, self-blame, behavioural self-blame, characterological self-blame, crime victim, rape victim, victim of sexual assault, physical violation, psychological violation, control, justice.

Handbook of Life Stress, Cognition and Health
Edited by S. Fisher and J. Reason
© 1988 John Wiley & Sons Ltd

7

Environmental and Nuclear Threats

JENNIFER BROWN
University of Surrey

INTRODUCTION

The physical environment has posed threats and caused pain and suffering to human beings since time immemorial. Natural disasters such as flooding, earthquakes or volcanic eruptions as well as famine and disease have always exacted their tolls in death or injury. As science and technology advanced, methods were developed to warn and mitigate the consequences of these dangers. Progressively, discovery and invention have resulted in a longer, safer and generally more comfortable existence.

However, paradoxically, technology has emerged as a major source of hazard to modern society. The development of the chemical and energy industries particularly, whilst bringing many benefits, has also wrought the tragedies of Bhopal and Chernobyl. Even the universally useful and apparently innocuous ballpoint pen has been responsible for the deaths by choking of at least ten children in Great Britain since the 1970s (Department of Trade and Industry, 1986).

This chapter will examine the *kinds* of threats posed by both the natural and technological environments and the *effects* these threats have on individuals. The central theme of the chapter will be to argue the case for an integrated approach, in which environmental threat is set in the context of cultural, societal and individual psychological circumstances. It is proposed that environmental threats challenge an individual's assumptions about personal relationships, social roles and behaviour as well as harming her or his physical well-being.

In addition, a detailed case example is provided of the threat associated with nuclear power plants and radioactive waste repositories. Of all environmental threats, nuclear power is one of the most complex, involving, as it does, polarized views as to its necessity, safety and cost. A nuclear power plant provokes strong public reactions during its planning, construction, operation and decommissioning stages. There are highly emotive, connotative social meanings attached to radiation and nuclear waste. Thus nuclear power provides a focus to discuss many of the conceptual and methodological difficulties in describing responses to environmental threats. It also demonstrates the effectiveness of taking an integrated approach when trying to explain how and why nuclear power generates adverse and stressful responses.

DEFINITIONS, CLASSIFICATIONS AND UNDERLYING DIMENSIONS

Environmental threats may be defined as the potential or actual disruption of the expected functioning of the natural or technological worlds. Many, such as car accidents, noise nuisance, air pollution or bad weather conditions, exist in everyday life. Others occur less frequently and may be thought of as low probability but high consequence events, such as fire or explosions. In the language of the stress literature, these hazards, dangers or threats are defined as 'stressors'. 'Stress' is assumed to be the intervening process resulting in an individual's coping or adaptive response.

Some sources of environmental threat have already been mentioned, and the examples can be expanded to include: (a) upheavals of geological or weather conditions, e.g. tornados, blizzards, flooding, earthquake, volcanic eruptions or drought (Leik et al., 1981; Quarantelle, 1978); (b) exposure to extreme conditions of wet, cold, dry, heat, high or differential pressures (space or underwater) for exploration, commercial exploitation, military or recreational purposes (Bachrach, 1982); (c) removal to unfamiliar environments such as hospitals (Leventhal et al., 1982), schools (Fisher et al., 1984; Brown and Armstrong, 1986), or new homes (Kasl, 1982); (d) impacts of the ambient environment such as the quality of water (Moser, 1984), air (Evans et al., 1982), noise (Cohen et al., 1982), and crowding (Sigal, 1980); (e) impacts of the siting of technological facilities, e.g. liquefied energy gas terminals (Kunreuther, 1983), toxic waste dumps (Edelstein, 1986), nuclear power plants (Baum et al., 1982a).

In order to understand the various dimensions underpinning these many types of environmental threat, a number of classification schemes have been proposed. The main purposes of categorizing the threats are the prediction, control, amelioration or mitigation of their potential or actual damaging consequences. Cvetkovitch and Earle (1985) find the most common distinction made is that between the natural and technological environments (e.g. Baum et al., 1983a). Four general types of environmental stressors have been described: cataclysmic events, stressful life events, daily hassles (Lazarus and Cohen, 1977) and ambient stressors (Campbell, 1983). Cataclysmic events are sudden, are preceded by little or no warning, are powerful and have overwhelming impacts. They tend to involve large numbers of people. Examples would include the Mexico earthquake disaster, and accidents at nuclear power plants. Stressful life events have powerful consequences but affect fewer people, e.g. car accidents, death in the family. Daily hassles occur in daily life but typically do not present great adaptive difficulties, e.g. noise, commuting problems. Ambient stressors are chronic but non-urgent, continuous conditions of the environment that may contribute to ill-health or worry, e.g. routine operation of a chemical plant.

Classifications can be useful if they are sensible and unproblematic. However, as Baum *et al.* (1982c, p. 25) point out: 'these various ways of classifying stressors do not always work. To different degrees some stressors cut across a number of distinctions.' Take the example of a nuclear reactor: it may produce a cataclysmic event if there is an accident, yet during its routine operation it may simply present one of life's daily hassles to those living within its environs. Similarly, it may only present a source of stress whilst it is being planned or built, and the threat may be adapted to once the plant is successfully operating. Also, clear-cut categories do not always reflect the blurring of definitions of real-life situations.

Another approach is to look at the differences engendered by impacts of ordinary versus exceptional circumstances. Kates (1981) proposes that life today might appear more secure, but this may be illusionary. Medical advances and improvements in safety, whilst preserving and increasing the longevity of life, may also endanger it. In the everyday context, scientific or technical advance, administrative oversight or regulatory failure may result in harm from ordinary objects, as with the children choking to death on ballpoint pens. Moreover, an environment that seems innocuous may not be, even in its routine operation. A cash dispenser or a lift button would not be considered an environmental threat except by an individual of restricted growth or skill. Against a background of possible insecurities created by daily life, there is also the occurrence of unexpected or exceptional events. Public concern tends to focus on the low probability, high consequence events such as accidents.

A corollary to the distinction between everyday and exceptional circumstances is the point elaborated by Murdock *et al.* (1987) in the context of a study of the proposed siting of a radioactive waste repository in Deaf Smith County, Texas. It is their contention that any new facility of whatever kind would pose threats to a community. These 'standard' threats would be recognized and consensually agreed, and include economic impacts on local employment, business activity and the income structure; population growth and settlement patterns of new migrants; use of community services; changes in community leadership patterns. In addition there are the 'special' effects of the particular environmental intrusion, in this case a radioactive waste repository. They identify four types of special effects: fear and anxiety, concern with equity, institutional concerns regarding security, and public participation and monitoring. The standard threats may be more objectively determined, whilst the special effects are more a function of individual assessment and judgement.

EFFECTS OF ENVIRONMENTAL STRESSORS

Broadly speaking, the impacts on individuals of environmental stressors can be categorized into physical, cognitive and affective. Numerous studies have shown that a wide variety of noxious environmental stimuli have physiological effects such as increasing blood pressure, respiration rates or muscle tension (Baum *et al.*, 1982c). Idzikowski and Baddeley (1983) present evidence of physiological reactions by soldiers under combat stress, reporting, for example, decreased levels of secretion of testosterone and other androgens in American soldiers fighting in Vietnam.

Certain cognitive deficits have also been demonstrated on task performance under stress. Broadbent (1963) reviewed a series of studies showing that monitoring tasks were more poorly performed as a consequence of high temperature, noise or sleep deprivation. Stress can also result in speech breakdown, e.g. increases in rate or pitch, or speech errors (reviewed by Argyle, 1975).

Affective and interpersonal behaviours, too, are affected by stressful environmental conditions and may show individuals in the best or worst lights. For example, Kasperson and Pijawka (1985) show that, in the context of 'therapeutic communities', in the immediate post disaster period there is a spontaneous expression of concern and helping behaviour by victims and non-victims alike before the institutional and organizational resources are summoned. On the other hand, Cohen and Spacapan (1984) show the more negative side of less altruism and co-operation and an increase in aggressive behaviours under stressful conditions

METHODOLOGICAL ISSUES

A number of methodological difficulties have been noted in relation to the impact of environmental stress. In the case of unfamiliar potential environmental threats, e.g. the siting of nuclear or toxic waste plants, the intervention of the investigator creates the first opportunity for respondents to formulate their views. Individuals may learn as much about issues of concern from the format and content of the questions (see Brown and White, 1987). There are conflicts between choice of individual differences or aggregate group responses. Individual variation is more difficult to explain and makes the theoretical work harder for the social scientist (see Evans and Cohen, 1987). Also, the use of open-ended self-report measures can be problematic because of the difficulties of validity and reliability, intentional and unintentional distortions. If a person is being asked about their views on ground-water contamination, their unfavourable response may be due to genuine concern, or a wish to facilitate compensation payments. Similarly, an apparently neutral reponse may be the consequence of successful denial or repression or a genuine appraisal that the contamination does not present a hazard. Measurements of responses in this area of research are sensitive to all the constraints of empirical investigation, e.g. demand characteristics of the questioner, setting, and temporal factors. There are also difficulties in relating the more objective indices of threat with subjective judgements. For example, physical measurable properties of stress, such as catecholamines or corticosteroid output may not correlate with psychological indices of a person's subjective feelings of stress. There are also ethical issues, discussed by Idzikowski and Baddeley (1983). Clearly, investigators should not subject people to threatening or frightening stimuli in order to study their responses. Avoiding this problem by studying naturally occurring disasters raises further difficulties, such as intrusion into private grief. Also, such events, by their nature, are unpredictable, and often inaccessible.

THEORETICAL BACKGROUND

Physiological Perspective

Evans and Cohen (1987) suggest that research on environmental stress falls within two research traditions: the physiological and the psychological. In an excellent review of biological models of environmental stress they focus on the physiological responses to noxious stimuli. Cannon (1932) argued that the body has an autonomic emergency response system of flight or fight from any potential challenging situation. Selye (1956) referred to the general adaptation syndrome (GAS), consisting of alarm (increased heart rate and adrenaline secretion), resistence (sweating or shivering), and exhaustion.

Evans and Cohen point out that one of the most problematic aspects of Selye's model has been what triggers the general adaptation syndrome in real-life situations. More especially, Evans (1982) notes three main issue of interest: (a) the importance of meaning—people live in a socially constructed as well as physical world (rock music may be both pleasurable or aversive, depending on one's musical taste); (b) the consideration of other impacts apart from the physical, e.g. disruption of one's personal or community relationships; (c) the limitations of laboratory-based research making extrapolation to real life problematic.

Psychological Perspectives

Several different approaches can be identified that derive from psychophysics, psychometrics, theories of attitude and social behaviour, and clinical psychology.

Psychophysics

Signal detection theory provides a methodology to examine the ability of people to detect stimulus objects. Responses are classified as correct hits, false hits, correct misses and false misses. Often it is used in conjunction with other explanatory frameworks to determine the sensitivity and accuracy of perception. Thus Evans *et al.* (1982) wished to separate observer response bias and perceptual sensitivity of individuals towards photochemical smog in Los Angeles. Their study revealed differences in response bias between residents with either recent or long-term experiences with poor ambient air quality.

Psychometrics

Differences in the perception of hazards have been the focus of much of the research effort by psychological risk analysts. Hitherto, engineering and actuarial studies of the risk of technological facilities concentrated on their physical and measurable properties. It was recognized that discrepancies existed between these objective indices and the subjective judgements of the lay public.

Risk perception studies are concerned with understanding differential judgements of the riskiness of various hazards. Fischhoff *et al.* (1978) asked people to judge some 90 hazards on different criteria. Factor analysis showed three underlying dimensions: 'dread' risks concerned with hazards that are judged to be fatal or catastrophic compared to those with less severe consequences; imposed, involuntary technological risks versus voluntary, known, technical risks; and a societal/personal consequences factor.

Slovic and his group have also highlighted the importance of biases in perception. They propose that lay people not only use qualitative criteria by which to judge hazards, but also are influenced by memorable instances. So a disaster graphically and dramatically portrayed, especially if it shows vulnerable individuals such as children at risk, may lead to erroneous beliefs about the likelihood of accidents. Slovic *et al.* (1982) illustrate this process with reference to nuclear power, showing it being particularly susceptible to perceptual biases.

Social Psychology

Theories of attitude developed by Fishbein and Ajzen (1975) provide important insights into psychological effects of environmental threat. Their expectancy–value model of attitude formation has been used widely in the study of public reactions to nuclear power. The approach broadly assumes that there are both positive, or beneficial, and negative, or adverse, attributes of an object. The greater the belief in positive attributes, the more likely it is that a person will be favourably inclined towards that object. Many studies adopt a factor analytic method to reveal the cognitive structure of beliefs (Lounsbury *et al.*, 1977; Otway *et al.*, 1978) which show that people think about nuclear energy in terms of economic factors, environmental consequences, sociopolitical implications, psychological risks and local impacts. As one might expect, public attitudes become progressively more 'anti' as the possibility increases of a nuclear power station being built in their own locality (Van der Plight *et al.*, 1985). Furthermore, those who are in favour, as compared with those who are opposed to nuclear power, show marked differences in the importance that they attach to socio-economic, environmental and health consequences of building a nuclear power station. This fits with the research showing that attitudes are important mediators in the response to environmental stressors. Baum *et al.* (1982c) reviewed a series of studies showing that fear of flying is a significant factor in the response to aircraft noise.

Within social psychology there are also formulations concerning the importance of the roles people adopt and the rules or patterns of behaviour that influence their actions (cf. Harré and Secord, 1972). These role rule models have been used by environmental psychologists to explain the relationships between people and their physical surroundings (Canter, 1985). Sime (1983) provides strong evidence to show how social relationships between individuals proved critical in their escape from a fire in 1973 at the Summerland Leisure complex on the Isle of Man, Great Britain. Some 3000 holidaymakers were in the building which caught fire and 30 people died. Sime's analysis of 148 police witness statements of survivors in the solarium part of the complex showed that most attempted to escape with family or group members. Canter (1985, p. 221) cites an example from the Kentucky Supper Club blaze in which waitresses apparently showed patrons at their own tables out of the building, often leaving customers at adjacent tables to their own devices.

Clinical Orientation

Two approaches may be subsumed under what is broadly defined as a clinical psychological approach: first, the work of Lazarus and his collaborators (Lazarus, 1966; Lazarus and Cohen, 1977; Lazarus and Launier, 1978), and, second, the work on clinical depression by Brown and Harris (1978).

Lazarus' model focuses on the individual's interpretation of the meanings of environmental events, and an appraisal of her or his ability to cope. Appraisal may be primary, i.e. evaluation of the stressor, or secondary, i.e. evaluation of personal coping resources. Primary appraisal takes into account both personal and situational variables, and includes beliefs about self-efficacy, centrality of goals or needs threatened by the stressor. Secondary appraisal may focus on problem-solving strategies on the one hand or emotional coping on the other. In other words, an individual may either change some aspect of the situation or redefine or redirect the anxiety provoked by the situation. Coping strategies include information seeking, direct action or palliative activity.

Evans and Cohen (1987) point out three important implications: the individuals' perceptions are the key to determining coping response; objective properties of the environment are important only to the extent that they inform the processes of appraisal; and both personal and social mediators can ameliorate or enhance the effects of stress. Thus environmental threats are not uniformly aversive. Moreover, the stressor can affect an individual's interpersonal relationships, cognitive functioning, and physical well-being.

Brown and Harris (1978) painstakingly evolved over several years a complex methodology for examining life events and psychiatric symptomology. They indicate (p. 83) the importance of examining environmental contexts as part of a detailed investigation of life events in relation to depression. In particular, they were interested in the interplay between the exceptional and the unusual. They state (p. 84) that the exceptional 'may deny to us a sense of reality'. Change, at least temporarily, challenges the person's 'assumptive world'. In other words, an event, action or crisis alters a person's views about her or himself, affecting aspirations about particular lifestyles. Having undermined, assumed or taken for granted relationships or behaviours, crises raise fundamental questions about cherished beliefs which force a critical reappraisal of an individual's life.

Brown and Harris have two indices of threat. The 'objective' index takes into account the observable events and surrounding circumstances. In essence, trained observers rate how most people might react to these circumstances. This is used in conjunction with the self-reported measures.

Main Conclusions

Each of these approaches has some insights to offer towards explaining human assessment of and response to environmental threats. The risk perception studies reveal important differences in the ranking of the riskiness of hazards among different social groups. However, the technique requires people to make somewhat arbitrary comparisons, e.g. between the risks of using pesticides or going skiing. The factor analytical studies which have identified the structure of risk perceptions as dread, familiarity and scale of exposure, have been the subject of a different interpretation (Wynne, in press). Wynne takes the case of the perception of nuclear energy, its association with the atomic bomb, and the unseen, all-penetrating power of radiation. Dread, he argues, is a code for the nature of the relationship between the knowable experts and the ignorant, 'irrational' public. In other words, experts who understand nuclear physics perceive nuclear power plants as technically controllable, the public, who do not, resort to dread. Thus dread is not an individual psychological response but rather the recognition of this social distance. Wynne's thesis, that a sociological level of analysis is necessary to examine the political conflicts and styles of risk-managing institutions, is reiterated by Short (1984). He argues convincingly that risk assessment takes place within the social fabric, and it is crucial to examine both group and institutional structures.

Approaches based on eliciting the structure of attitudes have found some important distinctions in the salience of beliefs of different groups in the assessment and response to environmental threats. Raynor (1984) and Raynor and Cantor (1987) take the notion of attitudes further, and propose a cultural hypothesis in stating that 'for different institutional settings each generates its own characteristic view of the world variously referred to as a cosmology or cultural bias. In turn it has been suggested that characteristic attributes of cultural bias, particularly preferred aesthetics, principles of social justice and perceived economic interest, will lead members of each type of institution to choose a particular liability distribution' (p. 5).

The cultural hypothesis also addresses the issue of why some people worry about certain hazards and not others (Douglas and Wildavsky, 1982). This question of selection of worry is not directly tackled by psychological models of stress. Sometimes stated as the 'worry bead' hypothesis (Kates, 1981), the suggestion is that groups or individuals have a small stock of worry beads to dispense on the many and various threats there are in the world. They are constrained in their choices by limitations of knowledge, cultural, ideological or personal aversions, or simply by the overwhelming number of threats about which to worry. Society's capacity to worry intelligently exceeds that of individuals, hence it is possible to divide the labour and distribute the anxiety. In some cases, worry may be deferred to the managing institution or even to the pressure group whose lobbying activity activates the managers.

Towards an Integrated Approach

The importance of considering contextual perspectives is illustrated by a longitudinal study of the impact of aircraft noise on elementary school children in Los Angeles by Cohen et al. (1986). They established that the child's school and home domains are interdependent, finding, for example, 'that noise abatement intervention was associated with a greater reduction of blood pressure among children living within quieter homes rather than in those within noisier areas' (p. 186). They argue that particular phenomena are embedded in and influenced by their surroundings, and suggest that research should be directed at identifying the salient contextual variables as well as the target phenomena. The first principle of their contextual analysis is that psychological phenomena should be viewed in relation to the spatial, temporal and sociocultural milieus in which they occur. Secondly, the focus on individuals' responses to discrete events in the short term should be replaced by molar and longitudinal analysis of everyday activities and settings. Thirdly, the search for lawful and general relationships between environment and behaviour should be counterbalanced by situation-specific phenomena. Finally, external as well as internal validity should be considered.

Contextual analysis emphasizes the importance of inextricable relationships between disciplines. Such a view is proposed by Canter (1985) in his plea for bridge building between the social and environmental psychologists to deal more effectively with the social and physical environments.

NUCLEAR THREATS

Nature is such that wealth can be wrested from her only by toil and often at great risk. Radium presents one of nature's toughest tasks, but for the sake of humanity workers toil in mine and laboratory regardless of danger or risk (*Children's new encyclopaedia*, 1947).

Introduction

This section will focus on the actual and potential threats of nuclear facilities, such as reactors and radioactive waste repositories. Nuclear installations pose threats at their planning, construction, operational and decommissioning stages. There is the physical harm to life and property through an actual accident; worry and concern anticipating accidents; socioeconomic and sociopolitical impacts on the local community and society at large. The Chernobyl tragedy confirmed that these are real and not just perceived threats. Moreover, Chernobyl demonstrated that the dangers are not confined spatially to the immediate locality of the plant, nor temporally to the immediate aftermath of the accident. For these reasons, together with its military connotations, nuclear power is a rather particular example of an environmental threat.

Richardson *et al.* (1987) suggest studies of impacts of nuclear power suffer from a lack of integrated theoretical underpinnings. They state (p. 17) 'case studies, instead of attempting to develop or test a theory, have focused on describing the peculiarities of response given the specific threat and incident.'

The remainder of this section will discuss a range of findings that represent the different layers of analysis, running from the broadest societal level to that of the individual.

Cultural Context

A number of investigators discuss the climate and prevailing societal trends within which the nuclear energy issue is embedded (Kates, 1981; Mitchell, 1982; Otway and Peltu, 1985; O'Riordan, 1983). These trends include: (a) increases in the scale of industrial accidents (e.g. Flixborough, Chernobyl, Bhopal); (b) revelations about the frailty or culpability of experts or multinational corporations (e.g. the Thalidomide tragedy or the shuttle disaster); (c) the political use of environmental issues highlighting problems of resource allocation and exploitation, or the centralization of decision making. (d) legislative responses; (e) the role played by the media not only in disseminating information but also in setting the agenda by giving extensive space to environmental disasters in a simplified but largely uncritical way.

Institutional Responses

Exceptional Circumstances

Accidents such as those at Three Mile Island and Chernobyl are examples of cataclysmic environmental threats. Under these circumstances, the managing and regulating institutions respond to mitigate or contain the physical as well as the psychological impacts of the accidents. Following the accident at Three Mile Island (TMI), the US Congress considered a moritorium on the operation of nuclear plants. President Carter instigated a special commission of inquiry, and the Nuclear Regulatory Commission sponsored over a hundred projects concerned with various aspects of the accident. As well as technical considerations, the social and political implications were considered. The American Civil Liberties Union was concerned by the threats to employees in nuclear power plants through surveillance and vetting procedures. The Federal, state and local authorities had reason to examine emergency preparedness. In particular, the role of the media and its dissemination of information and relationship with the utility, Edison Metropolitan, were closely scrutinized.

The President's Commission pinpointed the problems of TMI as human error rather than equipment failure as a major contributing factor. In particular they focused on the concept of 'mindset', i.e. managerial preoccupation with safety of equipment and serious underestimation of the human element (see Sills *et al.*, 1982).

Ordinary Circumstances

In more prosaic times, governmental and operating bodies attempt to provide information and communicate with the public about nuclear power. In the UK, the nuclear industry comprises the Atomic Energy Authority, the National Nuclear Corporation, the South of Scotland Electricity Board, the Central Electricity Generating Board, British Nuclear Fuels, as well as various governmental and independent regulatory and research bodies. Reviewing their institutional styles of handling information to the public, we found a number of distinctive strategies (Henderson *et al.*, 1986). They may ignore the problem and underwhelm people by giving little or no information, boring them with dull and uninteresting technical material, diffusing attention by announcing multiple potential sites or omitting crucial or controversial information. Another strategy involves attempts to allay anxiety by demonstrations such as crashing trains with (empty) radioactive waste containers to show they will not split open, providing educational material, or engaging in consultation. Most rarely, public sensitivities are accommodated by modification of their plans, cancellation of projects, or payment of compensation to affected individuals or communities. Recently, this strategy was used by the UK's Department of the Environment when it renounced its plans for shallow burial of low level radioactive waste, considering instead an above-ground storage option at nuclear power stations.

The General Public's Response

Exceptional Circumstances

To date the Three Mile Island accident has been the most extensively studied in terms of impact on public opinion. Research by Mitchell (1982) showed that, immediately following the accident, the percentage of the public in favour of nuclear power dropped from 52% to 44% and those opposed rose from 42% to 43%. A further 13% were uncertain, a difference of 7% compared with pre-TMI levels. By January 1981, measured opinion had returned to pre-TMI levels, i.e. 52% in favour, 39% against and 9% uncertain.

From Mitchell's analysis, it is evident that there was not a great upsurge of support for the anti-nuclear movement, nor was there an appreciable increase in the public's knowledge of nuclear power despite saturation coverage in the media. Previous studies had indicated that a good predictor of support or opposition to nuclear power is assessment of safety. There was hardly any shift after TMI. Mitchell reports that 30% of Americans thought nuclear power stations unsafe after TMI compared with 28% before, a non-statistically significant difference. Mitchell proposes this apparent lack of reaction can be explained by examining the sociopolitical and economic contexts.

The accident occurred during a petrol crisis which had served to heighten Americans' awareness of the nation's need for indigenous energy sources. President Carter had been critical of the nuclear industry, yet he supported it after the accident. No-one was actually killed as a direct consequence of the accident, and the estimates of possible cancer deaths following releases of radiation were low. The kind of accident, a loss of coolant, was a predicted credible accident, and the engineering system did contain the damage. Thus, people who were already opposed to or uneasy about nuclear power had their worst fears confirmed; those who supported nuclear power could be reassured that, in the event, a major catastrophe was averted. Hence, no major realignment of opinion occurred. It might also be added that the American nuclear industry was already suffering a decline in public support, which Greenhaulgh (1980) suggests was more to do with interest rates and other economic factors than with anti-nuclear feeling. At the time then, in 1979, there is support for the view that for the American public at large, TMI did not have a sustained effect. This is not to say that, taken as one in a series of serious or catastrophic accidents, it has not contributed, cumulatively, to erode belief in nuclear technology. That belief has been further eroded by that other cataclysmic accident, Chernobyl.

The impact of Chernobyl on the British public does present a somewhat different case. The sociopolitical climate within which the accident occurred was much more critical. A prestigious Parliamentary Committee, chaired by Sir Hugh Rossi, had severely criticized Britain's nuclear industry. In February, potential sites were announced for low and intermediate level radioactive waste disposal which aroused local hostility and were much vented in the national press. Moreover, Britain has large coal reserves as a major alternative to nuclear power. The Chernobyl disaster did kill a reported 31 individuals, and a further 200 are believed to be suffering the acute effects of radiation. Many more are expected to die prematurely from excess cancers.

Results of an attitude survey of 420 people (reported in Brown and White, 1987) indicate there was not only an increase in worry after Chernobyl (27% to 41%), but also an increase in the number of people who thought that nuclear power stations are dangerous (26% to 39%). Rather more interesting is the behavioural response of the British public following Chernobyl. Brown and White (1987) estimated, by contacting various organizations, that approximately 800 000 people telephoned some agency, such as the Department of the Environment, Friends of the Earth, National Radiological Protection Board, or the Sun newspaper help line, for information on, or to be given reassurance about, the dangers of radiation. This represents about 2% of the adult population of Great Britain.

Ordinary Circumstances

In the ordinary course of events, neither nuclear power stations nor radioactive waste are perceived as an environmental threat by the general public. Bearing in mind the methodological difficulties alluded to in an earlier section, empirical findings can be found to support this assertion. First, indicators of involvement in environmental issues in general, and nuclear energy controversies in particular, show low levels of membership of environmental organizations or complaints. An international study was carried out in 1982 by the International Insitute for Environment and Society. Results of the UK survey (n=438) indicated 4% to be members of an environmental group or at least interested in becoming a member, although 30% claimed to have complained at least once to someone in authority about an environmental problem. Watts (1988) compares European countries, and finds the British people to be characterized by low levels both of complaint and environmental awareness.

Secondly, self-reported answers to open-ended questions about the kinds of things that worry people (cf. the worry bead hypothesis) indicate a low level of spontaneous mentions of nuclear power—less than 4% (Cooper, 1984; Social and

Community Planning Research, 1982). In the latter study the highest proportion of answers—27%—related to fear of car accidents.

Thirdly, in an attempt to overcome the problem that non-response could be interpreted as denial or repression of anxiety, we conducted a perceptual defence experiment (Pollard, 1984). This was an exploratory study with 14 respondents from the University of Surrey volunteer panel. Individuals were shown a number of words, varying in length, that were nuclear related (e.g. nuclear power), anxiety provoking (e.g. heart attack), common (e.g. garden fence), or non-words, at subperceptual threshold. The duration of exposure was increased until correct recognition was achieved. The perceptual defence paradigm suggests that threatening words will take longer to recognize because individuals seek to protect themselves from the anxiety that the word generates. The word recognition test failed to provide a perceptual defence effect. Respondent's galvanic skin responses were also measured: greatest reaction was obtained from the non-nuclear anxiety-provoking words. Finally, on a semantic differential rating, the nuclear words were most often rated as frightening or worrying. Admittedly this was a small sample and an exploratory study, but it is tempting to conclude that the connotative meaning attached to the nuclear stimuli resulted in the cognitive appraisal of the words as threatening. Attempts to measure physical or emotional reactions showed greatest effects for the non-nuclear threatening stimuli. In other words, it is a social labelling response reminiscent of Wynne's conceptual analysis rather than an emotional psychological reaction.

The attitudinal literature, referred to in an earlier section, would suggest until an issue becomes salient or important to individuals, it is unlikely to have an impact on them. Richardson *et al.* (1987) demonstrated that sensitivity, defined as awareness, experience and preoccupation, was the greatest predictor of hostile attitudes towards nuclear power. Salience of the issue may be affected by either a national news story, such as an accident to a nuclear plant, or local communities being chosen as potential hosts for nuclear facilities.

Local Public's Reactions

Exceptional Circumstances

Of all environmental threats, radioactive waste invokes one of the strongest reactions from the public. Brown and White (1987) show that, from a national sample of 1511 UK citizens questioned in December 1984, 90% claimed they would oppose and take action against proposals to site a radioactive waste facility. This compares with 73% who claim they would oppose an airport, 59% a motorway, and 46% an industrial estate. Results from an unpublished quantitative survey (conducted by the Department of Psychology at the University of Surrey in 1986) of four villages proposed as potential sites for low level and intermediate short-lived radioactive wastes, indicated that nearly a quarter of the villagers spontaneously mentioned radioactive waste as an issue of social concern. The other concerns most frequently mentioned were violence (26%) and unemployment (56%). When specifically asked, 21% of the 1,966 respondents said they

were very worried, 24% quite a lot, and 21% somewhat worried about radioactive
waste. Over a third volunteered strong negative emotional reaction as their first
response to the announcement.

In the qualitative part of their study, four researchers spent 6 months monitoring local villagers' reactions. Space permits only outlining results for one of the
locations, Fulbeck, a village in rural Lincolnshire of about 2600 people. This
summary derives from a paper prepared by Howard (1986). He argued in favour
of reviewing the past social history of the village and surrounding communities in
order to understand present reactions. Fulbeck's community identity had been
progressively eroded with the loss of the village school and jobs, with commercial,
education, and entertainment needs being beyond the resources of the village.
Progressively, migrants from the professional classes had changed the social
composition of the village. The initial reactions are very reminiscent of the
challenge to the assumptive world hypothesis. This can most graphically be
illustrated by reference to a song recorded by a local band and which became the
theme song of the protesters.

> It's a little pretty village on a hillside by a stream,
> A place to bring your kids up and to realise your dream,
> There's cattle in the meadow and there's skylarks singing clear
> And radioactivity we don't want here.

> We don't want to move from Fulbeck and
> perhaps it's just as well,
> For now it's a fact that our houses won't sell
> So what will be our future here and what will be our world
> If Nirex dumps their everlasting poison in the earth.

For individuals, it was a time of crisis, challenging fundamental assumptions about
their lives and values. A notable example was the local squire, a former High
Sheriff of Lincolnshire, with parliamentary aspirations—a conviction and cradle
Conservative. The proposals profoundly shocked his political and philosophical
convictions. More generally, the proposals provided an opportunity to rediscover
community spirit and integrate the new migrants with the established residents.
There are examples of the personal growth outcomes highlighted by Edelstein
(1986) in his study of local people's reaction to ground-water contamination.
Howard (1986) notes, 'groups of the populous, both those born and bred in the
area, wives and/or mothers from across the social spectrum who did not have
specialised jobs outside the home, joined together for special events.'

Supportive evidence from the quantitative survey indicated an association
between spontaneous expressions of worry and concern, not only with anti-
nuclear attitudes, but also with the level of active protest. Of the total sample
(n=1966), less than 20% of those in favour of nuclear power expressed spontaneous feelings of worry, whilst nearly 30% of those against did so. Ninety per
cent of the self-declared unworried group did not take part in any protest action,
compared to 6% of those expressing worry; i.e. 94% (n=342) of worriers took at
least one action to register their protest.

What of local residents living near the scene of a nuclear accident. The most relevant series of students from the present point of view are those conducted by Andrew Baum and his colleagues, of people living in or near Harrisburg, scene of the Three Mile Island reactor accident (Baum, Fleming and Singer, 1982; Baum *et al.*, 1983; Fleming and Baum, 1985; Fleming *et al.*, 1985). They have undertaken an intensive and imaginative analysis of the appraisal and coping strategies of local residents: examining physiological measures of stress (urinary catecholamines), behavioural effects (cognitive performance), and affective response (rating on a standardized symptom checklist). They also looked at mediating factors such as influence of social support systems. Their results are 'not suggestive of severe hardship of debilitating stress, rather most are subclinical' (Baum *et al.*, 1982, p. 243).

This group of studies is informative in terms of both the methodological perspective and the analysis of the response to threat, but the findings, by the authors' own admission, are equivocal with respect to the generality and duration of debilitating effect of this accident on local residents. However, taken with other polls, there is no doubt the accident was disturbing to inhabitants in the immediate locality. Opinion polls of local residents conducted for the Nuclear Regulatory Commission found that just under half of those questioned thought the situation very serious, 19% serious, 21% somewhat serious, whilst 12% thought it posed no threat at all. Flynn (1982) concluded her review of the available evidence on local people's reactions by stating, 'the amount of stress experienced by people living near Three Mile Island was a function of the perceived amount of threat to physical safety and the reliability of information being used to ascertain the degree of danger'. (p. 55).

Ordinary Circumstances

People who live within the vicinity of a nuclear establishment have the opportunity to adapt to the potential threat. Evidence from surveys by the Department of Psychology at the University of Surrey, conducted in 1982 in the South West of England and in 1985 in East Anglia and Somerset, indicates that living near nuclear plant does not invoke self-reported anxiety. It may be that the residents feeling most anxiety move away, decline to participate in surveys, or successfully repress their emotional responses. We did conduct an analysis of the attitudes and self-reported worry of migrants versus indigenous populations, and found no significant differences in our Somerset and Avon populations, both localities hosting nuclear reactors. In Cornwall, a proposed green field site, the indigenous population were more antagonistic, and in Dorset, site of an experimental reactor, the migrants were more likely to oppose the building of a commercial reactor.

The refusal rate for the surveys averaged 20%, largely from respondents who were old, whose first language was not English, or who felt they knew nothing and could not comment on the topic. On the problem of our analyses being insensitive to respondents successfully denying or repressing anxiety, we can only report that generally speaking, spontaneous mentions that nuclear power was an issue of concern or worry was never greater than 15%. Information seeking was low. In one survey, around the Somerset Hinkley Point reactor, of 489 respondents, only 9% could be classified as active information seekers. Earle (1984) suggests that amongst consumers, active information seekers range between 10% and 20%. Thirty-five per cent of local people indicated they talked about the nuclear issue with family or friends, 7% indicated they were very worried when specifically asked, and 3% volunteered nuclear energy as a personal worry. It was our conclusion, from the survey evidence, numerous detailed interviews we carried out with local people, and the large numbers of apparently reassured local visitors to the Hinkley Point reactors, that during its routine operation the power plant is not perceived as a source of environmental threat.

SUMMARY AND CONCLUSIONS

There can be little doubt that the environment presents itself in a threatening form in some circumstances. So-called cataclysmic events such as large-scale natural or technological disaster cause death and injury and damage livelihoods and property. The effect on survivors may be long lasting. On a smaller scale, the quality of air, water, sound, and thermal comfort may also act as environmental stressors. Research suggests that people invoke both cognitive and emotional appraisal of the harmfulness of the threats and call upon various coping responses. They may take direct action to combat the threats or palliative actions to minimize or ignore them.

The degree to which people define something as threatening in the first place and subsequently cope with a threat, interacts with the broader social, political and cultural contexts, as well as their own individual resources. The risk perception literature of psychologists, sociologists and anthropoligists offers concepts and a framework into which environmental stressors and their meaning may be embedded.

Nuclear power is widely believed to be a universal environmental threat, yet the evidence suggests that under ordinary circumstances this is not so. It becomes so under unusual circumstances of accidents or siting proposals. However, it is difficult to separate the responses of people to the actual or potential threat of harm from nuclear installations and the symbolic meaning attached to it. Nuclear power has acted as a rallying point for aversion to centralized decision making, large-scale industrialization, and pre-eminent role of established expertise. Examining the impact of environmental stressors generally and nuclear power in particular is a complex task, best tackled by a contextual approach.

Acknowledgements

The research on public attitudes towards nuclear power station and radioactive waste sites in the Department of Psychology, University of Surrey, has been variously funded by the Central Electricity Generating Board, the Department of the Environment, United Kingdom Atomic Energy Authority, and the Health and Safety Executive. The overall director of the Research is Professor Terence

Lee, and members of the team include Joyce Henderson, Helen White, Cameron Adams, Keith Howard, Jenny Ward and Ian Waters. Judith Spencer is a post-graduate student attached to the project.

I would like to acknowledge Elizabeth Campbell and Gary Evans for their reading and helpful comments on earlier drafts of this chapter, Shirley Fisher for her thorough editorial suggestions, and Mary Banbury and Pauline Elliott for their patience in typing drafts of the manuscript.

REFERENCES

Argyle, M. (1975). *Bodily communication*. London: Methuen.

Bachrach, A.J. (1982). The human in extreme environments. In A. Baum, & J. Singer (eds), *Environment and health*, pp. 211–236. Hillsdale, NJ: Lawrence Erlbaum.

Baum, A., Fleming, R., & Davidson, L.M. (1983a). Natural disaster and technological catastrophe. *Environment and Behavior, 15*, 333–354.

Baum, A., Fleming, R., & Singer, J. (1982a). Stress at Three Mile Island; Applying psychological impact analysis. In L. Bickman (ed.), *Applied social psychology annual* (pp. 217–248). Beverly Hills, Calif.: Sage.

Baum, A., Gatchel, R.J., & Schaeffer, M. (1983b). Emotional, behavioural and physiological effects of chronic stress at Three Mile Island. *Journal of Consulting and Clinical Psychology, 51*, 565–72.

Baum, A., Grunberg, N., & Singer, J.E. (1982b). The use of psychological and neuroendocrinology measurements in the study of stress. *Health Psychology, 1*, 217–236.

Baum, A., Singer, J., & Baum, C. (1982c). Stress and the environment. In G. Evans (ed.), *Environmental Stress* (pp. 15–44). Cambridge: University Press.

Broadbent, D.E. (1963). Differences and interactions between stresses. *Quarterly Journal of Experimental Psychology, 15*, 201–211.

Brown, G., & Harris, T. (1978). *Social origins of depression*. London: Tavistock.

Brown, J., & Armstrong, M. (1986). Transfer from junior to secondary; The child's perspective. In M.B. Youngman (ed.), *Mid-schooling transfer: Problems and proposals* (pp. 29–46). Slough: NFER-Nelson.

Brown, J., & White, H. (1987). The public's understanding of radiation and nuclear waste. *Journal of the Society for Radiological Protection, (7)2*, 61–70.

Campbell, J.M. (1983). Ambient stressors. *Environment and Behaviour, 15*, 355–380.

Cannon, W.B. (1932). *The wisdom of the body*. New York: Norton.

Canter, D. (1985). Putting situations in their place. In A. Furnham (ed.), *Social behaviour in context* (pp. 208–239). Boston: Allyn and Bacon.

Children's new encyclopaedia (1947). London: Collins.

Cohen, S., & Spacapan, S. (1984). The social psychology of noise. In D.M. Jones & A.J. Chapman (eds), *Noise and society* (pp. 221–245). New York: John Wiley & Sons.

Cohen, S., Krantz, D.S. Evans, G.M., & Stokols, D. (1982). Community noise, behaviour and health; The Los Angeles Noise Project. In A. Baum & J. Singer (eds), *Environment and health* (pp. 295–317). Hillsdale, NJ: Lawrence Erlbaum.

Cohen, S., Evans, G.W., Stokols, D., & Krantz, D.S. (1986). *Behaviour, health and environmental stress*. New York: Plenum.

Cooper, I. (1984). Lay views of energy conservation in Britain. *Applied Energy, 18*, (261–300).

Cvetkovich, G., & Earle, T.C. (1985). Classifying hazardous events. *Journal of Environmental Psychology, 5*, 5–36.

Department of Trade and Industry (1986). *Home accidents. Home Accident Surveillance System*, Ninth Annual Report—1985 data. London: Consumer Safety Unit, Department of Trade and Industry.

Douglas, M., & Wildavsky, A. (1982). *Risk and culture*. Berkeley, Calif.: University of California.

Earle, T.C. (1984). Risk communication: A marketing approach. Paper prepared for NSF/EPA Workshop on Risk Perception and Risk Communication, Long Beach, California, December.

Edelstein, M.R. (1986). Psychosocial impacts of toxic exposure. An overview. In H.A. Becker & A.L. Porter (eds), *Impact assessment today* (pp. 761–776). Utrecht: Uitgeverij Jan Van Arkel.

Evans, G.W. (ed.) (1982. *Environmental stress*. New York: Cambridge University Press.

Evans, G.W., & Cohen, S. (1987). Environmental Stress. In D. Stokols & I. Altman (eds), *Handbook of environmental psychology*, Vol. I (pp. 571–610). New York: Wiley.

Evans, G.W., Jacobs, S.V., & Frager, N.B. (1982). Adaptation to air pollution. *Journal of Environmental Psychology*, 2, 99–108.

Fischhoff, B., Slovic, P., Lichtenstein, S., Read, S., & Combs, B. (1978). How safe is safe enough? A psychometric study of attitudes towards technological risks and benefits. *Policy Sciences*, 8, 127–152.

Fishbein, M., & Ajzen, I. (1975). Beliefs attitude, intention and behaviour. Reading, Mass: Addison-Wesley.

Fisher, J., Bell, P., & Baum, A. (1984). *Environmental psychology*, 2nd edn. New York: Holt, Rinehart and Winston.

Fisher, S., Frazer, N., & Murray, K. (1984). The transition from home to boarding school. *Journal of Environmental Psychology*, 4, 211–222.

Fleming, I., & Baum, A. (1985). The role of prevention in technological catastrophe. *Prevention in Human Services*, 4, 139–152.

Fleming, R., Baum, A., Gisriel, M., & Gatchel, R. (1985). Mediating influences of social support on stress at Three Mile Island. In A. Monat & R.S. Lazarus (eds) (pp. 96–106). New York: Columbia.

Flynn, C.B. (1982). Reactions of local residents to the accident at TMI. In D. Sills, C.P. Wolf & V.B. Shelanski (eds), *The accident at Three Mile Island: The human dimension* (pp. 49–61). Boulder, Colorado: Westview.

Greenhaulgh, G. (1980). *The necessity of nuclear power*. London: Graham and Trotman.

Harré, R., & Secord, P. (1972). *The explanation of social behaviour*. Oxford: Blackwell.

Henderson, J., Brown, J., & Spencer, J. (1986). Psychological impacts of the siting of nuclear facilities. In H. Becker & A. Porter (eds), *Impact assessment today* (pp. 777–804). Utrecht: Uitgeverij Jan Van Arkel.

Howard, K. (1986). *Crisis and community: a Lincolnshire village under threat from the nuclear industry*. Seminar paper. Department of Social Anthropology, Queen's University, Belfast, 4th November.

Idzikowski, C., & Baddeley, A.D. (1983). Fear and dangerous environments. In G.R.J. Hockey (ed.), *Stress and fatigue in human performance* (pp. 123–144). Chichester: John Wiley & Sons.

International Institute for Environment and Society (1984). *Ökologische Wertvorstellungen in Westlichen Industrienationen*. Berlin.

Kasl, S., Will, J., White, M., & Marcuse, P. (1982). Quality of the residential environment and mental health. In A. Baum & J. Singer (eds), *Environment and health*. Hillsdale, NJ: Lawrence Erlbaum.

Kasperson, R., & Pijawka, K.D. (1985). *Societal response to hazards and major hazard events: Comparing natural and technological hazards* (CENTED Reprint No. 45). Worcester, Mass.: Clark University Hazard Assessment Group Centre for Technology, Environment and Development.

Kates, R.W. (1981). *Risk assessment in environmental hazard scope Report 8*. Chichester: John Wiley & Sons.

Kunreuther, H.C. (1983). *Risk analysis and decision processes; The siting of liquefied energy gas facilities in four countries*. Berlin: Springer-Verlag.

Lazarus, R.S. (1966). *Psychological stress and the coping process*. New York: McGraw-Hill.

Lazarus, R.S., & Cohen, S. (1977). Environmental stress. In J. Wohlwill & I. Altman (eds), *Human behaviour and environment* (pp. 89–127). New York: Plenum.

Lazarus, R.S., & Launier, R. (1978). Stress related transactions between person and environment. In L. Pervin & M. Lewis (eds), *Perspectives in international psychology* pp. 287–327. New York: Plenum.

Leik, R.K., Carter, T.M., Clark, J.P., Kendall, S.D., Gifford, G.A., & Ekker, J. (1981). *Community response to natural hazard warnings*. University of Minnesota.

Leventhal, H., Nerenz, D.R., & Leventhal, E. (1982). Feelings of threat and private views of illness; Factors in dehumanization in the medical care system. In A. Baum & J. Singer (eds), *Environment and health* (pp. 85–114). Hillsdale, NJ: Lawrence Erlbaum.

Lounsbury, J., Sunderstrom, E., Schuller, C., Maltingly, T., & DeVault, R. (1977). Towards an assessment of the potential impacts of a nuclear power plant on a community. In K. Finterbusch & C.D. Wolf (eds), *Methodology of social impact assessment* (pp. 265–277). Stroudsburg, Penn./New York: Dowden Hutchinson and Ross/McGraw-Hill.

Mitchell, P.C. (1982). Public response to a major failure of a controversial technology. In D. Sills, C. Wolf & V. Schelanski (eds), *Accident at Three Mile Island* (pp. 21–38). Boulder, Colorado: Westview.

Moser, G. (1984). Water quality perception: a dynamic evaluation. *Journal of Environmental Psychology, 4*, 201–210.

Murdock, S., Hamm, R., & Leistritz, F.L. (1987). The social and special effects of siting high-level and low-level radioactive waste disposal facilities in rural areas. Paper presented to the Conference on Health and Behavioural Impacts of Environmental Hazards, University of California Symposium on Environmental Psychology, May 14–15.

O'Riordan, T. (1983). The cognitive and political dimensions of risk analysis. *Journal of Environmental Psychology, 3*, 345–354.

Otway, H.J., Maurer, D., & Thomas, K. (1978). Nuclear power, the question of public acceptance. *Futures, 10*, 109–118.

Otway, H.J., & Peltu, M. (1985). *Regulating industrial risks. Science, hazards and public protection*. London: Butterworths.

Pollard, P. (1984). Experiment on anxiety and nuclear power. Guildford: University of Surrey. (Mimeo.)

Quarantelle, E.L. (ed.) (1978). *Disasters: Theory and research*. Beverly Hills, Calif.: Sage.

Raynor, S. (1984). Disagreeing about risk: The institutional cultures of risk management and planning for future generations. In J. Haddon (ed.), *Risk analysis, institutions and public policy* (pp. 151–178). New York: Associated Faculty Press.

Raynor, S. & Cantor, R. (1987). How fair is safe enough? The cultural approach to societal technology choice. *Risk Analysis, 7*, 3–9.

Richardson, B., Sorensen, J., & Soderstrom, E.J. (1987). Explaining the social and psychological impacts of a nuclear power plant accident. *Journal of Applied Social Psychology, 17*, 16–36.

Selye, H. (1956). *The stress of life*. New York: McGraw-Hill.

Short, J. (1984). The social fabric at risk; Toward the social transformation of risk analysis. *Americal Sociological Review, 49*, 711–725.

Signal, J. (1980). Physical environmental stressors. In M. Gibbs, J. Rasic Lackenmeyer & J. Sigal (eds), *Community psychology theoretical and empirical approaches* (pp. 145–171). New York: Gardner Press, distributed by Halstead Press.

Sills, D., Wolf, C.P., & Shelanski, V.B. (eds), (1982). *The accident at Three Mile Island: The human dimension*. Boulder, Colorado: Westview.

Sime, J.D. (1983). Affiliative behaviour during escape to building exits. *Journal of Environmental Psychology, 3*, 21–42.

Slovic, P., Fischhoff, B. & Lichtenstein, S. (1982). Psychological aspects of risk perception in accidents at Three Mile Island. In D. Sills, C.P. Wolff & V. Shelanski (eds), *The human dimension*. Boulder, Colorado: Westview.

Thompson, M. (1983). *Postscript; A cultural basis for comparison*. In H.E. Kunreuther (ed.) *Risk analysis and decision processes* (pp. 232–262). Berlin: Springer-Verlag.

Van der Pligt, J., Eisner, J.R., & Spears, R. (1985). Social judgement in the field;
    Attitudes towards nuclear energy. In F.L. Denmark (ed.), *Social ecological psychology
    and the psychology of women* (pp. 333–346). Amsterdam: Elsevier North Holland.
Watts, N. (1988). Environmental complaint and concern in the countries of the European
    Community. In D. Canter, M. Krampen, & D. Stea (eds), *Environmental policy, assess-
    ment and communication*, Vol. 2. Ethnoscapes: current challenges to the social sciences,
    pp. 55–74.
Wynne, B. (in press). *The hazardous management of wastes; Implementation and the
    diatectics of credibility*. London: Springer-Verlag.

KEY WORDS

Chernobyl, nuclear power, cataclysmic events, daily hassles, ambient stressors, Three Mile
Island, radioactive waste, biological models, signal detection theory, risk perception,
dread, attitudes, mediators, role, rule models, appraisal, coping, information seeking,
assumptive word hypothesis, cultural theory, worry bead hypothesis, contextual analysis
perceptual defence.

Section IB:
Stressful Social Contexts

Handbook of Life Stress, Cognition and Health
Edited by S. Fisher and J. Reason
© 1988 John Wiley & Sons Ltd.

8

Marriage, Separation and Divorce

RAYMOND COCHRANE
University of Birmingham

The joys of marriage are the heaven on earth,
Life's paradise, great princess, the soul's quiet,
Sinews of concord, earthly immortality,
Eternities of pleasures . . .

John Ford (1586–1639)

No thorns go as deep as the rose's,
And love is more cruel than lust.
Time turns the old days to derision,
Our loves into corpses or wives;
And marriage and death and division
Make barren our lives.

Algernon Charles Swinburne (1837–1909)

There are clearly contrasting views about the benefit or otherwise of marriage. In popular lore there is a very deeply seated ambiguity in attitudes towards marriage, in much the same way as there is to work: it is seen as the 'natural' state for an adult and there is some suspicion of, and/or pity for, those who do not achieve it. But at the same time it is seen as a trap and a limit on individual freedom. What cannot be disputed is that in terms of health, at least, marriage is an unmixed blessing.

SOME BASIC DATA ON MARITAL STATUS AND HEALTH

It has long been observed that marital status is strongly correlated with health status, and that this relationship holds for physical, psychological and be-haviourally induced illnesses. The mortality rate for deaths from all causes is lower for the currently married than for the unmarried, whether they be single, widowed or divorced (Table 8.1). This is most dramatically the case for stress-related causes of death such as coronary heart disease and for deaths from behaviourally related disorders such as accidents, cirrhosis and lung cancer (Dominion, 1984; Gove, 1972; Koskenvuo *et al.*, 1986; Mergenhagen, Lee and Gove, 1985; Tcheng-Laroche and Prince, 1983). Morbidity rates and rates of

Table 8.1 Marital status, age-adjusted death rates and mental hospital admission rates per 100 000 population

| Marital status | Population[a] (1000s) | Rate per 100 000 | |
		Mental hospital admissions[b]	Deaths[c]
Single	8 317	770	1549
Married	22 765	260	1260
Widowed	3 249	980	1835
Divorced	1 286	1437	1639

[a] Aged 16 years and over for England, 1981.
[b] For year 1981, calculated from raw data suppled by DHSS, for England.
[c] For year 1984, for England and Wales, calculated from data in OPCS, *Mortality statistics 1984.*

utilization of medical services show a similar association with marital status (Riessman and Gerstel, 1985; Verbrugge, 1979). The pattern is even clearer when suicide and attempted suicide are considered, where the rates of both are far higher among the unmarried, particularly the divorced, than among the married (Carter and Glick, 1976; Holding *et al.,* 1977; Robinson *et al.,* 1986).

It is, however, in the area of mental illness that the most thorough examination of the relationship between marital status and vulnerability has been made. Marital status is, in fact, one of the strongest of all social correlates of mental hospital admissions (Cochrane, 1983; Gove *et al.,* 1983; Segraves, 1980). A recent analysis of data provided by the Department of Health and Social Security produced the results shown in Table 8.1, which provide clear evidence of the excess risk of the unmarried sections of the population to mental illness serious enough to warrant treatment as an in-patient in a mental hospital.

These data are, of course, not without their problems. For example, those people who are not legally married but who are co-habiting in a stable marriage-style relationship are counted as single, while those who are separated from their spouse, and who may be considered to have more in common psychologically with the divorced, are counted among the married. Also counted among the married are those who have experienced bereavement or divorce and who have remarried. However, the pattern is sufficiently robust to withstand these contaminations, and is by no means unique to Britain, also having been observed in the USA (Bachrach, 1975; Gove, 1972; Gove *et al.,* 1983), in Finland (Koskenvuo *et al.,* 1986), and in Norway (Odegaard, 1946).

When the mental hospital admission data are examined in more detail, and age, sex and diagnostic patterns taken into account, the picture becomes both more complex and more revealing (Table 8.2). First, there is the well known reversal of rates for men and women in the married compared to the unmarried categories. Among the single, the widowed and the divorced, men have the higher rates, but among the married it is women who are more likely to be admitted to mental hospitals. However, marriage is clearly 'protective' in this respect for both men and for women. It is only because among the adult population the married

Table 8.2   Mental hospital admissions in England, 1981, by sex, diagnosis and marital status. Age-adjusted rates per 100 000 population

Diagnosis	Age adjusted rates per 100 000 population							
	Single		Married		Widowed		Divorced	
	M	F	M	F	M	F	M	F
All diagnoses	785	755	198	323	1227	922	1552	1357
Schizophrenia and paranoia	264	191	19	34	166	101	205	201
Depression	165	234	57	133	284	317	330	461
Neuroses	44	63	21	44	70	147	142	210
Personality and behaviour disorders	62	70	13	19	219	70	219	163
Alcohol related	94	31	23	13	188	77	385	108

category is so much larger than the remaining three categories put together that women have higher rates overall than men. Although the risk of mental hospital admission for every diagnostic category is lowest among the married, the differences between the non-married and the married is greatest for the diagnosis of schizophrenia, where the ratios are greater than 10 : 1 for men and 6 : 1 for women.

Not only is marital status a good predictor of admission to mental hospital, but it is equally powerful as a predictor of treatment outcome. Bachrach (1975) quotes Garfield and Sundland (1966) as reporting that 'marital status alone is as good a prognostic indicator of length of hospital stay as any of the prognostic scales thus far developed'.Butler and Morgan (1977) found that, on average, the non-married spent much longer in hospitals when they were physically ill than did the married. These authors estimated that if the average duration of stay for the non-married was the same as that for the married, there would need to be about 24 000 fewer beds in non-psychiatric hospitals in England and Wales.

The evidence derived from analysis of out-patient treatment statistics and from community surveys on the relationship between marital status and mental health is, on the whole, consistent with the pattern found for mental hospital admissions. However, there have been some exceptions found to the general trend using both these indices of pathology (Bachrach, 1975; Cochrane and Stopes-Roe, 1980; Warheit et al., 1976). The issue of consistency of findings and the methodologies employed will be returned to later.

As is to be expected with such a wide range of findings which, although basically consistent, are derived from many studies in many locations, a variety of explanations has been put forward to account for the apparently poorer health of the unmarried. With one notable exception, all of these explanations employ the concept of stress in one way or another. The only types of explanations which do not employ this concept are the variants of the 'selection for marriage' hypothesis which will be considered in the 'marital process' section of this chapter. This is understandable enough, as the relationship between stress and disease has been well established for a long time and it is therefore logical to look at stress as the potential intervening variable between a social status, such as marriage, and an individual response, such as ill-health.

At its very simplest, the stress hypothesis is formed as follows: members of some social categories are exposed to more stress and, as a higher level of stress is related to elevated risk of illness, that social category will contain more ill members than alternative social categories whose members are exposed to less stress. Such a hypothesis has been invoked to explain the relationship between several social variables (e.g. social class, ethnicity, population density) and disease (Cochrane, 1983).

STRESS AND MARITAL STATUS

Can such an apparently simple explanation be all that is required to account for marital status differences in vulnerability to illness? In this section three issues will be examined before the question in the previous sentence is answered: how might stress and marital status be linked? what is meant by stress in this context? and what evidence exists that stress may vary with marital status? These three issues are clearly interrelated and they are the focus of many other contributions to this book, but each will be examined separately.

There are several ways in which stress levels might be related to marital status, both directly and indirectly. The most obvious direct association involves the stress usually assumed to accompany the transition from one status category to another (Kessler and Essex, 1982). Few would dispute that bereavement and divorce are almost always distressing events in themselves, so there is little surprise in the evidence that the widowed and the divorced are particularly vulnerable soon after the disruption of their marriages (Bachrach, 1975; Segraves, 1980; Stroebe and Stroebe, 1983). However, on many life events scales and checklists, 'getting married' is also included as a stressor. This results from the implicit definition of stress used by the authors of such scales which, in the main, derives from the Schedule of Recent Experience (SRE).

In the development of the SRE, Holmes and Rahe (1967) employed the concept of 'life change units', which refer to the degree of disruption to the ongoing life pattern that would be caused should an event befall an average person. While getting married is often undeniably disruptive to the life-style in this sense, the issue of whether it should be classed as a stressor in the more usual meaning of that term has been challenged. The 'positive' events which figure on life stress scales do not appear to be related to pathology in the same way as do the 'negative' events (Cochrane and Robertson, 1975; Dohrenwend, 1973; Vinokur and Selzer, 1975).

Excluding getting married as a stressful event neatly fits in with the observation of lower rates of illness among the married than among the separated and the divorced, but what about those people in the single category? Obviously some other intervening variable is required to account for their relatively high rates of illness.

Turning to the indirect ways in which marital status might be related to stress, there is a range of potential candidates. However, they do not all fit in so neatly with the hypothesis that the unmarried experience more stress than do the married. Indeed, many of the most commonly researched stressors would appear to be more likely to occur to those who have married. Children may be a blessing, but they also carry enormous potential as stressors in terms of illness, bereavement, schooling problems, legal difficulties and financial strains, to mention but a few. While not only the married will be caring for children, this role is more common in this category than in any of the other marital status categories. Again, if we look at the potential for role conflict which is associated with motherhood and career choices for many women, these too will be more likely to occur to married than to single, divorced or widowed women.

The problem identified here can be eased a little if a broader definition of stress is employed than that which necessarily is embodied in life events scales. In the construction of a typical inventory, a variety of judges are asked to rate, on an arbitrary scale of, say, 1 to 100, the stress which would be caused to an average person should an event befall them. A marker event is sometimes employed and given a central value, for example, in constructing the Life Events Inventory, Cochrane and Robertson (1973) set 'marriage' at 50 units and the other 54 items were rated by judges relative to this standard. On such an inventory, as has already been pointed out, apart from the core of universally relevant events, there are many items which are more likely to occur to the married (e.g. pregnancy, son or daughter leaving home) and some which can, by definition, only happen to those who are married (e.g. infidelity of spouse, increase in arguments with spouse). On the other hand, there are relatively few items which are only relevant to other status cateogries (e.g. divorce, death of spouse). This imbalance in the potential stressors to which the married and the unmarried appear to be exposed is due to the constraints of such measuring instruments rather than to any realistic assessment of the actual life circumstances of people in different marital status categories. The instructions to respondents associated with such devices give a clue to their limited range of content, e.g. 'Please indicate which of the following events has happened to you in the past year'.

Where there is an exclusive concentration on *events*, or changes in circumstances, that have a discrete and identifiable temporal onset (e.g. moving house, new job, death of relative, leaving home), there will inevitably be a very limited set of stressors tapped. Useful as this approach has proved to be in some circumstances, it is essential to consider a range of other types of potentially stressful experiences in order to gain a more complete picture of a person's life situation. Nowhere is this more relevant than when making comparisons between social groupings, such as the married and the unmarried, who, by definition, are likely to be in very different positions. Some of the other sources of potential stress will be outlined briefly.

The concept of *long-term difficulties* is employed by Brown and Harris (1978), among others, to describe ongoing and chronic problems that do not necessarily produce a particular and discrete crisis. Thus, conceptually, long-term difficulties are very different to life events but may be just as stress provoking. Examples of such difficulties include inadequate housing, long-term unemployment, a close relative who has been ill and bedridden for a number of years, and poverty. Some long-term difficulties may be more likely to affect the married (e.g. having a drunken husband), but some may be more common among the unmarried (e.g. very low income and children to support).

Life strains can be considered to be situations which are not inherently negative but which demand expenditure of psychic energy and the deployment of considerable coping resources and which can take their toll on those who live with them (Pearlin and Schooler, 1978; Mitchell *et al.*, 1983). Such strains may not produce attempts to escape, or even to mitigate the situation, by those involved in them. Examples include having a demanding job, parenting, studying for qualifications (taking exams would count as an event), and managing and maintaining a complex household. Presumably, such experiences will often have many beneficial aspects and produce positive affective states as well as stress. Clearly it is the balance between these which is important. Nevertheless, they are the kind of situations which are often overlooked in studies on the relationship between stress and illness.

Daily hassles, as a psychological concept, has a relatively short history, but subjectively we can all appreciate the irritation and stress they produce. Basically, hassles are events which are not major enough to figure on life event scales and which in and of themselves might be considered trivial or insignificant (Kanner *et al.*, 1981). However, if they are experienced repeatedly, in combination, or in a rapid sequence, they can be very stressful indeed. Daily hassles are legion, and choice of examples will reflect recent personal episodes rather than be representative in any sense, but we might include things such as a car which fails to start, a secretary becoming ill when a deadline is approaching, a burst water pipe, a pet cat being hurt in a road accident and requiring veterinary treatment on a day which already scheduled to be very busy! Zautra *et al.* (1986) have produced a scale to measure these 'small life events'. Probably for most people, for most of their lives, hassles are a more significant source of stress than are the undeniably traumatic, but fortunately quite rare, occurrences which appear on life events checklists.

Finally, in this context, we should consider the stress potential of *frustrations* or disappointments. These are of a somewhat different order to events, long-term difficulties, strains and hassles as they are characterized by something *not* happening rather than by something happening or being present chronically. A clear example might be living alone, not as a result of the dissolution of a relationship but where relationships had never been formed in the first place. The stress associated with loneliness can be very intense. An unrewarding occupation, even where not positively stressful in terms of the demands it makes upon the person doing it, can nevertheless be considered to be frustrating for the man or woman seeking job satisfaction. Failure to gain promotion for an ambitious person would be another example. So too would be failure to get married where this was considered a highly desirable aspiration by the person doomed to remain single and by the society in which they live. Equally, a marital relationship does not have to be characterized by rows, crises and periods of emotional blood letting to be experienced as unfulfilling by one or both partners. Perhaps because of inherent difficulties of measurement, disappointments and frustrations have rarely been considered explicitly in relation to stress and illness.

Is there any evidence that some marital status categories are more prone to stress experiences of any of the types listed above than are other marital categories? The answer to this question must be, 'very little'. Pearlin and Johnson (1977) showed that certain life strains were more likely to be experienced by an heterogeneous 'unmarried' group than by those who were married. Brown and Harris (1978), too, appear to show that unmarried women are more likely to experience a severe event or major difficulty than are married women, but do not report this directly. Kessler and Essex (1982) showed that the unmarried were more likely to have greater exposure to life strains, but only marginally so. They do, however, admit that they only considered a small and unrepresentative selection of possible life strains. Kandel *et al.* (1985) compared married and non-married women on levels of stress and strains which each group experienced associated with their work. Although married women scored lower on both the stress and the strain index than did unmarried women, the differences were not significant. Champion (1985) found that unmarried women scored significantly higher (mean = 259) on the Life Events Inventory than did married women (mean = 189), in her study of 300 women on a housing estate in Birmingham.

Thus the evidence in favour of the hypothesis that the marital categories at relatively high risk of physical and psychological illness are more prone to stress is, at present, rather tenuous to say the least. Even if it were not so, there is another difficulty in the way of providing an unambiguous answer to the question with which this section opened. The underlying model of the relationship being considered here can be represented as:

high risk category → more stress → more illness
(e.g. divorced)   (e.g. events)   (e.g. depression)

The problem is that, just as the link between different social categories and differential exposure to stress is tenuous, so is the link between stress and illness. While it is true that studies have consistently shown significant, albeit modest, correlations between higher stress levels and poorer health (Cochrane and Sobol, 1980), it is equally clear that the majority of people who are exposed to even very high levels of stress do not break down. On the other hand, some people in all categories who are exposed to apparently low stress levels do succumb. Referring back to Table 8.1, it can be seen that even in the highest risk social category, less than 1% of the group are admitted to mental hospitals each year. Even allowing for the fact that not all widows and widowers are exposed to particularly high stress levels, it is clear that other variables also need to be invoked to explain the observed relationship between marital categories and illness rates.

AN EXTENDED MODEL OF STRESS, COPING AND ILLNESS

In extending the oversimple model described above, several additional factors can be included in order to construct a more complete representation of the process by

144

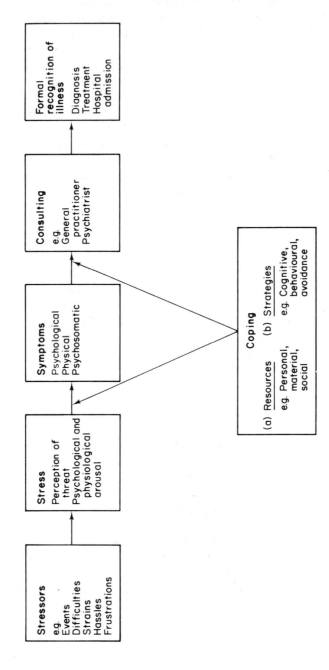

FIG. 8.1   A model of stress, coping and illness.

which stress may or may not result in illness, and how this relationship can vary with membership of social categories. Figure 8.1 contains the outlines of such a model taken from Cochrane (1983), with modifications introduced by McPherson (1987).

Initially, in this model a distinction is made between 'stressors' and 'stress', with the former referring to the objective occurrence of events, strains, hassles, frustrations and difficulties, and the latter to the subjective perception by an individual of these occurrences as being stressful or threatening. Where one person may find a particular happenstance (such as a critical comment from a superior at work) intensely arousing, another person may hardly notice a similar episode, or treat it with amusement or derision. The extent to which a potential stressor is, in fact, stressful will depend on such factors as the interpretation placed on its occurrence, the personality of the individual concerned, previous experiences of similar incidents etc.

Assuming that stressors are translated into subjectively experienced stresses in some circumstances, the person has to begin to respond to these stresses. This response is usually called 'coping' and can be defined as 'the cognitive and behavioural efforts made to master, tolerate, or reduce external and internal demands and conflict among them' (Folkman and Lazarus, 1980, p. 223). It has become clear that the way in which the term 'coping' has been used in fact encompasses at least two fairly distinct concepts, which can be separated out as coping *resources* and coping *strategies* (Menaghan, 1982; McPherson, 1987), and although the two are conceptually distinct, they are not totally independent of each other. Resources refer to personal, material and social assets that people have in varying quantities, while strategies refer to habitual behavioural and cognitive styles in aproaching problems.

Coping Resources

Turning first to coping resources, it is fairly obvious that in general the married will be at a considerable advantage over the unmarried. Several authors have attempted to catalogue resources for dealing with stress which may be available to people, and these attempts have produced good general agreement about what constitute the most valuable assets in this sense. In Cochrane's (1983) analysis, the four most desirable resources are listed as intrapsychic defence mechanisms, stress-opposing experiences, intimate personal relationships and informal helping networks.

Intrapsychic Defence Mechanisms

Intrapsychic defence mechanisms are personal characteristics which 'allow potentially threatening events to be misperceived or reinterpreted in such a way as to reduce, or entirely neutralize their impact' (Cochrane and Sobol, 1980, p. 169). Pearlin and Schooler (1978) found that the possession of a sense of self-mastery, positive self-esteem and the absence of self-denigrating attitudes were considerable advantages in combatting the effects of stress. Vaillant (1985) has reviewed a number of studies which have looked at the effectiveness of defence mechanisms in defending against psychological distress, and has developed his own typology which he employed in a 40-year follow-up study of nearly 400 boys/men. He found that fantasy and projection were used as more common defences in those who developed psychological problems, while altruism and suppression were more characteristic of men without any psychological problems. While being married is not a prerequisite for the development of these defences, and by no means all married couples will be able to mobilize them, it is likely that they will, on average, be more available to people within stable and affectionate relationships. Being loved and admired is bound to enhance self-esteem and to help to chase away self-doubt and feelings of inadequacy. Kessler and Essex (1982), in their study of 2300 respondents in Chicago, found clear evidence that the married people in their sample possessed significantly higher levels of mastery and self-esteem. What is more, these same authors showed that in explaining the significantly higher depression scale scores found for the non-married compared to the married, differential possession of mastery and self-esteem accounted for substantially more of the variance than did differential exposure to stress.

Stress-opposing Experiences

Stress-opposing experiences are not conceived of as preventing the occurrence of stressful events, or the occurrence of circumstances which directly resolve difficult situations, for example finding a good job immediately after being made redundant. Rather, the concept relates to positive experiences, events and situations which occur quite independently of any negative experiences. So getting promoted, praised, complemented, or securing a sense of achieving something in one context, reduces the impact of stressful experiences in another. Many of the situations and processes which are considered, conventionally at least, to be most fulfilling and satisfying are more likely to be accessible to the married. Sexual satisfaction, intimacy and security in personal relationships, home building, procreation and watching one's own children develop are not the exclusive prerogative of the married, but are normal expectations they might reasonably aspire to achieve.

The occurrence of these positive situations is a major contributor to what has become known as the quality of life, or psychological well-being. There is independent evidence that a better overall subjective quality of life, and a predominance of positive affect, is associated with having fewer psychological symptoms (Cohen et al., 1984; Cohen and Hoberman, 1983; Lazarus, Kanner and Folkman, 1980, Phillips, 1968; Reich and Zautra, 1981) and is considerably more likely to occur in married than in unmarried individuals. A meta-analysis of a large number of studies done in the USA found a significant correlation between subjective well-being and being married, especially for men (Haring-Hidore et al., 1985). This has been confirmed by recent exhaustive reviews of the correlates of subjective well-being by Diener (1984) and by Argyle (1987). The greater availability of stress-opposing experiences to the married might go some considerable way towards explaining the better health of married people of both sexes.

Intimate Personal Relationships

These have, as has been seen, a role to play in the maintenance of effective intrapsychic defence mechanisms and in providing stress-opposing experiences, but they also have enormous potential for providing direct and beneficial assistance in dealing with stress. There may be occasions when very close relationships may help combat the actual stress, for example a husband may give up work to look after the family if his wife is unable to fulfill this role and may, thereby, relieve secondary stress which would otherwise be associated with, let us say, an illness. Perhaps even more important is the use of such relationships as a refuge or source of solace if stressors prove intractable. The sharing of misery and the provision of psychological support may well prevent even extreme stress from resulting in physical or psychological disorder.

There is a vast research literature which attests to the potency of intimate and confiding relationships as buffers against stress, but perhaps the most detailed and convincing evidence has been provided by Brown and Harris (1978). They identified four 'vulnerability' factors which considerably and consistently increased the risk that women would become depressed in the face of stress. One of the most powerful of these factors was the absence of an intimate and confiding relationship. Without such a relationship, 41% of women who reported a severe event or major difficulty became depressed, compared to only 10% of those who did have such a relationship. Although in the Brown and Harris study, confidants could be found in other than marriage-type relationships, this very rarely occurred in fact. The most likely context in which to find these intensely involving and rewarding relationships is marriage. However, two caveats are in order here. First, being married is not a guarantee that such a confiding relationship will exist—many marriages have been found to be deficient in this respect. Second, it is just this kind of relationship which also provides the greatest potential for stress in most people's lives. Almost by definition, the loss of a person, whether by death or disloyalty, who has been such a source of intense gratification, will be personally devastating to the surviving spouse or partner. Tennyson's assertion that ''Tis better to have loved and lost, than never to have loved at all', expresses a sentiment that should be true, but there is precious little evidence for it!

Informal Helping Networks

Informal helping networks have some of the characteristics of intimate relationships but obviously lack their intensity. As with intimate relationships, there is an enormous body of evidence supporting the hypothesis that people with access to this resource are better able to deal with stress than are those without such access (Broadhead *et al.*, 1983; Kessler *et al.*, 1985), although there is some debate over the extent of the protection provided by more distant social support networks (Leavy, 1983). Again, it is almost inevitable that those who are married will have more relatives, such as sons, daughters, in-laws etc., than will the unmarried. Champion (1985) found that not only were married women more likely to have a confidant available, they also had better social support networks generally than did unmarried women. This also emerged very clearly in Pearlin and Johnson's (1977) study where a much larger proportion of the unmarried were categorized as being 'considerably' or 'fairly' isolated from social networks than were the married. Similar results have been produced by Veroff *et al.* (1981) and Fox (1984).

Coping Strategies

Turning now to coping strategies, there is again a large and growing body of evidence that people have consistent methods of attempting to deal with stress and that some methods are more effective than others (e.g. Billings and Moos, 1981; Menaghan, 1983; Parker and Brown, 1982; Pearlin and Schooler, 1978). Some authors have distinguished between coping strategies based on either approaching or avoiding problems (Roth and Cohen, 1986), others make the distinction between problem-focused coping strategies (for example, persuading someone to change their mind, standing one's own ground and arguing a case) and emotion-focused strategies (for example, looking on the bright side, trying to forget the whole thing) (Folkman and Lazarus, 1980). In general, the conclusion appears to be that the approaching and the problem-focused styles are more efficacious than the alternatives, although this does vary somewhat from situation to situation. Unlike the research with regard to coping resources, there is no evidence concerning the relationship between marital status and coping strategies, so it is not possible to say whether the married enjoy a similar advantage over the unmarried as they do so far as resources are concerned.

Two studies have examined the coping styles of married couples in an attempt to assess their effectiveness, however. Menaghan (1982) found that couples who attempted to negotiate and discuss conflicts, or who made optimistic comparisons of their own current situation with their past situation or with other people's situation, had fewer marital problems than those who tried to ignore (avoid) issues or who became resigned to them. Interestingly, those who employed the negotiation tactic in dealing with stress in the marriage did not have lower levels of subjective distress but did have fewer long-lasting problems.

Mitchell *et al.* (1983) compared marriages in which one partner was clinically depressed with those in which both partners were healthy. They found that the depressed patients had encountered more stress than the control group had, and also reported using fewer problem-oriented behaviours and more emotion-focused coping responses. The healthy spouses of patients were more like the control group in that they tended to employ problem-focused rather than emotion-focused coping strategies.

The relative availability of coping resources and the development of different coping strategies will help to determine whether the experience of stress results in symptoms of illness. They will also, to some extent, determine what the person who does develop symptoms does about them. It has already been mentioned that, at least as far as mental health goes, there is a greater discrepancy between the recorded rates of treated disorder between the marital status categories than there is for untreated disorder (e.g. Warheit *et al.*, 1976). One obvious reason for this is that a person who is married is likely to have an alternative source of help and nurturance to that provided by health professionals. An example of the strenuous attempts made by some spouses to keep their ill partner at home is supplied by the study of Yarrow *et al.*, (1955) of lengths to which wives went to prevent their husbands from being hospitalized for psychiatric treatment. It may indeed be that some of the differential in treatment rates evident for married men and women is accounted for by the greater willingness and ability of wives to care for sick husbands than vice versa. Even where treatment is sought, there is still the response of the physician to be considered. Goldberg and Huxley (1980) have documented some of the social variables (as distinct from clinical variables) which influence the decisions reached by GPs and psychiatrists about patients. They found, for example, that married men, in particular, were likely to be filtered out of the formal mental health system, while unmarried men were more likely to be referred on to the next stage of the treatment process.

THE MARITAL PROCESS

Some were married, which was bad, and some
did other things which were worse
Rudyard Kipling (1865–1936)

So far it has been convenient to discuss the marital statuses as though they were completely separate and internally homogeneous categories. In practice, they are not. There are transition stages from one to another, and there is great variability in the life experience of those within a single category. In addition, the social significance, and the potential for encountering stress, of each category varies over time and at different stages in a person's life.

In 1967, Wechsler and Pugh formalized the hypothesis that people with particular personal characteristics who are living in communities where those characteristics are less common should have higher rates of mental illness than people living in communities where those characteristics are more common—that is, people who do not 'fit in' in a community will be at a disadvantage.

This idea was applied to marital status variations in psychiatric morbidity by Martin (1976). He suggested that occupying an incongruous combination of sex × age × marital condition roles produces a form of socially induced stress. Where people occupy a combination of statuses which deviates from the expected pattern for people like them (e.g. being a very young divorcee, or a middle-aged single man), then more mental illness is expected to occur because, 'any combination of age, sex and marital statuses which is rarely held tends to be stressful' (Martin, 1976, p. 292). Martin found support for this hypothesis in an examination of age–sex–specific mental hospitalization rates for different marital conditions in the USA for the years 1930 and 1933.

Comparable data are available for England in the 1980s. Table 8.1 clearly shows that there is a perfect, negative rank order correlation between the number of people occupying a marital category and mental hospitalization rates, but this could have arisen for any number of reasons, as we have seen. What is required is

Table 8.3 Proportion of the population who are single or widowed in each age group, and age-specific rates of mental hospital admission per 100 000 population, England, 1981

Age group (years)	Single		Widowed	
	Proportion of population[a]	Admission rate[b]	Proportion of population	Admission rate
Males				
16–24	0.88	234	0.0001	2209
25–34	0.25	1067	0.001	2283
35–44	0.10	1602	0.004	1960
45–64	0.09	1249	0.03	1011
65+	0.08	773	0.17	879
Correlation[c]	−0.3		−0.9	
Females				
16–24	0.76	247	0.0005	1012
25–34	0.14	980	0.004	1629
35–44	0.06	1374	0.014	1318
45–64	0.07	1182	0.11	997
65+	0.12	933	0.49	988
Correlation[c]	−0.9		−0.7	

[a] In each age group.
[b] All diagnoses.
[c] Spearman's rho.

evidence of the relative rate of hospital admissions within status categories in different age cohorts. This evidence is provided in Table 8.3.

When the data are analysed in this way, there turns out to be a very strong negative rank order correlation between the percentage of an age group who are single and the age-specific hospital admission rates for women, with a lower correlation for men. For the widowed it is the other way round, with men showing the stronger correlation, but the correlation for women is still substantial. There was no relationship of this kind for the married or divorced categories. It does appear that remaining single when the overwhelming majority of one's peers are married, is related to poorer mental health, as is being widowed at a young age, as this is a relatively rare occurrence.

The data in Table 8.3, especially those pertaining to the single of both sexes, are also amenable to another interpretation, however. So far, the hypotheses considered have been that marital status, through some intervening variables (notably stress levels), causes variations in health status. These hypotheses are, in fact, only supported by correlational data, and the notorious difficulty in deriving causal relations from correlations has been ignored. Clearly the data are capable of sustaining other hypotheses, too. The most obvious alternative is that health status causes marital status in some way.

This proposition has received quite serious consideration and is known as the 'selection for marriage' hypothesis. Beginning with the assumption that marriage is a desirable objective and, to a certain extent, competitive, the selection hypothesis states that the reason there are relatively more ill people among the single than among the married is that illness, or predisposition to illness, reduces the likelihood of a person marrying. This could happen either because the unwell person is not inclined to marry and/or because they make an unattractive proposition for potential spouses. In this case they would find it difficult to marry even should they wish to do so. This means that those who do marry are selected, partly at least, on health status, and the resultant pool of the married contains a disproportionate number of healthy people, while the residual single pool contains a disproportionate number of unhealthy individuals. The selection effect might be stronger for men than for women as it has usually been the male who takes the lead in courtship and proposes marriage and, therefore, is required to demonstrate a certain degree of activity and competence. In addition, the traditional masculine stereotype is more incompatible with emotional disorder than is the traditional feminine stereotype, which even includes a certain element of emotional lability. Finally, it may be that women take more account of a suitor's psychological state when selecting a husband, on whom they may be economically dependent for some time, while men pay more attention to other (e.g. physical) characteristics when choosing a wife.

This hypothesis would certainly seem to be compatible with the data in Table 8.2 which pertain to schizophrenia. Of all the diagnoses, schizophrenia shows the largest single : married vulnerability ratio for both sexes. Given that the premorbid characteristics of schizophrenia are often said to include a low level of interest in sex, and the inability to form and maintain close relationships, it seems quite possible that those with incipient schizophrenia would be unlikely to marry.

The data in Table 8.3 are also relevant. As the proportion of the population who are single declines across age groups, and hence the single represent more and more a residual or rejected pool, the rate of treated mental illness tends to increase. Again, this can as easily be interpreted as support for the selection theory as it can for Martin's status integration theory.

There is still the need to explain the very high rates of psychological (and physical) disorder in the 'post married' groups—the widowed and the divorced. Here, it must be pointed out that we are also dealing with a residual category as it is quite common for remarriages to occur, so again selecting back into the married group certain individuals and leaving others in the less desirable status groups. In addition, it is not unreasonable to suggest that personality difficulties and emotional problems of one kind or another might contribute to a person getting divorced and thereby selecting into that category more such individuals.

Although this hypothesis has been around for some time, it has proved very difficult to test directly, as a thorough examination would require a longitudinal study of a cohort of men and women at least through their marriageable years (late teens and twenties). No such study appears to have been done. Instead, there have been studies of mental hospital admission rates (e.g. Rushing, 1979) and the duration of stay in hospitals (e.g. Eaton, 1975). These studies tend to support the selection hypothesis, at least as far as schizophrenia is concerned. In the absence of more definitive studies, however, it is not possible to determine the relative merits of the selection and the causation hypothesis at present.

Turning now to the married group itself, it is again clear that there is a great deal of variability from one married person to another in the experience of being married, the levels of stress likely to be encountered, and the resources available to deal with stress. It has already been pointed out that for many of the same reasons that a marriage, or a marital-type relationship, can be so fulfilling and beneficial, it also has the greatest threat potential of all relationships. Almost by definition, a failing or conflict-filled marriage is inevitably going to be very stress inducing, and there is considerable evidence to show that marital difficulties frequently precede severe psychological problems, including depression (Paykel et al., 1969), hypochondriasis (Kreitman, 1965), agoraphobia (Milton and Hafner, 1979), and psychosomatic disorders (Waring, 1977).

Even within reasonably well-functioning marriages, there is enormous variation in the type of relationships that exist between spouses. Waring and his colleagues (Waring, 1984; Waring and Reddon, 1983; Waring et al., 1981) have defined several dimensions of the quality of the marital relationship, which they have globally called intimacy. Marital quality was measured by taking self-reports of the degree of affection expressed by couples, the commitment to the marriage, sexual fulfilment, compatibility, sharing, ease of conflict resolution, etc. Thus, the composite variable of intimacy, as defined by Waring, bears only a small resemblance to the concept of an intimate and confiding relationship discussed earlier. Of the 250 marriages examined by Waring et al. (1986), only 20% displayed what the authors considered to be an optimal pattern of intimacy, while over 30% were rated as deficient in this respect. A further 35% of marriages were based on 'pseudo intimacy', which refers to couples who tried to portray their relationship as they thought it should have been rather than the way it actually was. Significantly, the prevalence of emotional distress varied directly with level of intimacy. Those marriages that were deficient in this respect yielded more than twice as many emotional difficulties as those that were optimal. Still, the important point to note is the relatively small proportion of marriages that achieved an optimal rating.

Two other aspects of stress within marriage have been examined in some detail: the impact of the stresses experienced by one partner on the psychological well-being of the other, and the consequences of occupying other roles which are potentially in conflict with the married role. Perhaps the most dramatic example of the impact of one person's stress on another occurs in the case where a spouse becomes mentally ill. Here there is a strong suggestion that the disorder is likely to be transmitted to the other partner, presumably because of the stress on them produced by being married to an emotionally disturbed person (Segraves, 1980).

Mitchell et al. (1983) suggest that it might be productive to examine stress levels in a total family context rather than just at the individual level. In their study of the interaction of the coping abilities of married couples, they found clear evidence that the greater the stress and strains experienced by one partner, the higher the level of depressive symptomatology that was reported by the other. More direct evidence of this was provided by Cochrane and Stopes-Roe (1981), who looked at the impact of unemployment of one spouse on the psychological health of the other. Wives of unemployed men were much more depressed than wives of employed men, and they were even more depressed than women who were themselves unemployed. It seemed that the presumably greater family and economic impact of male unemployment had more adverse consequences for women than their own lack of a job. Interestingly, the same relationship did not hold the other way round: while men who were out of work were more depressed than their working counterparts, the employment or unemployment of their wives made no differences to their own mental health.

This leads quite naturally on to a consideration of the interaction of marriage (and motherhood) with careers for women. One of the original attempts to explain the greater mental health risks of married women compared to married men (Gove, 1972; Gove and Tudor, 1973) suggested that men were protected because they were more likely to occupy two distinct roles, that of head of the household and a career role. Married women, on the other hand, were more likely to be confined to one role, that of housewife. Even if they did work, Gove suggested, it was likely they would, on average, have less intrinsically satisfying jobs than would men. The great majority of the evidence available in fact suggests that having a job is as beneficial to the psychological well-being of women as it is for men (e.g. Cochrane and Stopes-Roe, 1981; Tennant et al., 1982; Thoits, 1986), but this demonstration has lead to fears that married women who work may experience considerable stress from role conflicts, especially if they are the mothers of young children. This stress could derive both from physical demands on their time and energy made by the twin responsibilities of children and career, and from a fear that they were not fulfilling either role (especially the maternal role) adequately.

This has led to the concept of role overload, which is produced by occupying too many roles, or roles that are in some crucial way incompatible, which, it is hypothesized, in turn leads to stress and hence to illness. The evidence has not been kind to this theory! In fact, so overwhelming has been the evidence, and, it should be said, so strong the prevailing social attitudes of those involved in researching this topic, that the role overload concept has been completely reversed and the 'multiple role' hypothesis has taken its place (Barnett and Baruch, 1985). This posits that the more roles occupied the better, in health terms. There is no inevitable conflict between roles, and the positive gains from each role occupied cumulate to produce increments in well-being (Barnett and Baruch, 1985; Kandel et al., 1985; Thoits, 1983). So, in a sense, the wheel has turned full circle and we are back somewhere close to Gove's original explanation for the greater mental health risk of married women than married men. Although the proportion of married women who are economically active has grown rapidly since the Second World War, it is still lower than the participation rate of men. It could well be that the frustrations attendant on not having a job, where this is seen as a major source of personal fulfilment, accounts for some of the differences that exist between married men and women.

Recently, a new twist has been given to this line of research by the suggestion that men may encounter stress as a result of having a wife who works. The first study of this sort was conducted by Burke and Weir in 1976. They found that, among a sample of professional men, those with working wives suffered from poorer health and were less satisfied with their marriages, and their lives in general, than were the husbands of housewives, despite the likelihood of higher household income. There have been several other studies which have supported the main conclusions of the Burke and Weir study (Kessler and McRae, 1982; Rosenfield, 1980; Staines et al., 1985, 1986). The authors of these studies suggested that it was either the extra domestic burdens placed on husbands of employed wives or the feeling of having lost the sole breadwinner status in the family, which was contributing to husbands' dissatisfaction.

It should be pointed out that not all studies have supported the contention that it is bad for the health of married men to have working wives. A meta-analysis of several studies by Fendrick (1984) found no overall significant effect on husbands' health of wives' employment status. It is also important to note that the studies which have provided positive evidence for this relationship have been conducted in the United States. The only two studies so far conducted in Britain (Cochrane and Stopes-Roe, 1981; Newman and Cochrane, in press) have failed to show an association. Perhaps the differences in the relative positions of husbands and wives in the two countries account for the discrepancies in the findings.

Every marriage has to end. The majority of those who get married have to live through the dissolution of their marriage, whether by divorce or by bereavement. It is obvious, as has already been pointed out, that both of these processes are likely to be traumatic to the survivors. Divorce will almost always have been preceded by a period of deteriorated relationships, acrimony, antagonism and conflict. The actual divorce itself, in the legal sense, will very often follow a period of prolonged separation while the two parties technically remain married. Bereavement is much less likely to follow a breakdown in the relationship, but may come at the end of a long and very distressing illness. After divorce and bereavement have occurred there are some similarities in the situations of the survivors, such as the experience of loss and possibly loneliness; but there are also some significant differences in the cognitions they will retain about their erstwhile partner.

The data already presented in this chapter clearly show the much poorer health status of the divorced and the widowed than the married, and indeed it is usually taken for granted that these experiences contribute to an increase in psychological ill-health and physical disease. What is perhaps of more interest is the way in which people cope with these stressful events and the relative impact of them on different people at different times.

Bloom et al. (1978) point out that most of the literature on the problems faced by people whose marriages have been disrupted focuses on the divorced woman. This, they contend, is because of a widespread belief that marital disruption produces more stress for women than for men. This is perhaps not an unreasonable assumption, as economic hardship and continuing parental responsibilities are much more likely to befall women following divorce or bereavement than they are men. However, the data in Table 8.2 indicate quite clearly that both widowhood and becoming divorced are associated with a greater decline in the health status of men than of women. This was clearly confirmed in a review by Stroebe and Stroebe (1983) of the effects of widowhood for the two sexes on a variety of illness rates. Men clearly suffered more stress as a result of being widowed and this took a heavy toll in mental health terms. Although men are more likely to remarry after becoming widowed than are women, it seems they are much less able to cope with life while they remain alone. This is perhaps not surprising in the domestic sphere as it remains traditional for women to take the major responsibility in the household. However, it also appears true in the socio-emotional sphere that men adjust less well to partner loss than do women.

The same appears to be the case for divorce. Jacobs (1982), reviewing a number of studies, found that a significant proportion of divorced men initially experienced an excited sense of freedom immediately following their divorce and engaged in much phrenetic socializing and sexual activity in this period. However, after 6 months to 2 years, these same men, or at least those who had not remarried in the meantime, were very likely to be feeling left at a loose end, shut off from other people, rootless, and were experiencing symptoms of depression, anxiety and apathy. Divorced men increasingly also reported a newly found preference for a stable and loving heterosexual relationship rather than for casual affairs. A further stress for men who become divorced is the usual separation from their children. Greif (1979) found a clear association between the onset of depression after divorce and less than optimal access to children. Perhaps, as many women might confirm, men only realize what benefits they obtain from marriage after they have lost them.

These findings should not be taken to suggest that women do not experience stress following marital disruption. Riessman and Gerstel (1985) showed that separation prior to divorce had a much more negative impact on women than on men, particularly in terms of stress-induced physical illness. However, the pattern reversed itself when formal divorce was considered, and, in common with other studies, they found that this was worse, in health terms, for men. Lin *et al.* (1985) also showed that the period of separation (rather than actual divorce) and the recent experiences of widowhood produced far more depression in women than did actual divorce or a longer experience of being widowed. So, here there appears to be another important gender difference. Women appear to be able to adjust to marital dissolution over time, with the stressful effects gradually reducing as they become more acclimatized to their new-found state, while for men the opposite appears to be true. Although men may initially appear not to show signs of so many negative consequences as do women, over a prolonged period many more men develop severe problems and many more often fail to function altogether (Reissman and Gerstel, 1985, p. 631).

The major stress dimensions which account for the greater symptomatology of divorced women compared to married women appear to be related to material conditions. Gerstel *et al.* (1985) found that following divorce, women's stress derived mainly from economic hardship and lack of help and support with child rearing. Men, on the other hand, experienced much less economic hardship but were more likely to find that they lacked a sense of social integration and emotional support. These findings led these authors to speculate about the meaning of marriage as experienced by men and women. It is quite likely that marriage serves different stress-buffering effects for two sexes, and the break up of a marriage leaves them exposed to different sources of stress and with a need to make differential adjustments.

Before leaving this topic, it should, again, be pointed out that the health data presented are almost equally compatible with a selection for remarriage hypothesis as they are with the stress hypothesis. However, it seems unlikely in the extreme that such traumatic experiences as bereavement and divorce would not contribute directly to the poorer health status of those people in these categories.

SUMMARY AND CONCLUSIONS

Marital status is strongly related to health status, both physical and mental. Married people are healthier, happier and enjoy higher levels of social integration than do the single, widowed and divorced. They also experience less stress and are in a better position to resist the deleterious consequences of stress than are the unmarried.

Beginning with the observation of the noticeably poorer health status of the unmarried than the married, several explanations of this relationship have been explored. The most prominent of these is one that is based upon the idea that the unmarried are both exposed to high levels of stress in their lives, and have fewer resources with which to deal with this stress. They are, then, in a sense, doubly disadvantaged, and pay a heavy price in health terms. There are, however, other plausible explanations for the relationship between marriage and health, notably that which relies on a selection for marriage assumption. the relative merit of these explanations cannot at present be judged, but there appears to be more evidence for the stress hypothesis than for the selection hypothesis.

REFERENCES

Argyle, M. (1987). *The psychology of happiness*. London: Methuen.

Bachrach, L. (1975). *Marital status and mental disorders: An analytical review*. Washington, DC: Department of Health & Welfare.

Barnett, R.C., & Baruch, G.K. (1985). Women's involvement in multiple roles and psychological distress. *Journal of Personality and Social Psychology, 49*, 135–145.

Billings, A.G., & Moos, R.H. (1981). The role of coping responses and social resources in attenuating the stress of life events. *Journal of Behavioral Medicine, 4*, 139–157.

Bloom, B.L., Asher, S.J., & White, S.W. (1978). Marital disruption as a stressor: a review and analysis. *Psychological Bulletin, 85*, 867–894.

Broadhead, W.E., Kaplam, B.H., James, S.A., Wagner, E.H., Schoenbach, V.J., Grimson, R., Heyden, S., Tibblin, G., & Gehlbach, S.H. (1983). The epidemiologic evidence for a relationship between social support and health. *Amercian Journal of Epidemiology, 117*, 521–537.

Brown, G.W., & Harris, T. (1978). *The social origins of depression*. London: Tavistock.

Burke, R.J., & Weir, T. (1976). Relationship of wives' employment status to husband, wife and pair satisfaction and performance. *Journal of Marriage and the Family, 38*, 279–287.

Butler, J.R., & Morgan, M. (1977). Marital status and hospital use. *British Journal of Preventive and Social Medicine, 31*, 192–198.

Carter, H., & Glick, P.C. (1976). *Marriage and divorce: A social and economic study*. Cambridge, Mass.: Harvard University Press.

Champion, L.A. (1985). A psychosocial approach to the mental health of women:

depression, social support and self-help on a new housing estate. PhD Thesis, University of Birmingham.

Cochrane, R. (1983). *The social creation of mental illness*. London: Longman.

Cochrane, R., & Robertson, A. (1973). The Life Events Inventory: a measure of the relative severity of psycho-social stressors. *Journal of Psychosomatic Research, 17*, 135–139.

Cochrane, R., & Robertson, A. (1975). Stress in the lives of parasuicides. *Social Psychiatry, 10*, 161–171.

Cochrane, R., & Sobol, M. (1980). Life stresses and psychological consequences. In P. Feldman & J. Orford (eds), *The social psychology of psychological problems* (pp. 151–182). Chichester: John Wiley & Sons.

Cochrane, R., & Stopes-Roe, M. (1980). Factors affecting the distribution of psychological symptoms in urban areas of England. *Acta Psychiatrica Scandinavica, 61*, 445–460.

Cochrane, R., & Stopes-Roe, M. (1981). Women, marriage, employment and mental health. *British Journal of Psychiatry, 139*, 373–381.

Cohen, S., & Hoberman, H. (1983). Positive events and social supports as buffers of life change stress. *Journal of Applied Social Psychology, 13*, 99–125.

Cohen, L.H., McGowan, J., Fooskas, S., & Rose, S. (1984). Positive life events and social support and the relationship between life stress and psychological disorder. *American Journal of Community Psychology, 12*, 567–588.

Diener, E. (1984). Subjective well-being. *Psychological Bulletin, 95*, 542–575.

Dohrenwend, B.S. (1973). Life events as stressors: a methodological enquiry. *Journal of Health and Social Behavior, 14*, 167–175.

Dominion, J. (1984). *Marital breakdown and health: an overview*. Paper read at Marriage Research Centre Conference, Central Middlesex Hospital.

Eaton, W.W. (1975). Marital status and schizophrenia. *Acta Psychiatrica Scandinavica, 52*, 320–329.

Fendrick, M. (1984). Wives' employment and husbands' distress: a meta analysis and replication. *Journal of Marriage and the Family, 46*, 871–880.

Folkman, S., & Lazarus, R.S. (1980). An analysis of coping in a middle aged community sample. *Journal of Health and Social Behavior, 21*, 219–239.

Fox, J.W. (1984). Sex, marital status, and age as social selection factors in recent psychiatric treatment. *Journal of Health and Social Behavior, 25*, 394–405.

Garfield, S.L., & Sundland, D.M. (1966). Prognostic scales in schizophrenia. *Journal of Consulting Psychology, 30*, 18–24.

Gerstel, N., Riessman, C.K., & Rosenfield, S. (1985). Explaining the symptomatology of separated and divorced women and men: the role of material conditions and social networks. *Social Forces, 64*, 84–101.

Goldberg, D., & Huxley, P. (1980). *Mental illness in the community*. London: Tavistock.

Gove, W.R. (1972). The relationship between sex roles, marital status and mental illness. *Social Forces, 51*, 34–44.

Gove, W.R., Hughes, M., & Briggs-Style, C. (1983). Does marriage have positive effects on the psychological well-being of the individual? *Journal of Health and Social Behavior, 24*, 122–131.

Gove, W.R., & Tudor, J. (1973). Adult sex roles and mental illness. *American Journal of Sociology, 78*, 812–835.

Greif, J.B. (1979). Fathers, children and joint custody. *American Journal of Orthopsychiatry, 49*, 311–319.

Haring-Hidore, M., Stock, W.A., Okun, M.A., & Witter, R.A. (1985). Marital status and subjective well-being: a research synthesis. *Journal of Marriage and the Family, 47*, 947–953.

Holding, T.A., Buglass, D., Duffy, J.C., & Kreitman, N. (1977). Parasuicide in Edinburgh—a seven year review 1968–74. *British Journal of Psychiatry, 130*, 534–543.

Holmes, T.H., & Rahe, R.H. (1967). The social readjustment rating scale. *Journal of Psychosomatic Research, 11*, 213–218.

Jacobs, J.W. (1982). The effect of divorce on fathers: an overview of the literature. *American Journal of Psychiatry, 139*, 1235–1241.

Kandel, D.B., Davies, M., & Raveis, V.H. (1985). The stressfulness of daily social roles for women: marital, occupational and household roles. *Journal of Health and Social Behavior, 26*, 64–78.

Kanner, A.D., Coyne, J.C., Schaefer, C., & Lazarus, R.S. (1981). Comparison of two modes of stress measurement: daily hassles and uplifts versus major life events. *Journal of Behavioral Medicine, 4*, 1–39.

Kessler, R.C., & Essex, M. (1982). Marital status and depression: the importance of coping resources. *Social Forces, 61*, 484–507.

Kessler, R.C., & McRae, J.A. (1982). The effect of wives' employment on the mental health of married men and women. *American Sociological Review, 46*, 443–452.

Kessler, R.C., Price, R.H., & Wartman, C.B. (1985). Social factors in psychopathology: stress, social support and coping processes. *Annual Review of Psychology, 36*, 531–572.

Koskenvuo, M., Kaprio, J., Lonnqvist, J., & Sarna, S. (1986). Social factors and the gender differences in mortality. *Social Science and Medicine, 23*, 605–610.

Kreitman, N. (1965). Hypochondriasis and depression in out-patients in a general hospital. *British Journal of Psychiatry, 111*, 607–611.

Lazarus, R., Kanner, A., & Folkman, S. (1980). Emotions: a cognitive phenomenological analysis. In R. Platchik & H. Kellerman (eds), *Theories of emotions*. New York: Academic Press.

Leavy, R.L. (1983). Social support and psychological disorder: a review. *Journal of Community Psychology, 11*, 3–21.

Lin, N., Woelfel, M.W., & Light, S.C. (1985). The buffering effect of social support subsequent to an important life event. *Journal of Health and Social Behaviour, 26*, 247–263.

McPherson, I.G. (1987). Life stress and coping processes: a comparison of consulters for psychological problems with non-consulters in general practice. PhD thesis, University of Birmingham.

Martin, W.T. (1976). Status integration, social stress and mental illness: accounting for marital status variations in mental hospitalization rates. *Journal of Health and Social Behavior, 17*, 280–294.

Menaghan, E.G. (1982). Measuring coping effectiveness: a panel analysis of marital problems and coping efforts. *Journal of Health and Social Behaviour, 23*, 220–234.

Menaghan, E.G. (1983). Individual coping effects: moderators of the relationship between life stress and mental health outcomes, In H.B. Kaplan (ed.), *Psychosocial stress: Trends in theory and research* (pp. 157–191). New York: Academic Press.

Mergenhagen, P.M., Lee, B.A., & Gove, W.R. (1985). Till death do us part—recent changes in the relationship between marital status and mortality. *Sociology and Social Research, 70*, 53–56.

Milton, F., & Hafner, J. (1979). The outcome of behavior therapy for agoraphobia in relation to marital adjustment. *Archives of General Psychiatry, 36*, 807–814.

Mitchell, R.E., Cronkite, R.C., & Moos, R.H. (1983). Stress, coping and depression among married couples. *Journal of Abnormal Psychology, 92*, 433–448.

Newman, P.J., & Cochrane, R. (in press). Wives' employment and husbands' depression. *Social Behaviour*.

Odegaard, O. (1946). Marriage and mental disease: a study in social pathology. *Journal of Mental Science, 92*, 35–59.

Parker, G.B., & Brown, L.B. (1982). Coping behaviors that mediate between life events and depression. *Archives of General Psychiatry, 39*, 1386–1391.

Paykel, E.K., Myers, J.K., & Kienalt, M. (1969). Life events and depression. *Archives of General Psychiatry, 31*, 753–760.

Pearlin, L.I., & Johnson, J.S. (1977). Marital status, life strains and depression. *American Sociological Review, 42*, 704–715.

Pearlin, L.I., & Schooler, C. (1978). The structure of coping. *Journal of Health and Social Behavior, 19*, 2–21.

Phillips, D.L. (1968). Social class and psychological disturbance: the influences of positive and negative experiences. *Social Psychiatry, 31*, 41–46.

Reich, J., & Zautra, A. (1981). Life events and personal causation: some relationships with satisfaction and distress. *Journal of Personality and Social Psychology, 41*, 1002–1012.

Riessman, C.K., & Gerstel, N. (1985). Marital dissolution and health: do males or females have greater risk? *Social Science and Medicine, 20*, 627–636.

Robinson, A., Platt, S., Foster, J., & Kreitman, N. (1986). *Parasuicide in Edinburgh, 1985: a report on admissions to the Regional Poisoning Treatment Centre*. Edinburgh: Medical Research Council Unit for Epidemiological Studies in Psychiatry.

Rosenfield, S. (1980). Sex differences in depression: do women always have the higher rates? *Journal of Health and Social Behavior, 21*, 33–42.

Roth, S., & Cohen, L.J. (1986). Approach, avoidance and coping with stress. *American Psychologist, 41*, 813–819.

Rushing, W.A. (1979). Marital status and mental disorder: evidence in favor of a behavioral model. *Social Forces, 58*, 540–556.

Segraves, R.T. (1980). Marriage and mental health. *Journal of Sex and Marital Therapy, 6*, 187–198.

Staines, G.L., Pottick, K.J., & Fudge, D.A. (1985). The effects of wives' employment on husbands' job and life satisfaction. *Psychology of Women Quarterly, 9*, 419–424.

Staines, G.L., Pottick, K.J., & Fudge, D.A. (1986). Wives' employment and husbands' attitudes toward work and life. *Journal of Applied Psychology, 71*, 118–128.

Stroebe, M.S., & Stroebe, W. (1983). Who suffers more? Sex differences in health risks of the widowed. *Psychological Bulletin, 93*, 2, 279–301.

Tcheng-Laroche, F., & Prince, R. (1983). Separated and divorced women compared with married controls: selected life satisfaction, stress and health indices from a community survey. *Social Science and Medicine, 17*, 2, 95–105.

Tennant, C., Bebbington, P., & Hurry, J. (1982). Female vulnerability to neurosis: the influence of social roles. *Australian and New Zealand Journal of Psychiatry, 16*, 135–140.

Thoits, P.A. (1983). Multiple identities and psychological well-being: a reformulation and test of the social isolation hypothesis. *American Sociological Review, 48*, 174–187.

Thoits, P.A. (1986). Multiple identities: examining gender and marital status differences in distress. *American Sociological Review, 51*, 259–272.

Vaillant, G.E. (1985). An empirically derived hierarchy of adaptive mechanisms and its usefulness as a potential diagnostic axis. *Acta Psychiatrica Scandinavica, 71*, 171–180.

Verbrugge, L.M. (1979). Marital status and health. *Journal of Marriage and the Family, 41*, 267–285.

Veroff, J., Douvan, E., & Kulka, R.A. (1981). *The Inner American*. New York: Basic Books.

Vinokur, A., & Selzer, M.L. (1975). Desirable vs undesirable life events: their relationship to stress and mental distress. *Journal of Personality and Social Psychology, 32*, 329–337.

Warheit, G.J., Holzer, C.E., Bell, R.A., & Arey, S.A. (1976). Sex, marital status and mental health. *Social Forces, 55*, 459–480.

Waring, E.M. (1977). The role of the family in symptom selection and perpetuation in psychosomatic illness. *Psychotherapy and Psychosomatics, 28*, 253–259.

Waring, E.M. (1984). The measurement of marital intimacy. *Journal of Marital and Family Therapy, 10*, 185–192.

Waring, E.M., & Reddon, J.R. (1983). The measurement of intimacy in marriage: the Waring Intimacy Questionnaire. *Journal of Consulting and Clinical Psychology, 39*, 53–57.

Waring, E.M., McElrath, D., Lefcoe, D., & Weisz, G. (1981). Dimensions of intimacy in marriage. *Psychiatry, 44*, 169–175.

Waring, E.M., Patton, D., Neuron, C.A., & Linker, W. (1986). Types of marital intimacy and prevalence of emotional illness. *Canadian Journal of Psychiatry, 31*, 720–726.

Wechsler, H., & Pugh, T.F. (1967). Fit of individual and community characteristics and rates of psychiatric hospitalization. *American Journal of Sociology, 73*, 331–338.

Yarrow, M.R. Schwartz, C.G., Murphy, H.S., & Deasy, L.C. (1955). The psychological meaning of mental illness in the family. *Journal of Social Issues, 11*, 12–24.

Zautra, A.J., Guarnaccia, C.A., Dohrenwend, B.P. (1986). Measuring small life events. *American Journal of Community Psychology, 14*, 629–656.

KEY WORDS

Marriage, divorce, widowhood, mental illness, health stress, gender differences, coping, social support, employment.

Handbook of Life Stress, Cognition and Health
Edited by S. Fisher and J. Reason
© 1988 John Wiley & Sons Ltd

9

Family Stress

ABE FOSSON
University of Kentucky

THE IMPORTANCE OF FAMILY STRESS: AN INTRODUCTION

When stress and the family are considered together, it is generally in terms of the family as a supportive group of attached individuals that buffers members against a natural or man-made catastrophe, or at least a system that parcels out the stress of major life events as it supports distressed members. Quite the opposite seems to be equally true and clinically important. Some evidence indicates that family relationships are the most important source of stress for a large segment of the population (Ilfeld, 1982). Though these indolent stressors are common and probably associated with psychiatric disturbances, the appropriateness or usefulness of considering them together with life events and catastrophic stressors has been called into question (Garmezy and Rutter, 1985). In this chapter, the various permutations of stress generated within the family will be addressed, with emphasis on how a particular individual becomes stressed by the family. As the concepts unfold it will become obvious that stress of the catastrophic as well as the indolent type may be experienced because of membership in a particular family.

It has been asserted that stress placed upon an individual from family members and relationships (a persistently adverse situation) is sufficiently different from acute stressors, e.g. life events or catastrophic stress, conceptually or qualitatively, to make its grouping and discussion with these forms of stress unhelpful (Garmezy and Rutter, 1985). On the contrary, it can be argued that key aspects of a single event's impact on the respondent, i.e. distress, coping behavior and adjustment, vary from those of family stresses only in amount and not type. By this rationale, stress can be conceived to fall on a continuum of magnitude. This reasoning supports a convergent approach to family and other stressors which suits our purposes well.

The dissimilarities among stressors are numerous and important. Catastrophic and life event stressors are infrequent, major events of limited duration, usually originating outside the family. Family stressors are usually frequently recurring minor events, originating inside the family. Though the difference in magnitude of impact between an isolated stressful family event and a single major life event is great, actual findings of differences in the population are less than would be expected because stressful family events often occur in clusters or with great frequency. Since their impact is cumulative and their frequency high, family stressors are most important clinically (Kanner *et al.*, 1981). Family stress, then, is important because it is very prevalent and often accompanies problematic adjustments.

Evidence of the high prevalence of family stress in the general population is present from two sources. In a cross-sectional survey of 2299 Chicago households, gathering information on a range of life problems, Ilfeld (1982) found current social stressors to be significantly related to depressive symptoms. Of these, current marital stressors had the highest correlations with depression, followed by those related to parenting, employment and finances. Hall *et al.* (1985), investigating the association of social supports and stresses with depressive symptoms (prevalence 48%) in low-income mothers of young children, found among unmarried women in the samples that everyday stressors were strongly associated with depressive symptoms, while life events were weakly related. Blatt *et al.* (1979) reported that depressed normal young adults indicated that when they were children their parents were insensitive, unavailable, or overly intrusive and could not tolerate the child's strivings for autonomy. Again, Schwarz and Zuroff (1979), reporting on female college students, found significant relationships between depressive experiences and remembered parental conflict and inconsistency.

Despite the conviction of most clinicians that the family system plays a crucial role in the development of psychopathology, the results of empirical research have not been overwhelmingly in support of this. Some evidence for a high incidence of family stress among clients presenting for counselling may be mustered from children and adolescents with serious psychiatric conditions. Among 48 children presenting over a 20-year period with onset of anorexia nervosa before the age of 14, multiple adverse family characteristics were present in over 50% of the cases (Fosson *et al.*, 1987). Similarly, 18 cases of severely distorted family patterns of relating were found in the families of 20 children referred for admission to a psychiatric children's ward during a 4-month period in 1985 (Fosson and Lask, 1987). Systematic observations of selected children presenting with various symptoms have uncovered some seemingly consistent patterns of dysfunctional family organizations or habitual ways of interacting (Minuchin *et al.*, 1978).

WAYS THAT FAMILIES STRESS

Six general ways that families stress individual members will be addressed at this point: patterns of organization, transitions, role difficulties, personal attributes of an individual, flow of emotional material, and patterns of communication including the double bind.

PATTERNS OF ORGANIZATION

Families are organized according to hierarchy, alliances, age and stage of the family, rules or habits of relating, and recurrent patterns of communication (Glick and Kessler, 1980; Minuchin, 1974; Skynner, 1976; Walrond-Skinner, 1977). Transactual patterns (recurrent ways of interacting among members of a family) functionally define hierarchies, boundaries, subgroups and alliances. A dominant conceptual model for organizing thoughts and instructions in theoretical and clinical aspects of family systems has been structural family therapy (Minuchin, 1974). A brief discussion of the model must precede discussion of its utilization in exploring patterns of family interaction and individual stress.

The family is a group of attached individuals with certain characteristics. The family system has the characteristics of a partially closed system. Changes in one area are associated with compensatory changes in other areas so that set goals are achieved (e.g. getting the children off to school is accomplished even if one of the parents is unwell), and other constants characteristic of the particular family are maintained. Flow of information, emotions, etc. are subject to controlled access and egress to the family unit (a boundary). There is a hierarchy composed of one or two executives who have a strong attachment to each other and share information, at times to the exclusion of others. They set the precepts for others and have major responsibility for supporting, protecting and supervising other family members (Fig 9.1). The diagram in Figure 9.1, of an idealized nuclear family, illustrates the strength and closeness of the marital relationship (=); the *boundaries* which surround the family unit and separate parents from the sibling subgroup; the multiple roles of the parents (husband and wife as well are parents); and the more distant, weaker relationships between the children (−).

Boundaries are functionally defined by preferential communication, support etc., and tend to group individuals of similar developmental and age status (children, adolescents, adults, and grandparents). When boundaries are inadequately drawn, enmeshment is present. This may involve the boundary between two or more generations. It typically occurs when there are interactional problems among individuals within a homogeneous subgroup within the family, and is associated with cross-generational alliances and distancing within the peer group.

In Figure 9.2 example a(i), there is cross-generational enmeshment, or a very close relationship, between the mother and child. This often occurs in the postnatal period. Part of the father's function is to initiate the separation of the mother from her infant. The mother may resist this separation and if successful (father-dependent factors may also be associated with failure to initiate this process), the resulting distortion of family development is problematic and stress producing. The stress is felt by all three members of this interaction. The father usually feels frustrated and perhaps sad and/or angry over the partial loss of his wife. Though the mother may not feel frustration initially, eventually her constant companion, lack of privacy, absence of adult conversation etc., raise her level of frustration to a crisis point. When this finally happens a surrogate, usually the father, is requested to temporarily supervise the child and thus relieve her. The child frequently challenges the surrogate's (father's) right to supervise him by attempting to return to the mother or by breaking the rules. In the former scenario, the child soon returns to the mother's side, and in the latter instance the father usually must be firm to enforce the rules (because the child endows the

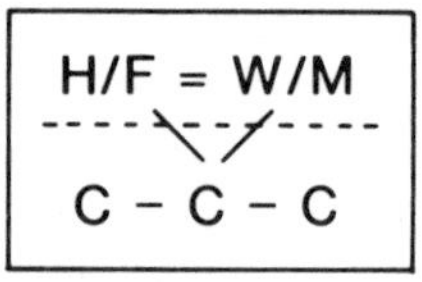

```
┌─────────────────┐
│   H/F = W/M     │
│  ----\--/----   │
│    \  /         │
│   C - C - C     │
└─────────────────┘
```

FIG. 9.1   Relationships within an idealized nuclear family.

father with few rights as an authority figure), and the child's protests involve the mother, who rescues him from the father's authority by returning him to her supervision. The father returns to more personally satisfying activities and the pattern of family organization remains unchanged, though much emotional energy and stress have been generated.

Figure 9.2a(ii) illustrates the situation when a child becomes overly involved in the marital dyad and in so doing brings about some, at least temporary, resolution of a conflict between his parents, thereby potentially saving his family. These behavioral patterns seem to originate from a serendipitous discovery by children who have had attention called to them (often because of acute serious illness, chronic relapsing illness, or acting-out behavior). The discovery, of course, is that the parents inhibit their conflict when the child commands their attention in times of personal distress. (An alternative conceptualization is that the parents relate to each other better in their roles of mother and father than in those of husband and wife.) Since most children want to save their families and most parents feel compelled to overlook difficulties and get along while their child is acutely ill or suffering, the pattern is perpetuated. Even this 'solution' to a stress-ladened

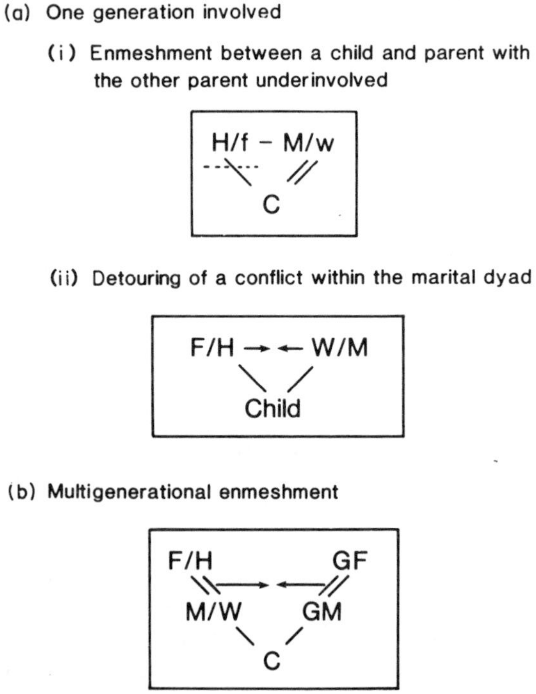

(a) One generation involved

(i) Enmeshment between a child and parent with
        the other parent underinvolved

```
┌─────────────────┐
│   H/f - M/w     │
│  --\---   //    │
│     \           │
│      C          │
└─────────────────┘
```

(ii) Detouring of a conflict within the marital dyad

```
┌─────────────────┐
│  F/H → ← W/M    │
│    \   /        │
│    Child        │
└─────────────────┘
```

(b) Multigenerational enmeshment

```
┌─────────────────┐
│  F/H        GF  │
│   \\──→ ←──//   │
│  M/W        GM  │
│    \   /        │
│      C          │
└─────────────────┘
```

FIG. 9.2   Examples of inadequate boundaries.

problem is stressful for the child, as he must remain distressed (stay in the sick or bad boy role) to effectively distract his parents from their emotionally loaded negative interactions (not an easy task).

The situation in Figure 9.2b is of multigenerational enmeshment, and in this situation the individuals feeling distress may be the parents or child. Generally the grandparents are confident that their actions in assistance of their grandchild are correct and feel little stress, except when in overt conflict with their own progeny. The parents are literally caught in the middle, with their own old authority figures undermining their authority with their child by countermanding their limits and precepts, often in the child's presence. This pattern is very common among adolescent mothers who reside as a single parent with their families of origin, and when the occupation of the role of mother is contested. Alternatively, the child may be torn by split loyalty to two sets of psychological parents.

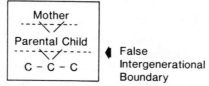

FIG. 9.3   The parental child.

The family system in Figure 9.3 illustrates a pattern of family organization which contains a boundary in an unusual position. In a very real sense, a false generation has been created and the individual in this position (usually the oldest girl among siblings) is delegated some of the mother's numerous responsibilities as a single head of a family. The 'promoted' individual might be stressed enough by this alone, but three confounding factors usually heighten the stress. Firstly, the responsibility usually involves supervising and caring for the younger siblings. Thus, a natural support group of the individual is lost to her. Secondly, little or no authority is granted to the individual (though she is held responsible for the consequences of the siblings' misconduct) by the mother or siblings, therefore cajoling and bribing are often utilized. Thirdly, the 'promoted' one often becomes a one-person support system for the mother. Children caught in these situations talk of worry and unfairness, while adult survivors bitterly complain of lost childhoods and inability to enjoy rearing their own offspring.

TRANSITIONS

Several periods of transition are important in the life of a family. Five of these are clinically important (major stress producing) and will be discussed. In approximate chronological order these are: establishment of a new family unit, addition of a significant family member, separation of significant family members, loss of a family member, and disintegration of the family unit. The mechanisms by which family stress emanates from transitions are few. The erection or destruction of boundaries can be associated with much stress for the individuals involved in the endeavor. Assumption of new roles involves added responsibilities, new work and different (generally more) commitments. These may be eventually comfortable or even comforting to the individual, but the adjustments always produce some stress. Similarly, attempts at establishing new alliances require reaching out, compromise, risk of being rejected, and (in short, much) work.

Establishing a New Family Unit

The tasks in initiating a new family unit are building a marital/family boundary, defining precepts, developing a system for making decisions, opening channels for effective communication of emotionally-laden material, and establishing comfortable roles in a dyadic relationship. The boundary is an extension and reinforcement of the intergenerational boundary which existed in their respective families of origin (Fig. 9.4). Its presence is manifest by various patterns of behavior which include emotional support, exclusive intimacy, sharing of various executive functions such as allocation of financial resources, and rules about when it is appropriate to breech the boundary, as in seeking advice from resources outside the family. The precepts for the family are negotiated within this boundary and any outside assistance may be experienced as an intrusion. Negotiating the rules and thereby establishing how to generate rules (make decisions) have been simplified by a process of matching during courtship on several (but not all) important relationship issues (Dick, 1967). The better the match in dyadic and family relationship styles within the couple (which correlates closely with similarities among the relationships, roles, communication patterns etc., in the couple's two families of origin), the fewer are the decisions, negotiations and compromises that must be worked out and the lower the stress. Relationship issues where differences occur are often not explicitly negotiated. Instead the dyadic member's affective response (which serves as feedback) may range from discomfort to rejection and anger when the partner does not provide the complementary behavior to theirs (meet their expectations). Various ways of interacting are tried until one that is fairly comfortable is found. For example, the wife's father might have helped with the Saturday cleaning as a communication of love and respect for his wife. If the new husband's father worked long hours for overtime pay so that he could provide nicer things for his wife and family as a communication of love, then the potential for misunderstanding and stress is obvious, and the amount of

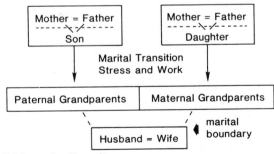

FIG. 9.4   Establishing a family unit.

discomfort, worry, and distress felt by the individuals will depend on their ability to communicate, understand and compromise with each other (or at least their willingness and speed in learning these skills). Faced with similar arrays of tasks at the various transitions, it is little wonder that these are times of high family stress.

Addition of a Significant Family Member

The addition of a significant family member is usually the next nidus of heightened family stress. As in the marital transition, boundaries must be amended, new roles assumed, as well as expectations and precepts carried over from the couple's separate families of origin integrated into the new system. As can be seen in Figure 9.5, the child's boundary with the mother is more diffuse than the corresponding boundary with the father. The integrity of this maternal portion of the intergenerational boundary is important clinically because it is the beginning of autonomy for the next generation and is adversely affected by many factors: marital discord and divorce, compromised intergenerational boundaries in the parents' families of origin, perceived or real vulnerability in the child, and threats to the mother.

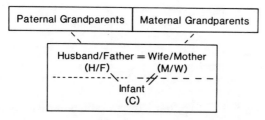

FIG. 9.5   Addition of a family member.

Separation, or Loss of a Significant Family Member

Above and beyond the individual grief work by family members at complete loss (i.e. death of a parent or child), loss to the family on permanent separation from an individual, and temporary loss of the individual who is expected to return, there is stress communicated from the distress of other individuals in the family, and the stress of role and boundary adjustments. Of these situations, the complete and permanent loss by death is most complex (Fig. 9.6a). If a spouse is involved, the stress may be so great that the family is driven to extremes and disintegrates, with the remaining parent and children entering other families, institutions or lifestyles, or the family may become very close, with individual members experiencing anxiety when attempting to separate. If the family stays together, the remaining parent, alone or with assistance (of another adult or an older child), must assume all the parent-executive roles and functions in the family. The transition to a single-parent family is associated with changes in personal habits, role assumptions and support (at least sources), which generate considerable stress (Pearlin and Johnson, 1977). (If one of the older children assumes some of

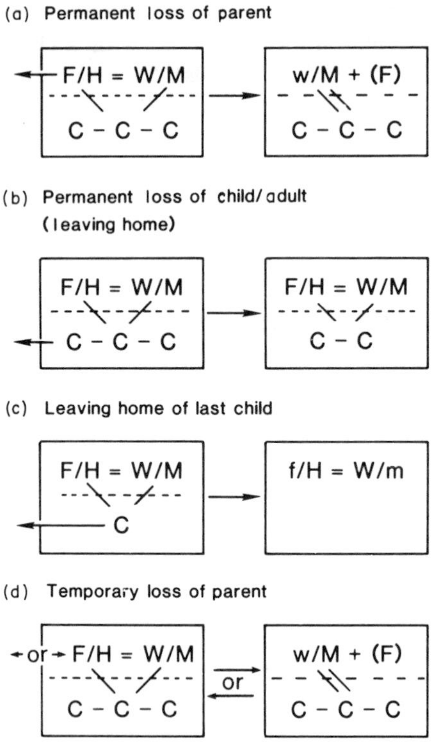

(a) **Permanent loss of parent**

F/H = W/M	w/M + (F)
C - C - C	C - C - C

(b) **Permanent loss of child/adult**
(leaving home)

F/H = W/M	F/H = W/M
C - C - C	C - C

(c) **Leaving home of last child**

F/H = W/M	f/H = W/m
C	

(d) **Temporary loss of parent**

F/H = W/M	w/M + (F)
C - C - C	C - C - C

FIG. 9.6   Loss of a significant family member.

the parent's responsibilities, a potentially stressful pattern is created for that child, which will be addressed under stress-provoking patterns of organization.) (The permanent complete loss of a parent without death—divorce—will be considered later as the main form of family disintegration.)

At one time the complete and permanent loss of a child occurred in most families. Though grief over loss (death) of a child may be great, the system changes and family stress are minor (Fig. 9.6b). The stress is usually manifest as a drawing of the family closer together by grieving parents and concerns of vulnerability by siblings.

Less stressful still is the permanent separation of an adult progeny from the family. This occurs in the life of most families when the children mature into young adults and leave home. (As illustrated in Fig. 9.6c, if it is the last child a new pattern of behavior and relating must be adopted, and therefore the stress is greater.) Even at this relatively common and lower stress transition, clinically important problems exist (Haley, 1980). The temporary loss or separation of a child from the family is often associated with little or no stress unless the presence of a dependent child is necessary to stabilize the mother in her role or the marital relationship. However, separation from the family of one of the parents, even with expected eventual reunion, may produce considerable stress because of temporary boundary, role, responsibility and task displacements (Fig. 9.6d).

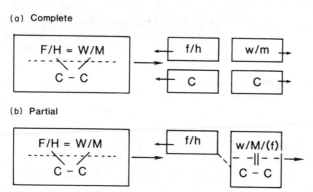

FIG. 9.7 Disintegration of a family unit.

Disintegration of the Family Unit

The disintegration of a family unit has the potential of producing the most system-related stress (Fig. 9.7a). In some ways it is the mirror image of establishing a family, especially if there is minimal survival of subsystems and cross-generational alliances. Beyond the loss of individuals and supportive relationships, new roles, boundaries, alliances and supportive systems must be developed (Pearlin and Johnson, 1977). Of course both parents are stressed, but the stress seems to fall heaviest on the children.

While complete disintegration of a nuclear family unit is unusual, except in cases of death of a mother or of governmental/judicial action, partial disintegration is quite common. A drawing together of the mother and remaining children is the most common result of divorce or a break in a co-habitation agreement (Fig. 9.7b). In this situation, the mother usually becomes responsible for the fathering role, including the financial aspects. This role assumption often is only partially successful, and discipline as well as the standard of living of the family slip a bit. Both of these are commonly associated with at least transient stress on the members of the now incomplete family. The altered and most commonly increased boundary with the father, usually with concurrent lessening of the boundary with the mother, fosters feelings of loss and encourages the children to take on some of the father's functions, i.e. the supervision of younger siblings, emotional support of the mother, and participation in adult level decisions.

Loss of a parent followed by substitution of a different adult in the parent role occurs too rapidly in divorce for most children to make a non-stressful adjustment. The rate of turnover of individuals in the parent role in family units based on co-habitation arrangements is so rapid that attachments between the father figure and the children are usually not formed. These latter families function essentially as single-parent families. In some societies the rate of co-habitation is so high that their frequent breakup may soon begin to represent an important stress factor for the entire population of children.

ROLE DIFFICULTIES

Roles induce stress in family members in several ways. Gradual evolution of role-specific behavior may necessitate stressful adjustments. Daily switching from career to family roles may be stressful because of large differences in levels of responsibility and respect. In the latter situation, the stressed individual may improve his own comfort, though not that of others in the family, by avoiding the more demanding or less prestigious of the discordant roles. This is often seen among professionals and executives who partially abandon the roles of ordinary husband and father to remain in their more prestigious career roles. Stress is also generated when differences between expectations among family members for role-appropriate behavior exist. This may involve only two people, or the discordance may be about the behaviour of a third (usually a child). If there is a general consensus among family members as to the appropriate role behavior in a specific situation, e.g. school, church or illness, the family member not following the accepted precepts will experience much pressure to conform, and will usually feel fairly stressed. Finally one family member may be stressed when necessity demands that they pick up the responsibilities and chores of a role abandoned by another family member.

PERSONAL ATTRIBUTES OF AN INDIVIDUAL FAMILY MEMBER

At times, personal aspects of individual family members may produce stress for others. These include: personal habits, physical deviances or symptoms, rigid personality traits, inappropriate dependency, and interactive styles supported by similar deviant styles in the individual's family of origin.

Children, and for that matter adults, with deviant and perhaps socially handicapping personal habits often produce frustration and stress for fellow family members. In the case of small children, their dependency and lack of socialized personal habits (inept feeding, incontinence, etc.) are confining, frustrating and stressful to their immediate caregivers (usually mother). When mothers also have a limited natural support system, their distress may be overwhelming (Richmond, 1976). Accordingly, the prevalence of depression is quite high among working class mothers with young dependent children (Brown *et al.*, 1975). When socially unacceptable personal habits (incontinence, etc.) persist later into childhood or reappear in old age, frustration and stress are once again common among family members. In some of these situations, the distressed individual may also feel guilty because of having such bad feelings about a family member.

Physical illness often increases the dependency needs of the ill and these are almost always met by family members. This usually does not represent significant stress in cases of acute illness but may in chronic disease. Recent evidence suggests that the prevalence of chronic illness in the general population is increasing. There are several medical conditions which only a decade ago produced a brief terminal illness and now quite regularly produce, in concert with medical intervention, prolonged relapsing illnesses which have a markedly adverse effect on families (Pless and Pinkerton, 1975; Walker *et al.*, 1987). With every relapse, healthy and ill family members alike experience frustration, anger, sadness and guilt. With every remission, affective responses improve but fears of the future, a sense of vulnerability, and sad feelings linger.

As with understandable dependency, inappropriate dependency can be very stressful to involved family members. A common example is that of children who are seen as vulnerable by their parents and therefore held close and dependent. As the children mature, they are reluctant to accept more responsibility (even for personal care) or abandon their dependent behavior, but demand more freedom and autonomy. This leads to much conflict and stress between the involved adults and children. Thus hostile–dependent relationships often develop out of parents' concern for their children's vulnerability. This parental concern may have originated from a family myth about 'fragile infants', or from more substantive but transient physical problems such as premature birth, maternal illness during gestation, threatened miscarriage, serious infections now resolved, etc. (Green and Solnit, 1964). This vulnerable child syndrome is such a common problem that, in surveys of large teaching hospital pediatric clinic waiting rooms, such cases constitute 27% of the children waiting to be seen (Levy, 1980).

Parents' families of origin play an important role in determining behavior within the parent's progenitive family. Many responses and actions taken by parents in day-to-day situations are not planned but automatic. These behaviors are often recapitulations or imitations of the behaviors of loved ones in similar situations in their past experience (Skynner, 1976). The right (comfortable) thing to do in a given situation, then, is determined by their past experience, and deviance from that creates some internal discomfort. To avoid the internal discomfort many parents insist on doing it their way. Since this often impacts on the deportment of others, interpersonal conflicts and individual stresses arise. The very prevalent and stressful interactions associated with child and spouse physical and sexual abuse may be an example of this type of multigenerational problem (Helfer and Kempe, 1974; Green, 1978; Tilelli et al., 1980). So the internalized family, by governing the actions of a current family member, may be indirectly causing current family stress.

FLOW OF AFFECT

When an individual within a family suffers a noxious event, family members not directly involved rally around and provide support. The physical and emotional benefits to the victim may be great, but as these resources are drawn from other family members they may feel drained, worried and distressed. Thus, part of the stress originally felt by the individual is now felt by other family members participating in the process, i.e. the stress and concomitant worry and anxiety have been transmitted. In this way the process that is so beneficial to the suffering individual becomes a source of stress for supporting members as the stress-triggered emotions flow through the family.

PATTERNS OF COMMUNICATION
The Double Bind

An example of this kind of a bind is illustrated by the story of a 12-year-old boy who developed a limp and then 'couldn't walk'. He had been the product of an adolescent pregnancy with the following outcomes. The parents entered into a long-term marital relationship and he was adopted by his maternal grandparents so that his parents could complete their educations. All went well enough until the mother, now in her early thirties and mother of three, began to grieve the loss of her first born. The two families lived in detached homes separated by a large lawn, and the sadness of the natural mother was daily witnessed by all but not openly discussed. Without an explicit discussion of their feelings and predicament, the two mothers negotiated a 'solution'. The 12-year-old could visit his natural mother and spend the night whenever he wanted. The boy held much affection for both these women and did not wish to hurt either. His problem was that when he visited his natural mother his grandmother became sad and hurt, and if he did not visit his natural mother, *she* became sad and hurt. A distressed young man caught in a double bind.

The double bind was an early conceptualization in the development of models addressing interpersonal interactions and families. In the double bind, the 'victim' is placed in a no-win position because a communication is coupled with another that makes a satisfactory response to the first very difficult or impossible. It requires two or more people and repeated similar experiences. The first statement might be, 'Don't do such and such or I'll punish you' coupled with, 'I'm not really your boss', or, 'Don't consider this punishment' (Sluzki and Ransom, 1976). So the double bind is one type of paradoxical communication like, 'Don't believe anything you read in this book' (Watzlawick and Weakland, 1974).

Confused Operational Definitions of Affect and Relationships

It has gradually become evident that the double bind is but one example of confused or mutually disqualifying and stress-producing communications that take place in families. One of the reasons these miscommunications arise so easily is that many or all communications between family members have important meanings on three levels. The most obvious level and least problematic is content that is what the words mean. This seems fairly straightforward, but within the same language the meaning of words varies from time to time and place to place. In fact, since many words are defined behaviorally during childhood, there is often an idiosyncratic component to the operational definitions of words used between family members. The second level of meaning is the affect which accompanies the words. This is conveyed by the voice tone, timbre, facial expression, etc., and is automatically processed by listeners most of the time. It lets them know how the speaker is feeling in the context of the communication, which is usually related to their feelings about the topic under discussion. Finally, there is communication about the relationship between the parties involved, e.g. the discussant is the boss of me and I accept that relationship as proper.

Communication which is clear, straightforward and concordant in its statements on all three levels is easiest to process and least stress provoking. Incongruence between the content of the discussion and affect of the discusser raises doubts in the listener's mind about the true feelings/emotions of the discusser. Discordances between explicit or implied verbal statements about the speaker and listener's relationship and other simultaneous verbal or action communications, which define their relationship, place the receiver of the communication in the position of having to make a choice as to how to respond. The situation can be very stressful (Haley, 1963).

SUMMARY

Families are important sources of stress as well as important resources in times of stress. Stress originating from sources within the family is common and associated with increased risk of psychological illness. Family members feel stressed when: roles are demanding, change is necessary, emotions emanating from a distressed sibling or parent are shared, expectations and performance are discordant, communication is ambiguous, boundaries are poorly drawn, cross-generational alliances are overly important, and members feel unsupported. This type of stress is the culmination of low-grade, high-frequency noxious events recurring on a daily basis.

This chapter is about family organization and how individual family members are stressed because they are part of a particular family. Stress may come about because the family: is in a transition, has a poorly functioning organizational pattern, contains individuals with difficult personal attributes, is involved in the sharing of noxious emotional material between members, disagrees on role issues, and has ambiguous communications.

REFERENCES

Blatt, S.J., Wein, S.J., Chevron, E., & Quinlan, D.M. (1979). Parental representations and depression in normal young adults. *Journal of Abnormal Psychology, 88*, 388–397.

Brown, G.W., Bhrolchain, M.N., & Harris T. (1975). Social class and psychiatric disturbance among women in an urban population. *Sociology, 9*, 225–254.

Dick, H. (1967). *Marital tension*. New York: Basic Books.

Fosson, A. & Lask, B. (1987). Pictorially displayed family patterns as an assessment instrument. Submitted for publication.

Fosson, A., Knibbs, J., Bryant-Waugh, R., & Lask, B. (1987). Early onset: anorexia nervosa. *Archives of Diseases of Childhood, 62*, 114–118.

Garmezy, N., & Rutter, M. Acute reactions to stress. In M. Rutter & L. Hersov (eds), *Child and adolescent psychiatry: Modern approaches* (pp. 152–176). Oxford: Blackwell Scientific.

Glick, I., & Kessler, D. (1980). *Marital and family therapy*. New York: Grune & Stratton.

Green, A.H. (1978). Psychiatric treatment of abused children. *American Academy of Child Psychiatry, 65*, 356–371.

Green M., & Solnit A.J. (1964). Reactions to the threatened loss of a child: A vulnerable child syndrome. *Pediatrics, 34*, 58–66.

Haley, J. (1963). *Strategies of psychotherapy*. New York: Grune & Stratton.

Haley, J. (1980). *Leaving home: the therapy of disturbed young people*. New York: McGraw-Hill.

Hall, L.A., Williams, C.A., & Greenberg, R.S. (1985). Supports, stressors and depressive symptoms in low-income mothers of young children. *American Journal of Public Health,* 75, 518–522.

Helfer, R.E., & Kempe, C.H. (eds) (1974). *The battered child,* 2nd edn. Chicago: The University of Chicago Press.

Ilfeld, F.W. (1982). Marital stressors, coping styles, and symptoms of depression. In L. Goldberger & S. Breznits (eds), *Handbook of stress: theoretical and clinical aspects* (pp. 482–494).

Kanner, A.D., Coyne, J.C., Schaefer, C., & Lazarus, R.S. (1981). Comparison of two modes of stress measurement: daily hassles and uplifts versus major life events. *Journal of Behavioral Medicine, 4,* 1–38.

Levy, J.C. (1980). Vulnerable children: Parents' perspectives and the use of medical care. *Pediatrics, 65,* 956–963.

Minuchin, S. (1974). *Families and family therapy.* Mass.: Harvard University Press.

Minuchin, S., Rosman, B., & Baker, L. (1978). *Psychomatic families, anorexia nervosa in context.* Mass: Harvard University Press.

Pearlin, L.I., & Johnson, J.S. (1977). Marital status, life-strains and depression. *American Sociological Review, 42,* 704–715.

Pless, I.B., & Pinkerton, P. (1975). Chronic childhood disorder-promoting patterns of adjustment. London: Henry Kimpton.

Richmond, N. (1976). Depression in mothers of preschool children. *Journal of Child Psychology and Psychiatry, 17,* 75–78.

Schwarz, J.C., & Zuroff, D.C. (1979). Family structure and depression in family college students: effects of parental conflict, decision-making power, and inconsistency of love. *Journal of Abnormal Psychology, 88,* 398–406.

Skynner, A.C.R. (1976). *One flesh–separate persons: principles of family and marital psychotherapy.* Edinburgh: Constable.

Sluzki, C., & Ransom, D. (1976). *Double bind, the foundation of the communicational approach to the family.* New York: Grune & Stratton.

Tilelli, J.A., Turek, D., & Jaffe, A.C. (1980). Sexual abuse of children: clinical findings and implications for management. *New England Journal of Medicine, 302,* 319–323.

Walker, L.S., Ford, M.B., & Donald, W.D. (1987). Cystic fibrosis and family stress: effects of age and severity of illness. *Pediatrics, 79,* 239–246.

Walrond-Skinner, S. (1976). *Family therapy, the treatment of natural systems.* London: The Lavenham Press Limited, 1977, pp. 10–32.

Watzlawick, P., Weakland, J., & Fisch, R. (1974). *Change principles of problem formation and problem resolution.* New York: W.W. Norton.

KEY WORDS

Additions, boundary, chronic illness, defining relationships, dependency of youth, divorce, double bind, enmeshment, emotional support, establishing a family, family disintegration, family organization, levels of communication, losses, parental child, patterns of communication, role difficulties, separations, transitions, vulnerable child syndrome.

Handbook of Life Stress, Cognition and Health
Edited by S. Fisher and J. Reason
© 1988 John Wiley & Sons Ltd

10

Women's Work and Family Roles: Sources of Stress and Sources of Strength

JANET E. MALLEY and ABIGAIL J. STEWART
Boston University

INTRODUCTION

It has been frequently suggested that the links between stress and physical and mental health are different for women and men (See Johnson, 1977; Nathanson, 1977). While it is impossible to be sure exactly why this should be so, a number of researchers have suggested that one explanation of this difference may lie in the differences in men's and women's social roles. Thus, for example, several researchers have argued that the general social devaluation of housework makes housewives vulnerable to depression, regardless of situational stresses (Oakley, 1974; Pearlin *et al.*, 1981). Alternatively, although a great deal of research suggests that, in general, employment is associated with positive health outcomes for women, Haynes and Feinleib (1982) found that women's employment in positions with little status or control, when they also had large families, was associated with stress-related illnesses. Similarly, Stewart and Salt (1981) showed that although the average level of psychological functioning in a sample of educated women did not vary as a function of their work and family roles, the *impact of stressful life events* did. Thus, married women with children but without careers seemed to become depressed in response to life changes, while single career women seemed to get physically ill (much as men do). The two groups who combined roles (married women with careers, and married women with careers and children) both showed no particular negative response to life changes.

Stewart and Salt speculated that single career women might be especially likely to experience life changes as posing challenges to their capacity for active coping, since they could not share responsibility either for the changes or the coping with other family members. In contrast, the mothers without careers might be especially likely to be faced with life changes imposed by the decisions of others (e.g. husband's career demanding family moves, etc.), and thus might lack a sense of control over the change, and be vulnerable to feelings of helplessness about coping with it. The two mixed role groups might, then, be buffered both from the stresses deriving from a sense of sole responsibility, and a sense of helplessness. The argument assumed that the different life structures might have different psychological risks and benefits, but the study was not grounded in a general theory of the link between work and family roles and psychological well-being.

In this chapter, we will present a theoretical description of the psychological experience of work and family roles which helps make clear how they might act as mediators of the stress–illness relationship. This theoretical account is intended to define how significant adult roles are typically experienced, in terms which are relevant to stress responses. In addition, it must leave room for the fact that there are large individual differences in the experience of those roles, since it seems unlikely that occupancy of particular roles *by itself* could account for different responses to stress. In developing this model, we assume that work and family roles can be sources of both stress and strength, and that the precise significance of events in any one role may depend importantly on one's experience in another one.

We will begin by sketching out our conceptual framework. We will then illustrate how it might be used in understanding existing findings by discussing some of the literature on the consequences of women's family and work roles for their mental and physical health. Our conceptualization may eventually be useful for understanding men's family roles and relationships as well as their work lives. However, the data on the relational aspects of men's lives are scarce, so a detailed exploration of the complex consequences of men's work and family lives must await further research.

AGENCY AND COMMUNION

We assume that two fundamental human needs, implied by the activities of loving and working, are crucial to most people's mental health and happiness. These needs have been named variously by different thinkers, but they were described clearly, for our purposes, by Bakan, in his discussion of 'the duality of human existence' (1966). Though Bakan is largely critical of what he calls 'agency', he defines it as a fundamental modality 'in the existence of living forms' (1966, p. 15), a modality which emphasizes the organism as an individual—separate and self-sufficient. Agency, then, is manifest in efforts at unconstrained self-expression as well as in efforts at self-control and self-direction. Autonomous pursuit of independent goals reflects agency in a direct, straightforward way. It is worth noting that Bakan argues that 'unmitigated agency', or agency with no communion, is always unhealthy. Thus, Bakan points out that agency can be expressed in ugly forms: 'Agency manifests itself in the formation of separations . . . in isolation, alienation, and aloneness . . . in the urge to master . . .' (p. 15). Moreover, Bakan suggests that it is the drive to assert the self without regard for others that results in illness. (See Jenkins (1976), Pleck and Sawyer (1974) and Wolf (1971) for evidence that he may be right.)

Some theorists (e.g. Lipman-Blumen and Leavitt, 1976) have noted that agency may be expressed indirectly, or vicariously. Thus, women's instrumental efforts have often been directed not toward pursuit of their own goals for themselves, but toward pursuit of their goals for others (e.g. their hopes for their children's achievement), or others' goals for themselves (e.g. their husbands' career aspirations). This indirect agency permits some gratification of the woman's wish to feel competent, but robs her of recognition and direct reward, diverts her from her own pursuits and goals, and may arouse jealousy and resentment in the person she aims to help (Hochschild, 1975; Miller, 1976). Thus, indirect agency is indeed a form of 'mitigated agency', but one with its own problematic potential.

Bakan proposes that the other 'fundamental modality' is communion, or 'the participation of the individual in some larger organism of which the individual is a part'. Bakan suggests that: 'communion manifests itself in the sense of being at one with other organisms . . . in the lack of separations . . . in contact, openness, and union . . . in noncontractual cooperation' (p. 15). Thus, communion includes a sense of affectionate and collaborative ties with others. These ties permit empathy, intimacy, and knowing and being known. It is clear that—unmitigated by agency—such ties can suffocate, depriving an individual of a sense of independent purpose or value. It is also clear that communion can be, and ideally is, experienced in a fully mutual relationship of intimate interdependence. However, intimacy can take place in an asymmetrical form, with one person providing more empathy and understanding than the other. Such relationships may leave the more empathic member depleted or drained (see Belle, 1982b).

Thus it is the simultaneous, or balanced, presence of opportunites for direct agency and mutual communion that provides women and men with the greatest satisfaction and mental health. Imbalance of agency and communion may lead to illness or tension (in the case of unmitigated agency), or to depression and despair (in the case of unmitigated communion). Moreover, direct agency is more satisfying than is indirect, both because it provides more social recognition and evokes less envy and resentment. Finally, mutual communion is more satisfying than is asymmetrical communion because it offers a sense of being understood and valued by an equal, as well as a sense of closeness and affection. In examining work and family roles, the concepts of balance, of direct agency, and of mutual communion, may provide useful ways of organizing what we know about the stresses and vulnerabilities of women in various kinds of relationships and employment situations.

FAMILY ROLES AND RELATIONSHIPS

Some of women's family roles (e.g. wife and mother) are defined in terms of the particular relationships that are at the center of the roles. While the social roles involved are defined in terms going well beyond the personal relationships, without the relationships the roles do not exist. In the next section we will explore how marriage and motherhood provide opportunities and make demands for agency (both direct and indirect) and communion (both mutual and asymmetrical). In this exploration we will rely on empirical studies of women's family roles and relationships; we do not pretend, though, that our review is in any way exhaustive. We will present the evidence we have found that is relevant to assessing our notion that it is the balance of direct and indirect agency, and mutual and asymmetrical communion that makes the most important difference to women's physical and psychological health, rather than the roles they occupy per se.

Marriage

The marital relationship is often viewed as the likeliest source of high levels of mutual communion. Many women indicate that they hope to find companionship in marriage (see, for example, Levinger, 1964; Rubin, 1976) and some report that companionship is a feature of their marraige that they value very highly indeed (see Veroff et al., 1981; Baruch et al., 1983).

In addition, in visions of the modern dual-career marriage, husbands and wives are often depicted as fully equal partners sharing fascinating careers, housework and child care, and a rich companionship of heart and mind (see, for example, Chafe, 1983). In this vision, husbands and wives support each other's agency (careers, goals, projects), and offer each other emotional support and caring (communion). This sort of balanced experience of direct and indirect agency and mutual communion does not seem to characterize everyone's experience of marriage, at least as that experience is described in the empirical literature.

First, wives make fewer claims on their husband's attention than their husbands make on theirs (Bernard, 1972; Warren, 1975). Moreover, wives are generally viewed by their spouses as having less right to demand emotional support (see Goode, 1982; Miller and Mothner, 1981). In fact, in traditional sex-differentiated marriages, self-disclosure of both husbands and wives is generally low (see Blood and Wolfe, 1960; Komarovsky, 1976; Rubin, 1976; Peplau and Gordon, 1985). 'Mutual communion' is, then, unlikely when spouses perceive themselves as unequal (see Miller and Mothner, 1981).

Even in relationships of equal status or power, marriage may not offer women mutual communion. A number of observers have pointed out that women's traditional and continuing family role is to act as the 'expressive' specialist, or the person 'in charge' of handling all family members' feelings and emotional needs (see Chodorow, 1978; Knupfer et al., 1966). In fact, Veroff et al. (1981) suggest that it is this role that takes its toll on women's mental health. Thus, while some early analyses assumed that perhaps the only thing women reliably found in marriage was companionship (see, for example, Bernard, 1972), recent arguments (Weiss, 1984) have stressed the extent to which wives must perform feats of nonverbal decoding, verbal cajoling, and multi-media 'stroking' in order to achieve any communication with their spouses. That communication then centers in a unilateral way on the disclosure and amelioration of the problems and pains of the husband (Jourard and Richman, 1963). Thus, because women are thought to be especially competent 'relationship partners', they may end up experiencing little mutual communion in their marriages, while providing considerable support to their husbands. The likely results of a long-standing pattern of asymmetrical communion with an adult include resentment of continuing demands and failure to reciprocate, erosion of the willingness to provide support, and a growing sense of isolation and separation (see Miller, 1976, Chapter 6).

The exercise of relational competence might, on the other hand, provide married women with a sense of competence or agency. However, this very competence itself renders women more vulnerable to interruptions of their agentic pursuits; thus, demands for emotional support can easily override the pursuit of women's own goals (see Miller's (1976) analysis of the case of Anne, p. 63). Thus, women's capacity for doing the 'work of relationships', when combined with the normative claims of marriage, puts women's opportunities for agency outside the marriage (e.g. in independent work) at risk.

Moreover, the pride and sense of competence a woman might feel as a result of her relational competence is likely to be rather small, since this talent is neither valued nor recognized socially, and reflects only an indirect form of agency—that is, agency on behalf of her husband's goals (see Papanek, 1973; Coser and Coser, 1974; Kanter, 1977; Seidenberg, 1975). There is ample evidence that though some women can take pride in this 'helpful' role, at least for a while, over time the lack of recognition and reward becomes frustrating, and resentment of being exploited or used grows (see Miller, 1976; Hochschild, 1975). Alternatively, the lack of confirmation may erode a woman's confidence to the point where she is no longer able to provide much help at all (Seidenberg, 1975; Rubin, 1979). Indirect agency, then, may provide some satisfactions, but when it continues over time without any opportunity for direct agency, it carries with it some important risks.

Motherhood

Parenting, like marriage, is normatively defined as a source of intense satisfaction and meaning; and many parents do find that their children are indeed a source of great joy (see Douvan, 1983). Nevertheless, becoming a parent has been regularly described as precipitating a 'crisis' (Rossi, 1968), and the demands of parenting are often identified as a source of marital strain (Belsky et al., 1983; Miller and Sollie, 1980) and individual stress (Guttentag, 1975). We believe that the mother–child relationship is one which can be understood as offering some potential for meeting women's needs for agency and communion; it offers, too, considerable potential for frustrating them.

First, some women do find that their relationships with their children are close and intimate (Balint, 1939; Chodorow, 1978); for these women, motherhood may offer some sense of mutual communion. Much of the time, though, motherhood offers the potential for closeness and connection, but without the possibility of mutuality, or being understood (see Weiss, 1979). In fact, the parent–child relationship is perhaps the quintessential relationship of legitimate asymmetrical communion. Such relationships may be experienced over time as draining and depleting, because they demand that much be given, in the absence of much in return (see Belle, 1982a, 1982b). Indeed, mothers do often report a sense that they are asked, as mothers, to give more than they have (see Baruch et al., 1983, Chapter 5).

Moreover, the absence of any mutuality in mothers' relationships has been identified as a source of low self-esteem, leading mothers to feel less able to seek or demand relationships with adult equals that might offer true mutual commun-ion (see Abernathy, 1973; Belle, 1982a, 1982b; Brown et al., 1975). Feeling unworthy of adult love and understanding, these depressed and depleted mothers in turn feel even less able to give to their children. Thus, having only relationships of asymmetrical communion can build toward despair.

Motherhood does provide women with some opportunity for agency. The acts involved in teaching and caring for children of all ages are acts which can and do promote a sense of competence (Chester, 1985). However, most women find that their own and others' expectations for their performance as mothers are so high that it is difficult to retain a stable sense of oneself as a 'good' or 'excellent' mother. Instead, many women find mothering arouses deep anxieties about their capacity to parent, and their children's resulting well-being (see, for example, Belle, 1982a; Grossman et al., 1980; Rapoport, et al., 1977).

Moreover, much of mothers' agency is indirect—in the service of their goals for their children (Siegler, 1976). Even if these goals feel, for a time, like a woman's own goals, eventually the separateness of the child must assert itself, precipitating those feelings of envy, resentment, and personal inadequacy that are always a risk of indirect agency. Thus, for women with little independent outlet for agency, the loss of children through normal development may precipitate a serious loss of a sense of value and purpose ('the empty nest syndrome'; Bart, 1971).

FAMILY ROLES DEFINED BY ABSENT RELATIONSHIPS

Some women occupy family roles that are defined socially in terms of the family relationships that are missing. Thus, 'single' women (women who have never married and have no children) are defined in terms of the marital relationships they lack, rather than in terms of the elements present in their lives. Similarly, widows and divorcees are defined in terms of the relationships they have willingly or unwillingly lost. These family roles—single woman, widow, divorcee—also may be understood in terms of their potential to allow women to meet their needs for agency and communion.

Unmarried Women

Women who have never married do not have institutionalized relationships with spouses and/or children. Instead, unmarried women must actively seek rela-tionships. The risk for these women, if they do not or cannot pursue a network of friends and intimates, is the absence of communal support. In fact, Stein (1976) reports that fear of loneliness is a major concern for single adults. In a society geared to married couples, singles can be made to feel inadequate and undesir-able. Moreover, a friendship network based solely upon nonfamily relationships may feel less secure than those formed by socially defined family relationships. On the other hand, it can be argued that single women, because of their autonomy, have more flexibility and independence to pursue friendships than married women (Baruch et al., 1983). Single women may even have an advantage over previously married women in that they lack both the experience of a public relational failure (of divorced women) and the sense of disloyalty (of widows) which might constrain their pursuit of new relationships. And because their relationships are with adults, are actively sought and sustained, and are not defined by social and legal norms, they are more likely to be reciprocal and mutually satisfying than those confined within the household.

However, it seems clear that pursuit of agency, not communion is relatively simple for women remaining single. Adams (1976) describes the advantages of single life as economic independence and social and psychological autonomy. Like divorced and widowed women who are reluctant to pursue new intimate relationships for fear of losing their new-found feelings of self-sufficiency and autonomy, single women describe themselves as more independent and achievement oriented, while viewing married women as concerned more with interpersonal relationships (Baruch et al., 1983). Thus, single women are at risk for lives of 'unmitigated agency' (Stewart and Salt, 1981).

Divorcees

Regardless of the quality of the married relationship, divorce represents the loss of a major potential source of companionship and/or intimacy. Baruch et al. (1983) report that loneliness is a major concern of divorced women. Not only do they miss the relationships they had with their ex-spouse and old friends, but when they are also single parents they have less free time to explore new relationships. Children can serve as a kind of 'communal buffer,' providing the women with some companionship (see Weiss, 1979). However, this is an asymmetrical relationship.

Very often, old friendships are no longer as satisfying as they had been before the divorce (Weiss, 1975). New friendships and an active social support network are consistently found to be related positively to adjustment to divorce in women (Smith, 1980; Weiss, 1975, 1979). One advantage of these new adult relationships is that they may be more mutually satisfying than previous ones, as the women are pursuing them to meet their own needs, and not just those of other family members. In fact, the divorced women in Miller's (1982) sample of low income single mothers felt that they were better able to develop and sustain friendships as they had more control over their time and greater flexibility in scheduling their day than their married counterparts.

Divorce can more generally provide women with new opportunities for personal growth. Married women have often operated in the traditional role of dependency expected in a marriage. With the divorce, and the loss of this dependent role, some can experience a sense of powerlessness and helplessness (Herman, 1977; Smith, 1980). Some women, though, do not respond to divorce or separation in the long term with feelings of helplessness and dependency, but rather take on a more active and instrumental role in their lives. They are better able to cope with the stress of that adjustment (Granvold et al., 1979), as well as with future stresses.

Miller (1982) found that the divorced women in her sample were compelled (particularly as a result of their financial situation) to take on new roles. They looked to themselves, rather than to their ex-husbands, to define and implement these roles and through their instrumentality developed a new sense of self-worth and competence. Baruch *et al.* (1983) also found that the employed, divorced women in their study experienced a strong sense of personal growth, competence and independence. However, they also found that women who were concerned about money were inhibited in developing a sense a mastery. Women who are trapped in poorly paying jobs and see these jobs only as a means of supporting their families may be agentic only for the benefit of others. In contrast, women who take from their jobs not only a paycheck, but also a sense of personal efficacy and competence, also increase their self-esteem. Finally, divorced women who do not need to establish financial independence, and continue to rely on their ex-spouse or other family members for support, may jeopardize this opportunity for growth and independence.

Although their life situation may in many ways be more difficult after a divorce—less money, less free time and flexibility, more demands upon their time—many women prefer their new situation because of the new sense of independence. Kohen *et al.* (1979) found in their study of divorced women that most of them were not seriously considering remarriage, despite the fact that many felt the loss of an intimate relationship. Their new-found freedom and independence were not worth risking for a new marriage. Similarly, Baruch *et al.* (1983) found the single mothers in their study to be torn about the conflict between their own needs for autonomy and the pleasure of an intimate relationship. Many concluded that they would not pursue an intimate relationship unless it could be achieved without the loss of their independence.

Widows

The issues for widows are similar to those for divorced women. However, the loss of communion implied by the loss of a spouse may be more painful for a widow than for a divorcee. When a woman's spouse dies, she may very well lose her principal source of intimacy and companionship (Barrett, 1981; Weiss, 1979). Even if the relationship was asymmetrical, and she was caring for her husband with very little support in return, she no longer has even the opportunity for that form of communion.

The loss of a spouse often also means the loss of a woman's principal role in life. This loss can be especially devastating for older women who were raised with the primary goals in life of wife and motherhood. Parkes and Weiss (1983) report that widows who were most dependent upon their spouses during their marriages have a poorer recovery rate after bereavement. They attribute this to the women's lack of independence and to an inability to form an identity outside of the marriage, coupled with low self-esteem and ability to succeed on their own.

Widows, like divorcees, may be able to redirect their communal needs to outside relationships. However, this takes time. Old friends may support them in their grief in the beginning, but friends are often uncomfortable with the constant reminder of their own and their loved one's vulnerability. And widows themselves may not find these friendships, based upon couple relationships, as rewarding as they had been. It becomes necessary to move on to someone who can relate to them in their new social role—often other widows (see Arling, 1976; Barrett, 1981). Parkes and Weiss (1983) say such understanding relationships can give the bereaved a sense of security. And as with divorced women, these new relationships, born of such a personal connection, may be even more mutually satisfying than what was experienced in their marriage, because they grow out of the woman's own needs.

Finally, some widows experience their widowhood as offering new opportunities for personal growth and development. About half of Lopata's (1973) widows reported positive aspects of widowhood, including independence. As Barrett (1977) indicates, 'Widowhood may be the first time in a woman's life that she is living alone. She is a member of a group that could wield substantial political power. She has the potential for self-mastery and discovery at a time of her life when new social roles can be pursued' (p. 868).

This new opportunity for agency is only available, of course, to widows with the health, education and resources to pursue independent goals. Many women are too constrained by limited financial resources, little job or educational experience, and poor health to capitalize on the new potential for agency that can be the compensatory 'benefit' of widowhood (see Barrett, 1977).

AGENCY, COMMUNION, AND THE WORK ROLE

Employment is strongly associated with women's increased sense of accomplishment, independence, and self-esteem (Baruch et al., 1983; Crosby, 1982). This is especially true for women who work in professional, better-paying jobs (Birnbaum, 1975) in which material and psychological rewards are high, but has been found to be so for lower class, blue-collar workers as well (Fox and Hesse-Biber, 1984; Tebbets, 1982).

Work is a source of communal benefits for women as well. As many as 42% of Crosby's (1982) middle-class, suburban workers found interpersonal relationships at work gratifying. Baruch et al. (1983) found that women, more than men, valued social contact at work. It is probable that these work associations can provide for increased social contacts and richer, more mutual communion than is likely to be readily available to housewives (Ferree, 1976; Oakley, 1974). Certainly, working women are found to be significantly less lonely than their counterparts who are not employed (Baruch et al., 1983; Crosby, 1982; Tebbets, 1982; Bernard, 1974b).

Clearly, then, the worker role can provide women with additional opportunities for experiencing both direct agency and mutual communion in their lives. The following is a discussion of the ways in which the worker role may enhance these opportunities and make demands for agency and communion for working women in various family structures.

Homemakers

The role of housewife may provide a balance of communion and agency for some women. However, the potential for this role to be insufficient is reflected in the overwhelming evidence of dissatisfaction of housewives in contrast to working women (Baruch et al., 1983; Crosby, 1982; Ferree, 1976).

The area of primary responsibility for the homemaker is housework. As with any job, housework carries with it the potential for a high degree of agency. However, unlike paid employment, performance of household tasks is difficult to assess, as there are no clear standards for evaluation (Piotrkowski, 1978; Bernard, 1974b) other than, perhaps, the unattainable standard of perfection. Thus, rather than gaining a sense of mastery or achievement from household work, women can experience frustration from feeling that their work is never good enough. Moreover, household chores are, for the most part, monotonous, repetitive, and boring (Bernard, 1974b), preventing women from developing new skills or abilities, or a sense of self-esteem (Piotrkowski, 1978). Similarly, housework is unpaid, and thus devalued (Bernard, 1974a; Oakley, 1974), minimizing any sense of satisfaction to be gained from its accomplishment. The limited opportunity it provides for satisfactory expression of agency may help account for Stewart and Salt's (1981) finding that stressed housewives are more depressed than stressed mothers employed outside the home.

The devaluing of housework may have ramifications for housewives' experience of communion as well. Caring for other family members provides a natural expression of communion. However, being unpaid, homemakers are dependent upon and subordinate to their salary-earning spouses (Piotrkowski, 1978). This unequal relationship may exacerbate the tendency for assymetrical communion between spouses and help to explain why employed men and women are more likely to take pleasure in their spouses than housewives (Crosby, 1982). In addition, the loneliness and isolation generally experienced by housewives (Baruch et al., 1983; Crosby, 1982; Tebbets, 1982; Bernard, 1974b) make other opportunities for mutual communion unlikely.

Moreover, the boundary between the agentic and communal areas of the housewife role are not clearly defined (Piotrkowski, 1978). This may enable the homemaker to satisfy both agentic and communal needs within the one role, but it may also create confusion and frustration when the two areas are in conflict. Thus, communal caring for children and wanting to make them happy can easily conflict with the simultaneous agentic goal of keeping the house clean (Oakley, 1974). Therefore, rather than balanced experience of both agency and communion, expression of both may be thwarted.

Married Workers

As has already been discussed, married homelife provides few opportunities for housewives' expression of direct agency and mutual communion. However, when both spouses work, relationships at home may take on a new quality. Attitudes toward work reflect and affect attitudes toward home (Piotrkowski, 1978). Thus, women who have developed a sense of independence, mastery and self-esteem at work may carry over this agentic posture into their activities at home. Employed wives have been found to enjoy a more egalitarian division of family roles and to play a more active part in family decision making (Steil and Turetsky, 1987).

Similarly, more mutually oriented communion experiences at work can redirect women's communal relations at home toward more symmetry. This phenomenon would help to explain Crosby's (1982) finding that employed women *and* men are more apt to take pleasure in their spouses than housewives. Weingarten (1978) similarly found in her study of 32 professional couples that the spouses were *mutually* responsive to each other's needs.

Employment, by providing an added dimension in a woman's life, can also function as a buffer against negative experiences at home (Baruch *et al.*, 1983; Crosby, 1982). With additional opportunities for agency and communion at work, unsatisfying experiences at home become less critical. Rather than suffering from role overload, working wives can benefit from expanded realms in which to meet their needs for agency and communion, enlarging the opportunities for a more balanced orientation. Generally speaking, women who work have been found to be more satisfied (Burke and Weir, 1976; Hoffman and Nye, 1974), physically healthier (Burke and Weir, 1976), and less depressed (Tebbets, 1982; Burke and Weir, 1976) than housewives. However, a critical variable in assessing working wives' seemingly more desirable state compared to housewives is whether or not the woman *wants* to work (Crouter and Perry-Jenkins, 1986). For example, working women with high job commitment have reported a higher degree of marital satisfaction than both working women with low job commitment and nonworking women (Safilios-Rothschild, 1971).

Married Working Mothers

Married working mothers have, in the past, been considered to be the most vulnerable to role strain, or overload (Fox and Hesse-Biber, 1984), especially if they have preschool children. More recently, though, it has been argued that multiple roles can actually increase women's life satisfaction (Stewart and Malley, 1987; Stewart and Salt, 1981). Baruch *et al.* (1983) found that those who scored *lowest* on their measure of mastery (similar to the concept of agency) were, in fact, women with the fewest roles—married housewives without children.

Moreover, as already noted, family roles of wife and mother, although principal sources of communion for women, tend toward asymmetry, and are, thus, intrinsically less satisfying. However, relationships with co-workers on the job can provide women with mutual, and thus more satisfying, communion experiences. With multiple roles, dissatisfaction in a specific role is not as critical, since it can be balanced by a more rewarding one. This may be especially true if one of the roles is that of paid worker, since a job brings with it the potential for more varied experiences than may be available in women's family roles (Ferree, 1976).

Multiple roles can enhance opportunities for a balance of agency and communion not only by providing more and varied life experiences, but also by curtailing those experiences which may be less satisfying (Epstein, 1987). Having a job provides a legitimate excuse for being unable, or refusing, to comply with demands related to other roles (Baruch *et al.*, 1983). For example, in the case of both men and women, the amount of time spent on housework decreases as working hours increase (Staines and Pleck, 1983). Working mothers are also found to be less anxious and worried about their children than full-time house-wives (Birnbaum, 1975). Thus, a working woman with multiple roles can easily dedicate less time and energy to those tasks which are not useful or satisfying to her in terms of agency and/or communion, freeing her time for other activities which encourage a better balance of the two orientations.

A problem, however, may arise for those working mothers who are unable to relax expectations of personal performance in all their roles, despite the addition of a new work role. Traditionally, women's primary commitment has been to the family (in contrast to men's principal commitment to the bread-winning role; Bailyn, 1978). As a result, mothers tend to be more accommodating to family needs, regardless of employment status, and demands of the family can intrude in and interfere with their work role (Pleck, 1977). When a child is sick or the babysitter is unexpectedly delayed, it is most often the mother who must provide the back-up care. Thus, it may be difficult for women to relinquish major responsibilities of family roles (Long and Porter, 1984), despite their less satis-fying qualities, and then potential benefits of a job in terms of agency and communion may not be realized.

The demands of the family can be even more difficult for low-income mothers who do not have the resources to purchase goods and services to meet family needs (Tebbets, 1982). For those women unable to afford adequate childcare, concerns about their children's welfare may be a constant stress, following them to work daily rather than just during times of crisis. In any case, for women who are still principally engaged in managing a household, agentic and/or communal benefits available through employment may be lost to the less personally fulfilling but more demanding task of household management.

Single Working Mothers

The same benefits of employment may accrue to single working mothers, in terms of increased agency and more balanced communion, as is the case for married working mothers. However, those benefits may be more difficult to attain. Having fewer financial resources to arrange management of the household in her absence may prevent a single mother from investing her full energy and attention in her job. Thus, the potential for agentic experiences in this arena may be eclipsed or not fully developed. Moreover, a single mother may be forced to choose a job which she does not like, but which pays better than one which would be more enjoyable and personally fulfilling.

However, improved opportunities for communion seem more likely to occur for single working mothers (see Gove and Zeiss, 1987). Adult relationships at work may allow for a more mutually satisfying expression of communion than is available in the parent–child relationship. Thus, although a rewarding agentic orientation may be difficult to attain from the employment role, a more satisfying communal orientation appears more readily achievable for single mothers who work than for those who do not.

Fully mutual relationships at work may, however, be difficult to attain, especially for women in high management or clerical positions (Fox and Hesse-

Biber, 1984; Long and Porter, 1984; Hennig and Jardim, 1977). In the case of managerial workers, women managers often find themselves the only female among all male peers and superiors. In response, they may focus on the business aspects of these work relationships, minimizing any social relationships which they feel may have negative consequences for their career advancement (Hennig and Jardim, 1977). Moreover, these highly career-oriented women may devote most of their time and energy to their careers at the expense of any outside social relationships, leaving them with few opportunities for communion (Hennig and Jardim, 1977).

Similarly, clerical workers, or female workers in any predominantly male setting, may find themselves in the role of 'mother' or 'office wife' at work (Fox and Hesse-Biber, 1984; Long and Porter, 1984). Thus, despite possible opportunities for mutual communion with female peers at work, women workers may find themselves experiencing the same asymmetrical communion with their male superiors that they find with their spouses at home.

Unmarried Workers

Because they have fewer family roles, unmarried women may be more likely to seek opportunities for expression of both agency and communion in their jobs. In fact, single workers tend to be most gratified at work by their interpersonal relations (Crosby, 1982). Surprisingly, they appear much less likely to gain a sense of accomplishment from their jobs as compared to other working women (Crosby, 1982). This difference, rather than reflecting a lack of agency at work for single working women, may represent the overabundance of agency in their lives and highlight the salience that work relationships have for these women as a primary source of communion. Women with their own families have more arenas in which to express communion than single women who must develop nonfamilial relationships. Thus, in contrast to married and/or maternal workers, single women may place a higher value on work relationships. The salience of these relationships is reflected in the fact that single women not only tend to be most gratified by interpersonal relationships at work, but also most bothered by them (Crosby, 1982).

SUMMARY AND CONCLUSIONS

Women's family roles demand indirect agency and asymmetrical communion, while offering relatively little opportunity for direct agency and mutual communion. On the other hand, the absence of family roles leaves women with relatively few resources for communion. Work roles, in contrast, usually provide opportunities for direct agency and, with some important exceptions, for mutual communion. This analysis may help explain some of the sex and intrasex differences in responses to stress. Different combinations of social roles, with their attendant opportunities and demands for agency and communion, may be crucial mediators for the relationships between stress and physical and mental health.

REFERENCES

Abernathy, V. (1973). Social network and response to the maternal role. *International Journal of Sociology of the Family, 3,* 86–92.

Adams, M. (1976). *Single blessedness.* New York: Basic Books.

Arling, G. (1976). The elderly widow and her family, neighbors and friends. *Journal of Marriage and the Family, 38,* 757–768.

Bailyn, L. (1978). Accommodation of work to family. In R. Rapoport & R. Rapoport (eds), *Working couples* (pp. 59–174). New York: Harper & Row.

Bakan, D. (1966). *The duality of human existence.* Boston: Beacon Press.

Balint, A. (1939). Love for the mother and mother-love. In M. Balint (ed.), *Primary love and psychoanalytic technique.* London: Hogarth Press.

Barrett, C.J. (1977). Women in widowhood. *Signs, 2*(4), 856–868.

Barrett, C.J. (1981). Intimacy in widowhood. *Psychology of Women Quarterly, 5*(3), 473–487.

Bart, P.B. (1971). Depression in middle-aged women. In V. Gornick & B.K. Moran (eds), *Women in sexist society* (pp. 163–186). New York: Basic Books.

Baruch, G., Barnett, R., & Rivers, C. (1983). *New patterns of love and work for today's women.* New York: New American Library.

Belle, D. (1982a). *Lives in stress.* Beverly Hills: Sage Publications.

Belle, D. (1982b). The stress of caring: Women as providers of social support. In L. Goldberger & S. Breznitz (eds), *Handbook of stress: Theoretical and clinical aspects* (pp. 496–505). New York: Free Press.

Belsky, J., Spanier, G., & Rovine, M. (1983). Stability and change in marriage across the transition to parenthood. *Journal of Marriage and the Family, 45,* 567–577.

Bernard, J. (1972). *The future of marriage.* New York: Bantam.

Bernard, J. (1974a). *The future of motherhood.* New York: Dial Press.

Bernard, J. (1974b). The housewife: Between two worlds. In P.L. Stewart & M.G. Cantor (eds), *Varieties of work experience* (pp. 49–66). New York: John Wiley & Sons.

Birnbaum, J. (1975). Life patterns and self-esteem of gifted family-oriented and career-committed women. In M. Mednick, S. Tangri & L.W. Hoffman (eds), *Women and achievement: Social and motivational analysis.* New York: Hemisphere-Halstead.

Blood, R.O., & Wolfe, D.M. (1960). *Husbands and wives: The dynamics of married living.* New York: Free Press.

Brown, G., Bhrolchain, M. & Harris, T. (1975). Social class and psychiatric disturbance among women in an urban population. *Sociology, 9,* 225–254.

Burke, R.J., & Weir, T. (1976). Relationship of wives' employment status to husband, wife and pair satisfaction and performance. *Journal of Marriage and the Family, 38,* 279–288.

Chafe, W.H. (1983). The challenge of sex equality: Old values revisited or a new culture? In M. Horner, C.C. Nadelson & M.T. Notman (eds), *The challenge of change: perspectives on family, work and education* (pp. 23–38). New York: Plenum.

Chester, N.L. (1985). Experiencing parenthood: A longitudinal study. Paper presented at Eastern Psychological Association, Boston.

Chodorow, N. (1978). *The reproduction of mothering: Psychoanalysis and the sociology of gender.* Berkeley, Calif.: University of California Press.

Coser, R.L., & Coser, L.A. (1974). The housewife and the greedy family. In L.A. Coser (ed.), *Greedy institutions.* New York: Free Press.

Crosby, F.J. (1982). *Relative deprivation and working women.* New Haven: Yale University Press.

Crouter, A.C., & Perry-Jenkins, M. (1986). Working it out: Effects of work on parents and children. In M. Yogman & T.B. Brazelton (eds), *In support of families* (pp. 93–108). Cambridge, Mass.: Harvard University Press.

Douvan, E. (1983). Family roles in a twenty-year perspective. In M. Horner, C.C. Nadelson & M.T. Notman (eds), *The challenge of change* (pp. 199–218). New York: Plenum.

Epstein, C.F. (1987). Role strains and multiple successes. In F.J. Crosby (ed.), *Women and men at home and at work: Studies in gender and role combinations* (pp. 23–35). New Haven: Yale University Press.

Ferree, M.M. (1976). Working-class jobs: Housework and paid work as sources of satisfaction. *Social Problems, 23,* 431–441.

Fox, M.F., & Hesse-Biber, S. (1984). *Women at work.* Palo Alto, Calif.: Mayfield.

Goode, W.J. (1982). Why men resist. In B. Thorne & M. Yalom (eds), *Rethinking the family: Some feminist questions* (pp. 131–150). New York: Longman.

Gove, W.R., & Zeiss, C. (1987). Multiple roles and happiness. In E.J. Crosby (ed.), *Women and men at home and at work: Studies in gender and role combinations* (pp. 125–137). New Haven: Yale University Press.

Granvold, D.K., Pedler, M.P., & Schellie, S.G. (1979). A study of sex role expectancy and female postdivorce adjustment. *Journal of Divorce, 2*(4), 83–393.

Grossman, F.K., Eichler, L.S., & Winicoff, S.A. (1980). *Pregnancy, birth, and parenthood.* San Francisco: Jossey-Bass.

Guttentag, M. (1975). Women, men and mental health. In L. Cater, A. Scott & W. Martyna (eds), *Women and men: Changing roles.* Palo Alto, Calif.: Aspen Institute for Humanistic Studies.

Haynes, S., & Feinleib, M. (1982). Women, work and coronary heart disease: Prospective findings from the Framingham Heart Study. *American Journal of Public Health, 70,* 133–141.

Hennig, M., & Jardim, A. (1977). *The managerial woman.* Garden City, NY: Anchor Press/Doubleday.

Herman, S.J. (1977). Women, divorce, and suicide. *Journal of Divorce, 1*(2). 107–117.

Hochschild, A.R. (1975). The sociology of feeling and emotion: Selected possibilities. In M. Millman & R.M. Kantor (eds), *Another voice: Feminist perspective on social life and social science* (pp. 280–307). Garden City, NY: Anchor Press/Doubleday.

Hoffman, L.W., & Nye, F.I. (1974). *Working mothers.* San Francisco: Jossey-Bass.

Jenkins, C.D. (1976). Recent evidence supporting psychologic and social risk factors for coronary disease. *New England Journal of Medicine, 194,* 987–994; 1033–1038.

Johnson, A. (1977). Sex differentials in coronary heart disease: The explanatory role of primary risk factors. *Journal of Health and Social Behavior, 18,* 46–54.

Jourard, S.M., & Richman, P. (1963). Disclosure output and input in college students. *Merrill-Palmer Quarterly of Behavioral Development, 9,* 141–148.

Kanter, R.M. (1977). *Men and women of the corporation.* New York: Basic Books.

Knupfer, G., Clark, W., & Room, R. (1966). The mental health of the unmarried. *American Journal of Psychiatry, 122,* 841–851.

Kohen, J.A., Brown, C.A., & Feldberg, R. (1979). Divorced mothers: The costs and benefits of female family control. In G. Levinger & O. Moles (eds), *Divorce and separation: Context, causes, and consequences* (pp. 228–245). New York: Basic Books.

Komarovsky, M. (1976). *Dilemmas of masculinity.* New York: Norton.

Levinger, G. (1964). Task and social behavior in marriage. *Sociometry, 27*(4), 433–448.

Lipman-Blumen, J., & Leavitt, H. (1976). Vicarious and direct achievement patterns in adulthood. *The Counseling Psychologist, 6*(1), 26–31.

Long, J., & Porter, K.L. (1984). Multiple roles of midlife women: A case for new directions in theory, research, and policy In G. Baruch & J. Brooks-Gunn (eds), *Women in midlife* (pp. 109–161). New York: Plenum.

Lopata, H.Z. (1973). *Widowhood in an American city.* Cambridge, Mass.: Schenkman.

Miller, B., & Sollie, D. (1980). Normal stresses during the transition to parenthood. *Family Relations, 29,* 459–465.

Miller, J.B. (1976). *Toward a new psychology of women.* Boston: Beacon.

Miller, J.B. (1982). Psychological recovery in low-income single parents. *American Journal of Orthopsychiatry, 52*(2), 346–352.

Miller, J.B., & Mothner, I. (1981) Psychological consequences of sexual inequality. In E. Howell & M. Bayle (eds), *Women and mental health* (pp. 41–50). New York: Basic Books.

Nathanson, A. (1977). Sex, illness, and medical care: A review of data, theory, and method. *Social Science and Medicine, 11,* 13–25.

Oakley, A. (1974). *Women's work.* New York: Vintage Books.

Papanek, H. (1973). Men, women and work: Reflections on the two-person career. *American Journal of Sociology, 78,* 852–870.

Parkes, C.M., & Weiss, R.S. (1983). *Recovery from bereavement.* New York: Basic Books.

Pearlin, L.I., Lieberman, M.A., Menaghan, E.G., & Mullen, J.T. (1981). The stress process. *Journal of Health and Social Behavior, 22,* 337–356.

Peplau, L.A., & Gordon, S.C. (1985). Women and men in love: Gender differences in close heterosexual relationships. In V.E. O'Leary, R.K. Unger & B.S. Wallston (eds), *Women, gender and social psychology* (pp. 257–291). Hillsdale, NJ: Lawrence Erlbaum.

Piotrkowski, C.S. (1978). *Work and the family system.* New York: Free Press.

Pleck, J.H. (1977). The work–family role system. *Social Problems, 24,* 417–427.

Pleck, J.H., & Sawyer, J. (eds), (1974). *Men and masculinity.* Englewood Cliffs, NJ: Prentice-Hall.

Rapoport, R., Rapoport, R.M., & Strelitz, Z. (1977). *Fathers, mothers and society: Perspectives on parenting.* New York: Vintage.

Rossi, A. (1968). The transition to parenthood. *Journal of Marriage and the Family, 30,* 26–39.

Rubin, L.B. (1976). *Worlds of pain.* New York: Basic Books.

Rubin, L.B. (1979). *Women of a certain age: The midlife search for self.* New York: Harper.

Safilios-Rothschild, C. (1971). Toward a conceptualization and measurement of work commitment. *Human Relations, 24,* 489–493.

Seidenberg, R. (1975). *Corporate wives—Corporate casualties?* Garden City, NY: Anchor Press/Doubleday.

Siegler, A. (1976). Anna Siegler. In S. Karmer (ed.), *The balancing act* (pp. 123–144). Chicago: Chicago Review Press.

Smith, M.J. (1980). The social consequences of single parenthood: A longitudinal perspective. *Family Relations, 29,* 75–81.

Staines, G.L., & Pleck, J.H. (1983). *The impact of work schedules on the family.* Michigan: University of Michigan Survey Research Center, Institute for Social Research.

Steil, J.M., & Turetsky, B.A. (1987). The relationship between marital equality and psychological symptomatology: Is equal better? In S. Oskamp (ed.), *Family process and problems: social psychological aspects. Applied Social Psychology Annual, 7,* 73–97.

Stein, P.J. (1976). *Single.* Englewood Cliffs, NJ: Prentice-Hall.

Stewart, A.J., & Malley, J.E. (1987). Role combination in women: Mitigating agency and communion. In F.J. Crosby (ed.), *Women and men at home and at work: Studies in gender and role combinations* (pp. 44–60). New Haven: Yale University Press.

Stewart, A.J., & Salt, P. (1981). Life stress, life-styles, depression, and illness in adult women. *Journal of Personality and Social Psychology, 40,* 1063–1069.

Tebbets, R. (1982). Work: Its meaning for women's lives. In D. Belle (ed.), *Lives in stress* (pp. 83–95). Beverly Hills: Sage.

Veroff, J., Douvan, E., & Kulka, R. (1981). *The inner American: A self portrait from 1957–1976.* New York: Basic Books.

Warren, R. (1975). The work role and problem coping: Sex differentials in the use of helping systems in urban communities. Paper presented at the annual meeting of the American Sociological Association, San Francisco.

Weingarten, K. (1978). The employment pattern of professional couples and their distribution of involvment in the family. *Psychology of Women Quarterly, 3*(1), 43–53.

Weiss, R.S. (1975). *Marital separation.* New York: Basic Books.

Weiss, R.S. (1979). *Going it alone: The family and social situation of the single parent.* New York: Basic Books.

Weiss, R.S. (1984). The husband's reactions. Paper presented at a conference on Modern Women: Managing Multiple Roles, Yale University, New Haven.

Wolf, S. (1971). Psychosocial forces in myocardial infarction and sudden death. In L. Levi (ed.), *Society, stress and disease.* Oxford: Oxford University Press.

KEY WORDS

Agency and communion as mediators of the relationship between stress and physical and mental health, family roles and relationships—marriage and motherhood, family roles defined by absent relationships—unmarried women, divorcees and widows, agency, communion and the work role—homemakers, married workers, married working mothers, single working mothers and unmarried workers.

Handbook of Life Stress, Cognition and Health
Edited by S. Fisher and J. Reason
© 1988 John Wiley & Sons Ltd

11

Psychosocial Factors in the Workplace

RUDOLF H. MOOS
*Stanford University and Veterans Administration Medical Centers,
Palo Alto, California*

INTRODUCTION

The work force in America is composed of more than 100 million persons, many of whom spend between one-third and one-half of their waking hours at work. A job can provide structure for a person's life, a sense of satisfaction and productivity that stems from completing meaningful tasks, a feeling of belonging to a valued reference group, a basis for self-esteem and personal identity, and a way to earn one's economic place in society. But many Americans are employed in bureaucratic organizations in which they pursue routine, predictable tasks and feel isolated and futile. Work stress, job dissatisfaction, and a sense of pressure and frustration are common.

These contrasting experiences and impacts of work are well known, but today they occur in the context of rising expectations about the quality of work life. Many people believe in the value of personal autonomy and the right to a hazard-free and reasonably satisfying work setting. Although the work force is more knowledgeable and better educated than ever before, technological developments such as automation and robotics make it possible to simplify and routinize many jobs. Such social 'progress' contributes to work stress, underutilization of individual abilities, and feelings of powerlessness and disaffection. Thus, there is a growing mismatch between the talents and aspirations of many individuals and the jobs available to them.

These issues are considered here in terms of some important environmental variables in the work setting, with emphasis on the social climate at work and its determinants and effects. A conceptual framework to help address long-standing questions about the quality and impact of work settings and newer concerns about how experiences at work can affect a person's spouse and children, choice of leisure activities, and general *weltanschauung* is presented elsewhere (Moos, 1986a).

THREE DOMAINS OF WORK CLIMATE

Based on research in a variety of social environments, the underlying facets of social climate can be organized into three domains: the way in which individuals in a setting relate to each other (relationship domain), the personal growth goals toward which a setting is oriented (personal growth or goal orientation domain), and the amount of structure and openness to change that characterize it (system maintenance and change domain; Moos, 1987). Similarly, Payne (1980) has divided aspects of organizational contexts into supports, demands, and constraints. The category of supports encompasses the quality of relationships with colleagues and supervisors and the adequacy of physical resources. Demands refer to aspects of an environment that stimulate employees to perform (goal orientation). The concept of constraint resembles that of system maintenance, but it is limited to conditions that confine or prevent an individual from fulfilling job demands.

The dimensions of several scales focused on work settings can be organized in terms of these three domains. As shown in Table 11.1, the six factors of Gavin and Howe's (1975) Psychological Climate Inventory reflect the three domains, as do the dimensions tapped by the Organizational Climate Index (Stern, 1970), the Psychological Climate Questionnaire (James & Sells, 1981), and the Quality of Employment Survey (Kahn, 1980). The Michigan Organizational Assessment Questionnaire (MOAQ) is a comprehensive procedure that covers employees' demographic characteristics, reactions to their job and organizational setting, and aspects of job morale and motivation as well as descriptors of the work environment (Camman et al., 1983). The facets of work group functioning, supervision, and job role characteristics tapped by the MOAQ fall into the three domains.

Some investigators have identified the goal orientation (demand, growth orientation) and system maintenance (structure, control) domains, but have tended to neglect the relationship domain. The five core job dimensions measured by the Job Diagnostic Survey reflect the personal growth or goal orientation area, but do not explicitly consider the relationship or system maintenance and change domains (Hackman and Oldham, 1980). All three work climate domains are important, because, for example, demanding jobs may be performed effectively in contexts that are rich in social support or high on autonomy and personal control. The three sets of dimensions help to describe and integrate the research to follow.

Describing and Comparing Work Climates

The Work Environment Scale (WES) has been developed to measure the three work climate domains (see Table 11.1). The scale is based on the idea that employees are participant observers in the work milieu and are uniquely qualified to appraise it. The WES relationship dimensions measure how much employee and managers are involved with and supportive of one another. The WES personal growth or goal orientation dimensions cover the goals toward which the work setting is oriented, that is, autonomy, task orientation, and work pressure

Table 11.1 Dimensions of work climate

Domain Instrument	Relationship	Goal/growth orientation	System maintenance and change
Psychological Climate Inventory (Gavin & Howe, 1975)	Esprit, managerial trust and consideration	Rewards, challenge and risk	Clarity of structure, hindrance structure
Organizational Climate Index (Stern, 1970)	Closeness, group life	Intellectual climate, personal dignity, achievement standards	Orderliness, impulse control (constraint)
Psychological Climate Questionnaire (James & Sells, 1981)	Work group cooperation and friendliness, leadership facilitation and support, organizational concern and identification	Job challenge, job importance, job variety	Role ambiguity, role conflict
Quality of Employment Survey (Kahn, 1980)	Relationships with co-workers, supervision	Task content (challenge), autonomy and control, working conditions (demand), promotions	Resource adequacy, wages
Michigan Organizational Assessment Questionnaire – Modules 3, 4 & 5 (Camman et al., 1983)	Work group cohesion, openness of communication, internal fragmentation, supervisor– subordinate communication and consideration	Participation in decision making, production orientation, role overload	Role conflict, role clarity, work group clarity, supervisor control, supervisor goal setting and problem solving, decision centralizations
Work Environment Scale (Moos, 1986b)	Involvement, peer cohesion, supervisor support	Autonomy, task orientation, work pressure	Clarity, control, innovation, physical comfort

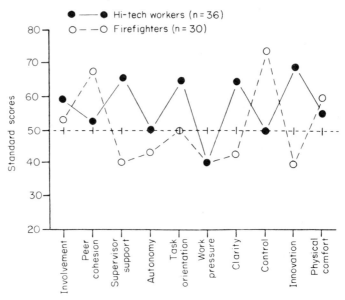

FIG. 11.1   Work environment scale (WES) Form R profiles for high-technology workers and firefighters.

The WES system maintenance and change dimensions deal with the amount of structure, clarity, and openness to change that characterize the workplace. These three sets of social climate factors typify different kinds of social settings (Moos, 1986b).

Scales such as the WES can be used to depict the perceptions of individual employees, compare employee and manager reports, and describe and contrast work settings. Figure 11.1 shows the WES profiles for 36 high-technology production workers and 30 firefighters from a county department. The production workers saw a supportive, task-oriented, and physically comfortable work milieu, characterized by clear expectations and innovation. Employees reported little work pressure. These findings were consistent with the employees' jobs, which were individually paced and highly independent. The plant was well known for its congenial work environment and low turnover.

The firefighters viewed their job setting as cohesive but rigidly controlled and lacking in clarity and innovation. They mistrusted their supervisors, who they saw as autocratic and arbitrary. In fact, the supervisors had instituted a strict timekeeping system and rigid job requirements. The unusually high supervisor control may have heightened co-worker cohesion by inducing the employees to stand up for each other. This type of information can be used to track changes in a work group, compare employees' actual and preferred job climates, and provide feedback to help improve work groups (Moos, 1986b).

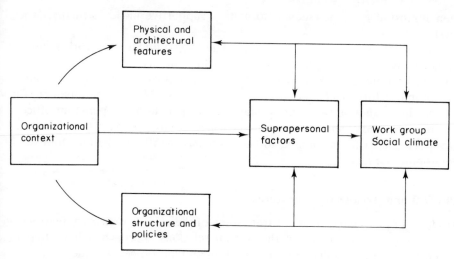

FIG. 11.2   A model of the interconnections among domains of work context factors.

THE DETERMINANTS OF WORK CLIMATE

Work groups vary widely in the quality of interpersonal relationships, the emphasis on task orientation and work pressure, and the level of clarity and organization. This finding raises an intriguing question. Why do social climates develop in such disparate ways; that is, what leads to an emphasis on supervisor support, or task orientation, or work pressure? How is social climate influenced by other domains of the environmental system and how does it mediate their impact?

To address this question, my colleagues and I have conceptualized the work environment as a dynamic system composed of physical and architectural features, organizational structure and policies, suprapersonal factors (employees' aggregate background and personal characteristics), and social climate. We have formulated a model of the relationships among these four sets of environmental factors and their connections to the organizational context (Fig. 11.2). The model posits that the impact of architectural, organizational, and suprapersonal factors stems in part from the social climate they help to promote. More specifically, the social climate can alter the impact of the other three domains on employee morale and performance.

According to the model, physical features can affect work group climate directly (open-plan offices may facilitate cohesion), or indirectly by altering organizational factors (greater distance between work groups may promote more flexible policies and autonomy). Organizational structure can influence social climate directly (small work groups tend to be more cohesive), and indirectly by altering the individuals who select a work group (hierarchical organizations may attract competitive persons who tend to create more task orientation and work demands). Human aggregate factors also can affect social climate. Compared to men, for instance, women seem to form more supportive and less structured social groups.

Each of these processes is reciprocal. The social climate of a work group can influence the type of people who select it (achievement-oriented individuals may favor task-oriented work settings), organizational policies (employee autonomy can promote formal channels for grievances), and physical parameters. Employees in a cohesive work group may elect to partition an open-plan office to control noise and create privacy. Finally, aspects of the company in which a work group is located (i.e. the organizational context) can affect each of the four sets of environmental factors.

Physical and Architectural Features

Studies of open-plan offices illustrate some of the effects of physical features on social climate. Proponents of the human relations approach believe that the absence of interior walls and barriers in open-plan offices will facilitate social relationships and promote job satisfaction and performance. The increased communication in open-plan offices is thought to enhance feedback by enabling employees and supervisors to share work-related and personal information. In contrast, the sociotechnical approach emphasizes the value of physical boundaries in constructing private, defensible space. Boundaries can clarify the nature of the work process, increase task identity and friendship formation, and create autonomy by making it less likely that co-workers and supervisors will constrict an employee's discretion.

Employees who move from conventional to open-plan offices describe an increase in non-work-related conversations while the amount of work-related conversation remains stable. But such offices may not provide enough privacy to support the formation of close friendships or to permit supervisors to offer candid evaluations to subordinates. Employees in open-plan offices report less job autonomy, fewer leadership opportunities, and a decline in co-worker and supervisor feedback. Thus, a change in physical features can alter the work climate and employee motivation and morale (Oldham and Brass, 1979). The impact of office physical features seems to depend on the opportunity for friendship and feedback and on employees' levels of autonomy and the types of tasks they perform (Oldham and Rotchford, 1983).

Organizational Structure and Policies

Some primary aspects of organizational structure are (a) organizational and work group size, (b) configuration, or the 'shape' of an organization, and the span of control (that is, how many employees each manager supervises), (c) centralization, or how much the locus of authority is vested in one or a small group of individuals, (d) specialization, or the extent to which each person performs different functions, and (e) formalization, or the degree to which rules and procedures are written and precisely defined. The first two aspects are seen as 'structural' qualities, whereas the other three are 'structuring' qualities in that they index policies that shape or constrain behavior. Some of these factors have been connected to work group climate or performance (see Berger and Cummings, 1979; Dalton *et al.*, 1980).

The most robust findings involve size and centralization. Large organizations typically are highly formalized and bureaucratic, and composed of work groups that are oriented toward rules, conventionality, and supervisor control. Employees in larger work groups tend to perform more specialized tasks and to report less group cohesion. Centralized organizations also are more formalized and emphasize task orientation and manager control more than autonomy or innovation. In general, the connection between a structural variable (such as size) and an outcome criterion (such as job involvement and motivation) is mediated by processes linked to size (formalization, centralization) and the social climate they create, as well as by personal characteristics of employees.

Suprapersonal Factors

When individuals come together in a social group, be it a work group, a college dormitory, or a congregate living unit for older people, they bring with them values, norms, and abilities. Because of selective mechanisms, groups draw their members in a non-random manner from the general population and produce distinctive blends of individual characteristics. The aggregate of the members' attributes (the suprapersonal environment) in part defines the subculture that forms in a group, and, in turn, the morale and behavior of its members. Thus, the type of work force attracted and retained by an organization can shape its culture and viability.

Holland (1985) theorizes that people's vocational choices are expressions of their personalities, and that occupations can be categorized into six groups. Since people in an occupational group have similar personalities, they should respond to situations in similar ways and create characteristic work climates. Thus, Holland describes six types of work settings linked to the six personality types: realistic, investigative, artistic, social, enterprising, and conventional. The type of environment is influenced by the modal personality of group members. In this way, an average background characteristic of a group (that is, the dominant vocational preference) creates a particular milieu with unique demands, rewards, and opportunities.

In a test of Holland's theory, we found that employees in realistic occupations (such as engineers and air traffic controllers) tend to see their work groups as high in control and lacking in autonomy and innovation. These groups also were low in involvement, cohesion, and supervisor support. In contrast, employees in social-type work settings (such as social workers and bartenders) reported relatively high emphasis on the relationship areas and on clarity and innovation. As expected, investigative work settings (such as those populated by physicists and computer operators) strongly accentuated autonomy and innovation and were espeically low in control. These findings support Holland's ideas and imply that modal personal characteristics can influence work group climate (Moos, 1986b).

Examining the Overall Model

Few, if any, studies have looked at all of the environmental domains and connected them with each other and with work group performance. Parasuraman and Alutto (1981) linked organizational factors to perceived work stressors in a food processing firm. Compared to administrative employees, those who were engaged in food production reported more technical problems and greater work demands and role frustration. This was thought to stem from their reliance on complex machinery and the presence of explicit performance criteria. Supervisors experienced more qualitative overload and time constraints, while employees in lower level positions experienced more role frustration. Task complexity and close supervision contributed to interunit conflict, role frustration, and efficiency problems, even after contextual and job level factors were considered. Thus, technical and social factors combine to produce work stressors.

Jones and James (1979) found that organizational structure and suprapersonal factors were predictably linked to the work climate on Navy ships. The types of work climates identified varied from cooperative and friendly, to enriched and warm but uninvolved, constricted and alienating, and ambiguous and conflicted. These climates seemed to reflect basic variations in group functions and in their technology and resources, structural factors, and personnel composition, and these factors were linked to group performance. Work groups with cooperative and friendly work climates performed most effectively, whereas those with cold and unsupportive climates functioned least well. The warm and friendly climates were associated with complex technology, little task specialization, flat configurations, small size, and more intelligent and well-educated work group members. In contrast, the cold and unsupportive climates were associated with routine technology, a broad span of control and large size, less interdependence with other work groups, and personnel who were less intelligent and well educated. Consistent with the model presented earlier, such findings imply that contextual, policy, and suprapersonal factors help to create certain social climates, which combine with them to influence work group effectiveness.

THE IMPACT OF WORK CLIMATE

A considerable body of research has examined the connections between work climate and employee morale, performance, and well-being. Most of the studies have tried to link characteristics of work settings directly to adaptation, but some have considered the role of personal factors and cognitive appraisal. (For a review of these issues in health care work settings, see Moos and Schaefer, 1987.)

Job Morale and Performance

As expected, work climates that are cohesive and accepting, oriented toward independence and autonomy, and provide meaningful and challenging tasks tend to produce good employee morale and to reduce turnover intentions. Considerate supervisors who specify clear goals and encourage participation in decision making also promote these outcomes, as well as employees' experience of being challenged and pleased, with intrinsic and extrinsic job rewards. Well-organized work settings in which individuals do not feel hindered by bureaucratic policies also tend to create better morale. Role ambiguity and overload and group conflict have the opposite impact, as do situational constraints and highly structured tasks and leaders (Fisher and Gitelson, 1983; Moos, 1986b).

Indices of Strain

Substance Use and Abuse

The work-related economic and social costs of substance abuse may be much greater than is commonly suspected. Alcohol consumption and adverse consequences of drinking have been associated with lack of challenge, role conflict and ambiguity, and high work demands. Employees who report more work-related problems tend to cite a wider variety of reasons for drinking, such as to relax and cope with job pressure. Thus, work problems may increase alcohol consumption by making an individual more likely to justify drinking as a response to job stressors.

Parker and Brody (1982) describe three models of risk factors associated with drinking in the workplace. The social control model posits that a weak occupational structure tends to promote deviant behavior and problem drinking. The alienation, or stress, model posits that lack of control over the job has a detrimental influence on morale and health. The social availability model posits that problem drinking is due to participation in group activities with heavy-drinking co-workers. When they tested these ideas, Parker and Brody (1982) found some support for the stress hypothesis: high work demands and routinization were associated with perceived job stress, which was related to more alcohol consumption and drinking problems.

Conway and his colleagues (1981) measured cigarette, coffee, and alcohol consumption among Navy petty officers. Smoking and drinking coffee were positively associated with perceived stress, but alcohol consumption tended to lessen under stress. This decline was attributed to the lack of easy access to alcohol: officers often remained on the base during peak demand periods. Individuals differed widely in whether they increased or decreased their habitual substance use in response to varying levels of stress. Such findings point to the need to consider the social context and individual variations in research on the impact of work.

Mental and Physical Symptoms and Medical Conditions

A substantial body of research has examined the links between work settings and health. Four aspects of work climate have been associated with employee strain and lack of well-being: high job demands, lack of opportunity to participate in decision making and to organize and pace the work, high supervisor control, and lack of clarity about the job and criteria for adequate performance (Moos, 1986a, 1986b).

Karasek (1979) has posited that strain is most likely to occur when job demands are high *and* the individual has little discretion in deciding how to meet them. When employees are allowed to make decisions about their work, high job demands can be stimulating and can promote problem solving and innovation. These ideas were tested among representative groups of working men in the United States and Sweden. Men who held jobs that were demanding and lacking in autonomy were more likely to report mental exhaustion, depression, and insomnia, to consume more sleeping pills and tranquilizers, and to take more sick leave. These problems declined among men who shifted to less stressful jobs. At every level of job demand, men who were able to use their skills to make decisions experienced less strain. Since these findings held when job characteristics were rated by experts as well as by the men themselves, they are not due to potential artifacts of self-report.

The Position Analysis Questionnaire (PAQ) provides a composite picture of job characteristics obtained from ratings conducted by personnel specialists, supervisors, or job incumbents. Shaw and Riskind (1983) found some predictable associations between the independently derived PAQ dimensions and work strains reported by individuals in a variety of blue-collar, clerical, and professional occupations. Employees in jobs rated as involved with controlled manual activities experienced more anxiety and depression, job dissatisfaction, and physical symptoms. Conversely, individuals located in responsible challenging jobs tended to report less negative affect and fewer symptoms and illnesses.

Mass psychogenic illness. Another set of studies has considered episodes of 'mass psychogenic illness' in work settings (Schmitt and Fitzgerald, 1982). These occur when employees experience symptoms such as headache, dizziness, and fatigue that cannot be traced to exposure to chemicals or other physical factors in the workplace. Employees who report high work pressure, lack of autonomy and clarity, and poor relationships with their peers and supervisors tend to complain of more symptoms during such episodes. Similarly, the average number of symptoms reported by employees is higher in work groups characterized by these social climate factors. Thus, a lack of co-worker and supervisor support may amplify the extent to which high work demands and low autonomy increase the prevalence of physical and mental symptoms.

Coronary heart disease and other medical conditions. High job demands and stress have been implicated in the development of varied medical conditions. After considering potential confounding factors (such as age, education, and smoking), House and his co-workers (1979) found that job stressors were related to self-reported angina, ulcers, and neurotic symptoms, and to medical evidence of hypertension and other heart disease risk factors. Job stressors were also associated with respiratory and dermatological symptoms, but only among workers who were exposed to potentially noxious physical-chemical agents. There were some logically consistent connections between specific stressors and symptoms. For instance, angina was linked to stressors involving performance and achievement, whereas ulcer symptoms were related primarily to interpersonal tension and lack of self-esteem.

In an extension of his earlier work, Karasek and his colleagues (1981) obtained six-year follow-up data on their sample of employed Swedish men. Initially, asymptomatic persons who developed a myocardial infarction (MI) or other signs of coronary heart disease (CHD) over the six years were matched with their asymptomatic peers who did not. The psychosocial characteristics of the work situation were indexed by the perceptions of working men from the nationwide interview survey rather than by the reports of the individuals who suffered CHD. High work demands and low job autonomy predicted new cases of CHD, even after considering such risk factors as age, obesity, and smoking. These associations were stronger among individuals whose work climate remained stable. Work demands may be especially harmful when environmental constraints prevent optimal coping or when coping does not increase the chance for personal growth.

Job Characteristics and Their Social Context

Hackman and Oldham (1980) believe that a job is more motivating when the task is unique and important, more skills are needed to perform it, and there is more autonomy and feedback. In fact, these aspects of jobs are linked to higher work satisfaction and performance, and less absenteeism. As noted earlier, these job conditions tap primarily the personal growth domain of work climate. Their impact should be moderated by social factors, such as the quality of relationships among employees and supervisors, as well as by individual growth needs. In an experimental test of these ideas, Orpen (1979) found that job enrichment had a stronger and more favorable impact on attitudes among clerical employees with high growth needs and among those who were satisfied with contextual and social job factors. Moreover, some of the effects of job enrichment were thought to be due to interpersonal factors: members of enriched groups worked together as a team more often than did their counterparts in unenriched jobs.

The social context may be more important than objective job conditions in determining how employees perceive and react to their job. Griffin (1983) conducted a field experiment in which jobs were enriched for one group of employees, and supervisors of another group were trained to provide positive feedback. A third group of employees received both enriched tasks and positive feedback. Feedback improved employees' views of their job tasks and their satisfaction with them as strongly as did job enrichment. More generally, social information such as job descriptions, role models, and praise from co-workers and supervisors can influence job motivation and performance as much as do presumably more concrete aspects of a job.

PERSONAL CHARACTERISTICS AS MODERATING FACTORS

Our discussion thus far implies that certain kinds of work climates typically have beneficial (or harmful) consequences. However, these consequences can be altered by personal factors. As noted earlier, job challenge and enrichment seem to benefit most employees, but those who have high personal growth needs react more positively to these aspects (Hackman and Oldham, 1980). Role clarity benefits the performance of competent employees more than that of their less competent counterparts. Conversely, work structure may be more important for individuals who have less well-developed growth needs. Such findings imply that an optimal match between person and environment can contribute to morale and reduce the dysfunctional consequences of some work settings.

Type A and Type B Managers

Type A managers presumably like a competitive, hard-driving style and enjoy exercising control over their environment. A bureaucratic work setting should present a special threat or challenge to such managers, since they wantto be in command of their environment. To test this idea, Chesney and Rosenman (1980) identified three groups of managers: a group in an internally controlled environment, a middle group, and a group in an externally controlled setting. As predicted, Type A managers in the externally controlled milieu reported more anxiety than did those in the freer one. Type B managers in the externally controlled setting reported less anxiety than did their Type B counterparts in more autonomous work situations. Type A employees who saw their work as cohesive and independent tended to have lower blood pressure than those who did not, whereas the reverse was true of Type Bs (Chesney *et al.*, 1981). An extroverted, assertive Type A person may feel congruent in a cohesive, independent setting. More introverted Type Bs seem to be more comfortable in a structured setting that does not emphasize autonomy or peer interaction.

Person–Environment Fit Theory

French and his colleagues (1982) have formulated a person–environment (P–E) congruence framework. Objective characteristics of the environment and the person index objective P–E fit. Similarly, indices of the perceived environment and of self-assessed personal characteristics can form a measure of subjective P–E fit. Measures of objective and subjective P–E congruence are only moderately related; perceived congruence is more closely linked to employee morale and health.

The studies conducted by these investigators point to a U-shaped relationship between some aspects of P–E fit and indices of morale and strain. For instance, depression tends to be lowest for employees with good fit on job complexity, and increases with both too little and too much complexity, either of which can prevent an individual from gaining a sense of self-esteem. Both too much and too little responsibility are associated with work-load dissatisfaction, anxiety, and anger. In general, measures of P–E fit account for as much or more of the variance in work strain as do the additive effects of the component person and environment indices. These studies need to be broadened to include observed aspects of work settings and to distinguish between two aspects of congruence: a person's ability in relation to job demands and a person's needs in relation to job opportunities.

Holland's Congruence Model

As noted earlier, Holland (1985) has proposed that people's personalities and occupations can be categorized into six types, each of which is associated with a distinctive work climate. Individuals who are congruent with their occupational environment (that is, who share the dominant interests and values of their work group) should be more satisfied and healthier than those who are not. Thus, realistic persons should feel better in realistic environments, investigative persons in investigative environments, and so on. Conversely, an investigative person who is relatively analytic and asocial may not fit well into a conventional environment that stresses conformity and control.

In general, processes of self-selection, job attrition, and gradual personality change seem to produce reasonably high P–E congruence. Individuals who are incongruent with their work settings tend to be less satisfied and productive in them. For instance, Furnham and Schaeffer (1984) found that employees with a poor P–E fit reported less job satisfaction and higher levels of mental distress. In contrast, correspondence between occupational needs and rewards has been associated with job satisfaction. Tziner (1983) asked one group of social workers to rate occupational rewards. Congruence between these rewards and the occupational needs of a second group of social workers was associated with their job satisfaction.

Job Longevity

Another approach to P–E congruence is to examine the influence of a person's longevity on the job. Sources of job satisfaction and performance may change systematically with the length of time a person is in a given job. In a perceptive analysis, Katz (1980) has formulated a three-stage framework of job longevity: a socialization stage, a period of innovation, and an adaptation phase. Employees in the socialization phase try to establish personal acceptance and are reactive to supervisor and peer feedback, but are not concerned about job independence or the variety of job tasks. Newcomers may profit more from directive structure than participation in setting performance goals, since knowledge of the supervisor's expectations helps to reduce uncertainty. In the innovation phase, employees respond more to the richness and challenge of their work and may react positively to job redesign. As employees move to the adaptation stage, even challenging jobs become routine; good job relationships and working conditions become more important.

FUTURE PROSPECTS

The growth of psychological research and a focus on the role of the individual in the workplace is a welcome trend that can complement the more established sociological focus on organizational processes. This person-oriented perspective can help to address emerging issues in the workplace, such as office automation, work-site intervention programs, and the active ways in which individuals shape and manage work.

Office Automation

Computer-assisted technology and robotics will grow rapidly in the next decade and beyond. Workplace automation can alter individuals' control over their jobs and affect the work climate and its links to performance and health. Alcalay and Pasick (1983) reason that technological innovations increase control for management and other professional workers but decrease it for clerical and blue-collar employees. Computer-based systems tend to heighten job challenge and productivity, but they also make the work environment more tense and demanding. Moreover, automation can lessen perceived control over work procedures and diminish the opportunity to interact with co-workers. Technology may also lead to a routinization of work, and eventually to intellectual rigidity and diminished self-efficacy.

We need to examine how complex technology alters job strain and employees' control over their jobs and inhibits the formation of social bonds at work. We should also identify preventive strategies, such as designing technical operations so that people can work in pairs of groups, establishing feedback channels, and allowing employees to help select equipment and work space design.

Work-site Intervention Programs

Poor job design and harsh work climates may create multiple problems, but job redesign and intervention programs can help to alleviate them. The organizational development (OD) and quality of working life (QWL) approaches provide two major perspectives on how to improve work settings. The OD perspective stems from Lewin's concepts of ecological psychology and his recognition of the open-system nature of persons and groups. The methods used to change organizations focus primarily on interpersonal and intragroup phenomena. In contrast, QWL programs tend to consider the entire work setting in a systems framework and to follow a sociotechnical approach.

Such intervention programs typically increase morale and job satisfaction and reduce absenteeism. Employees report that they have more responsible and complex work roles, are more involved in decision making, and enjoy more latitude and freedom in their work. Performance and productivity either remain stable or show moderate improvement. About 70% of OD interventions show positive effects, especially when they entail job redesign and are enhanced by system-wide commitment (Schneider, 1985). But enriched jobs may not have beneficial effects on employees in highly bureaucratic organizations. Moreover, short-term changes often fade out quickly over time. Attention to the interdependent role of contextual and personal factors may help to formulate more powerful intervention programs.

Individual and Group Coping Processes

Although there are some exceptions (e.g. Shinn and Morch, 1983), the essential thrust of research on work emphasizes the impact of organizational conditions on employees. We need to study how individuals select and shape their work. For example, there is an extensive body of research on how performance feedback affects employees. As noted by Ashford and Cummings (1983), however, seeking information and feedback also is a coping style that individuals use to reduce uncertainty, understand the probable outcome of their behavior, and learn how to achieve their goals. Both personal and contextual factors influence the use and efficacy of such coping processes.

New studies in the workplace can benefit from a broader consideration of stress and coping theory. In one example, Menaghen and Mervis (1984) consider the effectiveness of individual coping efforts on job distress and occupational problems. None of the coping strategies helped to reduce occupational problems. However, a propensity to use optimistic comparisons and to refrain from restricting one's expectations were associated with a decline in occupational distress over time. These two coping skills also help to lessen emotional distress that arises from marital and parental problems, implying that they may be generally effective. Future research on these issues should be anchored in a conceptual framework that considers work in relation to the family and other life contexts.

SUMMARY AND CONCLUSIONS

After a description of how work climates can be conceptualized in terms of relationship, personal growth or goal orientation, and system maintenance and change dimensions, this chapter focuses on how these dimensions can help to compare and contrast work settings. Some of the determinants of work climates are analyzed: physical and architectural features, organizational structure and policies, and suprapersonal factors; and some of the connections between work climate, employee morale and performance, and indices of strain such as mental and physical symptoms and medical conditions are examined. The findings imply that work climates can have beneficial or harmful consequences and that these consequences can be altered by personal factors. An optimal match between person and environment can contribute to morale, and reduce the dysfunctional consequences of some work settings.

REFERENCES

Alcalay, R., & Pasick, R. (1983). Psychosocial factors and the technologies of work. *Social Science and Medicine, 17,* 1075–1084.

Ashford, S., & Cummings, L.L. (1983). Feedback as an individual resource: Personal strategies of creating information. *Organizational Behavior and Human Performance, 32,* 370–398.

Berger, C., & Cummings, L. (1979). Organizational structure, attitudes and behaviors. In B.M. Staw (ed.), *Research in organizational behavior* Vol. 1 (pp. 169–208). Greenwich, CT: JAI Press.

Camman, C., Fichman, M., Jenkins, G.D., & Klesh, J. (1983). Assessing the attitudes and perceptions of organizational members. In S. Seashore, E. Lawler, P. Mirvis & C. Camman (eds), *Assessing organizational change: A guide to methods, measures and practices* (pp. 72–138). New York: John Wiley & Sons.

Preparation of the manuscript was supported by NIAAA Grants AA02863 and AA0699, and Veterans Administration Medical and Health Services Research and Development Service research funds. Portions of the manuscript were adapted from Moos (1986a).

Chesney, M., & Rosenman, R. (1980). Type A behavior in the work-setting. In C.L. Cooper & R. Payne (eds), *Current concerns in occupational stress* (pp. 186–212). New York: John Wiley & Sons.

Chesney, M., Sevelius, G., Black, G., Ward, M., Swan, G., & Rosenman, R. (1981). Work environment type A behavior and coronary heart disease risk factors. *Journal of Occupational Medicine, 23*, 551–555.

Conway, T., Vickers, R., Ward, H., & Rahe, R. (1981). Occupational stress and variation in cigarette, coffee and alcohol consumption. *Journal of Health and Social Behavior, 22*, 155–165.

Dalton, D., Todor, W., Spendolini, M., Fielding, G., & Porter, L. (1980). Organization, structure and performance: A critical review. *Academy of Management Review, 5*, 49–64.

Fisher, C., & Gitelson, R. (1983). A meta-analysis of the correlates of role conflict and ambiguity. *Journal of Applied Psychology, 68*, 320–333.

French, J.R.P., Caplan, R., & Van Harrison, R. (eds) (1982). *The mechanisms of job stress and strain*. New York: John Wiley & Sons.

Furnham, A., & Schaeffer, R. (1984). Person–environment fit, job satisfaction and mental health. *Journal of Occupational Psychology, 57*, 295–307.

Gavin, J., & Howe, J. (1975). Psychological climate: Some theoretical and empirical considerations. *Behavioral Science, 20*, 228–240.

Griffin, R. (1983). Objective and social sources of information in task redesign: A field experiment. *Administrative Science Quarterly, 28*, 184–200.

Hackman, J.R., & Oldham, G. (1980). *Work redesign*. Reading, MA: Addison Wesley.

Holland, J. (1985). *Making vocational choices: A theory of careers*. Englewood Cliffs, NJ: Prentice-Hall.

House, J., McMichael, A., Wells, J., Kaplan, B., & Landerman, L. (1979). Occupational stress and health among factory workers. *Journal of Health and Social Behavior, 20*, 139–160.

James, L., & Sells, S. (1981). Psychological climate: Theoretical perspectives and empirical research. In D. Magnusson (ed.), *Toward a psychology of situations: An interactional perspective* (pp. 275–295). Hillsdale, NJ: Erlbaum.

Jones, A., & James, L. (1979). Psychological climate: Dimensions and relationships of individual and aggregated work environment perceptions. *Organizational Behavior and Human Performance, 23*, 201–250.

Kahn, R. (1980). *Work and health*. New York: John Wiley & Sons.

Karasek, R. (1979). Job demands, job decision latitude, and mental strain: Implications for job redesign. *Administrative Science Quarterly, 24*, 285–307.

Karasek, R., Baker, D., Marxer, F., Ahlbom, A., & Theorell, T. (1981). Job decision latitude, job demands, and cardiovascular disease: A prospective study of Swedish men. *American Journal of Public Health, 71*, 694–705.

Katz, R. (1980). Time and work: Toward an integrative perspective. In. B. Staw & L. Cummings (eds), *Research in organizational behavior* Vol. 2 (pp. 81–127). Greenwich, CT: JAI Press.

Menaghan, E., & Mervis, E. (1984). Coping with occupational problems: The limits of individual efforts. *Journal of Health and Social Behavior, 25*, 406–423.

Moos, R. (1986a). Work as a human context. In M.S. Pallak & R.O. Perloff (eds), *Psychology and work: Productivity, change, and employment* (pp. 9–52).

Moos, R. (1986b). *Work Environment Scale manual;* 2nd edn. Palo Alto, CA: Consulting Psychologists Press.

Moos, R. (1987). *The Social Climate Scales: A user's guide*. Palo Alto, CA: Consulting Psychologists Press.

Moos, R., & Schaefer, J. (1987). Evaluating health care work settings: A holistic conceptual framework. *Health Psychology: An International Journal, 1*, 97–122.

Oldham, G. & Brass, D. (1979). Employee reactions to an open-plan office: A naturally occurring quasi-experiment. *Administrative Science Quarterly, 24*, 267–284.

Oldham, G., & Rotchford, N. (1983). Relationships between office characteristics and employee reactions: A study of the physical environment. *Administrative Science Quarterly*, *28*, 542–556.

Orpen, C. (1979). The effects of job enrichment on employee satisfaction, motivation, involvement, and performance: A field experiment. *Human Relations*, *32*, 189–217.

Parasuraman, S., & Alutto, J. (1981). An examination of the organizational antecedents of stressors at work. *Academy of Management Journal*, *24*, 48–67.

Parker, D., & Brody, J. (1982). Risk factors for alcoholism and alcohol problems among employed women and men. In *Occupational alcoholism: A review of research* (National Institute on Alcohol Abuse and Alcoholism Research Monograph No. 8; pp. 99–127). Washington, DC: US Government Printing Office.

Payne, R. (1980). Organizational stress and social support. In C.L. Cooper & R. Payne (eds), *Current concerns in occupational stress* (pp. 269–298). New York: John Wiley & Sons.

Schmitt, N., & Fitzgerald, M. (1982). Mass psychogenic illness: Individual and aggregate data. In M. Colligan, J. Pennebaker & L. Murphy (eds), *Mass psychogenic illness: A social psychological analysis* (pp. 87–100). Hillsdale, NJ: Erlbaum.

Schneider, B. (1985). Organizational behavior. *Annual Review of Psychology*, *36*, 573–611.

Shaw, J., & Riskind, J. (1983). Predicting job stress using data from the position analysis questionnaire. *Journal of Applied Psychology*, *68*, 253–261.

Shinn, M., & Morch, H. (1983). A tripartite model of coping with burnout. In B.A. Farber (ed.), *Stress and burnout in the human service professions* (pp. 227–240). New York: Pergamon Press.

Stern, G. (1970). *People in context: Measuring person–environment congruence in education and industry*. New York: John Wiley & Sons.

Tziner, A. (1983). Correspondence between occupational rewards and occupational needs and work satisfaction: A canonical redundancy analysis. *Journal of Occupational Psychology*, *56*, 49–56.

KEY WORDS

Dimensions of work climate, determinants of work climate, physical and architectural features, organizational structure and policies, suprapersonal factors, impact of work climate, job morale and performance, substance use and abuse, mental and physical symptoms, medical conditions, social context, personal characteristics as moderating factors, person–environment congruence.

Handbook of Life Stress, Cognition and Health
Edited by S. Fisher and J. Reason
© 1988 John Wiley & Sons Ltd

12

The Experience of Unemployment in Social Context

DAVID FRYER
University of Stirling, Scotland

WHAT IS THE EXPERIENCE OF UNEMPLOYMENT?

During half a century of research, a very large number of mental and physical states, referred to by an even larger number of terms, has been ascribed to unemployed people. Below, some of the major findings are presented in terms of a small number of widely used headings.

Demoralization

One of the most widespread early generic terms is 'demoralization'. The Royal Commission on the Poor Laws and on the Relief of Distress from Unemployment (1905–1909) carried a minority report summarized by Sydney Webb (Taylor, 1909). This emphasized the 'demoralisation of prolonged unemployment', creating problems which allegedly eventually arrived at the doors of 'medical officers of health'. In a seminal paper summarizing evidence from research carried out in Britain during the depression of the 1930s, Eisenberg and Lazarsfeld (1938) reviewed 112 sources and summarized the findings of 'all writers' as demonstration that 'there is a general lowering of morale with unemployment.'

A non-specific descriptive term like 'demoralization' may seem a quaint, even unacceptable, anachronism to modern, operationally attuned ears. However, although terms have changed since the 1930s, the concept of 'psychological well-being' is perhaps not all that different as a general term. Both can be broken down into affective, conative, cognitive, anomic and physical health components, each with subjective and behavioral indicators. Although the social scientific terminology has changed, the foci of research attention have remained remarkably stable over five decades of investigation.

Affect

Poulot (1872) remarked that unemployment is a 'terrible calamity', at the thought of which the person 'feels strangled, shakes, trembles with emotion' (cited in Garraty, 1978); these are common psychosomatic symptoms of emotional anxiety. Eisenberg and Lazarsfeld (1938) summarized the belief of 'all writers' that 'unemployment tends to make people more emotionally unstable than they were previous to unemployment'.

Recently, Warr (1984a) has summarized the evidence collected by means of standardized, well-validated questionnaires designed to investigate affective reactions. These studies allow the comparison of mean scores derived from large numbers of respondents in differing subpopulations. Impressive cross-sectional evidence is now available concerning: positive and negative affect (Bradburn, 1969; Warr, 1978); happiness (Bradburn and Caplovitz, 1965; Bradburn, 1969); present life satisfaction (Campbell *et al.*, 1976; Donovan and Oddy, 1982; Gaskell and Smith, 1981; Hepworth, 1980; Miles, 1983; Schlozman and Verba, 1979); experience of pleasure and of strain (Warr and Payne, 1982). In all studies reported above, groups of *unemployed* people exhibited higher mean levels of experienced strain and negative feelings and lower mean levels of happiness, present life satisfaction, experience of pleasure and positive feelings, than *employed* people selected as far as possible to be comparable in all other relevant respects.

Anxiety

In 1932 the Chief Medical Officer at the Ministry of Health wrote that the 'pervading and ubiquitous' effects of unemployment included 'prolonged worry and anxiety (which) may impair normal bodily functions, such as digestion, or aggravate existing states of mental irritability or instability, and thus engender various forms of psycho-neurosis' (Newman, 1932). Beales and Lambert (1934) summarized their study as presenting on every page a 'melancholy record of worry neurosis', and Pilgrim Trust (1938) repeatedly referred to anxiety, restlessness and nervousness: 'when a man is out of work, anxiety is part of a vicious circle, and the more he worries, the more he unfits himself for work.'

Research in the last decade has also focused on anxiety, but is characterized by the use of self-report measures designed to detect potential cases of minor psychiatric morbidity in community surveys (Banks and Jackson, 1982; Cochrane and Stopes-Roe, 1980; Donovan and Oddy, 1982; Estes and Wilensky, 1978; Henwood and Miles, 1987; Hepworth, 1980; Jackson and Warr, 1984; Jackson *et al.*, 1983; Levi *et al.*, 1984; McKenna and Fryer, 1984; McKenna and Payne, 1985; Miles, 1983; Payne, 1986; Pearlin and Lieberman, 1979; Warr *et al.*, 1985; Warr and Jackson, 1985). Many of these investigations have used the twelve-item version of the General Health Questionnaire (GHQ-12; Goldberg, 1972, 1978). The GHQ-12 may reasonably be regarded as an index of general anxiety since, when used with unemployed samples, it correlates highly (about 0.90) with the anxiety subscale of the longer 28-item version of the GHQ, designed to differentiate sets of symptoms (Payne and Hartley, 1984). It is not, of course, totally independent of depression, psychosomatic symptoms etc. However, it does have the considerable merits of established reliability and validity. GHQ scores significantly predict outcomes of, for example, the Present State Examination (Banks, 1983; Henderson *et al.*, 1979).

Results are consistent. The mean scores of unemployed samples are reliably about double those of comparable employed samples (14 or 15 as opposed to 8 or 9 out of 36), a larger score implying more anxiety.

Employment status accounts for about 14% of the variance of GHQ-12 (Fryer and Payne, 1986). Warr (1984b), examining a number of GHQ studies, showed that for four unemployed groups, between 54% and 62% of each sample scored above the cut-off point which Goldberg (1972) suggests indicates repondents to be 'at risk' of being diagnosed as psychiatric cases if they were to undergo detailed psychiatric assessment. By comparison, Wing (1980) found 9% in a general population survey to be 'cases'. However, the criteria for deciding those at risk used by Goldberg and Wing are difficult to compare. This, compounded by the fact that a number of GHQ items might be disproportionately likely to be checked by unemployed people irrespective of mental health (e.g. 'Felt that you are playing a useful part in things', 'Been able to enjoy your normal day to day activities'), counsels caution in considering Warr's high percentage 'at risk'.

Depression

Depression is routinely cited as a consequence of unemployment throughout its long psychological literature. For example, the pioneering investigators of an Austrian village, (Marienthal) stricken by mass redundancy assigned each of the unemployed families to one of four categories of 'attitude'. One category, those 'in despair', was characterized by 'despair, depression, hopelessness, and a feeling of futility of all effort' (Jahoda *et al.*, 1972). For the Pilgrim Trust (1938) researchers, their overriding impression was of 'the depression and apathy which finally settles down in many of the homes'.

Finlay-Jones and Eckhardt (1981) found 43% of young unemployed Australians claimed depressive symptoms which had only started after becoming unemployed and in the absence of any other precipitating cause. Many modern studies use well-validated measures of depression. Where they do, they consistently report higher mean levels of depressive symptoms in unemployed than in employed groups. This is true using both the depression subscale of the GHQ-28 (Payne and Hartley, 1984) and the Beck Depression Inventory (Feather, 1982). In the latter study, Feather found unemployed respondents to score around 11 (out of a maximum possible score of 63) and employed respondents to score around 5.5. Broadly consistent findings have been reported by Cobb and Kasl (1977); Feather and Bond (1983); Figuerra-McDonough (1978); Kasl (1979); Radloff (1975); and Tiggemann and Winefield (1980).

Hopelessness

One state of mind sometimes regarded as associated with, or even a component of, depression is feeling hopeless. The Royal Commission (1905–1909) claimed that 'the man from a permanent situation', when unemployed, 'ultimately loses hope and goes under in one way or another' (Taylor, 1909), and Bakke (1933) wrote of the 'physical and mental exhaustion' which results from, what one of his interviewees expressed as, 'the hopelessness of every step you take when you go in search of a job you know isn't there'. Israeli (1935), in a study comparing unemployed, student and mental patient respondents on three short question-naire measures, found the unemployed sample to have the most negative future expectations of failure of all.

Few modern studies have yet attempted to measure hopelessness as opposed to depression. However, the cognate notions of future orientation and planning are currently the focus of considerable theoretical attention in the field (Adams, 1986; Bolton and Oatley, 1985; Fryer, 1986; Fryer and McKenna, 1987; Jahoda, 1986b; McKenna and Fryer, 1984). Empirical work using operationalizations of hopelessness, perhaps including Beck's Hopelessness Scale (Beck *et al.*, 1974), would be valuable.

Self-esteem

Bakke (1933) wrote of his research informants that 'practically every man who had a family showed evidence of the blow his self-confidence has suffered', and a study of young unemployed men, interviewed five times over three years between 1936 and 1939, revealed maintenance of self-respect as the main problem (Carnegie UK Trust, 1943).

Modern research on self-esteem produced initially puzzling inconsistency of findings. Cobb and Kasl (1977) and Kasl (1979) detected no difference in self-esteem, as operationalized in a six-item measure, between employed and unemployed samples. Gaskell and Smith (1981) and Hartley (1980), using Rosenberg's 1965 scale and a measure of global self-esteem respectively, were equally unable to detect differences in self-esteem between employed and unemployed samples. However, Donovan and Oddy (1982) did find that young unemployed people had significantly lower group mean scores, i.e. lower self-esteem, than a comparable employed sample, and Gurney (1980) reported significantly lower self-esteem for unemployed compared with employed females, though not for males.

The variability in results may, according to Warr and Jackson (1983), arise because positive and negative aspects of self-esteem are semi-independent, with unemployment affecting negative but not positive aspects. This claim emerged from research in which they used separate measures for negative and positive self-esteem. Levels of positive self-esteem which were not statistically different in samples of employed and unemployed young people were reported. However, the unemployed sample exhibited significantly worse levels of negative self-esteem. This study also allowed the tracking of the samples longitudinally in and out of employment. Negative self-esteem changed in the predicted direction with change in employment status; positive self-esteem did not alter.

Resignation

Aspects of demoralization repeatedly reported in the 1930s' literature concern resignation, apathy and fatalism. In the Marienthal investigation, 70% of families were assigned to the 'resigned' category, characterized incidentally by 'hopelessness' (Jahoda *et al.*, 1972). Eisenberg and Lazarsfeld's (1938) third and final summarizing claim to be given the authority of 'all writers' ' agreement, was of an inevitable progression towards fatalism and resignation. The most direct behavioral indicator of resignation is, perhaps, decreasing activity.

Inactivity

Modern research, in general, confirms the inhibition of activity with unemployment. Stokes (1983) reported that a large proportion of his young unemployed sample had become lethargic and apathetic. Fagin and Little (1984) reported that the proportion of unstructured to structured time in the lives of their interviewees increased by a factor of 20 with unemployment. Since sitting around, watching television and chatting were categorized as 'unstructured', whilst time preparing for and travelling to and from employment was categorized as 'structured', this increase is hardly surprising, but it underlines the magnitude of change involved in unemployed people's activities and is consistent with several studies showing an increase in 'passive' and 'domestic' activities for many unemployed people (Kelvin *et al.*, 1985; Kilpatrick and Trew, 1985; Warr and Payne, 1983).

Importantly, there is a demonstrated negative association between the extent to which behaviour is passive and psychological well-being for unemployed samples. Warr and Payne (1983) reported a correlation between domestic and other pastimes such as television watching and psychological distress, and Kilpatrick and Trew (1985) showed inactivity and withdrawal to be associated with worsening mental health. Conversely, Fryer and Payne's (1984) sample of people coping extremely well with unemployment was characterized by extremely high levels of self-initiated activity. In general, activity level has repeatedly been shown to moderate psychological distress in unemployed samples (Feather and Bond, 1983; Fryer and McKenna, 1987; Henwood and Miles, 1987; Hepworth, 1980; Swinburne, 1981).

Social Isolation

A noxious repercussion of reduced activity is the associated diminishing social contact (Bakke, 1940; Jahoda *et al.*, 1972). The Pilgrim Trust researchers wrote in 1938 of their 'impression of isolation and loneliness', and Beales and Lambert (1934) remarked upon 'the effects of isolation from friends and dependence on relatives'.

Recently, Henwood and Miles (1987) have reported studies which operationalized Jahoda's latent function, 'imposed social contact', which she maintains is a necessary consequence of employment but not of unemployment. For both men and women, the researchers reported unemployed groups to be experiencing significantly less social contact than either employed or retired groups. McKenna and Payne (1985) showed that men unemployed for between 6 and 18 months had greater problems reflected in the social isolation component of the Nottingham Health Profile than men re-employed after a similar period of unemployment.

That declining social contact accompanies unemployment for many mature unemployed people has also been confirmed by a number of self-report (e.g. Warr, 1984b) and time budget (e.g. Trew and Kilpatrick, 1984) studies.

Cognitive Changes

Although the psychological literature generally links affect to cognitive performance, little investigation of cognitive change has yet been reported. However, Fryer and Warr (1984) elicited reports on cognitive difficulties from a sample of 954 working-class men stratified by age and length of unemployment. About one in three respondents reported taking longer over things, having difficulty concentrating, and felt they were getting 'rusty'. Ten out of the twelve items showed a significant length effect, with men unemployed longer reporting more cognitive difficulties. Five items showed an age effect, middle-aged men reporting greatest difficulty.

Anomic Change

In the 1930s, some 'claimed that unemployment makes people immoral, makes them radicals, atheists etc.' (Eisenberg and Lazarsfeld, 1938). There was little reliable evidence however, and what there was suggested no marked effect. Bakke (1940) was typical in discovering no evidence for an effect of unemployment on religious belief, respect for the law, or political radicalization: 'talk of revolution is conspicuous by its absence'. Recently, however, Banks and Ullah (1987) have used survey data to support a claim of increasing detachment from the main political systems of some unemployed young people, and Stokes (1983) reported a disinclination to participate in society in his sample of young unemployed people (but see also Clark, 1985; Gaskell and Smith, 1985). Likewise, despite impressionistic claims to the contrary (Williams, 1933), the little actual evidence suggested a decrease in sexual activity with unemployment, where there was an effect at all (Komarovsky, 1940).

Physical Health

The Pilgrim Trust (1938) reported 'nervous anxiety, and in some cases physical deterioration', in both unemployed and employed respondents. For unemployed families on unemployment assistance there was 'almost invariably definite want': in a quarter of families, children were suffering ill-health.

More recently, Warr (1984a) reports that between 25% and 30% of unemployed men in recent studies asserted their health had deteriorated since unemployment. Cross-sectional studies (e.g. Verbrugge, 1983) reveal poorer reported health amongst unemployed than employed samples, and O'Brien and Kabanoff (1979) reported that an unemployed subsample of a larger Australian population survey had more symptoms of bronchitis, allergies, nose and throat problems than the employed subsample. On the other hand, Cobb and Kasl (1977) found no evidence of deteriorating physical health in their longitudinal study. However, their sample was small, the length of unemployment brief and the labour market buoyant. Given the multicausal nature of illness and the relatively long periods of time likely for effects of stressors and material hardship to translate into physical illness, longitudinal studies of large samples over long time periods using robust indicators of physical health are clearly required to settle the issue. Beale and Nethercott (1986) provide such persuasive evidence. They analyzed the medical records of 129 patients in the first author's medical practice over an eight-year period, which embraced their involuntary redundancy. Both threatened and actual redundancy had a negative impact on health, in terms of frequency of medical consultations, bouts of illness and attendance at hospital as out-patients, compared to non-redundant controls' health records. Aggregate epidemiological studies of health are also useful. Many of these suggest a link between unemployment and health (e.g. Brenner, 1987), parasuicide and suicide (e.g. Platt, 1984).

Stages of Response to Unemployment

Some researchers have combined attention to the whole range of psychological and physical health states associated with unemployment with description of change over time to develop 'stage' or 'phase' accounts. These involve the prediction of an ordered succession of qualitatively distinct behaviours and mental states consequent upon employment. Much of the evidence, however, is of poor quality, internally contradictory, non-specific as to domain, and grossly individualistic. There have been at least seventeen different publications during the last half century commending stage accounts of unemployment, but the proponents differ amongst themselves not only in the definition of each stage but even in the number of stages they posit. Some writers offer phases within stages, others allow the same mental states to characterize different stages, and where writers suggest time bands for stages, suggestions diverge (for further detailed criticisms see Fryer, 1985).

This is not to say an acceptable version of a stage account will never be articulated. There is a reasonable expectation that the experience of unemployment would change over time, and this is supported by evidence concerning the mediating effect of the length of unemployment on unemployment experience.

Jackson and Warr (1984) systematically sampled six lengths of unemployment: less than a month, 1–2 months, 2–3 months, 3–6 months, 6–12 months, and more than 12 months. The study used GHQ-30, with a sample of 954 men. Within the first month of unemployment, psychological health was worse for the unemployed men than for a group of comparable employed men. A small but significant mean increase in psychological health was detected at 2–3 months, followed by a decrease at 6 months, and subsequent stabilization. This was a cross-sectional study, but its results are consistent with a stage account. However, a more widespread view is of gradual deterioration in well-being over about 3 months, then levelling out to remain fairly stably low (Warr and Jackson, 1985), or even slightly improving (Payne et al., 1984). Re-employment seems to be reflected in a drop in GHQ-30 scores by about half (37 to 19) (Warr and Jackson, 1985), although Fineman (1987), on the basis of following up and reinterviewing participants in an unemployment study after 6 years of re-employment, doubts that re-employment resets the 'psychological equation'. Unemployment, Fineman asserts, leaves a legacy of perceived stigma, self-doubts, cautiousness and wariness.

HOW MUCH CONFIDENCE CAN BE PLACED IN THE FINDINGS?

Research evidence comes from the whole gamut of available methods. These include the qualitative approaches of: informal interviewing (e.g. Marsden 1982); structured interviewing (e.g. Fagin and Little, 1984); depth interviewing (e.g. Fryer and Payne, 1984); personal document analysis (e.g. Beales and Lambert, 1934); public document analysis (e.g. Jahoda *et al.*, 1972); participant observation (e.g. Jahoda, 1987); and ethnography (e.g. Bostyn and Wight, 1987). Methods used also include: objective observational methods such as time budget diaries (e.g. Henwood and Miles, 1987); survey methods using well-validated quantitative psychological measures such as the SAPU studies (see Warr (1987b) for examples); psychiatric community studies (e.g. Bebbington *et al.*, 1981); psychiatric diagnosis (e.g. Roy, 1981); practice-based physician studies (e.g. Beale and Nethercott, 1986); physiological measurement techniques (e.g. Cobb and Kasl, 1977); and sophisticated epidemiological methods (e.g. Dooley and Catalano, 1980). Thirdly, methods used have embraced action research (e.g. Cassell *et al.*, in press).

It would be inaccurate to claim that the history of psychological research on unemployment comprises a shift from less to more sophisticated and confidence-inspiring methods. The Marienthal study (Jahoda *et al.*, 1972) is still unrivalled today in its exemplification of thorough-going triangulation (Fryer, in press). The Pilgrim Trust (1938), employing a team of researchers to interview a random sample of 1086 people, whose names were drawn on a single day in 1936 from the live file of the Unemployment Assistance Board in six towns selected to sample equally prosperous, average and 'specially distressed' areas, achieved a remarkable success rate of 81%, collecting at each interview material on a wide range of topics.

These early studies are not easily surpassed. Undeniably, however, the most compelling research evidence concerning *causes* is that of the recent longitudinal investigations. Cross-sectional studies showing an association between poor psychological health and unemployment are open to the interpretation that the poor well-being is the cause rather than the result of unemployment. This is, admittedly, an unpersuasive argument during periods of rapid recession. It is unlikely, for example, that the record British levels of unemployment in the 1980s are the result of rapid increases in poor mental health.

However, it takes longitudinal studies following groups of people in and out of employment to settle the matter convincingly. There is now such persuasive longitudinal evidence, using well-validated measures, in respect of: happiness (e.g. Tiggemann and Winefield, 1980); present life satisfaction (e.g. Cohn, 1978); experience of pleasure and of strain (e.g. Payne, 1985); satisfaction with self (e.g. Cohn, 1978); general health questionnaire (e.g. Banks and Jackson, 1982);

negative self-esteem (e.g. Warr and Jackson, 1983); depression (e.g. Tiggemann and Winefield, 1980; Feather and O'Brien, 1986); and physical health (e.g. Beale and Nethercott, 1986). Groups who became unemployed during the course of these longitudinal studies exhibited means which deteriorated compared with continuously employed groups. Groups which became employed during the course of the studies exhibited means which improved compared with continuously unemployed groups.

Systematic research on unemployment straddles half a century and three continents. It has been carried out by a variety of researchers, basing their work on a variety of assumptions. It has been achieved by the use of a wide range of methods, using many different designs, and analysed at every level and type of sophistication. Yet, there is a remarkable consistency of findings and themes: 'the evidence for the 1970s . . . presents apparently much the same impact of unemployment as in the earlier period' (Jahoda, 1979). It is no longer reasonable to doubt that unemployment *causes* psychological change.

VARIATIONS IN THE EXPERIENCE OF UNEMPLOYMENT AND FOCUS OF RESEARCH

The experience of unemployment is sometimes portrayed as homogenously negative. Yet wide within-group variation in the experience of unemployment has always been recognized in the primary literature.

In Marienthal, for example, the investigators discovered 23% of the unemployed families to be 'unbroken', characterized by 'maintenance of the household, care of the children, subjective well being, activity, hopes and plans for the future, sustained vitality, and continued attempts to find employment' (Jahoda *et al.*, 1972, p. 53). Moreover, this group had already been depleted by the emigration of 'the most active and energetic families'. Pilgrim Trust (1938) likewise reported that 'there are unemployed men who not only enjoy their leisure but have found in unemployment the opportunity to develop aspects of their personalities which during employment have never had a chance'.

A number of qualitative studies emphasize exceptions to the general picture of apathy, inactivity and depression (Fagin and Little, 1984; Fryer and Payne, 1984; Fineman, 1979, 1983; Harrison, 1976; Marsden, 1982; Walter, 1985).

Other, quantitative, research similarly shows a range of reactions to unemployment—including positive ones (e.g. Evans, 1986; Hartley, 1978; Huczynski, 1978). Summarizing several large quantitative studies, Warr (1984a) suggests that about 15% of unemployed men actually report an improvement in physical health, and between 5% and 10% report an improvement in psychological health since becoming unemployed: 'not everyone is affected negatively when they become unemployed'. Why is this?

This reviewer believes that the experience of unemployment is constituted by the dynamic intersection of personal agency (such as values, purposes, perceptions, degrees of self-directedness) with powerful social contexts (such as social institutions, expectations, norms, environmental and material circumstances).

Most, especially recent, research focuses on individuals (usually males) taken out of the social contexts which make their behaviour and experience meaningful to themselves and understandable to the researcher. Throughout the literature, however, a minority of researchers have radically shifted the focus of attention from the individual male to the family, community or subculture. Moreover, in order to tease apart systematically the variety of unemployment experience, more orthodox survey researchers have gradually focused attention on particular subpopulations of respondents on the basis of gender, social class, age, race, personal vulnerability—so-called mediating variables. Whilst the particular focus, assumptions and methods of the two approaches to heterogeneity differ substantially, the evidence generated can be considered complementary and therefore research evidence from both approaches is here summarized together.

Focus on the Family and Gender Expectations

Women's Unemployment

Most psychological research on unemployment has focused on males (Callender, 1985; Jackson and Walsh, 1987; Griffin, 1986; Hurstfield, 1986). However, there is a minority literature dealing with the impact of unemployment on women—both those who lose paid jobs (redundant women) and those whose expectations of employment are unmet (especially female school leavers).

Despite the title of its publication (*Men without work*), the Pilgrim Trust (1938) did investigate women's unemployment too, concluding that job loss was a blow to women on both social and financial grounds. A recent review agrees that unemployment and high levels of psychological distress are associated for both single and married women living in deprived environments (Warr and Parry, 1982). Similar evidence exists concerning satisfaction with self (Cohn, 1978) and emotional strain (Warr and Payne, 1982).

Regarding female school leavers, a number of studies have reported large differences in both GHQ and negative self-esteem scores between unemployed and employed women, with the former showing more distress (Banks and Jackson, 1982; Warr and Jackson, 1983; Warr et al., 1985). Longitudinally, significant differences in scores of well-being of unemployed and employed young women are found, even though no such differences can be detected between the groups' scores when at school (Banks and Jackson, 1982).

As with most measures of affect in general population surveys, women tend to exhibit poorer well-being than men. Warr et al. (1985) found, in a study of teenagers, that females exhibited lower well-being than males on the GHQ-12 (13 for females, 11 for males), the Zung depression inventory and the Zung anxiety scale (Zung, 1974). The reasons are unclear. However, the most impressive differences in these studies are not by gender, but by employment status. Unemployment seems to affect well-being 'in all cases where, male or female, are in effect principal wage earners' (Warr, 1984b, p. 275).

The claim about principal wage earners receives empirical support from a number of studies. Finlay-Jones and Burville (1979) found that a negative association between well-being and unemployment for single women was not apparent for married women. Cohn (1978) could demonstrate no association between employment status and satisfaction with self for women with children, whilst Warr and Parry (1982) could find no evidence for an association between employment and well-being for mothers, unless living in very adverse home environments.

'His Unemployment: Her Problem'? (McKee and Bell, 1986)

Another approach looks at the impact of unemployment on women not themselves made redundant but as affected by men's redundancy. Kelvin and Jarrett (1985, p. 66) express this succinctly: 'though women do feature in the literature on unemployment, they do so first and foremost as the wives of unemployed men, and the mothers of such men's children'.

McKee and Bell's insightfully titled study points to the repercussions, for a woman, of a male partner's unemployment in terms of managing on reduced · income, nurturing the partner, coping with his sometimes intrusive presence, and its effect on the household division of labour (see also Laite and Halfpenny, 1987). Their most general conclusion was that 'recognition should be paid to the impact of unemployment on the family rather than the unemployed as individuals' (see also Allatt and Yeandle, 1986; Bakke, 1961; Binns and Mars, 1984; Cavan and Ranke, 1938; Clarke, 1987; Fagin and Little, 1984; Jackson and Walsh, 1987).

Summarizing her research in Marienthal in 1931/2, Jahoda (1982) writes: 'While family relations continued in established patterns longer than other relations and activities, there was some evidence that they, too, deteriorated and family quarrels increased'. Modern research can be cited in support of Jahoda's claims. Schlozman and Verba (1979), for example, concluded from a telephone study that unemployment and family strain are related, especially for those previously in poor jobs and those longer unemployed (see also Binns and Mars; 1984, Fagin and Little, 1984; Liem and Liem, 1979; Tausky and Piedmont, 1967). Komarovsky (1940) was, however, more cautious in concluding that unemployment was an exacerbator of pre-unemployment problems rather than the origin of problems, and Bakke (1940) agreed: 'unemployment does not destroy family harmony it merely acts as an irritant on whatever tendencies are already present'. Thomas et al. (1980), after conducting two small-scale studies and a literature review, concluded that, 'for a majority of families, including white and blue collar workers, crisis does not accompany husbands' unemployment'.

Several studies have emphasized how 'the household as a unit of analysis can obscure individual degrees of disadvantage, suffering and equality' (McKee and Bell, 1986, p. 136). The Pilgrim Trust (1938) had reported that 'in most unemployed families the parents, and in particular the wives, bore the burden of want, and in many instances were literally starving themselves in order to feed and clothe the children reasonably well'. In one-third of these families, the mother was suffering from anaemia and/or nervous debilitation.

We have looked at the impact of unemployment on women who were 'principal wage earners' and also on women who are 'wives and mothers' of unemployed men. However, these two approaches may be seen as exemplifying the criticisms of some researchers: 'the few studies that do incorporate women . . . are either gender blind or gender bound. They assume that women's experiences are either the same as men's or that they can be explained solely in terms of the sexual division of labour and women's domestic role' (Callender, 1987, p. 23).

There is a sense in which the 'principal wage earner' approach treats women's own unemployment seriously only to the extent that the women are 'honorary males' in terms of signing on, job search, commitment to employment, etc. However, many women may perceive themselves neither as unemployed nor employed (Cragg and Dawson, 1984), might not 'actively' seek employment (Callender, 1987), nor even believe they have a legitimate right to a job in terms of a 'queue' of priority candidates (Martin and Wallace, 1984), yet still both wish to be employed and suffer psychologically as a result of not being employed.

Callender (1987) has much justification for claiming that 'prevailing ideas surrounding employment and unemployment are male dominated and . . . inappropriate for understanding the position of women in the labour market' (p. 23). Henwood and Miles (1987) are amongst those beginning to tease apart gender and employment status by systematically comparing the experience of full-time and part-time employed women, housewives, retired and unemployed women, with variations on male employment status.

Unemployment and Children

In a summary of 150 case studies of unemployed families from cities spanning the USA, Elderton (1931) provided an awesome catalogue, copiously illustrated by case material, of repercussions of unemployment upon children: 'cruelty towards wife and children', 'anxious attitude of children', 'children put in homes', 'delinquency', 'food trimmed', 'milk supply cut down', give an idea of the contents. Whilst this study is one of the most disquietingly graphic, it was by no means unique in its claims. Other studies reported ragged misery, poor educational achievement, emotional instability, insecurity and anxiety, as well as malnutrition and child abuse (see also Eisenberg and Lazarsfeld, 1938, pp. 379–308; Save the Children International Union, 1933).

A fairly recent review (Madge, 1983) presents evidence that many children in unemployed families still suffer not only materially and economically but also socially, educationally and psychologically compared with peers in employed families. Disturbingly, many recent findings echo the 1930s. Cater and Easton (1980), for example, found one in three fathers of abused children to be unemployed (see also Dhooge and Popay, 1987).

Piachaud (1986) reports that one in every nine children in Britain are in unemployed families. Given what we know about the impact of unemployment on adults, i.e. their parents, it seems unlikely that many children in unemployed families will remain totally unscathed (see also Fryer, 1987).

Focus on Collectivities

Communities

The most famous community study is that of Marienthal, Austria, carried out in

1931/2. A team of fourteen social scientists and physicians, directed by Lazarsfeld and Jahoda, conducted an extraordinarily intensive investigation of the community of 1486 people; 77% of families had no member in employment. The study exemplified thorough triangulation, combining quantitative data gathering, qualitative interviewing, unobtrusive and participant observation, action and evaluation research. 'Sampling' was impressive: for some data, every inhabitant and every family was investigated. A summary by the main researchers concluded that unemployment causes 'a diminution of expectation and activity, a disrupted sense of time, and a steady decline into apathy through a variety of stages and attitudes' (Jahoda *et al.*, 1972, p. 2).

A more recent community study took place in 1981 on the Isle of Sheppey, Kent, UK. By means of a one in nine random survey of the entire community, with a 79% response rate, Wallace and Pahl investigated 'all forms of work', whether inside or outside an employment relationship, and showed convincingly that the black economy, where it operates at all, is overwhelmingly the province of the employed rather than unemployed people, who were found to be 'poor, isolated and unable to engage in any more than marginal informal activities' (Wallace and Pahl, 1986, p. 130).

An intensive sociographic study over a period of two years was conducted by Bostyn and Wight (1987) whilst living in a council flat in an ex-mining Scottish village where 30% of men and 60% of women were not employed. The researchers used questionnaires, interviews, participant and unobtrusive observation to describe in detail a community of people 'deprived of meaning in their lives' by lack of money and of a clear time structure.

Social Interventions

Six years after the Marienthal study, Jahoda conducted an equally impressive collective level investigation in Wales. This study, conducted in 1937/8, was of a 'co-operative enterprise manned by the unemployed to produce goods and service for their own consumption' (Jahoda, 1987). It was a pioneering venture designed by an Order of friends to 'overcome the disastrous economic and human consequences of unemployment' and of previous poor quality employment. Jahoda conducted the research alone, working in turn in each of the twelve departments of the enterprise whilst living in turn in the family homes of nine of the 'unemployed workers'. Her methods, again, were immersion and triangulation. The enterprise failed due to resignation, poverty and 'the overwhelming influence of the industrial tradition . . . on every sphere of life' (Jahoda, 1987).

More recently a number of other action research/evaluation projects have been conducted. Stafford (1982) and Branthwaite and Garcia (1985) have evaluated British job creation schemes from a psychological perspective, with conflicting findings. Buss *et al.* (1983) conducted a study of use made of community mental health and 'human service' facilities in a US steel community ravaged by the loss of over 4000 jobs. More non-redundant than redundant workers sought help from every source except the loan agency. Winfield (1981) broached the issue of how psychologists could help members of unemployed workers' centres help themselves. One answer is being provided by Cassell *et al*. (in press), who report an action/evaluation research project engaged in providing unemployed people with access to information technology in local community centres and making available to them opportunities to acquire skills necessary to develop computer applications relevant to their own communities.

Subcultures

Ullah (1987), following both a large quantitative longitudinal survey of unemployed black and white youths and a detailed ethnographic investigation, concluded that for young blacks, 'their experience of unemployment needs to be viewed within the wider context of their individual and collective experience of being black in a predominantly white society' (p. 111). A fundamental finding was that 'many of the black people did not strongly identify themselves as unemployed', rather, 'being unemployed was simply another feature of being black, in much the same way that bad housing and limited educational opportunities' were viewed to be.

Such insights go some way to making sense of the available survey data on ethnicity. Warr *et al*. (1985) compared 1150 black and white young people of both sexes on GHQ-12, the Zung anxiety scale and the Zung depression scale. Whites, both male and female, scored higher than blacks on the GHQ and depression measures, i.e. were more distressed. The mean differences did reach the 5% statistical confidence level but the clinical significance of what were, in real terms, very small differences (10.8 vs 11.28 for males; 12.24 vs 13.56 for females) is probably not great. In a multiple regression, whilst ethnicity did predict depression, it was the weakest of all predictors; employment commitment and variables measuring time filling and varied social life were much stronger. It may be, counterintuitively, that belonging to a subcultural ethnic group actually helps, but only slightly, in coping with unemployment. Whilst ethnicity does affect unemployment experience, other personal and social variables seem to have stronger roles.

Labour Market Contexts

The significance of the local labour market for employment prospects at the individual level of the psychological experience of unemployment is clear. Relevant research is reported by Jackson and Warr (1987) and Raffe (1986). Labour market effects, when aggregated up, may be accessible through 'proxy' variables such as *age* and *social class*, since different employers may have differing preferences for the age of new employees in terms of labour and training costs, compliance, attitude, etc., and social class is conventionally operationalized in terms of Registrar General occupational classification.

The relationship between age and psychological well-being is curvilinear for unemployed groups (Daniel, 1974; Hepworth, 1980). This is systematically demonstrated by Jackson and Warr (1984) who, based on a sample of men stratified by age and length of unemployment, reported mean GHQ-30 scores of

31 for 20 years old, 37 for those aged between 20 years and 59 years, and a mean score of 26 for those between 60 years and 64 years. Being in the middle group still predicted poorer mental health, even when variables such as the proportion of family income lost since unemployment and number of dependents were entered into a multiple regression.

The impact of unemployment on white-collar and professional workers has been investigated by several researchers (Fineman, 1979, 1983; Hartley, 1980; Kaufman, 1982; Little, 1976). All agree there is wide variation in responses in such groups but *dis*agree as to whether white-collar workers are generally more or less severely affected than blue-collar workers. Hartley, Little and Fineman argue that the consequences are less traumatic, Kaufman that they are more traumatic. Payne *et al.* (1984) conducted a study with 399 men aged 25–39, unemployed for between 6 and 11 months. Half of the sample's previous jobs were white-collar and half blue-collar. In the general population there is a reliable and sizeable difference in mean GHQ scores between such groups (Goldberg, 1978). However, although in this study the blue-collar group reported greater financial anxiety and more difficulty filling time than the white-collar group, there was no significant difference on any of the physical or psychological health measures.

Focus on Personal Vulnerability

A major assumption underlying the review in this chapter is that the experience of unemployment is constituted by a conjunction of material circumstances, social institutions and unique aspects of individual agents.

It is important not to exaggerate the role of the individual, and thus err into psychologism, by suggesting that an explanation of unemployment experience can be provided simply in terms of the individual characteristics of the unemployed person. This perspective was a regrettable feature of some work in the 1960s and 1970s conducted in buoyant economies on so-called, 'hard core unemployed'. Tiffany *et al.* (1970), for example, used the term 'work inhibited' to describe people 'physically capable of work . . . but prevented from working because of psychological difficulties'.

On the other hand, it is important to acknowledge that unique aspects of individual agents do have a role in explaining the experience of unemployment and the documented variations in it. An explanation entirely at the level of social structures misses this.

A number of individual-level personality-related factors which might make a person more or less vulnerable to unemployment distress have been discussed in the literature, including hardiness (Kobasa *et al.*, 1982); neuroticism (Payne, in press); pro-activity (Fryer and Payne, 1984; Evans, 1986; Haworth and Evans, 1987); attributional style (Feather and Davenport, 1981; see also Chapter 23, this volume).

By far the most systematically researched, apparently individual, factor, however, is employment commitment. A person highly attached to employment seems likely to be more severely affected by loss of employment than one less attached, whether because of the so-called protestant work ethic or for other more secular reasons such as the standard of living it enables.

The notion has, in recent times, been considered a relatively stable dispositional variable and has gone through a number of operationalizations: work
involvement (Warr and Lovatt, 1977) and employment commitment (Jackson et
al., 1983). Employment commitment, so measured, moderates the association
between employment status and GHQ-12 score. Employed people higher on
employment commitment have fewer symptoms, unemployed people higher on
employment commitment have more symptoms (Stafford et al., 1980; Banks and
Jackson, 1982; Jackson et al., 1983; Payne and Hartley, 1984; Warr et al., 1985).
Longitudinally, young people with higher employment commitment showed
greater increases in psychological distress scores when they became unemployed
(Jackson et al., 1983).

It is worth noting that employment commitment as a measure is very highly
skewed. Mean scores are about 4.70 on a scale with a maximum of 5.0, with
standard deviations of only 0.50, i.e. almost everyone tested is committed to
employment (for further discussion of the measure see Fryer and Payne, 1986, pp.
257–258).

WHAT IS IT ABOUT UNEMPLOYMENT WHICH CAUSES PSYCHOLOGICAL DISTRESS?

Two main approaches to explaining unemployment experience, based on differing assumptions and with differing emphases, can be found in the literature. These
involve absence of latent functions, and agency restriction.

Absence of Latent Functions

Jahoda (1979, 1982) and Jahoda and Rush (1980) have provided the currently
dominant model in the field. Jahoda claims that employment as a social institution
has both manifest (intended) and latent (unintended) consequences. Most people
enter an employment relationship for financial reasons: 'earning a living is taken
for granted as the manifest consequence of employment' (Jahoda, 1981). However, according to Jahoda (1986a), there are also six latent functions of employment: time structure; social contact; activity; status; purposefulness; and control.
The step from an account of employment to one of unemployment is short:
'unemployment of more than a very short period is psychologically destructive
because of the absence of the latent consequences of employment' (Jahoda and
Rush, 1980).

Jahoda's latent functions approach finds striking echoes in the work of Fagin
and Little (1984), Hartley (1980), Hayes and Nutman (1981), Kelvin (1981), Miles
and Henwood (1987), Murray-Parkes (1972), O'Brien (1986), Warr (1987a & b),
most of whom cite her as a source.

Two variations on a latent functions approach deserve mention. O'Brien (1986)
places a central explanatory emphasis on the content of work tasks in the entire
field of 'work and unemployment' and is avowedly critical of Jahoda because,
according to him, she 'omits the crucial element of employment—the content of

the tasks' in her latent functions account, and he criticizes her 'simple psychological deprivation theory that will lead only to descriptive studies'. Both of these criticisms are off target. Jahoda (1942, 1987) investigated task traction, and careful hypothesis testing based on her latent functions explanation is reported (e.g. Miles, 1983; Henwood and Miles, 1987; Fryer and McKenna, 1987). In fact, O'Brien's own account is itself more or less a pared down version of Jahoda's latent functions account: 'unemployment . . . is a state where the individual is dramatically deprived of job income and the opportunity to use valued skills' (O'Brien, 1986, p. 185). It is an elaboration of just one of Jahoda's latent functions ('activity'), and her manifest one (income)—although O'Brien subsequently places little explanatory emphasis on the latter.

Warr's (1987a) nine-factor framework can be interpreted as a cultivation, rather than a paring down, of Jahoda's essential insights. His framework includes: opportunity for control, skill use and interpersonal contact; goal and task demands; variety; environmental clarity; availability of money; physical security; and valued social position. It can be seen that this is essentially Jahoda's absence of manifest and latent functions model; it is a 'model in terms of unemployment causing decrements in nine environmental features' (Warr, 1987a). There are some differences: 'imposition' of experience has been softened to 'opportunity'; the manifest function has been expanded to embrace explicitly not only income but also the physical security it usually allows; 'environmental clarity' has been added; and 'activity' has been interpreted as skilled activity.

The latent functions approach to explaining the experience of unemployment, in both its original and elaborated versions, is a considerable achievement with valuable integrative, predictive and policy relevant features. However, Jahoda's approach has been criticized on pragmatic, methodological, empirical and theoretical grounds. Moreover, the assumptions upon which it rests have been criticized as implying a rather passive, retrospective model of the person and giving insufficient explanatory emphasis to the role of poverty in the experience of unemployment (see Fryer, 1986; Fryer and Payne, 1986, for further details). For these and other reasons, an account with an emphasis on personal agency, future orientation and poverty has been proposed.

Agency Restriction

The agency restriction approach rests on the basic assumption that people are agents who strive to assert themselves, initiate and influence events, are intrinsically motivated and live in perceived worlds in which what they attempt depends on their views of the future as well as on their memories of the past. These characteristics are claimed to be routinely limited, restricted, frustrated, discouraged and undercut by the social context of unemployment.

A number of particular aspects of agency restriction have been highlighted in the literature: the frustrated search for meaning in the arbitrary, exceedingly complex or intrinsically distressing reality of unemployment and its seemingly fathomless bureaucracy; the restriction of choices; blocking of need satisfactions; stymying of hopes; confrontation with threatening novel problems without appropriate skills and with inadequate resources. The likelihood of failure under these conditions, with consequent effects on well-being, self-esteem and perceived efficacy, is great.

Future orientation and the role of planning are aspects of agency restriction currently receiving research attention (Bolton and Oatley, 1985; Fryer, 1986; Fryer and McKenna, 1987). However, it is frustration of agency by relative poverty, and associated social, psychological repercussions, which is at the core of the approach.

Financial hardship has repeatedly been mentioned throughout this review. It recurs in empirical reports but is generally treated as an economic consequence of unemployment which goes along with psychological distress. Jahoda, O'Brien and Warr all include poverty in their explanatory accounts. However, none of these gives poverty a central explanatory role. Jahoda and Rush (1980) are quite explicit: '*beyond financial problems* unemployment of more than a very short period is psychologically destructive because of the absence of the latent consequences of employment *even when adequate redundancy payments are available*' (my emphasis). O'Brien emphasizes skill exercise deprivation in explaining contemporary unemployment distress, whilst Warr (1987a) places 'availability of money' sixth in his list of nine factors.

In general, there has been a remarkable lack of emphasis on poverty in the recent psychological literature on unemployment experience (Fraser, 1981; Gurney and Taylor, 1981). There are a number of very persuasive reasons for believing that poverty is a crucial aetiological factor in unemployment experience.

Firstly, unemployed people repeatedly tell us so. Shortage of money is consistently reported by unemployed respondents as the greatest source of personal and family difficulties (e.g. Daniel, 1974; Smith, 1980; Warr, 1987a). Secondly, we know that unemployment is, in fact, associated with substantial drops in income. Davies *et al.* (1982) found that nearly 50% of their unemployed respondents were receiving less than half, in state benefits, of what they had previously received in wages. Only 6% reported actually receiving more in state benefits than they had in wages. Warr and Jackson (1984) reported an even bleaker picture: 66% of their unemployed respondents reported a total household income of between a third and a half of their previous household income when employed. Finlay-Jones and Eckhardt (1981) found two-thirds of their sample were in debt after 10 months of unemployment, and 50% of Smith's (1980) sample had been unable to keep up repayments, whilst 8% had had fuel supplies cut off. Cooke (1987) shows that poverty of unemployment extends beyond low income to inferior or inexistent credit, low asset wealth and debt—all of which contribute to low living standards. Ironically, as household income and general standard of living decline with unemployment, in many respects financial demands go up. Heating and lighting of homes, food and drink during 'working time' are all expensive. The search for employment may involve expense in fares, postage, telephones, newspapers, self-presentation etc. At the same time, subsidised facilities of the work place—canteens, clubs, sport and leisure facilities—frequently become unavailable, credit is hard to come by, and less benign in case of non-repayment than conventional sources.

Thirdly, the literature consistently finds a relationship between indicators of financial distress and measures of psychological distress (e.g. Schlozman and Verba, 1979). Warr and Payne (1983) found that reported financial problems correlated around 0.40 with GHQ scores. Little (1976) found professional workers in worse financial circumstances reported job loss as more negative. Estes and Wilensky (1978) reported psychological morale to be related negatively to both objective and subjective indices of economic deprivation, but interestingly found no significant differences in psychological morale between employed and unemployed respondents not suffering financial problems. Klandermans (1979) found the extent to which an unemployed sample had had to economize was correlated with boredom. Many studies have reported a sharp decline, with unemployment, of activities, particularly those involving expense (Dewbury, 1985; Miles, 1983; Morley-Bunker, 1982; Warr and Payne, 1983).

Apart from difficulties encountered due to the low level of income, the source of it and combinations of these factors with social norms, expectations and representations seems to produce a psychologically still more noxious result. The actual process of claiming benefit is widely viewed by unemployed people as an uncomfortable situation because of poor conditions, intrusion of privacy, experienced dismissive passive processing, and sense of humiliation (Kay, 1984). Moreover, the very process of being 'maintained' may contain its own stressors. As early as 1938, the Pilgrim Trust had noted that 'real distress' is caused by 'the maintenance of the same dead level . . . with no hope of an extra at any time'. Thoits and Hannan (1979) review the income maintenance literature, noting small but significant negative effects of income maintenance per se on psychological distress, divorce and geographical mobility.

The fulfilment of one's own and others' role expectations can be restricted not only by reduction in disposable income, but by widely held beliefs about the appropriateness of certain forms of expenditure for differing role incumbents. Conspicuous spending, particularly on social drinking, is an important part of working class male culture in the UK, for example. This may be restricted, with resulting social isolation, for reasons of perceived entitlement—what a claimant is 'entitled' to spend benefit on—as well as by penury (Bostyn and Wight, 1987). Poverty and social expectation also restrict the unemployed person in the roles of consumer as well as of breadwinner/provider (Campbell, 1984; Seabrook, 1982).

More generally still, in contemporary society being a wage earner, as opposed to benefit recipient, is a legitimate social role, with wages being a symbol of the value and status of the individual's contribution to society (Marsden, 1982). On the other hand, society is riddled with norms and expectations regarding the appropriate way to fulfill the role of unemployed person. People in receipt of unemployment benefit are expected to live frugally, look diligently for employment, and exhibit gratitude and humility (Furnham, 1983). Indeed, to receive unemployment benefit at all is in some eyes a sign of inadequacy (Kelvin, 1984); 40% of Bakke's (1940) New Haven unemployed men waited 2 years or even longer before applying for relief, allegedly to avoid stigma (see also Ginsburg, 1942). More recently, Liem (1983) claims that unemployed people fail to seek help from formal agencies in order to maintain a sense of dignity, commenting 'when help receiving is actually stigmatised, resistance to seeking this help is a positive assertion of one's humanity'.

SUMMARY AND CONCLUSIONS

There is good evidence that unemployment causes a wide range of largely negative psychological repercussions. This is demonstrated by means of many different methodologies, across half a century of research, in differing countries and cultures. Explanation of these repercussions has been dominated by a powerful model: Jahoda's latent functions approach. The role of material poverty, whilst widely acknowledged as an economic effect of unemployment concurrent with its psychological consequences, has received little emphasis as a psychological factor explaining the personal and social effects. Poverty restricts personal agency, both economically via its direct effects on the pocket, but also, in combination with social expectations and social representations, social psychologically: this is a central tenet of an agency restriction approach. Interpretations of the agency restriction and latent functions approaches are, perhaps, complementary emphases: recall that Jahoda's full approach is couched in terms of manifest and latent functions. Gradually, historically, the latent functions received the explanatory emphasis, whilst the manifest function, earning a living, fell into its shadow.

Since Jahoda both conducted the seminal 1933 field study at Marienthal, and developed the influential latent functions approach (e.g. Jahoda, 1979), there is a tendency to assume the former provides the empirical grounding for the latter. However, empirically, the 1938 study in Monmouthshire (Jahoda, 1987) seems here more influential in her thought. Certainly, the Marienthal study itself scarcely supports the latent functions account, but rather very heavily endorses the view that the majority of distress of unemployed people stemmed ultimately from poverty.

The study is, rightly, remembered for the general decline in activity: 'the unemployed decreased their attendance of clubs and voluntary organizations' (Jahoda, 1982). But close reading of the text reveals three organizations which went against this trend: the Workers' Cycling Club membership remained unchanged; 'Happy Childhood' 'grew considerably' (Jahoda et al., 1972); and a third club, 'The Flames', actually grew in membership by 11%. The clue to popularity lay in finance. The cycling club facilitated legally required cycle insurance, 'Happy Childhood' ran a nursery school, and 'The Flames' was a cremation society which helped out with funeral expenses. The researchers concluded: 'as privation increases organization membership becomes less a matter of conviction and more a matter of financial interest' (Jahoda et al., 1972).

The Marienthal study is also rightly remembered for its categorization of unemployed families by degrees of demoralization of 'attitude'. However, it is seldom appreciated that the researchers found a direct 'connection between a family's attitude and its economic situation' (Jahoda et al., 1972). The investigators concluded that 'a process of psychological deterioration . . . runs parallel to the narrowing of economic resources and the wear and tear on personal belongings. At the end of this process lies ruin and despair' (Jahoda *et al.*, 1972). This, regrettably, is still as true today.

REFERENCES

Adams, J. (1986). *Psychic tomorrows: explorations in the psychology of planning with special reference to unemployment and education*. London: Tangent Charitable Trust.

Allatt, P., & Yeandle, S. (1986). It's not fair is it?: youth unemployment, family relations and the social contract. In S. Allen, A. Waton, K. Purcell & S. Wood (eds), *The experience of unemployment* (pp. 98–115). Basingstoke: Macmillan.

Bakke, E.W. (1933). *The unemployed man*. London: Nisbet.

Bakke, E.W. (1940). *Citizens without work*. Newhaven: Yale University Press.

Bakke, E.W. (1961). The cycle of adjustment to unemployment. In W. Bell & E.F. Vogel (eds), *A modern introduction to the family* (pp. 145–197). London: Routledge & Kegan Paul.

Banks, M.H. (1983). Validation of the General Health Questionnaire in a young community sample. *Psychological Medicine, 3*, 349–353.

Banks, M.H., & Jackson, P.R. (1982). Unemployment and risk of minor psychiatric disorder in young people: cross-sectional and longitudinal evidence. *Psychological Medicine, 12*, 789–798.

Banks, M.H., & Ullah, P. (1987). Political attitudes and voting among unemployed and employed youth. *Journal of Adolescence, 10*, 201–216.

Beale, N., & Nethercott, S. (1986). Job-loss and health—the influence of age and previous morbidity. *Journal of the Royal College of General Practitioners, 36*, 261–264.

Beales, H.L., & Lambert, R.S. (1934). *Memoirs of the unemployed*. Wakefield: E.P. Publishing.

Bebbington, P., Hurry, J., Tennant, C., Sturt, E., & Wing. J.K. (1981). Epidemiology of mental disorders in Camberwell. *Psychological Medicine, 11*, 561–579.

Beck, A.T., Weissman, A., Lester, D., & Trexler, L. (1974). The measurement of pessimism: the hopelessness scale. *Journal of Consulting and Clinical Psychology, 42*, 6, 861–865.

Binns, D., & Mars, G. (1984). Family, community and unemployment: a study in change. *The Sociological Review, 32*(4), 662–695.

Bolton, W., & Oatley, K. (1985). Plans, depression and the experience of time. *Teorie & Modelli, II*, suppl. 1, 183–197.

Bostyn, A.M., & Wight, D. (1987). Inside a community: values associated with money and time. In S. Fineman (ed.), *Unemployment: personal and social consequences* (pp. 138–154). London: Tavistock.

Bradburn, N.M. (1969). *The structure of psychological well-being*. Chicago: Aldine.

Bradburn, N.M., & Caplovitz, D. (1965). *Reports on happiness*. Chicago: Aldine.

Branthwaite, A., & Garcia, S. (1985). Depression in the young unemployed and those on Youth Opportunities Schemes. *British Journal of Medical Psychology, 58*, 67–74.

Brenner, M.H. (1987). Economic change, alcohol consumption and heart disease mortality in nine industrialized countries. *Social Science and Medicine, 25*, 2, 119–132.

Buss, T.F., Stevens Redburn, F., & Waldron, J. (1983). *Mass unemployment*. Beverly Hills: Sage.

Callender, C. (1985). Unemployment: the case for women. In C. Jones & M. Brenton (eds), *The yearbook of social policy in Britain 1984–5*. London: Routledge & Kegan Paul.

Callender, C. (1987). Women seeking work. In S. Fineman (ed.), *Unemployment: Personal and social consequences* (pp. 22–46). London: Tavistock.

Campbell, A., Converse, P.E., & Rodgers, W.L. (1976). *The quality of American life*. New York: Russell Sage Foundation.

Campbell, B. (1984). *Wigan Pier revisited*, London: Virago Press.

Carnegie UK Trust (1943). *Disinherited youth: a survey 1936–39*. London: Constable.

Cassell, C., Fitter, M. Fryer, D.M., & Smith, L. (in press). The development of computer applications by unemployed people in community settings. *Journal of Occupational Psychology*.

Cater, J., & Easton, P. (1980). Separation and other stress in child abuse. *Lancet, 1*, 972–973.

Cavan, R.S., & Ranke, K.H. (1938). *The family and the Depression*. Chicago: University of Chicago Press.

Clark, A.W. (1985). The effects of unemployment on political attitude. *Australian and New Zealand Journal of Sociology, 21*(1), 100–108.

Clark, D.Y. (1987). Families facing redundancy. In S. Fineman (ed.), *Unemployment: Personal and social consequences* (pp. 97–117). London: Tavistock.

Cobb, S., & Kasl, S.V. (1977). *Termination: The consequences of job loss*. Cincinatti: US Department of Health, Education and Welfare.

Cochrane, R., & Stopes-Roe, M. (1980). Factors affecting the distribution of psychological symptoms in urban areas of England. *Acta Psychiatrica Scandinavica, 61*, 445–460.

Cohn, R.M. (1978). The effect of employment status change on self-attitudes. *Social Psychology, 41*, 81–93.

Cooke, K. (1987). The living standards of unemployed people. In D.M. Fryer & P. Ullah (eds), *Unemployed people: Social and psychological perspectives* (pp. 148–173). Milton Keynes: Open University Press.

Cragg, A., & Dawson, T. (1984). *Unemployed women: A study of attitudes and experiences*, Research Paper No. 47. London: Department of Employment.

Daniel, W.W. (1974). *A national survey of the unemployed*. London: Political and Economic Planning Institute.

Davies, R., Hamill, L., Moylan, S., & Smee, C.H. (1982). Incomes in and out of work. *Employment Gazette, 90*, 237–243.

Dewbury, C. (1985). Unemployment and use of time. Paper presented to the Annual Conference of the British Psychological Society, Swansea.

Dhooge, Y., & Popay, J. (1987). Social services and unemployment: impact and responses. In S. Fineman (ed.), *Unemployment: Personal and social consequences* (pp. 157–177). London: Tavistock.

Donovan, A., & Oddy, M. (1982). Psychological aspects of unemployment: an investigation into the emotional and social adjustment of school leavers. *Journal of Adolescence, 5*, 15–30.

Dooley, D., & Catalano, R. (1980). Economic change as a cause of behavioural disorder. *Psychological Bulletin, 87*, 450–468.

Eisenberg, P., & Lazarsfeld, P.F. (1938). The psychological effects of unemployment. *Psychological Bulletin, 35*, 258–390.

Elderton, M. (1931). *Case studies of unemployment*. Philadelphia: University of Philadelphia Press.

Estes, R.J., & Wilensky, H.L. (1978). Life cycle squeeze and the morale curve. *Social Problems, 25*, 277–292.

Evans, S. (1986). *Variations in activity and psychological well-being in unemployed young adults*. Unpublished PhD thesis, University of Manchester.

Fagin, L., & Little, M. (1984). *The forsaken families*. Harmondsworth: Penguin.

Feather, N.T. (1982). Unemployment and its psychological correlates: A study of depressive symptoms, self-esteem, protestant ethic values, attributional style, and apathy. *Australian Journal of Psychology, 34*, 309–323.

Feather, N.T., & Bond, M.J. (1983). Time structure and purposeful activity among employed and unemployed university graduates. *Journal of Occupational Psychology, 56*, 241–254.

Feather, N.T., & Davenport, P.R. (1981). Unemployment and depressive affect: a motivational analysis. *Journal of Personality and Social Psychology, 41*, 422–436.

Feather, N.T., & O'Brien, G.E. (1986). A longitudinal study of the effects of employment and unemployment on school leavers. *Journal of Occupational Psychology, 59,* 121–144.

Figuerra-McDonough, J. (1978). Mental health among unemployed Detroiters. *Social Service Review, 52,* 383–399.

Fineman, S. (1979). A psychosocial model of stress and its application to managerial unemployment. *Human Relations, 32,* 323–345.

Fineman, S. (1983). *White collar unemployment.* Chichester: John Wiley & Sons.

Fineman, S. (1987). Back to employment: wounds and wisdoms. In D.M. Fryer & P. Ullah (eds), *Unemployed people: Social and psychological perspectives.* Milton Keynes: Open University Press.

Finlay-Jones, R.A., & Burvill, P.W. (1979). Women, work and minor psychiatric morbidity. *Social Psychiatry, 14,* 53–57.

Finlay-Jones, R.A., & Eckhardt, B. (1981). Psychiatric disorder among the young unemployed. *Australian and New Zealand Journal of Psychiatry, 15,* 265–270.

Fraser, C. (1981). The social psychology of unemployment. In M. Jeeves (ed.), *Psychology Survey No. 3,* (pp. 172–186). London: Allen & Unwin.

Fryer, D.M. (1985). Stages in the psychological response to unemployment; a (dis)integrative review article. *Current Psychological Research and Reviews, 4*(3), 257–273.

Fryer, D.M. (1986). Employment deprivation and personal agency during unemployment. *Social Behaviour, 1,* 1, 3–23.

Fryer, D.M. (1987). Unemployment and the Scottish child. *The Scottish Child, 1,* 2, 6–7.

Fryer, D.M. (in press). The Marienthal study of unemployment. In S. Greif, H. Holling & N. Nicholson (eds), *European Handbook of Work and Organizational Psychology.* Munich: Urban and Schwarzenburg.

Fryer, D.M., & McKenna, S. (1987). The laying off of hands—unemployment and the experience of time. In S. Fineman (ed.), *Unemployment: Personal and social consequences* (pp. 47–73). London: Tavistock.

Fryer, D.M., & Payne, R.L. (1984). Proactivity in unemployment: findings and implications. *Leisure Studies, 3,* 273–295.

Fryer, D.M., & Payne, R.L. (1986). Being unemployed: a review of the literature on the psychological experience of unemployment: In C.L. Cooper & I. Robertson (eds), *International review of industrial and organizational psychology 1986,* (pp. 235–278). Chichester: John Wiley & Sons.

Fryer, D.M., & Warr, P.B.W. (1984). Unemployment and cognitive difficulties. *British Journal of Clinical Psychology, 23,* 67–68.

Furnham, A. (1983). Attitudes towards the unemployed receiving social security benefits. *Human Relations, 36,* 2, 135–150.

Garraty, J.A. (1978). *Unemployment in history, economic thought and public policy.* New York: Harper & Row.

Gaskell, G., & Smith, P. (1981). 'Alienated' black youth: an investigation of 'conventional wisdom' explanations. *New Community, 9,* 182–193.

Gaskell, G., & Smith, P. (1985). An investigation of youth's attributions for unemployment and their political attitudes. *Journal of Economic Psychology, 6,* 65–80.

Ginsburg, S.W. (1942). What unemployment does to people. *American Journal of Psychiatry, 99,* 439–446.

Goldberg, D.P. (1972). *The detection of psychiatric illness by questionnaire,* Oxford: Oxford University Press.

Goldberg, D. (1978). *Manual for the General Health Questionnaire.* Windsor: National Foundation for Educational Research.

Griffin, C. (1986). It's different for girls: the use of qualitative methods in a study of young women's lives. In H. Beloff (ed.), *Getting into life,* (pp. 95–117). London: Methuen.

Gurney, R.M. (1980). Does unemployment affect the self-esteem of school-leavers? *Australian Journal of Psychology, 32,* 175–182.

Gurney, R.M., & Taylor, K. (1981). Research on unemployment: defects, neglect and prospects. *Bulletin of the British Psychological Society, 34,* 349–352.

Harrison, R. (1976). The demoralising experience of prolonged unemployment. *Department of Employment Gazette*, *84*, 339–348, London.

Hartley, J.F. (1978). *An investigation of psychological aspects of managerial unemployment*. Unpublished PhD thesis, University of Manchester.

Hartley, J.F. (1980). The impact of unemployment upon self-esteem of managers. *Journal of Occupational Psychology*, *53*, 147–155.

Haworth, J.T., & Evans, S.T. (1987). Meaningful activity and unemployment. In D.M. Fryer & P. Ullah (eds), *Unemployed people: Social and psychological perspectives* (pp. 241–267). Milton Keynes: Open University Press.

Hayes, J., & Nutman, P. (1981). *Understanding the unemployed: The psychological effects of unemployment*. London: Tavistock.

Henderson, S., Duncan-Jones, P., Byrne, D.G., Scott, R., & Adcock, S. (1979). Psychiatric disorder in Canberra: A standardised study of prevalence. *Acta Psychiatrica Scandinavica*, *60*, 335–374.

Henwood, F., & Miles, I. (1987). The experience of unemployment and the sexual division of labour. In D.M. Fryer & P. Ullah (eds), *Unemployed people: Social and psychological perspectives* (pp. 94–110). Milton Keynes: Open University Press.

Hepworth, S.J. (1980). Moderating factors of the psychological impact of unemployment. *Journal of Occupational Psychology*, *53*, 139–145.

Huczynski, A. (1978). Unemployed managers—a homogeneous group? *Management Education and Development*, *9*, 21–25.

Hurstfield, J. (1986). Women's unemployment in the 1930s: some comparison with the 1980s. In S. Allen, A. Waton, K. Purcell & S. Wood (eds), *The experience of unemployment* (pp. 29–44). Basingstoke: Macmillan.

Israeli, N. (1935). Distress in the outlook of Lancashire and Scottish unemployed. *Journal of Applied Psychology*, *19*, 67–69.

Jackson, P.R., & Walsh, S. (1987). Unemployment and the family. In D.M. Fryer & P. Ullah (eds), *Unemployed people: Social and psychological perspectives* (pp. 194–216). Milton Keynes: Open University Press.

Jackson, P.R., & Warr, P.B. (1984). Unemployment and psychological ill-health: The moderating role of duration of age. *Psychological Medicine*, *14*, 605–614.

Jackson, P.R., & Warr, P.B. (1987). Mental health of unemployed men in different parts of England and Wales. *British Medical Journal*, 29 August, *295*, 525.

Jackson, P.R., Stafford, E.M., Banks, M.H., & Warr, P.B. (1983). Unemployment and psychological distress in young people; the moderating role of employment commitment. *Journal of Applied Psychology*, *68*, 525–535.

Jahoda, M. (1942). Incentives to work—a study of unemployed adults in a special situation. *Occupational Psychology*, *16*, 1, 20–30.

Jahoda, M. (1979). The impact of unemployment in the 1930s and the 1970s. *Bulletin of the British Psychological Society*, *32*, 309–314.

Jahoda, M. (1981). Work, employment and unemployment: values, theories, and approaches in social research. *American Psychologist*, *36*, 2, 184–191.

Jahoda, M. (1982). *Employment and unemployment*. Cambridge: Cambridge University Press.

Jahoda, M. (1986a). The social psychology of the invisible: an interview with Marie Jahoda by David Fryer. *New Ideas in Psychology*, *4*, 1, 107–118.

Jahoda, M. (1986b). In defence of a non-reductionist social psychology. *Social Behaviour: International Journal of Applied Social Psychology*, *1*, 25–29.

Jahoda, M. (1987). Unemployed men at work. In D.M. Fryer & P. Ullah (eds), *Unemployed people: Social and psychological perspectives*, (pp. 1–73). Milton Keynes: Open University Press.

Jahoda, M., Lazarsfeld, P.F., & Zeisel, H. (1972). *Marienthal: The sociography of an unemployed community*. New York: Aldine-Atherton.

Jahoda, M., & Rush, J. (1980). *Work, employment and unemployment*. Occasional paper Series, No. 12, Science Policy Research Unit, Sussex University.

Kasl, S.V. (1979). Changes in mental health status associated with job loss and retirement. In J.E. Barrett, R.M. Rose & G.L. Klerman (eds), *Stress and mental disorder*. New York: Raven Press.

Kaufman, H.G. (1982). *Professionals in search of work: Coping with the stress of job loss and underemployment*. New York: John Wiley & Sons.

Kay, D. (1984). *Counter benefits: Making contact with the DHSS*. Scottish Consumer Council Working Paper 7, Glasgow. ISBN 0 905653 90 4.

Kelvin, P. (1981). Work as a source of identity: The implications of unemployment. *British Journal of Guidance and Counselling*, 9, 1, 2–11.

Kelvin, P. (1984). The historical dimensions of social psychology: The case of unemployment. In H. Tajfel (ed.), *The social dimension* (pp. 405–424). Cambridge: Cambridge University Press.

Kelvin, P., & Jarrett, J.E. (1985). *Unemployment: Its socal psychological effects*. Cambridge: Cambridge University Press.

Kelvin, P., Dewberry, C., & Bunker, N. (1985). Unemployment and the use of time. Paper presented at the BPS Annual Conference, Swansea.

Kilpatrick, R., & Trew, K. (1985). Life-styles and psychological well-being among unemployed men in Northern Ireland. *Journal of Occupational Psychology*, 58, 207–216.

Klandermans, P.G. (1979). Werklozen en de Werklozenbeweging. *Mens en Maatschappij*, 54, 5–53 (cited in Warr, 1984).

Kobasa, S.C., Maddi, S.R., & Kahn, S. (1982). Hardiness and health: a prospective study. *Journal of Personality and Social Psychology*, 42, 168–177.

Komarovsky, M. (1940). *The unemployed man and his family*. New York: Dryden.

Laite, J., & Halfpenny, P. (1987). Employment, unemployment and the domestic division of labour. In D.M. Fryer & P. Ullah (eds), *Unemployed people: Social and psychological perspectives* (pp. 217–240). Milton Keynes: Open University Press.

Levi, L., Brenner, S., Hall, E.M., Hjelm, R., Salovaara, H., Arnetz, B., & Pettersson, I. (1984). The psychological social and biochemical impacts of unemployment in Sweden. *International Journal of Mental Health*, 13, 1, 18–34.

Liem, R. (1983). Reconsidering the concept of social victim: the case of the unemployed. Paper presented at the Annual Meeting of the American Psychological Association, Anaheim, California.

Liem, R., & Liem, J. (1979). Social support and stress: some general issues and their application to the problem of unemployment. In L. Ferman & K. Gordus (eds), *Mental Health and the Economy* (pp. 347–379). Kalamazoo: Upjohn Institute.

Little, C.B. (1976). Technical– professional unemployment: Middle-class adaptability to personal crisis. *The Sociological Quarterly*, 17, 262–274.

Madge, N. (1983). Unemployment and its effects on children. *Journal of Child Psychology and Psychiatry*, 24, 311–319.

Marsden, D. (1982). *Workless*. London: Croom Helm.

Martin, R., & Wallace, J. (1984). *Working women in recession: Employment, redundancy and unemployment*. Oxford: Oxford University Press.

McKee, L., & Bell, C. (1986). His unemployment, her problem: the domestic and marital consequences of male unemployment. In S. Allen, A. Waton, K. Purcell & S. Wood (eds), *The experience of unemployment* (pp. 134–149), Basingstoke: Macmillan.

McKenna, S.P., & Fryer, D.M. (1984). Perceived health during lay-off and early unemployment. *Occupational Health*, 36, 201–206.

McKenna, S.P., & Payne, R.L. (1985). A comparison of The General Health Questionnaire and The Nottingham Health Profile in a study of unemployed and reemployed men. *MRC/ESRC Social and Applied Psychology Unit Memo No. 696*, University of Sheffield.

Miles, I. (1983). *Adaptation to unemployment*. Science Policy Research Unit Technical Report, University of Sussex.

Morley-Bunker, N. (1982). Perceptions of unemployment. Paper to the British Psychological Society Annual Occupational Psychology Conference, Brighton.

Murray-Parkes, C. (1972). *Bereavement*. London: Tavistock.

Newman, G. (1932). *On the state of public health*. Annual Report of the Chief Medical Officer of the Ministry of Health, London.

O'Brien, G.E. (1986). *Psychology of work and unemployment*. Chichester: John Wiley & Sons.

O'Brien, G.E., & Kabanoff, B. (1979). Comparison of unemployed and employed workers on work values, locus of control and health variables. *Australian Psychologist, 14*, 143–154.

Payne, R.L. (1985). Predictors of affective reactions to long-term unemployment: a longitudinal study. MRC/ESRC Social and Applied Psychology Unit Memo No. 727, University of Sheffield.

Payne, R.L. (in press). A longitudinal study of the psychological well-being of unemployed men and the mediating effect of neuroticism. *Human Relations*.

Payne, R.L., & Hartley, J. (1984). Financial situation, health, personal attributes as predictors of psychological experience amongst unemployed men. *Journal of Occupational Psychology, 60*, 31–47.

Payne, R.L., Warr, P.B., & Hartley, J. (1984). Social class and the experience of unemployment. *Sociology of Health and Illness, 6*, 152–174.

Pearlin, L.i., & Liebermann, M.A. (1979). Social sources of emotional distress. *Research in Community and Mental Health, 1*, 217–248.

Piachaud, (1986). *Poor children: A tale of two decades*. London: Child Poverty Action Group.

Pilgrim Trust, (1938). *Men without work*. Cambridge: Cambridge University Press.

Platt, S. (1984). Unemployment and suicidal behaviour: a review of the literature. *Social Science and Medicine, 19*, 93–115.

Poulot, D. (1872). *Le sublime: ou le travaileur comme il est au 1870 et ce qu'il peut être*. Translated and cited in J.A. Garraty (1978), p. 115.

Radloff, L. (1975). Sex differences in depression: The effects of occupation and marital status. *Sex Roles, 1*, 249–265.

Raffe, D. (1986). Change and continuity in the youth labour market: a critical review of structural explanations of youth unemployment. In S. Allen, A. Waton, K. Purcell & S. Wood (eds), *The experience of unemployment* (pp. 45–60). Basingstoke: Macmillan.

Roy, A. (1981). Vulnerability factors and depression in men. *British Journal of Psychiatry, 138*, 75–77.

Save the Children International Union (1933). *Children, young people and unemployment: A series of enquiries into the effects of unemployment on children and young people*. Geneva: SCIU.

Schlozman, K.L., & Verba, S. (1979). *Injury to insult: Class and political response*. Cambridge, Mass.: Harvard University Press.

Seabrook, J. (1982). *Unemployment*. London: Quartet Books.

Smith, D.J. (1980). How unemployment makes the poor poorer. *Policy Studies, 1*, 20–26.

Stafford, E.M. (1982). The impact of the Youth Opportunities Programme on young people's employment prospects and psychological well-being. *British Journal of Guidance and Counselling, 10*, 1, 12–21.

Stafford, E.M., Jackson, P.R., & Banks, M.H. (1980). Employment, work involvement and mental health in less qualified young people. *Journal of Occupational Psychology, 53*, 291–301.

Stokes, G. (1983). Work, unemployment and leisure. *Leisure Studies, 2*, 269–286.

Swinburne, P. (1981). The psychological impact of unemployment on managers and professional staff. *Journal of Occupational Psychology, 54*, 47–64.

Tausky, C., & Piedmont, E.B. (1967). The meaning of work and unemployment. *International Journal of Social Psychiatry, 14*, 44–49.

Taylor, F.I. (1909). *A bibliography of unemployment and the unemployed*. London: P.S. King and Son.

Thoits, P., & Hannan, M. (1979). Income and psychological distress: the impact of an income-maintenance experiment. *Journal of Health and Social Behavior, 20,* 120–138.

Thomas, L.E., McCabe, E., & Berry, J.E. (1980). Unemployment and family stress: a re-assessment. *Family Relations, 29,* 517–524.

Tiffany, D.W., Cowan, J.R., & Tiffany, P.M. (1970). *The unemployed: A social psychological portrait.* Englewood Cliffs, N.J.: Prentice-Hall.

Tiggemann, M., & Winefield, A.H. (1980). Some psychological effects of unemployment in school leavers. *Australian Journal of Social Issues, 15,* 269–276.

Trew, K., & Kilpatrick, R. (1984). *Daily life of the unemployed: Social and psychological dimensions.* Belfast: Queen's University Psychology Department.

Ullah, P. (1987). Unemployed black youths in a northern city. In D.M. Fryer and P. Ullah (eds), *Unemployed people: Social and psychological perspectives* (pp. 111–147). Milton Keynes: Open University Press.

Verbrugge, L.M. (1983). Multiple roles and physical health of women and men. *Journal of Health and Social Behavior, 24,* 16–30.

Wallace, C., & Pahl, R. (1986). Polarisation, unemployment and all forms of work. In S. Allen, A. Waton, K. Purcell & S. Wood (eds), *The experience of unemployment* (pp. 116–133). Basingstoke: Macmillan.

Walter, T. (1985). *Hope on the dole.* London: SPCK.

Warr, P.B. (1978). A study of psychological well-being. *British Journal of Psychology, 69,* 111–121.

Warr, P.B. (1984a). Economic recession and mental health: a review of research. *Tijdschrift voor Sociale Gezondheidzorg, 62,* 298–308.

Warr, P.B. (1984b). Job loss, unemployment and psychological well-being. In V. Allen & E. van de Vliert (eds), *Role transitions* (pp. 263–285) New York: Plenum Press.

Warr, P.B. (1987a). Workers without a job. In P.B. Warr (ed.), *Psychology at work,* (pp. 335–356). Harmondsworth: Penguin.

Warr, P.B. (1987b). *Work, unemployment and mental health.* Oxford: Oxford University Press.

Warr, P.B., Banks, M.H., & Ullah, P. (1985). The experience of unemployment among black and white urban teenagers. *British Journal of Psychology, 76,* 75–87.

Warr, P.B., & Jackson, P.R. (1983). Self-esteem and unemployment among young workers. *Le Travail Humain, 46,* 335–366.

Warr, P.B., & Jackson, P.R. (1984). Men without jobs: some correlates of age and length of unemployment. *Journal of Occupational Psychology, 57,* 77–85.

Warr, P.B., & Jackson, P.R. (1985). Factors influencing the psychological impact of prolonged unemployment and re-employment. *Psychological Medicine, 15,* 795–807.

Warr, P.B., & Lovatt, J. (1977). Retraining and other factors associated with job finding after redundancy. *Journal of Occupational Psychology, 50,* 67–84.

Warr, P.B., & Parry, G. (1982). Paid employment and women's psychological well-being. *Psychological Bulletin, 9,* 498–516.

Warr, P.B., & Payne, R.L. (1982). Experience of strain and pleasure among British adults. *Social Science and Medicine, 16,* 1691–1697.

Warr, P.B., & Payne, R.L. (1983). Social class and reported changes after job loss. *Journal of Applied Social Psychology, 13,* 206–222.

Williams, J.M. (1933). *Human aspects of unemployment and relief.* Chapel Hill, Carolina: University of North Carolina Press.

Winfield, I. (1981). Psychology and centres for the unemployed: challenge or chimera? *Bulletin of the British Psychological Society, 34,* 353–355.

Wing, J.K. (1980). The use of the present state examination in general population surveys. *Acta Psychiatrica Scandinavia, 62,* 231–240.

Zung, W.W.K. (1974). The measurement of affects: depression and anxiety. In P. Pichot & R. Oliver-Martin (eds), *Psychological measurement in psychopharmacology.* Basel: Karger.

Acknowledgement

I would like to thank Roy Payne and Marie Jahoda for substantial contributions to this chapter.

KEY WORDS

Unemployment, health, psychological well-being, deprivation, poverty, agency, depression, social psychology, occupational psychology.

Section II
Life Events and Disorder

Handbook of Life Stress, Cognition and Health
Edited by S. Fisher and J. Reason
© 1988 John Wiley & Sons Ltd.

13

Life Events and Mental Disorder

E.S. PAYKEL
University of Cambridge, England
and
D. DOWLATSHAHI
St George's Hospital Medical School, London

METHODOLOGICAL ASPECTS

The belief that recent life events cause mental disorder is of long standing. Empirical research involving an acceptable methodology into the issue is more recent. The first step was the development of schedules of life events. The earliest studies employed self-report questionnaires (Holmes and Rahe, 1967), but later studies have moved towards semistructured interview schedules (e.g. Brown and Birley, 1968; Paykel *et al.*, 1969) because of recognition of the problems inherent in the retrospective reporting of events. There may be bias in recall, particularly compounded in the psychiatric patient by likely attempts to explain illness in terms of preceding stress. This 'effort after meaning' may lead to events being over-reported or exaggerated both by patients and their relatives.

Self-report questionnaires are vulnerable to these effects since most do not provide space to describe each item fully, and unless some key words are defined there may be ambiguity. Thus, without specific definitions of, for example, what constitutes a 'major personal injury or illness', the category can include anything from influenza to cancer. However, if full definitions are provided, the speed and convenience of questionnaires are lost.

An additional problem concerns accurate recall of the time of occurrence of an event. In our own experience, using semistructured interviews, it has been necessary to give frequent reminders and indications of the relevant time periods otherwise subjects report events outside the relevant period. Such a procedure is not possible wih a self-report checklist.

Several semistructured interview schedules are available. Among these, Brown's is the most detailed, involving a lengthy and comprehensive interview, with tape recording and later full rating of events and their qualities (Brown *et al.*, 1973a; Brown and Harris, 1978). Paykel (1983) provided a shorter and less detailed questionnaire which is easier to use if time is limited; it covers 64 events and makes judgements of two central aspects—the degree of independence of the event, and its objective negative impact.

Whilst some events may be independent of the individual's behaviour, in some cases the individual creates them, for example illness might cause loss of a job. Therefore it is important to separate out dependent and independent events. Brown et al. (1973a) pointed out that with detailed scrutiny of circumstances it is possible to identify events which are unlikely to have been self-produced or influenced by illness, and which are therefore of causal significance. Determining the timing of symptom onset in order to confine attention to time periods preceding it may be an additional technique.

Even for independent events, a way of assessing the level of associated stress is necessary. Life events are not equal in effect and it is not enough to say that a patient has experienced a life event; it is necessary to distinguish level of stressful effect. Holmes and Rahe (1967) used an additive scale derived from consensus rating to produce weighted scores and total stress scores. Brown and Harris (1978) have argued that events cannot be assumed to be additive unless they are severe and clearly unrelated to each other. However, different methods of estimating stress tend to produce similar findings. Brown et al. (1973a) used a judgements context based on rater judgements of the stressfulness of an event to the average person. Paykel et al. made use of a similar rating, but in addition categorized events into different types, such as 'exits' and 'entrances', 'undesirable' and 'desirable' (Paykel et al., 1969; 1975; 1976). An undesirable method involves the subjective judgement of stress, because experience of psychiatric disorder may contaminate the judgements of the stressful qualities of preceding events. The contextual method of rating events avoids this problem.

The ultimate aims are reliability and validity. A review of reliability studies (Paykel, 1983) has shown that self-report schedules produce low test–retest reliability, whilst those employing interview methods lead to moderately high reliabilities. Inter-rater reliability has also been found to be high with use of a semistructured interview—95% for specific event and 85% for month of occurrence (Paykel, 1983).

Another method of testing reliability is to examine fall-off in the mean number of events per month reported in the general population as time periods extend back into the past. Ill subjects may be expected to show a peak of events in recent months as compared with a random distribution of events in the general population. Self-report studies have shown substantial fall-off of as much as 4%–5% per month (Paykel, 1983), but studies using interview techniques have found considerably lower fall-off, of between 1% and 3% per month (Brown and Harris 1978; Paykel, 1980; Brown and Harris, 1982).

Validity in life event research can be tested by comparing the information gained from the patient with that gained from another informant, usually a close relative. Generally, much higher agreement has been found when interview methods have been employed. Brown et al. (1973a) and Brown and Harris (1982 reported about 80% agreement for individual events.

When studying the role of life events in psychiatric disorder the control group must be chosen with care. In early studies, psychiatric patients were compared with medical or surgical patients. There is some risk that event rates may be raised in such controls, either because of the consequences of illness (early studies did not eliminate these) or because events may be associated with, for example, deterioration or hospitalization. It is preferable to compare psychiatric patients with normal control groups, taken from the same population and matched on factors such as age, sex, marital status and social class, because of the established relationship of these variables with the frequency of events.

Brown et al. (1973b) have pointed out that large differences in the rate of life events in patient and control groups, occurring over short time periods before the onset of disorder, can be completely masked if long time periods are used. The most marked effects will be found by employing the appropriate time period. There are advantages in analysing multiple time periods to examine the pattern of effects.

LIFE EVENTS AND ONSET OF DEPRESSION

Life events have been studied extensively with respect to onset of psychiatric disorder. This review will focus on subjects receiving psychiatric treatment, since studies of milder disorders in the community raise additional issues as to whether qualitatively different disturbance is being studied. Studies have been concerned with anxiety disorders, obsessive–compulsive neurosis, mania, schizophrenia, attempted and completed suicide, but the disorder most studied has been depression.

Table 13.1 summarizes the findings of 25 published retrospective comparisons of psychiatrically treated depressed patients with control groups. Twelve studies (from the USA, England, Italy, Poland, Kenya and India) employed general population controls, including one study of elderly patients (Murphy, 1982). All found more events reported prior to depressive onset, although in one study, with small numbers, the difference did not reach significance. Two studies compared depressives with medical patient controls: both found more events reported by depressives but the differences were not very striking or clearly attributable to causes rather than effects of depression.

Comparisons of depressives and other psychiatric patients are also summarized in the table. Depressives have been found to report more events than schizophrenics. In one study, however (Leff and Vaughn, 1980), differences for independent events were suggestive but not significant, and there was no difference in terms of undesirable events. Two additional studies not shown in the table failed to find differences between depressives and schizophrenics, but life event methodologies were limited (Eisler and Polak, 1971; Lahniers and White, 1976).

Some comparisons with mixed psychiatric patients have also suggested greater effects in depressives, but not consistently. On the other hand, three comparisons of suicide attempters with depressives found more events in the former group.

Some other studies using different designs or samples are not shown in the table. In a small study (Paykel, 1974) using patients as their own controls, we found that event rates in depressives dropped on follow-up but not fully to the

Table 13.1 Controlled comparisons of life events at onset of clinical depression

Nature of controls	Author	Excess any events	Excess separations	Excess other types of events
General population	Paykel et al. (1969)	Yes	Yes	Various, especially undesirable events
	Thomson & Hendrie (1972)	Yes	Not reported	More stress overall
	Cadoret et al. (1972)	Suggestive	Suggestive	Not reported
	Brown et al. (1973b)	Yes	Not reported	Markedly and moderately threatening events
	Fava et al. (1981)	Yes	Yes	Undesirable, negative impact
	Vadher & Ndetei (1981)	Yes	Yes	Suggestive only
	Chatterjee et al. (1981)	Yes	Yes	Health, interpersonal
	Bebbington et al. (1981)	Yes, males only	Not reported	Events of severe and moderate threat
	Murphy (1982)	Yes	Suggestive	Health
	Billings et al. (1983)	Yes	Yes	Various negative events
	Bidzinska (1984)	Yes	No	Marital and family conflicts, work overload, failures
Medical patients	Roy et al. (1985)	Yes	No	Undesirable events
	Forrest et al. (1965)	Yes, weak	No	Social factors
	Hudgens et al. (1967)	Yes, weak	No	Moves, interpersonal discord
Other psychiatric patients	**Schizophrenics**			
	Beck & Worthen (1972)	Yes	Suggestive	Events of higher rated hazard
	Brown et al. (1983b)	Yes	Not reported	Events/moderate and marked threat over longer time
	Jacobs et al. (1974)	Yes	Yes	Undesirable, health, financial, interpersonal discord
	Suicide attempters			
	Paykel et al. (1975)	Fewer events in depressives	No	Fewer events in depressives, especially undesirable, upsetting
	Slater & Depue (1981)	Fewer events in depressives	No, fewer exits	Fewer independent events
	Cohen-Sandler et al. (1982)	Fewer events in depressives	Fewer deaths, separations	Case note study in children
	Mixed psychiatric patients			
	Sethi (1964)	Yes	Yes	Not reported
	Levi et al. (1966)	Yes	Yes	Not reported
	Malmquist (1970)	No	No	No
	Uhlenhuth & Paykel (1973)	No	No	No

244

general population level. One study has shown heroin addicts with secondary depression to have more stressful events than those without depression (Prusoff *et al.*, 1977), while another obtained similar findings for depressed compared with non-depressed schizophrenics (Roy *et al*, 1983), as did a questionnaire study of secondarily depressed and non-depressed alcoholics (Fowler *et al.*, 1980). A follow-up study of drug addicts found events to be associated with continuing depression and failure of recovery (Beck Depression Inventory), but the direction of causation was not clear (Kosten *et al.*, 1983).

A specific causal hypothesis would suggest that depression and only depression is induced by certain types of events. The research literature indicates the prominent role of loss. The concept of loss is somewhat diffuse, including, amongst other types, interpersonal separations and deaths, and loss of self-esteem.

Interpersonal losses of various kinds have received the most attention. As shown in Table 13.1, in eleven out of nineteen studies concerned with recent separations, depressives reported more than the control groups (which included both general population and other psychiatric patients), suggesting some specificity. There was, however, no excess over medical patients. Two studies not only found that exit events were related to depression, but also that their converse, entrance events, were not (Paykel *et al.*, 1969; Fava *et al.*, 1981). However, one study (Slater and Depue, 1981) found that primary depressives making a suicide attempt had experienced more exits than those who did not attempt suicide, indicating a greater relationship between the two. Some additional studies (not shown in the table) have found a relationship between depression and recent bereavements (Paykel, 1982).

Also common in the studies are arguments and discord with various key interpersonal figures; they may involve the threat of separation. Blows to the self-esteem and failures have not usually been explicitly correlated. As can be seen from the table, a wide variety of events is involved. In general, the studies suggest only weak specificity. There is some relationship between depression and interpersonal losses, but these also precede other disorders, and many depressions are not preceded by them. The strongest relationship appears when events are categorized in rather broad terms such as 'threatening' or 'undesirable'. This extends well beyond interpersonal loss.

All the studies in Table 13.1 were of clinical levels disorder and thus provide evidence against the view that life events are only important for milder disorders identified in community surveys.

ENDOGENOUS DEPRESSION

A further issue involves the distinction between endogenous and neurotic depression. About 20% of depressive episodes are not preceded by life events. As the term is usually employed, endogenous depressions are also regarded as showing a specific symptom pattern, including greater severity, psychomotor retardation or agitation, occasional depressive delusions, early morning wakening, and diurnal variation with morning worsening (Rosenthal and Klerman, 1966).

Several recent studies using careful life event methods have shown that life events and symptom pattern are only weakly related. In our first New Haven study, symptoms were rated by one rater and life event information collected blind by another. *Absence of life stress showed only a low correlation*, although in the predicted direction, with an endogenous symptom factor (Paykel *et al.*, 1969). In a subsequent study in London (Paykel, 1979), using a more crude clinical judgement as to whether the depression was precipitated, there was no relationship with symptom pattern. Finally, Paykel *et al.* (1984) reported a non-significant weak relationship between life events and symptoms in 146 out-patients.

Other studies have produced similar findings. Brown *et al.* (1979) found that depressives characterized as psychotic or neurotic on the basis of their symptoms showed only a very small difference in the proportions of illnesses attributed to a severe event or major difficulty. When the depressions were divided into those with and those without such an event or difficulty, relatively few individual symptoms distinguished the groups. Benjaminsen (1981) compared neurotic and non-neurotic depressives and found that almost equal proportions had experienced a stressful event. Katschnig and Berner (1984) obtained similar findings. Matussek and Neuner (1981) found differences between neurotic and endogenous depression only for separations from an important partner. Bebbington *et al.* (1981), in a small study, did find fewer life events in patients with endogenous symptom patterns, but found little evidence of this in a larger sample (Bebbington *et al.*, in press). Roy *et al.* (1985) compared the frequency of life events in endogenous and neurotic depressives, and a third group of normal controls who were matched on age and sex. When the depressives were taken together and compared with the control group, they showed more life events than controls. A further analysis looked at the subdivided depressives and found that the neurotic depressives had significantly more life events than endogenous depressives.

Overall, however, it would appear that life events bear only a weak relationship to symptom pattern, and that the latter is predominantly determined by some other mechanism.

BIPOLAR MANIC DEPRESSIVE DISORDER

One aspect not yet adequately studied is that of elated affective disorder. Bipolar manic depressives in many respects appear to be a separate group, distinguished by family history, personality, course, and some biological aspects (Perris, 1982).

Mania is a disorder producing increased activity and disinhibition, and readily leading to new dependent events such as job changes, financial problems, arguments and disruptions of old relationships and initiation of new ones. Particular care therefore needs to be taken to define independent events in such studies.

Three studies have examined mania. Ambelas (1979) studied a time period of 4 weeks preceding admission and found that manic patients had four times as many stressful life events as a surgical control group. Information on manic subjects was mainly based on case notes, but most of the events listed did appear to be independent. Ambelas found that the events experienced were mostly unpleasant ones. Whenever a pleasant event was found, an element of threat or loss was also strongly suspected. Stresses were categorized into two types, losses and threats; losses were present twice as often as threats, and bereavement was found in five out of fourteen cases. In the second study, Kennedy *et al.* (1983) looked at the 4 months before onset in manic patients, using both a matched control group and patients as their own controls. They found a twofold increase in life events during the 4-month period. The within-patient control comparison was used to test whether or not these patients might have more life events in any 4-month period, for reasons such as personality traits, but this was not found to be the case. A third recent case note study (Ambelas, 1987) gave similar findings, with a much more marked effect for first attacks. This is consistent with the finding of another study in a lithium clinic that fluctuations in treated manic depressives were not stress related (Hall *et al.*, 1977). A major life crisis may contribute to the onset of a disorder for which subsequent attacks are much more biologically determined. One study (Glassner and Halidpur, 1983) found more evidence of stressful life events in bipolars with onset over the age of 20 than under, suggesting that constitutional factors might be more important in the latter.

LIFE EVENTS AND OUTCOME OF DEPRESSION

The relationship between life events and outcome of depression has also been investigated. Lloyd *et al.* (1981) carried out a drug trial of two tricyclic anti-depressants and found that presence or absence of life events at onset did not influence outcome. In another drug trial (Rowan *et al.*, 1982) comparing phenelzine, amitryptyline and placebo, there was found to be a weak trend for outcome to be worse where a major life event had occurred (unpublished analyses). In a somewhat different third study, Billings and Moos (1984) compared depression with either a recurrent or a non-recurrent illness. The authors proposed that as chronic patients in general seem to be more alienated from their surroundings, stressors should have less influence on them. However, a comparable proportion of each of the depressed groups were found not to have experienced any life event at onset.

Events concurrent with treatment might be expected to have greater effects. In the study cited earlier, Lloyd *et al.* (1981) found that patients who had a poor outcome after 4 weeks were more likely to have experienced undesirable events, physical illnesses, illnesses in family members, and events outside the patient's control. Rowan *et al.* (1982) found that events occurring during a 6-week treatment period had no significant effect on outcome, but few major independent events occurred. Tennant *et al.* (1981), in a study of community cases, found that remission was more likely over a 1-month period if a 'neutralizing' event had taken place. They defined a neutralizing event as one which caused minimal threat but which counteracted the effect of an earlier threatening event or chronic difficulty.

Two studies have examined concurrent events over follow-up periods of between 6 and 8 months. The first (Surtees, 1980) used a mixed sample of depressives and found that greater event stress was associated with worse outcome. The second (Paykel and Tanner, 1976) examined relapse. The patients were women who had responded to amitriptyline and were then either continued on or withdrawn from medication. Life events were assessed concurrently, and relapse was found to be associated with undesirable life events in the 3 months prior to relapse. These relapses appeared to be separate from those related to drug withdrawal.

Two longer term follow-up studies (Murphy, 1983; Giel et al., 1978) both provided evidence supporting the hypothesis that outcome is worse if a threatening event has occurred.

The picture emerging from these studies is that life events at onset do not greatly effect outcome. However, where events recur concurrently with treatment, negative events lead to worse outcome, and neutralizing events to better outcome.

NEUROTIC DISORDERS

There have been relatively few retrospective controlled studies of the relationship between life events and neurotic disorders. Life events do appear to be implicated in anxiety disorders. Faravelli (1985) studied 23 patients with panic disorder and compared them with 23 normal matched controls. Significantly more life events occurred in the patient group, due almost entirely to the excess of events in the month prior to onset. Both loss events and threatening events played a part. Whether different kinds of events are involved in anxiety and depression is not clear. Uhlenhuth and Paykel (1973) found no difference in amount or type of life event stress between predominantly depressed and anxious patients in a mixed neurotic sample. Barrett (1979), in a similar study with symptomatic volunteers, found more exit events and undesirable events in depressives but it was not clear whether this simply reflected a general excess of stressful types of events in this group. Finlay-Jones and Brown (1981), in a study involving general practice patients, found more 'loss' events preceding depression, and 'danger' events preceding anxiety.

Although a number of descriptive studies have reported precipitating life events in obsessive–compulsive neurosis, adequate controlled studies have been limited by the relative paucity of cases with a recent onset, and only one such study has been reported. McKeon et al. (1984) interviewed patients who had developed the illness within the last 10 years and who consented to having a close relative interviewed for the study. The comparison group was drawn from the general population. Onset was defined by the researchers as a change from normality or non-obsessive–compulsive symptoms. Events were examined in the year preceding onset. For the 6 months prior to onset the patient group had a significantly higher rate, peaking in the last month. This study also looked at personality traits and found that those with premorbid abnormal personalities had experienced significantly fewer life events.

SCHIZOPHRENIA

In the aetiology of schizophrenia, twin and adoption studies provide evidence of a

Table 13.2   Controlled studies of life events at schizophrenia

Controls	Author	Findings in schizophrenics Excess events
General population	Brown & Birley (1968) Jacobs & Myers (1976) Schwartz & Myers (1977a,b) Al Khani *et al.* (1986)	Three weeks before onset Yes, relatively weak Yes, minor symptoms in community Yes (Saudi Arabia). Only significant for married women
Non-relapsing schizophrenics	Leff *et al.* (1973)	Yes: relapses on placebo
Neurotics	Hendrie *et al.* (1975)	No: more male schizophrenics in low stress category
Depressives	See Table 13.1	See Table 13.1

moderately strong genetic element. Nevertheless, concordance rates in mono-zygotic twins leave considerable room for environmental influences, and there is strong evidence that social factors have important effects on the course.

Several studies have examined recent life events. Findings are shown in Tables 13.1 and 13.2. Brown and Birley (1968) found more independent events than in general population controls but only in the 3 weeks before onset or relapse. The differences were considerably less than in Brown's later studies of depression. Jacobs and Myers (1976), using our methods, found more life events in the year before first onset than in the general population, but here too differences were relatively weak, and for a small group of events categorized as likely to be independent of the subject's control, they did not reach significance. The studies by Schwartz and Myers (1977a, 1977b) involved schizophrenics in the community not undergoing major relapse. Life events were more common in those showing minor symptoms, particularly of depression and anxiety, than in the general population. Al Khani *et al.* (1986) compared Saudi Arabian schizophrenics and controls for the 6 months before onset. Differences were only significant for married women but were suggestive for other groups.

Among studies using other kinds of control groups, Leff *et al.* (1973) found life events to be more common in schizophrenics who relapsed than in those who did not, but only in placebo rather than active drug groups from two maintenance drug trials. In extension of these findings, Leff and Vaughn (1980) later found that life events tended to occur in relapsing schizophrenics whose families did not show high expressed emotion. Hendrie *et al.* (1975) compared schizophrenics with neurotics and personality disorder patients using the Holmes–Rahe question-naire. Among males but not females, schizophrenics were predominantly char-acterized by low stress, neurotics by high stress. Comparisons with depressives have already been shown in Table 13.1. They tend to show fewer events, or fewer subjects having a major event, in the schizophrenics.

One other study used different methods. Steinberg and Dureli (1968), in an epidemiological study, found the inception rate for schizophrenia to be signifi-cantly raised in the early months of military service.

Overall, life events do appear to contribute to schizophrenic onset and relapse, but to a much lesser extent than to depression.

ATTEMPTED SUICIDE

Suicide attempters comprise a special group of patients who need to be distinguished from depressives. Although some show the clinical picture of a persistent depressive syndrome, many do not, and they are predominantly younger in age. A number of studies have examined the role of recent life events in the genesis of the attempt. These are summarized in Table 13.3. Paykel *et al.* (1975) interviewed suicide attempters with respect to life events in the 6 months before the attempt. Comparisons were made with matched general population controls and with matched depressives who were interviewed concerning the 6 months prior to onset. Suicide attempters reported four times as many events as did the general population, and one and a half times as many events as did depressives in the period prior to onset. There was a marked peak of events in the month before the attempt, and often in the week before. The excess over general population controls involved most types of life events.

Table 13.3 Controlled comparison of life events and suicide attempts

Controls	Author	Findings in suicide attempts
General population	Paykel *et al.* (1975)	Excess events, 6 months, especially last month. Most types of event
	Cochrane & Robertson (1975)	Higher stress scores and number of life events over 1 year. Especially unpleasant events, disrupted interpersonal relationships
	Isherwood *et al.* (1982)	Higher stress
	Jacobs (1971)	Adolescents. Excess of events in weeks/months before attempt, particularly break of relationship, physical illness, injury, pregnancy
Medical patients, other psychiatric patients	O'Brien & Farmer (1980)	Higher rates in previous 6 weeks for most events. Fall off on 1-year follow-up
	Levi *et al.* (1966)	More separations in last year
	Stein *et al.* (1974)	More separations in last year. Significant except for black women, where suggestive
	Greer *et al.* (1966) (controls also included medical patients)	Controls also included medical patients. More disruptive relationships in last 6 months than either group. Psychiatric controls intermediate
Depressives	See Table 13.1	See Table 13.1

Cochrane and Robertson (1975) used a less satisfactory method, a self-report checklist, and studied only male subjects. In the year before the attempt, total stress scores and the number of life events were much higher in depressives than in matched general population controls. The excess particularly involved unpleasant events and disrupted interpersonal relationships. Isherwood *et al.* (1982) also used a modified Holmes–Rahe methodology. Suicide attempters showed much higher stress scores than did general population controls or a second control group of drivers involved in automobile crashes.

One study was limited to adolescents aged 14–18 years. Jacobs (1971) compared suicide attempters and normal controls for events throughout their lifetimes. The time periods nearer the attempt showed an excess of events, particularly the few months preceding it, when there were more break-ups of relationships, illnesses, injuries and pregnancies.

O'Brien and Farmer (1980) compared life events in the 6 weeks before the interview of suicide attempters who had taken overdoses of medication, compared with young people visiting general practitioners for various complaints, a type of medical patient control. Most life events were much more frequent for the suicide attempters. Patients were followed up at 3 months and a year. At 3 months there was no decrease in life event rates, but at 12 months there was a decrease. This was in the only study in which subjects served as their own controls, confirming that not all the life event elevation prior to the attempt was due to persistent lifestyles rather than recent increase in life events.

Studies making comparisons with depressives have been summarized in the section on depressive onset and in Table 13.1. Among studies making use of other psychiatric control groups, Luscomb *et al.* (1980) used a self-report inventory to study male suicide attempters admitted to Veterans Administration hospitals and patients with no history of suicide attempts. Using number of events, scores for perceived stress, frequency of events rated high in stress, exit events, desirable events, and undesirable events, the researchers found some differences, with a particularly high rate of exit events.

Three studies have been limited to separations, both recent and early. Levi *et al.* (1966) examined actual or threatened disruptions of interpersonal relationships in the preceding year among suicide attempters, patients with suicidal thoughts, and non-suicidal patients. Suicide attempters experienced more separations than the non-suicidal group, while those with suicidal thoughts were intermediate. In a replication study, Stein *et al.* (1974) found more recent separations among suicide attempters than among psychiatric controls. Greer *et al.* (1966) found that disrupted interpersonal relationships were more common in the last 6 months in suicide attempters than in psychiatric or medical controls.

In some other relevant, uncontrolled studies, Power *et al.* (1985) found that severe events, ascertained over a 6-month period, peaked in the month before a suicidal attempt, but non-severe events did not. Suicidal intent, assessed subjectively and objectively, correlated with total life event stress, but lethality of attempt did not. Katschnig (1980) found a peak of threatening events in the 3 weeks before the attempt.

In a controlled study, but of a less recent event, Birtchnell (1970) found that more psychiatric patients with a recent suicide attempt had experienced death of a parent in the preceding 1–5 years than had non-suicidal psychiatric controls. In another controlled comparison, Paykel *et al.* (1974) studied suicidal feelings in the general population. Subjects reporting suicidal feelings in the last year experienced more life events, particularly undesirable events.

COMPLETED SUICIDE

Completed suicides need to be studied by methods other than direct subject interview, such as case records or interview with relatives. A small number of studies have looked at recent events and these are summarized in Table 13.4.

Bunch (1972) interviewed informants concerning bereavement in the previous 5 years for suicides and general population controls. There was a significant excess among suicides in their last 2 years, particularly involving the deaths of mothers and spouses. Men, especially if unmarried, appeared more vulnerable to the loss of a mother. MacMahon and Pugh (1965) used death certificates to compare the timing of deaths from suicides and other causes in widows and widowers. Suicides showed a clustering in the few years following death of a spouse, and particularly in the first year.

Hagnell and Rorsman (1980) compared recent events among suicides from the prospective Lundby cohort study, matched non-violent deaths, and general

Table 13.4   Studies of recent life events and completed suicide

Controls	Author	Findings in suicide Excess events
General population	Bunch (1972)	Bereavement only. More in previous 2 years
	MacMahon & Pugh (1965)	Bereavement only; comparison group natural death. Clustering of subject death by suicide in 4 years following spouse death, especially previous year
	Hagnell & Rosman (1980)	Comparison also with natural death. More changes of living conditions, work problems and object loss than general population in last year; more object loss than natural death
Psychiatric patients	Humphrey (1977)	More losses, not all recent, than in neurotics; homicides intermediate
	Pokorny & Kaplan (1976)	More adverse events after discharge, particularly where higher defenseless during hospitalization
	Borg & Stahl (1982)	No significant difference although tendency to more deaths
	Fernando & Storm (1984)	More losses

population controls. Seven of twenty suicides experienced stressful life events in the 2 weeks before death, compared with none of the people who had natural deaths. Viewed over the year before death, the suicides showed more changes of living conditions, work problems, and object losses than the normal controls, and more object losses than the people with natural deaths, for whom work was not relevant because of the nature of their terminal illness. Some of the events in the suicides appear to have been consequences of psychiatric illness, rather than being independent.

Other studies have used psychiatric patient controls. Humphrey (1977) studied male suicides, homicidal offenders, and patients hospitalized with neurotic disorders. The study examined losses over a lifetime rather than purely recent ones. Excluding early losses, the suicides had significantly more evidence of occupational, marital and parental loss than did the neurotic patients; homicides tended to be intermediate. Information on neurotic patients was obtained from hospital charts, which might not be comparable with the psychological autopsies on the suicides.

Pokorny and Kaplan (1976) interviewed relatives of psychiatric in-patients at a Veterans' Administration hospital who subsequently committed suicide. Suicides were more likely to have had adverse life events between discharge and suicide than patients who, over a comparable time period, did not commit suicide, particularly when scores during hospitalization had been high on a measure of defenselessness, mainly reflecting depressive content. However, Borg and Stahl (1982) also compared psychiatric patients who committed suicide in varying time periods up to 2 years following presentation, with matched psychiatric controls. There were no significant differences for the individual life events analysed from case notes, and, overall, the controls had experienced more events, although the suicide victims had reported more deaths. Fernando and Storm (1984) undertook a similar comparison. They found a significantly greater frequency of losses in the last year; these included divorce, separation, illness or death of a first degree relative or friend and loss of job.

New Haven and St George's Hospital Studies

The general trend of findings in studies of life events in psychiatric patients is illustrated by the findings of our own studies. Starting in New Haven, Connecticut, three patient samples were studied: depressed patients attending psychiatric facilities (Paykel et al., 1969); first admission schizophrenics (Jacobs et al., 1974; Jacobs and Myers, 1976); suicide attempters (Paykel et al., 1975). Comparisons were made with matched controls from a large general population survey. All subjects were interviewed with a systematic life event interview, for events over a 6-month period preceding onset of disorder, or, in the general population, the interview. Interview with patients was postponed until acute psychiatric disturbance had subsided, to improve the accuracy of information.

Overall, a ranking of mean event frequencies was found, reflecting, in the retrospective frame, the magnitude of causative effects. Schizophrenics reported twice as many events as did general population controls, depressives three times

Table 13.5   Percentage of subjects in New Haven studies reporting events in each category at least once in 6 months (modified from Paykel, 1979)

	Suicide attempters	Depressives	Schizo-phrenics	General population control
Number of events[a]	3.3	2.1	1.5	0.8
Exits	21[a]	25	14	9
Entrances	34[a]	13	16	11
Undesirable	60[b]	40[b]	42[b]	21
Desirable	13[b]	4	8	11
Interpersonal arguments (full event list)	75[b]	62[a]	18	3
Major (scaling study)	68[b]	45[b]	—	23
Intermediate	53[b]	26[b]	—	4
Minor	49[b]	45[b]	—	25
Uncontrolled	66[b]	40[a]	—	21
Controlled	34[b]	32[a]	—	17

[a] Mean number of events in 6 months.
[b] Significantly more common in patient group than general population.

as many, suicide attempters four times as many (see Table 13.5). Depressives tended to have a peak of events in the month before onset, but the rate was still elevated 6 months before; suicide attempters showed a very pronounced peak in the month before the attempt (Paykel *et al.*, 1975).

Table 13.5 summarizes findings for event types in these studies. Events were divided where possible into contrasting dichotomies. Depressives showed a particular excess of exit events but not entrances, undesirable events but not desirable events (Paykel *et al.*, 1969), indicating some selectivity in the effects of different events. There was limited selectivity by disorder. All disorders were preceded by exit events, but for schizophrenics the effect was borderline; suicide attempts were also preceded by an excess of entrance events. However, all disorders were preceded by undesirable events and none by desirable events. When compared with depressives, suicide attempters had experienced more events rated as major in a scaling study, and more events outside the subject's control (Paykel *et al.*, 1975); this may have simply reflected a greater occurrence of all the more threatening types of events. Another group of events reported in all disorders, but particularly before suicide attempts and depression, were interpersonal arguments and difficulties with other people. They were omitted from most analyses because it is harder to define them, ensure their reporting reliably and to the same extent in patients and controls, and be confident that they are independent of illness and personality. Clinically they do appear very important.

These findings illustrate general trends in the literature regarding event specificities. To some extent the empirical evidence supports the implication of loss events in depression, but the specificity is weak. Detailed scrutiny of the events preceding depression reveals a wide variety of threatening, unpleasant and challenging occurrences. Moreover, the same events may precede other disorders. What does emerge is that different disorders relate to events to differing extents; the effects are highest for suicide attempters; depression is intermediate; the excess of events is least for schizophrenia, and it extends back only short time periods before onset or relapse.

What also emerges is that the events relating to psychiatric disorder show a general tendency to be regarded as stressful in everyday experience. In scaling studies of perception of life events carried out both in New Haven (Paykel *et al.*, 1971) and London (Paykel *et al.*, 1976), the disorder-related event categories of exits, undesirable events, and uncontrolled events, were scaled as more stressful than their opposites—entrances, desirable events, and events under the subjects' control (Paykel *et al.*, 1976). There is a general quality of stressfulness in some events, paralleled in psychiatric disorder and everyday life. Depending on other factors, the same event can precede depression, another psychiatric disorder, a medical psychosomatic disorder, or no disorder at all.

In other studies the role of events in depression was confirmed by comparison of subjects relapsing or not relapsing on follow-up (Paykel and Tanner, 1976) and by a fall in events from onset to follow-up in recovering subjects, using patients as their own controls (Paykel, 1974). In a series of studies into endogenous depression in New Haven (Paykel, 1974) and London (Paykel, 1979; Paykel *et al.*, 1984), the weakness of the relationship between symptom pattern and life stress was consistently confirmed.

In a study of suicidal feelings in the general population (Paykel *et al.*, 1974), stressful life events were found to be strongly associated. In a London study of puerperal depression (Paykel *et al.*, 1980) the importance of life events was shown once again. The strongest predictor of puerperal depression was the occurrence of a recent stressful life event, unrelated to the pregnancy. Other associated factors were absence of marital support, presence of previous history of psychiatric disorder, and early postpartum blues. In a recent study (Sireling, unpublished), undesirable and threatening life events were also found to precede appendicectomy, both for histologically confirmed acute appendicitis and for abdominal pain found histologically not to be due to an inflamed appendix, compared with general population controls. Discussion of the occurrence of life events before physical disorder is outside the immediate ambit of this review; there is a considerable literature, but many studies do not use adequately rigorous methods.

EFFECT SIZE AND MODIFYING FACTORS

The life events implicated in psychiatric disorder, although stressful and unpleasant, are not usually of catastrophic magnitude. They are often experienced by the general population without disorder following. Brown *et al.* (1973b) attempted to quantify the causative effect by using the concept of 'brought forward time': an estimate of the average time from an onset brought about by an event to the time a spontaneous onset would have occurred if no event were present. They concluded that the effect was large in magnitude and formative for depression, but smaller and only triggering for schizophrenia.

An epidemiological measure which can be used in this context is the relative risk (Paykel, 1978). This is the ratio of the rate of disease among those exposed to a causative factor to the rate among those not exposed. When this was applied to some of our own studies, it was found that the risk of developing depression in the 6 months after the most stressful classes of events was approximately 6 : 1, falling off rapidly with time after the event. Other studies have produced similar findings. The relative risks for schizophrenia were much lower, at only 2–3 : 1 over 6 months, but for suicide attempts they were higher.

Relative risks of this magnitude indicate an effect which is important, but not overwhelming (Paykel, 1979). They are consistent with follow-up findings of subjects in the community undergoing single major events, such as bereavement. In these circumstances, although distress is usual and help from family doctors and community agencies may be common, overt presentation of major disorder to the psychiatrist is relatively rare.

These findings suggest disorders with multifactorial causation, in which any single factor may account for only a relatively small proportion of the variance. Although events are important, a large part in determining whether an event is followed by disorder must be attributed to other modifying factors. There may be a whole host of these, both genetic and environmental, ranging from biochemical, through personality and coping mechanisms, to social.

Brown and Harris (1978) studied the moderating effects of other social vulnerability factors in determining whether or not depression developed after a life event in women in a working class area of London. Vulnerability factors associated with depression were presence of several young children at home, absence of a confidant, lack of employment, and early loss of mother. In a subsequent study in the contrasting rural social environment of the Outer Hebrides, only the first two of these replicated, but there was one additional vulnerability factor indicative of non-integration: absence of churchgoing (Brown and Prudo, 1981). In a further London study in Islington (Brown et al., 1986), low self-esteem and poor social support acted as vulnerability factors. Brown's seminal studies have mainly concerned disorder in the community rather than treated disorder, and therefore lie largely outside the focus of this review, but are described elsewhere in this volume (see chapter 24).

There is an extensive published literature on social support and psychiatric disorder, which also lies outside the immediate scope of this review. Most studies suggest that absence of support predisposes to disorder, either by modifying event stress, or as an independent factor. The effect in severe psychiatric disorder is less well studied, and the independence of social network and support from one's own personality resources is also less clear-cut (Paykel, 1984).

THE FUTURE OF LIFE EVENT RESEARCH IN PSYCHIATRY

After 20 years the general outlines of the relationship between life events and mental disorder are now well established. Life events precede and contribute to a variety of psychiatric disorders. Type of life event is only weakly related to type of disorder: those events which are more generally stressful are also more likely to produce disorder. Some disorders are certainly much more likely to be produced by life events and other psychosocial stresses than are others, which presumably are more genetically, biochemically and physically determined. However, in most psychiatric disorders, life events make only a partial contribution and aetiology is multifactorial, even in the individual case. Stress interacts with personality, cognitive style, genes, social support, and neurochemical mechanisms.

There are some lacunae in this picture. Some psychiatric disorders have not yet been adequately studied in relation to life events; the spotlight has only moved slowly from depression. The field of psychosomatic disorders is outside this review, but, even from the limited standpoint of psychiatric disorders, it would be valuable to have better comparative data from somatic disorders, studied by means of the same methodology of life event interview and elimination of illness-caused events. It is at present unclear whether the cluster of somatic disorders traditionally regarded as psychosomatic show effect magnitudes for life events at onset at all comparable to those of the psychiatric disorders.

Beyond this, the basic life event descriptive work is done, and the field needs to move more towards exploration of the underlying mechanisms and interactions with other factors. In the area of interactions, relationships with social support are reasonably well studied: whether the effect is independent and additive, or interactive, social support clearly does buffer stress. The 'independence' of social support is unclear: there is a complex interrelationship between personality, capacity to forge social ties, and the amount of social support available. Interactions of stress with personality and cognitive factors need further exploration, particularly outside the experimental laboratory. Are obsessional personalities particularly vulnerable to events involving major changes of life patterns? Are work failures Achilles' heels for Type As? These and other similar linkages appear possible, but there is virtually no overt evidence in relation to psychiatric disorder.

Perhaps the most important area for future research, and the greatest present gap, lies in relationships between psychological and biological factors, including underlying neurobiological mechanisms. Life events do not produce effects in the absence of a brain. Social events make their impacts through psychological perceptions and these have their substrates and concomitants in brain function: neurophysiological functional state and psychological state are simply different aspects of the same phenomenon. In these terms it is easy to see how life events, via psychological effects, may be translated into reduced or increased firing in systems mediating depression, anxiety, or the disturbances associated with schizophrenia, and may interact with genetic variants of neurotransmitter synthesizing or metabolizing enzymes, structural changes, and incipient disease processes.

Easy, that is, in theory. In practice there have been few such studies and the approach has many difficulties. Among the more clinically ascertainable factors, previous history of psychiatric disorder tends to predict future disorder, perhaps reflecting some form of predisposition. In one study it was associated with puerperal depression irrespective of the occurrence of stressful life events (Paykel *et al.*, 1980). Patrick *et al.* (1978) hypothesized an inverse relationship between presence of life events and degree of family history loading at onset of the first episode of bipolar disorder, assessed retrospectively, but failed to find it. McGuffin *et al.* (in press), in a recent careful study of unipolar cases, obtained similar findings.

Calloway *et al.* (1984a, 1984b), in the neuroendocrine field, found no relationship between the presence of life events and dexamethasone non-suppression, but the presence of difficulties on Brown's interview was associated with blunted TSH response to TRH. Few other studies have employed life event measures with biological markers, either state or trait related. It is clear that biological factors are important in most psychiatric disorders, and that future studies will have increasingly to look simultaneously at psychosocial and biological elements. Such studies may in the long run illuminate both causes and mechanisms.

SUMMARY AND CONCLUSIONS

Studies using careful interview methodology have shown elevated rates of recent life events prior to a range of psychiatric disorders, particularly depressive disorders, suicidal behaviours, neurotic disorders and schizophrenia. Type of life event is only weakly related to type of disorder. In depression, the most extensively studied disorder, recent studies indicate that events also precede illnesses with endogenous symptom patterns, and that events occurring during follow-up influence outcome. Causative effects are moderate in magnitude, being greatest for parasuicidal acts, and least for schizophrenia. However, in most functional psychiatric disorders, aetiology appears multifactorial. Further studies are needed of the interactions between recent life events and other factors, including social support, personality, cognitive style, genes, neurochemical mechanisms and other biological factors.

REFERENCES

Al Khani, M.A.F., Bebbington, P.E., Watson, J.P., & House, F. (1986). Life events and schizophrenia: a Saudi Arabian study. *British Journal of Psychiatry, 148*, 12–22.

Ambelas, A. (1979). Psychologically stressful events in the precipitation of manic episodes. *British Journal of Psychiatry, 135*, 15–21.

Ambelas, A. (1987). Life events and mania. A special relationship? *British Journal of Psychiatry, 150*, 235–240.

Barrett, J.E. (1979). The relationship of life events to onset of neurotic disorders. In J.E. Barrett (ed.), *Stress and mental disorder* (pp. 87–109). New York: Raven Press.

Bebbington, P.E., Tennant, C., & Hurry, J. (1981). Adversity and the nature of psychiatric disorder in the community. *Journal of Affective Disorders, 3*, 345–366.

Bebbington, P.E., MacCarthy, B., Brugha, T., Potter, J., Sturt, E., Wykes, T., Katz, R., & McGuffin, P. (1981). The Camberwell collaborative Depression Study. I. Adversity and the form of depression (in press).

Beck, J.C., & Worthen, K. (1972). Precipitating stress, crisis theory and hospitalization in schizophrenia and depression. *Archives of General Psychiatry, 26*, 123–129.

Benjaminsen, S. (1981). Stressful life events preceding the onset of neurotic depression. *Psychological Medicine, 11*, 369–378.

Bidzinska, E.J. (1984). Stress factors in affective diseases. *British Journal of Psychiatry, 144*, 161–166.

Billings, A.G., Cronkite, R.C., & Moos, R.H. (1983). Social–environment factors in unipolar depression: comparisons of depressed patients and nondepressed controls. *Journal of Abnormal Psychology, 92*(2), 119–133.

Billings, A.G., & Moos, R.H. (1984). Chronic and nonchronic unipolar depression. The differential role of environment stressors and resources. *Journal of Nervous Diseases, 172*, 65–75.

Birtchnell, J. (1970). The relationship between attempted suicide, depression and parent death. *British Journal of Psychiatry, 116*, 307–313.

Borg, S.E., & Stahl, M. (1982). Prediction of suicide. A prospective study of suicides and controls among psychiatric patients. *Acta Psychiatrica Scandinavica, 65*, 221–232.

Brown, G.W., Bhrolchain, N.I.M., & Harris, T.O. (1979). Psychotic and neurotic depression. Part 3. Aetiological and background factors. *Journal of Affective Disorders, 1*, 195–211.

Brown, G.W., & Birley, J.L.T. (1968). Crises and life changes and the onset of schizophrenia. *Journal of Health and Social Behaviour, 9*, 203–214.

Brown, G.W., & Harris, T. (1978). *The social origins of depression: a study of psychiatric disorder in women.* London: Tavistock.

Brown, G.W., & Harris, T. (1982). Fall off in the reporting of life events. *Social Psychiatry, 17*, 23–28.

Brown, G.W., Harris, T.O., & Peto, J. (1973b). Life events and psychiatric disorders. Part 2. Nature of causal link. *Psychological Medicine, 3*, 159–176.

Brown, G.W., & Prudo, R. (1981). Psychiatric disorder in a rural and urban population: I. Aetiology of depression. *Psychological Medicine, 11*, 581–599.

Brown, G.W., Sklair, F., Harris, T.O., & Birley, J.L.T. (1973a). Life-events and psychiatric disorders. Part I. Some methodological issues. *Psychological Medicine, 3*, 74–87.

Brown, G.W., Andrews, B., Harris, T., Adler, Z., & Bridge, L. (1986). Social support, self-esteem and depression. *Psychological Medicine, 16*, 813–831.

Bunch, J. (1972). Recent bereavement in relation to suicide. *Journal of Psychosomatic Research, 16*, 361–366.

Cadoret, R.J., Winokur, G., Dorzab, J., & Baker, M. (1972). Depressive disease: life events and onset of illness. *Archives of General Psychiatry, 26*, 133–136.

Calloway, S.P., Dolan, R.J., Fonagy, P., de Souza, V.F.A., & Wakeling, A. (1984a). Endocrine changes and clinical profiles in depression: I. The dexamethasone suppression test. *Psychological Medicine, 14*, 749–758.

Calloway, S.P., Dolan, R.J., Fonagy, P., de Souza, V.F.A., & Wakeling, A. (1984b). Endocrine changes and clinical profiles in depression: II. The thyrotropin-releasing hormone test. *Psychological Medicine, 14*, 759–765.

Chatterjee, R.N., Mukherjee, S.P., & Nandi, D.N. (1981). Life events and depression. *Indian Journal of Psychiatry, 23*, 333–337.

Cochrane, R., & Robertson, A. (1975). Stress in the lives of parasuicides. *Social Psychiatry, 10*, 161–171.

Cohen-Sandler, R., Berman, A.L., & King, R.A. (1982). Life stress and symptomatology: determinants of suicidal behaviour in children. *Journal of American Academy of Child Psychiatry, 21*, 178–186.

Eisler, R.M., & Polak, P.R. (1971). Social stress and psychiatric disorder. *Journal of Nervous and Mental Disease, 153*, 227–233.

Faravelli, C. (1985). Life events preceding the onset of panic disorder. *Journal of Affective Disorders, 9*, 103–105.

Fava, G.A., Munari, F., Pasvan, L., & Kellner, R. (1981). Life events and depression. A replication. *Journal of Affective Disorders, 3*, 159–165.

Fernando, S., & Storm, V. (1984). Suicide among psychiatric patients of a district general hospital. *Psychological Medicine, 14*, 661–672.

Finlay-Jones, R., & Brown, G.W. (1981). Types of stressful life event and the onset of anxiety and depressive disorders. *Psychological Medicine, 11*, 803–815.

Forrest, A.D., Fraser, R.H., & Priest, R.G. (1965). Environmental factors in depressive illness. *British Journal of Psychiatry, 111*, 243–253.

Fowler, R.C., Liskow, B.I., & Tanna, V.L. (1980). Alcoholism, depression and life events. *Journal of Affective Disorders, 2*, 127–135.

Giel, R. Ten Horn, G.H.M.M., Ormel, J., Schudel, W.J., & Wiersma, O. (1978). Mental illness, neuroticism and life events in a Dutch village sample: a follow-up. *Psychological Medicine, 8*, 235–243.

Glassner, B., & Halidpur, C.V.G. (1983). Life events and early and late onset of bipolar disorder. *American Journal of Psychiatry, 140*, 215–217.

Greer, S., Gunn, J.C., & Koller, K.M. (1966). Aetiological factors in attempted suicide. *British Medical Journal, 2*, 1352–1357.

Hagnell, O., & Rosman, B. (1980). Suicide in the Lundby study: a controlled prospective investigation of stressful life events. *Neuropsychobiology, 6*, 319–332.

Hall, K.S., Dunner, D.L., Zeller, G., & Fieve, R.R. (1977). Bipolar illness: a prospective study of life events. *Comprehensive Psychiatry, 18*, 497–502.

Hendrie, H.C., Lachar, D., & Lennox, K. (1975). Personality trait and symptom correlates of life change in a psychiatric population. *Journal of Psychosomatic Research, 19*, 203–208.

Holmes, T.H., & Rahe, R.H. (1967). The social readjustment rating scale. *Journal of Psychosomatic Research, 11*, 213–218.

Hudgens, R.W., Morrison, J.R., & Barchha, R. (1967). Life events and onset of primary affective disorders. A study of 40 hospitalised patients and 40 controls. *Archives of General Psychiatry, 16*, 134–145.

Humphrey, J.A. (1977). Social loss: a comparison of suicide victims, homicide offenders and non-violent individuals. *Disorders of the Nervous System, 38*, 157–160.

Isherwood, J., Adam, K.S., & Hornblow, A.R. (1982). Life event stress, psychosocial factors, suicide attempt and auto-accident proclivity. *Journal of Psychosomatic Research, 26*, 371–383.

Jacobs, J. (ed.) (1971). *Adolescent suicide*. New York: Wiley-Interscience.

Jacobs, S., & Myers, J. (1976). Recent life events and acute schizophrenic psychosis: a controlled study. *Journal of Nervous and Mental Disease, 162*, 75–87.

Jacobs, S.C., Prusoff, B.A., & Paykel, E.S. (1974). Recent life events in schizophrenia and depression. *Psychological Medicine, 4*, 444–453.

Katschnig, H. (1980). Measuring life stress: a comparison of two methods. In H. Farmer & S. Hirsch (eds), *The suicide syndrome* (pp. 116–123). London: Croom Helm.

Katschnig, H., & Berner, P. (1984). The poly-diagnostic approach in psychiatric research. In *Proceedings of the International Conference on Diagnosis and Classification of Mental Disorder and Alcohol and Drug-Related Problems*. Geneva: World Health Organisation.

Kennedy, S ., Thompson, R., Stancer, H.C., Roy, A., & Persad, E. (1983). Life events precipitating mania. *British Journal of Psychiatry, 142*, 398–403.

Kosten, T.R., Rounsaville, B.J., & Kleber, H.D. (1983). Relationship of depression to psychosocial stressors in heroin addicts. *Journal of Nervous and Mental Disease, 171*, 97–104.

Lahniers, C.E., & White, K. (1976). Changes in environmental life events and their relationship to psychiatric hospital admissions. *Journal of Nervous and Mental Disease, 163*, 154–158.

Leff, J., & Vaughn, C. (1980). The interaction of life events and relatives expressed emotion in schizophrenia and depressive neurosis. *British Journal of Psychiatry, 136*, 146–153.

Leff, J., Hirsch, S.R., Gaind, R., Rohde, P.D., & Stevens, B. (1973). Life events and maintenance therapy in schizophrenic relapse. *British Journal of Psychiatry, 123*, 659–660.

Levi, L.D., Fales, C.H., Stein, M., & Sharp, V.H. (1966). Separation and attempted suicide. *Archives of General Psychiatry, 15*, 158–165.

Lloyd, C., Zisook, S., Click, M., & Jaffe, K.E. (1981). Life events and response to antidepressants. *Journal of Human Stress, 7*, 2–15.

Luscomb, R.L., Clum, G.A., & Patsiokas, A.T. (1980). Mediating factors in the relationship between life stress and suicide attempting. *Journal of Nervous and Mental Disease, 168*, 644–650.

MacMahon, B.R., & Pugh, T.F. (1965). Suicide in the widowed. *American Journal of Epidemiology, 81*, 23–31.

McGuffin, P., Katz, R., & Bebbington, P. (in press). The Camberwell collaborative depression study III—depression and adversity in the relatives of depressed probands.

McKeon, J., Rao, B., & Mann, A. (1984). Life events and personality traits in obsessive–compulsive neurosis. *British Journal of Psychiatry, 144*, 185–189.

Malmquist, C.P. (1970). Depression and object loss in psychiatric admissions. *American Journal of Psychiatry, 126*, 1782–1787.

Matussek, P., & Neuner, R. (1981). Loss events preceding endogenous and neurotic depressions. *Acta Psychiatrica Scandinavica, 64*, 340–350.

Murphy, E. (1982). Social origins of depression in old age. *British Journal of Psychiatry, 141*, 135–142.

Murphy, E. (1983). The prognosis of depression in old age. *British Journal of Psychiatry, 142*, 111–119.

O'Brien, S.E.M. & Farmer, R.D.T. (1980). The role of life events in the aetiology of episodes of self-poisoning. In R. Farmer & S. Hirsch (eds), *The suicide syndrome*. London: Croom Helm.

Patrick, V., Dunner, D.L., & Fieve, R.R. (1978). Life events and primary affective illness. *Acta Psychiatrica Scandinavica, 58*, 48–55.

Paykel, E.S. (1974). Recent life events and clinical depression. In E.K. Gunderson & R.H. Rahe (eds), *Life stress and illness* (pp. 134–163). Springfield, Illinois: Charles C. Thomas.

Paykel, E.S. (1979). Causal relationships between clinical depression and life events. In J.E. Barrett (ed.), *Stress and mental disorder* (pp. 71–86). New York: Raven Press.

Paykel, E.S. (1978). Contribution of life events to causation of psychiatric illness. *Psychological Medicine, 18*, 245–253.

Paykel, E.S. (1980). Recall and reporting of life events. *Archives of General Psychiatry, 37*, 485.

Paykel, E.S. (1982). Life events and early environment. In E.S. Paykel (ed.), *Handbook of affective disorders* (pp. 146–161). Edinburgh: Churchill-Livingstone.

Paykel, E.S. (1983). Methodological aspects of life events research. *Journal of Psychosomatic Research, 27*, 341–352.

Paykel, E.S. (1984). Life events, social support and clinical psychiatric disorder. In I.G. Sarason & B.R. Sarason (eds), *Social support: Theory, research and applications* (pp. 321–347). NATO ASI Series. The Hague: Martinus Nijhoff.

Paykel, E.S., McGuinness, B., & Gomez, J. (1976). An Anglo-American comparison of the scaling of life events. *British Journal of Medical Psychology, 49*, 237–247.

Paykel, E.S., Prusoff, B.A., & Myers, J.K. (1975). Suicide attempts and recent life events: A controlled comparison. *Archives of General Psychiatry, 32*, 327–333.

Paykel, E.S., Prusoff, B.A., & Uhlenhuth, E.H. (1971). Scaling of life events. *Archives of General Psychiatry, 25*, 340–347.

Paykel, E.S., Rao, B.M., & Taylor, C.M. (1984). Life stress and symptom pattern in out-patient depression. *Psychological Medicine, 14*, 559–568.

Paykel, E.S., & Tanner, K. (1976). Life events, depressive relapse and maintenance treatment. *Psychological Medicine, 6*, 481–485.

Paykel, E.S., Myers, J.K., Dienelt, M.N., Klerman, G.L., Lindenthal, J.J., & Pepper, M.P. (1969). Life events and depression: a controlled study. *Archives of General Psychiatry, 21,* 753–760.

Paykel, E.S., Myers, J.K., Lindenthal, J.J., & Tanner, J. (1974). Suicidal feelings in the general population: a prevalence study. *British Journal of Psychiatry, 30,* 771–778.

Paykel, E.S., Emms, E.M., Fletcher, J., & Rassaby, E.S. (1980). Life events and social support in puerperal depression. *British Journal of Psychiatry, 136,* 339–346.

Perris, C. (1982). In E.S. Paykel (ed.), *Handbook of affective disorders* (pp. 45–58). Edinburgh: Churchill Livingstone.

Pokorny, A.D., & Kaplan, H.B. (1976). Suicide following psychiatric hospitalization. *Journal of Nervous and Mental Disease, 162,* 119–125.

Power, K.G., Cooke, D.J., & Brooks, D.N. (1985). Life stress, medical lethality and suicidal intent. *British Journal of Psychiatry, 147,* 655–659.

Prusoff, B., Thompson, W.D., Sholomskas, D., & Riordan, C. (1977). Psychosocial stressors and depression among former heroin-dependent patients maintained on methadone. *Journal of Nervous and Mental Disease, 165,* 57–63.

Rosenthal, S.H., & Klerman, G.L. (1966). Content and consistency in the endogenous depressive pattern. *British Journal of Psychiatry, 112,* 471–484.

Rowan, P.R., Paykel, E.S., & Parker, R.R. (1982). Phenelzine and amitriptyline: effects on symptoms of neurotic depression. *British Journal of Psychiatry, 140,* 475–483.

Roy, A., Thompson, R., & Kennedy, S. (1983). Depression in chronic schizophrenia. *British Journal of Psychiatry, 142,* 465–470.

Roy, A., Breier, A., Doran, A.R., & Pickar, D. (1985). Life events in depression. Relationship to subtypes. *Journal of Affective Disorders, 9,* 143–148.

Schwartz, C.C., & Myers, J.K. (1977a). Life events and schizophrenia. I. Comparison of schizophrenics with a community sample. *Archives of General Psychiatry, 34,* 1238–1241.

Schwartz, C.C., & Myers, J.K. (1977b). Life events and schizophrenia. II. Impact of life events on symptom configuration. *Archives of General Psychiatry, 34,* 1242–1245.

Sethi, B.B. (1964). Relationship of separation to depression. *Archives of General Psychiatry, 10,* 186–195.

Slater, J., & Depue, R.A. (1981). The contribution of environmental events and social support to serious suicide attempts in primary depressive disorder. *Journal of Abnormal Psychology, 90,* 275–285.

Stein, M., Levy, M.T., & Glasberg, M. (1974). Separations in black and white suicide attempters. *Archives of General Psychiatry, 31,* 815–821.

Steinberg, H.R., & Durell, J. (1968). A stressful social situation as a precipient of schizophrenia symptoms: an epidemiological study. *British Journal of Psychiatry, 114,* 1097–1105.

Surtees, P.G. (1980). Social support, residual adversity and depressive outcome. *Social Psychiatry, 15,* 71–80.

Tennant, C., Bebbington, P., & Hurry, J. (1981). The short-term outcome of neurotic disorders in the community: the relation of remission to clinical factors and to 'neutralizing' life events. *British Journal of Psychiatry, 139,* 213–220.

Thomson, K.C., & Hendrie, H.C. (1972). Environmental stress in primary depressive illness. *Archives of General Psychiatry, 26,* 130–132.

Uhlenhuth, E.H., & Paykel, E.S. (1973). Symptom configuration and life events. *Archives of General Psychiatry, 28,* 743–748.

Vadher, A., & Ndetei, D.M. (1981). Life events and depression in a Kenyan setting. *British Journal of Psychiatry, 139,* 134–149.

KEY WORDS

Stress, life events, loss, depression, neurosis, endogenous depression, bipolar manic depressive disorder, schizophrenia, attempted suicide, completed suicide, modifying factors, life event research and psychiatry.

Handbook of Life Stress, Cognition and Health
Edited by S.Fisher and J. Reason
© 1988 John Wiley & Sons Ltd.

14

Lethal Stress: A Social–Behavioral Model of Suicidal Behavior

Marsha M. Linehan and Edward N. Shearin
University of Washington

INTRODUCTION

Suicidal behaviors are remarkably ubiquitous, occurring in almost all known societies. There are numerous theoretical perspectives on suicidal behavior, which Linehan (1981) has classified into five categories: sociological, biological, psychodynamic, cognitive, and learning. Common to all the theories is the notion that suicidal behaviors represent a dysfunctional outcome of some sort of intense internal or environmental distress. Theoretical differences generally revolve around which factors have primary etiological significance in determining suicidal behavior. Importance has been attributed to environmental, biological, and behavioral (affective, cognitive, overt action) events. The factors posited as primary depend more on the theoretical stance of the investigator than on any persuasive data one way or the other.

More sophisticated, recent theories attempt to integrate person variables with social/environmental factors. Braucht (1979) suggested that 'there is something special not only about the people who are cases of suicide or merely about the areas in which there are high rates of suicidal behavior, but about the interactions between individuals and their environments' (p. 658). De Catanzaro (1980, 1981) proposed a diathesis–stress model of suicidal behavior in which it is situated within a context of evolutionary and cultural adaptation and individual predispositions to suicide. Linehan (1981) presented a social–behavioral theory which stressed the interaction of environmental, organismic, and behavioral variables in understanding suicidal behaviors.

The purpose of this chapter is to present an updated version of the social–behavioral theory of suicidal behavior, emphasizing the diathesis–stress interaction. We will then examine the data relevant to the theory (space limitations preclude a complete review).

DEFINITIONS AND METHODOLOGICAL ISSUES

Suicidology

A continuing controversy in the field of suicidology has been how to define and label the subject under study. The generic term 'suicidal behavior' may refer to completed suicide, non-fatal deliberate self-harm (e.g. suicide attempts, suicide gestures, parasuicide, self-injury, self-poisoning, self-harm) with or without suicidal intent, suicide communications including suicide threats, and/or suicide ideation. It is not unusual to find research studies where subjects are mixed together from each of these categories, with little attention to differences that might exist between the groups. Less common but still too frequent is the practice of studying one group, e.g. individuals who deliberately harm themselves but do not die, and drawing conclusions about another group, e.g. suicide. This terminological and methodological confusion reflects a similar confusion about the nature of the population under study.

Fatal Self-Harm

The definition of suicide is largely out of the control of the scientific community, since classification is a legal rather than a scientific decision. Thus, the scientific study of individuals who commit suicide is limited by the particular decision rules used in the community of the suicide. There have been few attempts to compare what different individual official classifiers (coroners, medical examiners, physicians filling out death certificates, etc.) mean by the term suicide or what inclusion and exclusion criteria they actually use. The few scientific definitions, such as the six semi-independent dimensions of Douglas (1967), currently offer little in the way of guidelines to this classification process.

Parasuicide

The problems in defining suicide may be legion; problems classifying and labeling non-fatal suicidal behavior are a methodological nightmare. At a minimum, all investigators require that the individual have some knowledge or belief that the activity engaged in poses a risk to life or to health. Most investigators also require the execution of an overt act that is either believed to be harmful or is potentially so. Controversies have typically been framed in terms of the role of intent to die in defining non-fatal self-injury as suicidal or not. At least two other motivations, however, are also relevant: the intent to engage in the act in question, and the intent to incur harm. Investigators differ on how much intent is required to label behavior suicidal. Furthermore, how to define and measure suicide intent is not clear, and there appears to be little consensus (e.g. Fox and Weissman, 1975; Kovacs *et al.*, 1975a). The validity of different assessment methods is unknown, but they are not likely to be interchangeable. For instance, Bancroft *et al.* (1979) reported substantial disagreement both between psychiatric opinion of suicide intent for a group of overdosers and the overdosers' self-reports of intent, and between free-form self-reports and selections of various intent statements from a list provided by the investigators.

Kreitman (1977) introduced the term *parasuicide* as a label for non-fatal, intentional, self-injurious behavior, suggesting that the term replace the more common designation of such behaviors as suicide attempts. His reasoning was that not only is suicide intent difficult to infer but also many non-fatal intentional self-injurious acts do not appear to be motivated by an intent to die, and thus are improperly viewed as unsuccessful attempts at suicide. This usage also avoids the perjorative connotation usually associated with terms like suicide gesture. Dyer and Kreitman (1984) defined parasuicide as 'a non-fatal act in which an individual deliberately causes self-injury or ingests a substance in excess of any prescribed or generally recognized therapeutic dosage' (p. 3). They included all instances of drug poisoning with non-therapeutic drugs, excluding alcohol but including illegal recreational drugs, to which toxic reactions have been as much as 26% of emergency room admissions for drug reactions (Petersen and Chambers, 1975).

Some sort of inference about intent seems indispensable in defining suicidal behavior. At least, it must be differentiated from accidental self-harm. Furthermore, different labels are needed to differentiate different levels and types of intent. As can be seen in Figure 14.1, differing definitions result in quite different inclusion levels. The problems in drawing comparative conclusions among studies with such diverse entrance restrictions are obvious.

Suicide Ideation

Compared to suicide and parasuicide, there are very few studies of suicide ideation and suicide communications. What data exist suggest that individuals with suicide ideation enough to come to professional attention may differ little from parasuicides or suicides (Fowler *et al.*, 1979; Marks and Haller, 1977; Meyers, 1982; Paykel *et al.*, 1974; Schwab *et al.*, 1972). When differences are found between ideators and parasuicides, the ideators are generally more disturbed than the parasuicides in terms of a number of variables. The very minimal

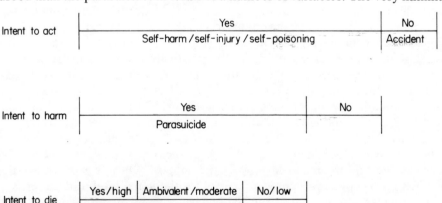

FIG. 14.1 Different definitions and inclusions of suicide.

data on subjects defined as threateners suggest they are also more disturbed than parasuicides. There is a serious definitional problem here, however. To qualify as an ideator in most studies, the individuals had to communicate their suicide intent, but since the line between communicating suicide ideation and threatening suicide is very murky, it is unclear whether the populations in some suicide ideation studies are threateners or ideators.

Present Approach

In summary, the policies across much of the suicidal literature of providing ambiguous definitions for the behavior in question and mixing groups of varying levels of suicidal behavior in one analysis make firm conclusions extremely difficult to draw. Furthermore, these problems are matched by statistical issues in many instances. Innumerable studies not only include more dependent variables than subjects but also fail to utilize multivariate statistics. Some empirical articles do not even report statistical analyses. Others fail to include control groups. Although we have included only the better studies, the reader must still consider these problems before accepting the conclusions.

Since many investigations of deliberate, non-fatal self-harm include individuals of varying levels of intent, in the remainder of this chapter we will use the broader term parasuicide, regardless of the terms used by the original authors of each study. The term 'suicidal' can refer to persons who engage in any type of suicide-related behavior. An effort will be made in this chapter to specify which class of behavior is meant. The more generic term will be used when all categories of suicidal behavior are meant to be included.

STRESS

Model Assumptions

Depue and Monroe (1986) have noted that while the most common model of stress–disorder interaction is what might be termed a stress-initiation model, few researchers have taken the precautions to insure that this model can actually be applied to their study samples. The underlying assumption of the stress-initiation model is that the stressing event and a putatively related disorder must be sufficiently independent that the disorder is not causing the stressful event. This can be done by insuring that events clearly precede any onset of disorder and are not generated by aspects of the disorder itself, or, in a more statistical fashion, controlling for the initial level of disorder before associating events with subsequent variation in disorder. The infrequency of these techniques was noted by Cohen and Wills (1985) in their review of 43 studies reporting significant associations between disorder and level of social support. Only five of the studies included prospective procedures to control for the initial level of disorder.

In particular with respect to suicidal behavior, a loss of key individuals who were probably providing social support has both been associated with subsequent suicidal behavior (Borg and Stahl, 1982; Fernando and Storm, 1984) and viewed

s a consequence of the suicidal behavior (Slater and Depue, 1981). Obviously,
research designs which do not allow these to be distinguished only contribute to
he confusion.

Measurement Timing and Overlap

A problem in much of stress research is that infrequent measurement of both
stress and levels of disorder leads to lowered associations between stressors and
disorder (Depue and Monroe, 1986). Such widely spaced measurements, typically
5 months to a year apart, are at best imprecise as to the timing of stressing events,
and may miss subsequent fluctuations in disorders which last for comparatively
shorter periods of time or have delayed onset. This is especially significant for
stress-maintenance models because many chronic disorders do not show large
fluctuations. Thus, without frequent measurement, the time association of a
stressor to changes in the disorder is rendered more uncertain by a lack of
distinctiveness regarding the level of the disorder. Furthermore, the smaller
changes both in magnitude and duration associated with chronicity are more likely
to be missed.

Measurement overlaps are another potential source of confusion in the untangling of causality (Monroe and Steiner, 1986). An event may be given a
particular label but share significant features of a different variable. For instance,
conflict with a spouse may be identified as a stressful event, but it could also be
seen as a lack, or even loss, of social support. To the degree that it is measured as
both, the correlation between stress and lack of social support will be misleading.
Such confounding is inherent in the nature of the variables, but failing to make
conceptual distinctions or have proper controls can only decrease the likelihood of
understanding the nature of the relationships.

Present Approach

Although we will point out these problems as they arise in the following literature,
the reader will do well to resist simplistic either–or interpretations of the effects.
In most cases, the methodological untangling could have been done only by
proper initial design of the study, and so these outcomes will represent a blend of
the relevant factors. As yet, there is nothing in suicide research to compare with
the recent advances in degree of control found in such areas as depression (e.g.
Monroe et al., 1986).

SOCIAL–BEHAVIORAL THEORY OF SUICIDAL BEHAVIORS

The developmental, situational, and behavioral pathways leading to suicide and
parasuicide are multiple and complex. It is unlikely that there is a single behavioral or situational characteristic common to all parasuicides or suicides. Studies
using cluster and component analysis procedures have found several typologies of
both parasuicide and suicide (Bagley et al., 1976; Colson, 1973; Henderson et al.,
1977). Nor is it likely that the locus of causality for suicidal behavior will be found

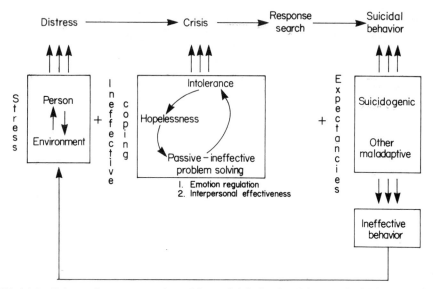

FIG. 14.2   Schematic representation of the social–behavioral theory of suicidal behaviors.

in an analysis of either the situation or the person alone. The few studies using multivariate analyses have demonstrated that it is the combination of particular situational characteristics together with specific person factors that best predict future suicidal behavior. The model presented by Linehan (1981) suggests that suicidal behavior is the result of a dynamic interaction between the individual and the environment as well as among forces interacting within both the environmental system (e.g. negative life changes in one area affecting social support) and the person/behavioral systems (e.g. the effects of cognitive processes on physiological responses and their effect on overt behaviors).

The model we are presenting here reorganizes somewhat the previous model, and adds an outline for the developmental progression of a suicidal episode. It is represented schematically in Figure 14.2. Briefly, the model suggests that suicidal behaviors are a result of (a) environmental and person-generated stresses, combined with (b) individual vulnerability factors of inadequate problem-regulating capacities, negative life expectancies, and low tolerance for distress, together with (c) suicidogenic expectancies about the effectiveness of suicidal as compared to other strategies, as a means of solving the individual's problems and distress.

Our point of view is based on the notion that suicidal behaviors, including parasuicide and suicide, represent an individual's attempt at problem solving (Applebaum, 1963; Grollman, 1971; Levenson and Neuringer, 1971; Linehan, 1981; Maris, 1971; Neuringer, 1961; Schotte and Clum, 1982; Stengel and Cook, 1958). In this attempt, the individual tries to get rid of problems by death or 'manipulation' of events rather than accommodate to them (Applebaum, 1963; Basescu, 1965; Kovacs *et al.*, 1975b; Olin, 1976; Sifneos, 1966; Stengel, 1960, 1964). The theory we are presenting is a diathesis–stress model in that it presumes that suicidal behaviors are the outcome of the interaction between particular stressful events and the individual's unique vulnerability to such stresses.

ORIGINS OF STRESS

At a particular point in time, the problem to be solved, or precipitating stress, might originate in the environment, within the person, or be due to some interaction between the person and the environment. We will consider these in turn.

External Environmental Events

The major environmental stresses related to suicidal behavior, particularly those stemming from the social milieu, are a primary focus of this chapter. The idea that suicidal behavior is a result of stressful environmental events has consistently been a part of attempts to explain suicidal behaviors (Hankoff, 1979; Paykel, 1979), but a lack of control groups and multivariate statistics as well as dubious independence of events and the suicidal person's behavior hamper most studies.

We have divided environmental stresses into three categories: a lack of social support, negative life events including interpersonal loss, and social conflict. These categories are interactive rather than exclusive. For example, social support serves as a buffering factor which, when present, can mitigate the effects of negative life events or life changes that otherwise can be direct precipitants of suicidal behavior. Conversely, the loss of social support can act independently as a stress, or exacerbate the stress due to other categories. Furthermore, it would seem difficult for one to sustain a significant interpersonal loss without some loss of social support.

Lack of Social Support

The interpersonal environment has traditionally been accorded great importance in studies of suicide. For example, numerous sociological theories stress the person's role and status in the social system. The classic sociological theory is that proposed by Emile Durkheim (1951), who suggested that two characteristics of society, social integration and social regulation, together or singly determine social conditions, which in turn influence the suicide rate. Later sociological theories introduced concepts such as the stability and durability of social relationships, social restraints and social meaning as important in suicidal behavior (Henry and Short, 1954; Gibbs and Martin, 1964; Douglas, 1967).

Psychological theories have begun to place much importance on the social environment, and a variety of negative outcomes have been related to a lack of interpersonal support. Blazer (1982) found the risk of mortality (all causes) in a group of elderly men and women to be related to a lack of social support. Sandler and Barrera (1984) found that measures of anxiety, depression, somatization, and psychological disorder were negatively related to social support satisfaction. However, the symptomatology indexes were positively related to a measure of the number of network members who were perceived as sources of interpersonal problems. This last finding illustrates the point noted earlier that care is required to avoid confounding measures of support and conflict. Furthermore, as is evident from the preceding studies, research involving social support has not achieved uniformity of measurement. Indeed, detection of effects is very dependent upon the measure employed (Cohen and Wills, 1985; Sarason et al., 1987). Thus, it is very important to consider the measures used when comparing studies.

Topol and Reznikoff (1982) found that among adolescents, lack of a confidant, particularly among the females, distinguished parasuicidal adolescents from normal but not psychiatric controls. Using a different measure, Taylor and Stansfeld (1984) compared 8–17-year-old parasuicidal children in London to an age- and sex-matched group of psychiatric outpatients and found that a lack of warmth was significantly more common in the parasuicides' families preceding the parasuicide. Among adults, Greer et al. (1966) found that parasuicides were more socially isolated than medical controls but not more than psychiatric controls. Slater and Depue (1981) found more parasuicides without confidant support than depressive controls, although most cases arose due to a loss during the study period.

In early studies of completed suicide, Sainsbury (1955) noted that compared to the general population, more suicides in London had been living alone, and Stengel (1957) found higher rates of suicide in areas of London characterized by social isolation. Numerous suicide studies have documented unstable work and living situations (e.g. Hagnell and Rorsman, 1980) or restricted social access due to unemployment or retirement (Bagley et al., 1976; Kreitman, 1977) which were likely to have resulted in lower social support.

As can be seen from the preceding studies, evidence linking low social support to parasuicide or suicide, as opposed to pathology in general, is either weak or indirect. For the indirect evidence, the assumption that environmental changes alone will lead to low social support is not tenable since social support levels have been shown, at least for some groups, to be more a characteristic of the person than the changing situation (Sarason et al., 1986). Resolution of this relationship will require both more precise, consistent definitions and instruments, and a separation of social support levels from the confounds of loss and conflict.

Negative Events

In a particularly well-controlled design, Hagnell et al. (1981) conducted a prospective study of 28 suicides over a 25-year period. More in the suicide group than in two control groups of normals and individuals dying of natural causes experienced object loss (loss of a loved one or of property) during the year preceding the suicide. Borg and Stahl (1982) compared 34 suicides over a 2-year period to a group of non-suicidal psychiatric patients matched for age, sex, diagnosis, and patient status. Loss of a key person by death had been judged a significant precipitating factor in their psychiatric disorder more often among the suicides than among the controls. In a 5-year review, Fernando and Storm (1984) found significantly more losses among 22 suicides than among controls matched for treatment setting, admission status, therapeutic team, sex, admission date, and ge. Loss was defined as a divorce or separation, illness or death of a first-degree relative or close friend, or loss of a job.

Data on negative events occurring prior to parasuicide are considerably more extensive. In their classic 1975 study, Paykel *et al.* examined the frequency, type, and patterning of life events for 53 parasuicides admitted to an emergency room compared to age- and sex-matched non-suicidal psychiatric patients and members of the general population. During the previous 6 months, they found that parasuicides experienced more major events that were upsetting and uncontrollable than either of the control groups. Rates were relatively constant over the 6-month period for the general population controls, peaked during the month before onset of depression among the depressed controls, and peaked during the month prior to the parasuicide for the group of interest. However, the implications of this study are somewhat limited since the parasuicides were predominantly young females.

The importance of age differences was highlighted in the study of Luscomb *et al.* (1980). They compared male parasuicides with male non-suicidal psychiatric patients and found more total events, stressful events, and exit events (interpersonal losses) during the preceding year among only the older subjects. Among younger subjects there were no differences but, like Paykel, they found a higher number of highly stressful events occurring among all parasuicides.

Slater and Depue (1981) also found no overall difference in number of events reported by depressed parasuicides compared to depressed non-suicidal inpatients for the previous year or before the onset of depression. At both points in time, however, parasuicides reported more interpersonal losses than did the depressed controls. Furthermore, after the onset of the depressive episode, the parasuicides reported more total events leading up to parasuicide. When only the events which could be considered independent of the patients' symptomatology were considered, parasuicides reported more events than non-parasuicides for each time period. The importance of interpersonal losses in the time period before parasuicide is further highlighted by Levi *et al.* (1966), who found more separations from people in the prior year for parasuicides admitted to an emergency room compared to non-suicidal admissions. The parasuicides, however, did not differ from suicide ideator control subjects.

Kosky (1983) examined 10–11-year-old psychiatric inpatients. Physicians (problematically not blind to the child's status) rated loss as related to the child's problems more often for parasuicides than for non-suicidal children. Cohen-Sandler *et al.* (1982) studied children between the ages of 5 and 14. During the previous year, they found that suicidal children (suicide ideators and parasuicides combined, unfortunately) experienced more stressful events and more temporary and permanent losses of a parent or grandparent.

Taken together, these studies support the commonsense observation that suicidal actions (suicide, parasuicide) are a response to prior negative events occurring in the environmental milieu. In particular, they suggest that interpersonal loss is a potent precipitator of suicidal behavior. Psychological theories have long stressed the importance of interpersonal losses and conflict in the etiology of suicidal behaviors. Additionally, this view is consistent with the importance placed upon loss developmentally (Bowlby, 1980).

Social Conflict

As noted before, interpersonal conflict has been viewed from perspectives of both loss and external stress. Additionally, it can be seen as either an environmental provision by which individuals are exposed to an additional source of stress, or as something which interacts with, or is even generated solely by, the person in question. An early example of this range was described by Wolfgang (1958), who found upon investigation that over a quarter of Philadelphia homicide 'victims' had actually sought out the fatal conflict and/or drawn a weapon first. Thus, an interactionist position, particularly for adults, seems a more plausible position unless otherwise ruled out.

Miller et al. (1982) found, in comparing parasuicidal to non-suicidal adolescents within a delinquent US population of 13–15 year olds, that conflict with parents was the third most significant factor associated with parasuicide. Only suicidal ideation and depression were more highly associated. Given the cross-sectional design, however, the causal direction cannot be determined. Taylor and Stansfeld (1984), in their London child study described before, found both more discord in the parasuicides' families preceding the parasuicide than in psychiatric outpatient controls, and also more prior disturbances in the parasuicidal children's relationships with parents, particularly with the father.

Kosky (1983) found, in comparing a group of parasuicidal children to psychiatric controls, that the suicidal children had been more exposed to both violent interactions between parents and physical abuse from the parents. Similarly Asarnow et al. (1987) discovered that parasuicidal children aged 8 to 14, when compared to depressed psychiatric controls, rated their families as higher on conflict and lower on cohesion and control as measured by the Moos Family Environment Scale. In a comparison with medical controls, Deykin et al. (1985) found a higher incidence of previously reported child abuse and neglect among parasuicidal adolescents.

In an interesting comparison of cultural effects, Kitamura (1985) found that family and love problems were the dominant reasons given for a suicide attempt by group of West German children and adolescents, whereas school problems were the most frequent for a Japanese adolescent sample. Thus, in the Western samples considered, family conflict has been cited more frequently, whereas in Japan, an external issue of school problems was given. Some caution should be observed in interpreting this East–West difference, however, since it is possible that it represents, at least in part, a difference in willingness to criticize the family (DeVos, 1980, p. 129). On the whole, then, a higher level of conflict, both between parents and between parent and child, has been a significant factor differentiating parasuicidal behavior from other problematic behaviors for children and adolescents.

Turning to adults, Greer et al. (1966) found more interpersonal conflicts in close relationships within 6 months of hospitalization for an English sample of 15 parasuicides than for similar numbers of psychiatric or medical patients. Kiev

(1974), in a 1-year prospective study of 300 inpatient and outpatient parasuicides, found that higher levels of interpersonal conflict as well as unstable families were associated with no improvement following treatment. In contrast, both the much improved and those who committed suicide during the study year had lower levels. Along the same lines in a Greenland study, Grove and Lynge (1979) noted a conflicted family of origin and more interpersonal conflict for parasuicides in comparison to normal controls.

Again, in a New Zealand study, Adam *et al.* (1980) reported more conflict as well as more separations and emotional deprivation and less stability in parasuicides than in a matched group of medical outpatients. It is important to note, however, that while many parasuicides have such conflict, not all do. Kiev (1976), in a cluster analysis of the 300 subjects reported above, found interpersonal conflict to be high in only half of the clusters identified. Whereas conflict appeared to be the major problem for some groups, for others, depression, general dysfunction, or characterological problems were central.

In summary, interpersonal conflict is a frequent environmental factor in parasuicide and suicide, and is especially significant in connection with parasuicidal behavior in children and adolescents. Viewing such conflict as a major source of stress appears reasonable, but differences between adult and child status and the heterogeneity of the suicidal population suggest that in a more fine-grained analysis of conflict causation and interaction, no one model is likely to fit most situations. Furthermore, despite the frequency of conflict, only a few studies (e.g. Nelson *et al.*, 1977; Neuringer, 1964a) have attempted such an analysis, and these have not been very explanatory. The variability in parasuicides noted above makes an exploration of this question difficult, but such a step would now add significantly to understanding of this group.

Internal Within-Person Events

Within-person negative events such as illness, affective lability, negative emotions, and uncontrollable thought processes and behavior are intimately related to environmental stress. They increase vulnerability to such stress, can be caused by exposure to prior environmental stresses, and can, in turn, precipitate further stressful environmental events.

Illness

In various studies, from 25% to 70% of persons who committed suicide were in poor health immediately prior to the act (Andress and Corey, 1977; Bagley *et al.*, 1976; Dorpat and Ripley, 1960). A type of person characterized as focusing on medical symptoms has emerged in several typologies of suicide (e.g. Bagley *et al*, 1976; Farberow and McEvoy, 1966). Others have found that poor health as a precipitant of suicide increases with age (Dorpat and Ripley, 1960). Hagnell *et al.* (1981) found that illness during the preceding year was greater for suicides than for a matched control group, and comparable to a matched group of individuals dying of natural causes. The association between poor health and parasuicide is less clear. An association has not been found in some studies (Slater and Depue, 1981), the relevant analyses were not reported in others (Luscomb *et al.*, 1980), and control groups have been lacking in other relevant studies.

Psychiatric Disorder

The relationship between psychiatric disorder and suicidal behavior is strong and convincing. Robins *et al.* (1959) found evidence of a psychiatric disorder in 94% of US suicides. Barraclough *et al.* (1974) reported similar rates in Britain, and Martin *et al.* (1985) reported a suicide rate among psychiatric outpatients fifteen times higher than in a matched non-psychiatric control group. The suicide rate for male alcoholics is 75 times greater than for the general male population (Kessel and Grossman, 1961), and for opiate addicts it is estimated at five to twenty times that of the general population (Murphy *et al.*, 1983). Up to 13% of schizophrenics commit suicide, most during the first 10 years of the illness in the context of a severe, chronic relapsing from of the disorder with many exacerbations and hospitalizations by the time of the suicide (Roy, 1982). Interestingly, most schizophrenics show clinical improvement prior to their suicidal act, or do not appear to be acutely relapsed at the time of suicide (Brier and Astrachan, 1984; Otto, 1967; Seeman, 1979; Shneidman *et al.*, 1962; Yarden, 1974), suggesting that in many cases the current symptoms of the disorder are not direct precipitants of impulsive suicides. However, it is possible that suicide within this population is a planned escape from the painful sequelae of the disorder. The data currently do not allow an answer to this question.

Suicide rates among individuals diagnosed as having a bipolar affective disorder range from 9% to 60%, with a modal figure in the 10%–30% range (Jamison, 1986). In 20% of the studies Jamison reviewed, at least 50% of the bipolar patients had committed suicide. Other studies indicate that between 25% and 50% of bipolar patients attempt suicide (parasuicide). Bipolars are unlikely to commit suicide during a manic phase; the highest risk is in the depressed or mixed stages (Kotin and Goodwin, 1972; Robins *et al.*, 1959; Winokur *et al.*, 1969). Suicide in bipolars is related to severe depressive symptoms but is also at times related to apparent improvement (Keith-Speigel and Spiegel, 1967; Weeke, 1979). As with schizophrenia, however, it is difficult to know if the individual is responding to the stress of the bipolar symptoms themselves or whether the disorder produces a heightened vulnerability to other stresses.

VULNERABILITY FACTORS

Not everyone experiencing negative life events or person-generated life stress, even in the absence of social support systems, engages in suicidal behavior. Something else is needed. The middle portion of Figure 14.2 outlined suicidogenic person vulnerability factors which are related to an individual's inability to cope with stress. Specifically, we are suggesting that the personal vulnerabilities most highly related to suicidal behaviors can be summarized as occurring in one of three categories: (a) problem-solving skills for reducing both environmental stress and regulating affective distress, (b) hope and reasons for living, even in the face of seemingly intolerable stress, and (c) tolerance for high levels of distress.

Problem-Solving Skills

A number of studies suggest that parasuicides are more rigid in their thinking (Levenson, 1972; Neuringer, 1964b; Patsiokas et al., 1979; Vinoda, 1966), less capable of abstract and interpersonal problem solving (Goodstein, 1982; Levenson and Neuringer, 1971; Schotte and Clum, 1987), and possibly more field dependent (Levenson, 1972) than psychiatric control populations. In our own work, we have found that inpatient parasuicides are more passive and less active interpersonal problem solvers than are both inpatient suicide ideators and non-suicidal psychiatric inpatients (Linehan et al., 1987). In this study we demonstrated that inadequate problem-solving skill is a trait of parasuicides which is stable over time, rather than a characteristic of high stress states associated with parasuicide and hospital admission. Finally, in the first such finding for children, Asarnow et al. (1987) compared suicide ideators and parasuicides to depressed psychiatric controls and discovered that the ideators but not the parasuicides were less likely to generate active cognitive coping strategies.

Cognitive rigidity, field dependence, and poor problem-solving capabilities may be functionally related to parasuicide by limiting the range of problem solutions open to these people. When faced with seemingly catastrophic life problems and environmental stresses, those who eventually become parasuicides may be unable to generate alternative solutions to effect outcomes preferable to suicidal outcomes. A rigid cognitive style also suggests that in the face of changing environmental contingencies these people will be unable to change their expectancies. Thus they may experience even more negative changes than would be the case if they could monitor contingencies more effectively and change overt behavior accordingly.

Levenson and Neuringer (1971) commented that 'problem solving incapacity is of lethal consequence' (p. 435). However, problem-solving inadequacies among suicides are yet to be determined empirically. For instance, in reviewing literature relevant to their diathesis–stress model of suicidal behavior, Schotte and Clum (1987) do not even mention data on completed suicides.

A deficit in skills for regulating emotions, or affect problem solving, is suggested by the relationship of negative affective states with suicidal behavior. Empirical studies have focused, for the most part, on interpersonal emotional responses, including hostility, friendliness, and comfort with people, and feelings of depression, apathy, and dysphoria. With very few exceptions, these studies indicate that, at least after the fact, parasuicides appear to be more angry, hostile and irritable than non-suicidal psychiatric patients and general population control groups (Crook et al., 1975; Lester, 1968; Nelson et al., 1977; Richman and Charles, 1976). These findings hold even when sex, age, and depression are controlled (Weissman et al., 1973). Some support for the view that the hostility is not a function of the parasuicidal behavior itself or of the survival from an attempt to die is suggested by Paykel and Dienelt (1971), who followed depressed inpatients for 10 months after discharge. They found that prior psychiatrists' ratings, self-ratings, and mood rating of high hostility levels were more characteristic of those who subsequently became parasuicidal. In contrast, persons who later commit suicide are often characterized as less angry (Dean *et al.*, 1967; Litman, 1974) and more often apathetic and/or indifferent (Dean *et al.*, 1967; Farberow and MacKinnon, 1974; Farberow and McEvoy, 1966; Farberow *et al.*, 1970; Virkkunen, 1976). A large percentage of suicides are diagnosed, either prior to the act or retrospectively, as depressed. The same is true for parasuicides; Weissman (1974) reviewed diagnostic studies from 1960 to 1971 and found that depression accounts for 35% to 79% of all cases.

These negative emotional states can be viewed as indications that suicidal individuals lack the skills necessary to regulate and alter negative emotions, although the sources of these emotions are not clear. Perhaps, given the data cited on the frequency of negative external events for suicidal groups, these individuals are overwhelmed by a higher than usual number of events in combination with their regulation deficits. Studies addressing both these areas are greatly needed to clarify the picture.

Hope, Reasons for Living, and Distress Tolerance

One of the strongest findings to date has been the consistent positive relationship of hopelessness with both suicide intent and with suicidal behaviors. Studies by Farberow and MacKinnon (1974), Farberow and McEvoy (1966) and Barraclough *et al.* (1974) suggest that general hopelessness is frequent among suicides. In an important 10-year prospective follow-up study, Beck *et al.* (1985) demonstrated that hopelessness scores are a powerful predictor of suicide. These results were cross-validated in a restrospective study of patients previously given the same scale (Beck, 1986).

The relationship of hopelessness to parasuicide is not clear. The suicidal intent measure positively related to hopelessness is negatively related to parasuicide as compared with suicide (Beck *et al.*, 1974). Weissman *et al.* (1973) found controls to be equal to parasuicides in terms of hopelessness, whereas other investigators found parasuicides to be more hopeless (Paykel and Dienelt, 1971; Wetzel, 1976). In a mixed sample of suicide ideators, parasuicides, and non-suicidal psychiatric controls, Schotte and Clum (1987) found both that the non-suicidal patients were lower on hopelessness than the suicidal patients, and that suicidal intent was best predicted by hopelessness.

Linehan *et al.* (1983) reasoned that in the face of overwhelming stress, individuals who had important reasons for living rather than committing suicide would be less likely to engage in suicidal behaviors. In studies of both a general population sample and psychiatric patients, they found that parasuicides compared to non-parasuicides have fewer important reasons for living. In addition, the positive coping beliefs scale not only predicted suicide intent but was a stronger predictor than was hopelessness (Strosahl *et al.*, submitted for publication).

Little has been studied regarding the relationship of distress tolerance to suicidal behavior. In a study of female college students, Cantor (1976) found an inability to tolerate frustration as measured by the Edwards Personal Preference Schedule Endurance scale, and a much lower threshold for psychological pain and stress when she compared parasuicides and high suicide ideators to a group of low ideators and normals. There were no differences between the parasuicides and high ideators on these variables, however. Farberow *et al.* (1970) have reported a similar intolerance of frustration for suicides.

Indirect evidence comes from a variety of sources. Nelson *et al.* (1977) found parasuicides to be less tolerant of others than psychiatric controls, as measured by the California Personality Inventory Tolerance scale. The findings cited earlier (e.g. Crook *et al.*, 1975), that parasuicides are in general more angry, hostile, and irritable, may arise in part due to a lower tolerance for frustration and other negative emotions.

Expectancies

We would expect that an individual exposed to significant stress with inadequate coping skills will resort to some sort of dysfunctional behavior to ameliorate the stress, but why would it be suicidal behavior instead of drinking, drugs, or other forms of escape behavior? Research into other areas of problematic behavior such as alcohol addiction (Marlatt, 1978) suggests that expectancies about the outcomes of specific problem-solving behaviors may be particularly important in determining an individual's response to a stressful situation. The research described above on positive and negative expectancies, e.g. reasons for living and hopelessness, demonstrated that general life expectancies can be related to suicidal behaviors. More specifically, Linehan *et al.* (1987) found both suicide ideators and parasuicides to have higher expectancies than psychiatric controls for suicide as a solution to life's problems. McCutcheon (1985) also found a similar relationship among Veterans Administration psychiatric patients.

Thus, from our theoretical perspective, to the degree that individuals have important reasons for living and beliefs that they can cope with stressful events, suicidal behavior is less likely. Furthermore, for a given level of hopelessness among parasuicides, the presence of such positive reasons may discriminate between those less and more likely to proceed with parasuicidal behavior. However, the presence of positive suicide expectancies and a low level of distress tolerance are likely to be significant factors which make engaging in suicidal behavior a more appealing option than enduring what seems comparatively intolerable.

SUMMARY AND CONCLUSIONS

Definitional and methodological issues related to suicidology and stress research were reviewed and their relevance to the studies to follow was clarified. The definition of parasuicide was chosen as the label for all non-fatal deliberate self-injurious behavior, and the interactive nature of suicidal behavior and environmental events was stressed.

A diathesis–stress model of suicidal behavior was advanced in which suicidal behaviors result from the interaction of environmental and person-generated stresses with the vulnerability factors of inadequate problem solving, negative life expectancies, and low tolerance for distress in conjunction with individual expectancies of the differential efficacy of suicidal behavior. Using this model as an outline, the literature relevant to each point was reviewed.

Environmental events associated with suicidal behavior were divided into the categories of lack of social support, negative life events including interpersonal loss, and social conflict. The evidence for lack of social support as a specific factor in suicidal behavior above and beyond its role as a general factor in many types of pathology was weak, and complicated by inconsistent definitions and confusion with interpersonal loss and conflict. In contrast, the data for negative life events, particularly interpersonal loss both developmentally and in the immediate time frame, strongly implicated these factors as precipitators of both suicide and parasuicide. Similarly, social conflict was highly related to suicidal behavior, with children and adolescents being the most vulnerable.

The within-person events were divided into illness and psychiatric disorder. Illness and poor health were related to suicide, with the association increasing with advancing age, but the relationship of illness and parasuicide has not been clearly demonstrated. In contrast, the relationship between psychiatric disorder and suicide was strong and convincing.

Turning to the vulnerability factors comprising the diathesis component of the model, the evidence for the relationship between deficits in problem-solving skills and parasuicide was extensive. Cognitive rigidity, field dependence, and inadequate, passive approaches were all related to both parasuicide and suicide ideation. In spite of long-standing assumptions of a relationship, however, there are no data connecting these deficits to suicides. There were strong data relating hopelessness to suicide and, on the flip side, emerging data indicating that positive reasons for living are a deterrent to parasuicide. Only a few studies have investigated distress tolerance and suicidal behavior, and while these are supportive, better definitions and more research are needed to clarify this vulnerability component. Finally, suicidal expectancies also appear to be important, but more research is needed on different samples to clarify the relationship between deficits in problem solving versus efficacy of beliefs about suicidal behavior.

Thus, there is evidence for a stress–diathesis model of suicidal behavior incorporating most of the components outlined above. As noted, however, the interaction of most of these components and the variability within the suicidal population make extensive, careful research a necessity further to define these elements.

Preparation of the manuscript was supported in part by National Institute of Mental Health Grant NIMH No. 5 ROI MH34486–03 to Marsha M. Linehan.

REFERENCES

Adam, K.S., Bouckoms, A., & Scarr, G. (1980). Attempted suicide in Christchurch: a controlled study. *Australian and New Zealand Journal of Psychiatry, 14,* 305–314.

Andress, V., & Corey, D. (1977). Suicide motives: Comparison of assignment of motives by coroners and psychologists. *Psychological Reports, 40,* 11–14.

Applebaum, S.A. (1963). The problem-solving aspect of suicide. *Journal of Projective Technology, 27,* 259.

Asarnow, J.R., Carlson, G.A., & Guthrie, D. (1987). Coping strategies, self-perceptions, hopelessness, and perceived family environments in depressed and suicidal children. *Journal of Consulting and Clinical Psychology, 55,* 361–366.

Bagley, C., Jacobson, S., & Rehin, A. (1976). Completed suicide: a taxonomic analysis of clinical and social data. *Psychological Medicine, 6,* 429–438.

Bancroft, J., Hawton, K., Simkin, S., Kingston, Cumming, & Whitwell. (1979). The reasons people give for taking overdoses: a further inquiry. *British Journal of Medical Psychology, 52,* 353–365.

Barraclough, B., Bunch, J., Nelson, B., & Sainsbury, P. (1974). A hundred cases of suicide: Clinical aspects. *British Journal of Psychiatry, 125,* 355–373.

Basescu, S. (1965). The threat of suicide in psychotherapy. *American Journal of Psychotherapy, 19,* 99.

Beck, A.T. (1986). Hopelessness as a predictor of eventual suicide. In J.J. Mann & M. Stanley (eds), *Psychobiology of suicidal behavior. Annals of the New York Academy of Sciences, 487,* 90–96.

Beck, A.T., Steer, R.A., Kovacs, M., & Garrison, B. (1985). Hopelessness and eventual suicide: a 10-year prospective study of patients hospitalized with suicidal ideation. *American Journal of Psychiatry, 142,* 559–563.

Beck, R.W., Morris, J.B., & Beck, A.T. (1974). Cross-validation of the suicidal intent scale. *Psychological Reports, 34,* 445–446.

Blazer, D. (1982). Social support and mortality in an elderly community population. *American Journal of Epidemiology, 115,* 684–694.

Borg, E.S., & Stahl, M. (1982). A prospective study of suicides and controls among psychiatric patients. *Acta Psychiatrica Scandinavica, 65,* 221–232.

Bowlby, J. (1980). *Loss: sadness and depression.* New York: Basic Books.

Braucht, G.N. (1979). International analysis of suicidal behavior. *Journal of Consulting and Clinical Psychology, 47,* 653–669.

Brier, A., & Astrachan, B.M. (1984). Characterization of schizophrenic patients who commit suicide. *American Journal of Psychiatry, 141,* 206–209.

Cantor, P.C. (1976). Personality characteristics found among youthful female suicide attempters. *Journal of Abnormal Psychology, 85,* 324–329.

Cohen, S., & Wills, T.A. (1985). Stress, social support, and the buffering hypothesis. *Psychological Bulletin, 98,* 310–357.

Cohen-Sandler, R., Berman, A.L., & King, R.A. (1982). Life stress and symptomatology: Determinants of suicidal behavior in children. *Journal of the American Academy of Child Psychiatry, 21,* 178–186.

Colson, C. (1973). An objective analytic approach to the classification of suicide motivation. *Acta Psychiatrica Scandinavica, 49,* 105–113.

Crook, T., Raskin, A., & Davis, D. (1975). Factors associated with attempted suicide among hospitalized depressed patients. *Psychological Medicine, 5,* 381–388.

Dean, R.A., Miskimins, W., Cook, R., Wilson, L.T., & Maley, R.E. (1967). Prediction of suicide in a psychiatric hospital. *Journal of Clinical Psychology, 23,* 296–301.

de Catanzaro, D. (1980). Human suicide: a biological perspective. *Behavior and Brain Sciences, 3,* 265.

de Catanzaro, D. (1981). *Suicide and self-damaging behavior: a sociobiological perspective.* New York: Academic Press.

Depue, R.A., & Monroe, S.M. (1986). Conceptualization and measurement of human disorder in life stress research: the problem of chronic disturbance. *Psychological Bulletin, 99,* 36–51.

DeVos, G. (1980). Afterword. In D.K. Reynolds (ed.), *The quiet therapies: Japanese pathways to personal growth.* Honolulu: University Press of Hawaii.

Deykin, E.Y., Alpert, J.J. & McNamarra, J.J. (1985). A pilot study of the effect of exposure to child abuse or neglect on adolescent suicidal behavior. *American Journal of Psychiatry, 142,* 1299–1303.

Dorpat, T.L., & Ripley, H.S. (1960). A study of suicide in the Seattle area. *Comparative Psychiatry, 1,* 349–359.

Douglas, J.D. (1967). *The social meaning of suicide.* Princeton, NJ: Princeton University Press.

Durkheim, E. (1951). *Suicide.* Translated by J.A. Spaulding & G. Simpson. Glencoe, Illinois: Free Press.

Dyer, J.A.T., & Kreitman, N. (1984). Hopelessness, depression and suicidal intent in parasuicide. *British Journal of Psychiatry, 144,* 127–133.

Farberow, N.L., & MacKinnon, D. (1974). Prediction of suicide in neuropsychiatric hospital patients. In C. Neuringer (ed.), *Psychological assessment of suicidal risk.* Springfield, Illinois: Charles C Thomas.

Farberow, N.L., & McEvoy, J.L. (1966). Suicide among patients with diagnoses of anxiety reaction or depressive reaction in general medical and surgical hospitals. *Journal of Abnormal Psychology, 71,* 287–299.

Farberow, N., McKelligott, J., Cohn, S., & Darbonne, A. (1970). Suicide among cardiovascular patients. In E.S. Shneidman, N.L. Farberow & R.E. Litman (eds), *The psychology of suicide.* New York: Science House.

Fernando, S., & Storm, V. (1984). Suicide among psychiatric patients of a district general hospital. *Psychological Medicine, 14,* 661–672.

Fowler, R.C., Tsuang, M.T., & Kronfol, Z. (1979). Communications of suicidal intent and suicide in unipolar depression: a forty year follow-up. *Journal of Affective Disorders, 1,* 219–225.

Fox, K., & Weissman, M. (1975). Suicide attempts and drugs: Contradiction between method and intent. *Social Psychiatry, 10,* 31–38.

Gibbs, J.P., & Martin, W.L. (1964). *Status integration and suicide: a sociological study.* Eugene: University of Oregon Press.

Goodstein, J. (1982). Cognitive characteristics of suicide attempters. Unpublished doctoral dissertation, The Catholic University of America.

Greer, S., Gunn, J.C., & Koller, K.M. (1966). Aetiological factors in attempted suicide. *British Medical Journal, 2,* 1352–1355.

Grollman, E.A. (1971). *Suicide prevention, intervention, postvention.* Boston: Beacon Press.

Grove, O., & Lynge, J. (1979). Suicide and attempted suicide in Greenland. *Acta Psychiatrica Scandinavica, 60,* 375–391.

Hagnell, O., Lanke, J., & Rorsman, B. (1981). Suicide rates in the Lundby study: Mental illness as a risk factor for suicide. *Neuropsychobiology, 7,* 248–253.

Hagnell, O., & Rorsman, B. (1980). Suicide in the Lundby study: a controlled prospective investigation of stressful life events. *Neuropsychobiology, 6,* 319–332.

Hankoff, L.D. (1979). Situational categories. In L.D. Hankoff & B. Einsidler (eds), *Suicide: Theory and clinical aspects* Littleton, Mass.: P.S.G. Publishing.

Henderson, A.S., Hartigan, J., Davidson, J., Lance, G.N., Duncan-Jones, P., Koller, K.M., Ritchie, K., McAuley, H., Williams, C.L., & Slaghuis, W.A. (1977). Typology of parasuicide. *British Journal of Psychiatry, 131,* 631–641.

Henry, A.F., & Short, J.F. (1954). *Suicide and homicide.* London: Free Press.

Jamison, K.R. (1986). Suicide and bipolar disorders. In J.J. Mann & M. Stanley (eds), Psychobiology of suicidal behavior. *Annals of the New York Academy of Sciences, 487,* 301–316.

Keith-Speigel, P., & Spiegel, D.E. (1967). Affective states of patients immediately preceding suicide. *Journal of Psychiatric Research, 5,* 89–93.

Kessel, N., & Grossman, G. (1961). Suicide in alcoholics. *British Medical Journal, 2,* 1671–1672.

Kiev, A. (1974). Prognostic factors in attempted suicide. *American Journal of Psychiatry, 131,* 987–990.

Kiev, A. (1976). Cluster analysis profiles of suicide attempters. *American Journal of Psychiatry, 133,* 150–153.

Kitamura, A. (1985). Suicide and attempted suicide among children and adolescents: a transcultural study. *Pediatrician, 12,* 73–79.

Kosky, R. (1983). Childhood suicidal behaviour. *Journal of Child Psychology and Psychiatry, 24,* 457–468.

Kotin, J., & Goodwin, F.K. (1972). Depression during mania: Clinical observations and theoretical implications. *American Journal of Psychiatry, 129,* 679–686.

Kovacs, M., Beck, A.T., & Weissman, A. (1975a). Hopelessness: an indicator of suicidal risk. *Suicide and Life-Threatening Behavior, 5,* 98–103.

Kovacs, M., Beck, A.T., & Weissman, A. (1975b). The use of suicidal motives in the psychotherapy of attempted suicides. *American Journal of Psychotherapy, 29,* 363–368.

Kreitman, N. (1977). *Parasuicide.* Chichester: John Wiley & Sons.

Lester, D. (1968). Suicide as an aggressive act: a replication with a control for neuroticism. *Journal of General Psychology, 79,* 83–86.

Levenson, M. (1972). Cognitive and perceptual factors in suicidal individuals. Unpublished doctoral dissertation, University of Kansas.

Levenson, M., & Neuringer, C. (1971). Problem-solving behavior in suicidal adolescents. *Journal of Consulting and Clinical Psychology, 37,* 433–436.

Levi, D., Fales, C., Stein, M., & Sharp, V. (1966). Separation and attempted suicide. *Archives of General Psychiatry, 15,* 158–164.

Linehan, M.M. (1981). A social behavioral analysis of suicide and parasuicide: Implications for clinical assessment and treatment. In H.G. Glazer & J.F. Clarkin (eds), *Depression: Behavioral and directive intervention strategies* (pp. 229–294). New York: Garland Press.

Linehan, M.M., Goodstein, J.L., Nielsen, S.L., & Chiles, J.A. (1983). Reasons for staying alive when you are thinking of killing yourself: the reasons for living inventory. *Journal of Consulting and Clinical Psychology, 51,* 276–286.

Linehan, M.M., Camper, P., Chiles, J.A., Strosahl, K., & Shearin, E.N. (1987). Interpersonal problem solving and parasuicide. *Cognitive Therapy and Research, 11,* 1–12.

Litman, R.E. (1974). Models for predicting suicide risk. In C. Neuringer (ed.), *Psychological assessment of suicidal risk.* Springfield, Illinois: Charles C Thomas.

Luscomb, R.L., Clum, G.A., & Patsiokas, A.T. (1980). Mediating factors in the relationship between life stress and suicide attempting. *Journal of Nervous and Mental Disorders, 169*(11), 644–650.

Maris, R.W. (1971). Deviance as therapy: the paradox of the self-destructive female. *Journal of Health and Social Behavior, 12,* 113–124.

Marks, P.A., & Haller, D.L. (1977). Now I lay me down for keeps: a study of adolescent suicide attempts. *Journal of Clinical Psychology, 33,* 390–400.

Marlatt, G.A. (1978). Alcohol, stress, and cognitive control. In P.E. Nathan & G.A. Marlatt (eds), *Experimental and behavioral approaches to alcoholism.* New York: Plenum Press.

Martin, R.L., Clonninger, C.R., Guze, S.B., *et al.* (1985). Mortality in a follow up of 500 psychiatric outpatients. II. Cause-specific mortality. *Archives of General Psychiatry, 30,* 737–746.

McCutcheon, S.R. (1985). Understanding attempted suicide: a decision theory approach. Unpublished doctoral dissertation, University of Washington.

Meyers, E.D. (1982). Subsequent deliberate self-harm in patients referred to a psychiatrist: a prospective study. *British Journal of Psychiatry, 140,* 132–137.

Miller, M.L., Chiles, J.A., & Barnes, V.E. (1982). Suicide attempters within a delinquent population. *Journal of Consulting and Clinical Psychology, 50,* 491–498.

Monroe, S.M., & Steiner, S.C. (1986). Social support and psychopathology: Interrelations with preexisting disorder, stress, and personality. *Journal of Abnormal Psychology, 95,* 29–39.

Monroe, S.M., Bromet, E.J., Connell, M.M., & Steiner, S.C. (1986). Social support, life events, and depressive symptoms: a 1-year prospective study. *Journal of Consulting and Clinical Psychology, 54,* 424–431.

Murphy, S.L., Rounsaville, B.J., Eyre, S., & Kleber, H.D. (1983). Suicide attempts in treated opiate addicts. *Comprehensive Psychiatry, 241,* 79–88.

Nelson, V.L., Nielsen, E.C., & Checketts, K.T. (1977). Interpersonal attitudes of suicidal individuals. *Psychological Reports, 40,* 983–989.

Neuringer, C. (1961). Dichotomous evaluations in suicidal individuals. *Journal of Consulting Psychology, 25,* 445–449.

Neuringer, C. (1964a). Reactions to interpersonal crises in suicidal individuals. *Journal of General Psychology, 71,* 47–55.

Neuringer, C. (1964b). Rigid thinking in suicidal individuals. *Journal of Consulting and Clinical Psychology, 28,* 54–58.

Neuringer, C. (1974). Self- and other-appraisals by suicidal, psychosomatic and normal hospitalized patients. *Journal of Consulting and Clinical Psychology, 42,* 306.

Olin, H.S. (1976). Psychotherapy of the chronically suicidal patient. *American Journal of Psychotherapy, 30,* 570–575.

Otto, U. (1967). Suicide attempts made by psychotic children and adolescents. *Acta Paediatrica Scandinavica, 56,* 349–356.

Patsiokas, A., Clum, G., & Luscomb, R. (1979). Cognitive characteristics of suicide attempters. *Journal of Consulting and Clinical Psychology, 47,* 478–484.

Paykel, E.S. (1979). Life stress. In L.D. Hankoff & B. Einsidler (eds), *Suicide: Theory and clinical aspects,* Littleton, Mass.: P.S.G. Publishing.

Paykel. E.S., & Dienelt, M.N. (1971). Suicide attempts following acute depression. *Journal of Nervous and Mental Disorder, 153,* 234–243.

Paykel, E.S., Prusoff, B.A., & Meyers, J.K. (1975). Suicide attempts and recent life events. *Archives of General Psychiatry, 32,* 327–333.

Paykel, E.S., Meyers, J.K., Lindenthal, J.J., & Tanner, J. (1974). Suicidal feelings in the general population: a prevalence study. *British Journal of Psychiatry, 124,* 460–469.

Petersen, D.M., & Chambers, C.D. (1975). Demographic characteristics of emergency room admissions for acute drug reactions. *International Journal of the Addictions, 10,* 963–975.

Richman, J., & Charles, E. (1976). Patient dissatisfaction and attempted suicide. *Community Mental Health Journal, 12,* 301–305.

Robins, E., Gassner, S., Kayes, J., Wilkinson, R.H., & Murphy, G.E. (1959). The communication of suicidal intent: a study of 134 consecutive cases of successful (completed) suicide. *American Journal of Psychiatry, 115,* 724–733.

Roy, A. (1982). Suicide in chronic schizophrenics. *British Journal of Psychiatry, 141,* 171–177.

Sainsbury, P. (1955). *Suicide in London: an ecological study.* London: Chapman & Hall.

Sandler, I.N., & Barrera, M., Jr (1984). Toward a multimethod approach to assessing the effects of social support. *American Journal of Community Psychology, 12,* 37–52.

Sarason, I.G., Sarason, B.R., & Shearin, E.N. (1986). Social support as an individual difference variable: Its stability, origins, and relational aspects. *Journal of Personality and Social Psychology, 50,* 845–855.

Sarason, B.R., Shearin, E.N., Pierce, G.R., & Sarason, I.G. (1987). Interrelations of social support measures: Theoretical and practical implications. *Journal of Personality and Social Psychology, 52,* 813–832.

Schotte, D.E., & Clum, G.A. (1982). Suicide ideation in a college population. *Journal of Consulting and Clinical Psychology, 50,* 690–696.

Schotte, D.E., & Clum, G.A. (1987). Problem-solving skills in suicidal psychiatric patients. *Journal of Consulting and Clinical Psychology, 55,* 49–54.

Schwab, J.J., Warheit, G.J., & Holzer III, C.E. (1972). Suicidal ideation and behavior in a general population. *Diseases of the Nervous System, 33,* 745–748.

Seeman, M.V. (1979). Management of the schizophrenic patient. *Canadian Medical Association Journal, 120,* 1097–1103.

Shneidman, E.S., Farberow N.L., & Leonard, C.V. (1962). Suicide: evaluation of treatment of suicide risk among schizophrenic patients in psychiatric hospitals. *Medical Bulletin of Veterans Administration, 8,* 1–20.

Sifneos, P. (1966). Manipulative suicide. *Psychiatric Quarterly, 40,* 525–537.

Slater, J., & Depue, R.A. (1981). The contribution of environmental events and social support to serious suicide attempts in primary depressive disorder. *Journal of Abnormal Psychology, 90,* 275–285.

Stengel, E. (1957). *Attempted suicide.* London: Chapman & Hall.

Stengel, E. (1960). The complexity of motivations to suicidal attempts. *Journal of Mental Science, 106,* 1388.

Stengel, E. (1964). *Suicide and attempted suicide.* Baltimore: Penguin.

Stengel, E., & Cook, N. (1958). *Attempted suicide.* London: Oxford University Press.

Strosahl, K., Linehan, M.M., Chiles, J.A., & Ivanoff, A. (submitted for publication). Prediction of suicide intent in hospitalized parasuicides: Reasons for living, hopelessness, and depression.

Taylor, E.A., & Stansfeld, S.A. (1984). Children who poison themselves: I. a clinical comparison with psychiatric controls. *British Journal of Psychiatry, 145,* 127–135.

Topol, P., & Reznikoff, M. (1982). Perceived peer and family relationships, hopelessness and locus of control as factors in adolescent suicide attempts. *Suicide and Life-Threatening Behavior, 12,* 141–150.

Vinoda, K.S. (1966). Personality characteristics of attempted suicides. *British Journal of Psychiatry, 112,* 1143–1150.

Virkkunen, M. (1976). Attitude to psychiatric treatment before suicide in schizophrenia and paranoid psychoses. *British Journal of Psychiatry, 128,* 47–49.

Weeke, A. (1979). Causes of death in manic-depressives. In M. Schou & E. Stromgren (eds), *Origin, prevention and treatment of affective disorders.* London: Academic Press.

Weissman, M.M. (1974). The epidemiology of suicide attempts 1960 to 1974. *Archives of General Psychiatry, 30,* 737–746.

Weissman, M., Fox, K., & Klerman, G.L. (1973). Hostility and depression associated with suicide attempts. *American Journal of Psychiatry, 130,* 450–454.

Wetzel, R.D. (1976). Semantic differential ratings of concepts and suicide intent. *Journal of Clinical Psychology, 32,* 11–12.

Winokur, G., Clayton, P., & Reich, T. (1969). *Manic-depressive illness: 108.* St Louis, Miss.: Mosby.

Wolfgang, M.E. (1958). *Patterns in criminal homicide.* New York: John Wiley & Sons.

Yarden, P.E. (1974). Observations on suicide in chronic schizophrenics. *Comprehensive Psychiatry, 154,* 325–333.

KEY WORDS

Suicide, diathesis–stress model, stress, parasuicide, suicide intent, suicide ideation, social support, vulnerability factors, negative life expectancies, suicidogenic expectancies, negative life events, interpersonal loss, social conflict, illness, psychiatric disorder, problem-solving skills, reasons for living, hopelessness, distress tolerance.

Handbook of Life Stress, Cognition and Health
Edited by S. Fisher and J. Reason
© 1988 John Wiley & Sons Ltd.

15

Life Events, Stress and Addiction

FIONA O'DOHERTY and JOHN BOOTH DAVIES
University of Strathclyde, Glasgow, Scotland

INTRODUCTION

The association between stressful events and illness has already been discussed in other chapters. In areas such as heart disease and cancer, the focus of the work is, in principle at least, clear, and at some level of discrimination it is possible to say with confidence that cardiac malfunction or tumour has occurred or is present, and that it presents a health problem. In other areas, however, there is more ambiguity. For example, in studies of life events and 'depression', the picture is complicated by the fact that the distinction between ill and not ill is less well defined. Thus any work touching on the relationship between life events and illness (however defined) becomes more open to individual bias and interpretation.

Nowhere is this more true than in the area of research which examines the link between life events and addiction. Whilst historically a disease notion of the nature of addiction has held sway throughout the earlier part of this century, it has become increasingly plain that such a view is somewhat misplaced. Recent research has shown how even such cornerstones as withdrawal symptoms, dependence, irresistible craving, and rapid reinstatement of symptoms after periods of withdrawal, are very much dependent on social and psychological factors. Indeed, the often disputed ability of 'alcoholics' to return to normal patterns of drinking has a literature in its own right, and strikes at the very heart of the notion of alcoholism-as-disease. The position taken here is one which has been increasingly advocated in the field of addiction over the past 10 or 15 years, namely that the blanket application of a disease model creates more problems than it solves. Instead, the attempt to understand addicted behaviour has increasingly concentrated on social, behavioural and cognitive factors. It is not disputed that there are pharmacological effects of drug use, that people come to depend on their drug of choice, and that sometimes their drug use results in serious health consequences. Nonetheless, drug use is fundamentally a form of voluntary behaviour. Voluntary because, in the early stages at least, the reasons for use are in most cases hedonistic. Thus most drug users start using drugs not as an escape from a cruel world, but primarily because it is a very pleasurable experience for them. Most people drink for precisely that reason. Voluntary, also, because at various stages during the course of their addiction, many users show a degree of control and choice with respect to their pattern of use which many would find surprising, a picture which is markedly different from the one usually portrayed in the media. (On this point the reader is referred to the recent Royal College of Psychiatrists' report (1987) in which it is noted that deaths due to illicit drug use number some 200–300 annually, though this is increasing. By contrast, deaths attributable to alcohol number some 25 000 and those due to smoking in the region of 100 000. In terms of mortality, the socially sanctioned drugs, alcohol and tobacco, present by far the biggest problem, a fact which again seldom emerges in media coverage. Secondly, the term 'drug abuse' is now, in the addiction literature, habitually taken to include all drugs, and not merely the illicit ones. Some readers may be surprised, therefore, to find in the following paragraphs that all problems of substance misuse are referred to as 'drug misuse', since it is popularly assumed by many that the term refers only to the misuse of illicit drugs.)

The relegation of the disease model to a less prominent position has certain consequences for the study of life events and addiction. Firstly, rather than looking for links between stressful or other events and some medically diagnosable condition, one is seeking links between events and a type of behaviour. Whilst there are obvious factors which specifically characterize the area of drug abuse, in principle the task is the same as looking for links between events and *any* type of behaviour. Furthermore, in the area of addiction, when one talks of predispositions or vulnerability factors, one needs to be aware that the words have slightly different connotations than usual. The questions 'Predisposition to what?' and 'Vulnerability to what?' might equally well be asked in connection with many other voluntary acts, especially those involving risk or sensation seeking. Consequently, such factors emerge not at the level of individual characteristics such as personality (for which there is no convincing evidence) or genetic make-up (for which there is very limited and unsatisfactory evidence), but at the level of variables such as area of residence, choice of friends, source of income, attitudes and values, and so forth.

In an area such as coronary heart disease, there is a strong commonsense basis for a 'theory' of the relationship between stress and illness. If a researcher found that heart disease was *most common* amongst individuals experiencing *no* stressful events, and *lowest* amongst those experiencing the *most* stress, it would be apparent that something was wrong. However, in the area of addiction research, there is no comparable commonsense theory. On the one hand, one can argue that drug use is a response to stress, poor social conditions, unemployment, and so forth; and on the other hand, it is clear that some drug use, for instance the illegal use of cocaine, is associated with a comfortable, upwardly mobile, middle-class lifestyle. It also appears to be the case that stresses and trauma associated with illicit use of hard drugs are frequently the very factors that lead many users to give up; consequently coming *off* drugs is also associated with the experience of stressful events. There is evidence for all these positions, and indeed some workers have proposed exactly opposite motivational theories to explain contradictory findings.

For example, in studies of smokers, Gunn (1983) found that recent life stress, occurring prior to treatment, was a predictor of later failure at giving up cigarettes. The author concluded that stressful life events were responsible for 'poor motivation in men who come to "stop smoking" clinics'. For comparison, it is interesting to consider Prochaska and Lapsanski's (1982) study, in which it was found that *positive* life events were associated with failure to stop smoking. In this case the authors suggested that motivation to maintain abstinence was eroded because things got better prior to treatment so that subjects no longer had a reason to give up. Clearly, these two sets of findings can only be reconciled with difficulty, and then only at the level of some higher-order (and as yet non-existent) theoretical statement about how stressful and non-stressful events influence addictive behaviour. The absence of any compelling theoretical development dealing with the problem of how stress and addiction are related is, however, one of the major shortcomings in this area. Consequently, given these and many other similar findings, if one were to ask the question 'Is there a connection between the experience of stressful life events and addiction?', the answer would probably be 'Yes'. If one then asked 'What is the nature of the relationship?', the answer, on the basis of the available evidence, would have to be 'It's difficult to say'. The lack of an obvious commonsense directionality to the theory is what prompted Edwards (1984) to remark that there was as yet little understanding of the 'natural history' of addiction, and the lack of such an account is only now being remedied.

Finally, by way of introduction, it is worth pointing out that the failure of a clear-cut consensus to emerge from the literature throws into relief a number of methodological problems which might not otherwise come to light. The absence of such a consensus raises problems of non-comparability between studies in terms of methods, and also leads to greater methodological scrutiny. These issues are covered in detail in a paper by O'Doherty and Davies, (1987a) but may be summarized as problems of sampling, of control groups, problems of retrospective recall (which is known to be unreliable, particularly with respect to recollection of timing of events), and absence of a testable theory. The interested reader might like to pursue these issues further by examining the literature, but some of them are highlighted in the partial review that follows.

THE EVIDENCE

Drug Misuse as a Response to Stress

The idea that drugs provide an effective means of tension reduction has been fairly well explored. In relation to the particular stresses caused by life events, it has been proposed that the use of drugs (a) can alleviate the stressful effects of life events, and therefore (b) are taken for that purpose. Not everyone agrees however. Within the life events literature there are studies which conclude that high stress leads to increased consumption or increased likelihood of starting drug use, but there are also a number of studies showing that life stress *reduces* the likelihood of use.

Two studies have examined stress and how it is related to continued problem drinking amongst alcohol abusers (Moos *et al.,* 1979; Billings and Moos, 1983). Both studies found that less stress in the family environment was associated with better treatment outcome amongst drinkers, i.e. there was decreased incidence of relapse. Furthermore, stress at work was also related to poorer treatment outcome in the second study. It seems therefore that these studies support the idea that people drink more when their family and work environments are highly stressful. However, Miller *et al.* (1983) found that the longer a problem drinker remained abstinent from alcohol, the greater the reduction in family problems and consequently in associated stresses in the family environment. There is thus an alternative explanation for the results of the two studies above, namely that excessive alcohol use creates tension and stress and that abstaining from it reduces tension and stress. In these studies there was no examination of the direction of the causal link between stress and drinking.

In order to clarify whether family stress is predictive of drinking or merely a result of that drinking, prospective studies need to be carried out. Unfortunately this type of study is extremely rare in addiction research. Krueger (1981), however, did use a prospective design to study heroin addicts on a methadone maintenance regimen. The Holmes and Rahe (1967) Social Readjustment Rating Scale (SRRS) was administered to 270 subjects and readministered to those who subsequently relapsed (n=48). Comparisons were made between the relapsers' second scores and non-relapsers' scores at the earlier time. Once again higher life stress was found for those who relapsed. Note, though, that the interpretation of these results as supporting the 'addiction as a response to stress' argument, is crucially dependent on the assumption that scores of the non-relapsers remained the same, and this was not in fact examined. However, in another study, Reinecker and Zauner (1983) attempted to overcome the problem of retrospective data collection by examining life stress in the lives of a group who were 'at risk' for developing problem drinking, but who were not yet addicted. When these people were compared with a group who were 'not at risk', increased levels of life stress were found in the 'at risk' group. This is an impressive result and does support the hypothesis that drinking follows stressful life situations.

On the other hand, the actual number of stressful events was found by Rosenberg (1983) to be similar in both relapsers and non-relapsers in an alcohol treatment programme. The relapsers were more likely, however, to perceive the events as negative and the non-relapsers were more likely to perceive the events as positive. It is suggested that those who relapsed were more susceptible to stress than those who did not relapse, but, unfortunately, this is one of several studies in which the results could be explained by the fact that the data were collected after subjects had relapsed. With hindsight, the relapsers may have interpreted their lives more negatively because they had relapsed, and the results could thus be due to 'making sense' of their situation. A similar type of comparison of life stress in a group of alcohol abusers and a group of heroin users was made in two studies by Dudley *et al.* (1974; 1976). High levels of life stress were found in both groups.

Again the authors were interested not only in the amount of stress experienced, but also in the way in which the drinkers and heroin users perceived that stress. Their first study showed that the alcohol group underestimated the amount of stressfulness and life change which would result from certain events, but the heroin addicts were more like a normal or non-addict group. However, the later study did not confirm these differences. The results of the earlier study support the hypothesis that alcohol reduces the impact of stressful events, but a stress reduction role for heroin was not supported by either of the studies and no explanation was offered for the fact that the differences between the groups were not maintained at the later follow-up.

Neff and Husaini (1982) approach the problem from a different angle. They hypothesized a functional role for alcohol in ameliorating the effects of stressful life events. The underlying assumption in their work is that the occurrence of stressful life events is associated with an increase in depression, and that alcohol 'buffers' the stress and thereby reduces the risk of depression. Hence, increased alcohol consumption will be associated with *lower* indices of depression. However, the evidence is equivocal. First, in confirmation of the hypothesis, a positive correlation between the number of negative life events and level of depression was reported for an abstinent group, and this was not found in a moderate drinking group. However, a positive relationship between life events and depression reappeared when a heavy drinking group was examined. One possibility is that moderate and heavy drinking groups are fundamentally different. Perhaps the short-term ameliorating effect is swamped by the penalties of *heavy* drinking and these penalties create further events which propagate depression. Thus the authors may be implicitly proposing an interaction between the capacity of alcohol to ameliorate stress, and level of consumption, though this is highly speculative. The study is notable, however, for the attempt to provide theoretical insight into the relationship of life stress to drinking by hypothesizing a counter-intuitive relationship with consumption (i.e. depression will be lower amongst drinkers, and higher amongst non-drinkers). The relationship between life events and depression was also studied amongst heroin users in two studies by Kosten *et al.* (1983; 1986). In the first of these studies, addicts who reported low numbers of life events were less likely to become depressed. In the second, a follow-up of the same addicts 2.5 years later, it was found that depression at the initial interview (and therefore higher life stress at the initial interview) was associated with continued heroin use. Interestingly, however, it was also found that recent stressful events at the second interview (i.e. in the 5 months prior to follow-up) were associated with better treatment outcome. This means that stressful events were associated both with maintaining use and with remission. It appears that support for the stress-buffering role of heroin is equivocal, and that the impact of a stressful event might vary with the pattern and extent of drug use at the time.

Pathways into Drug Use

A number of authors have examined pathways into alcohol, tobacco and opiate use, and the role of stress in initiating use.

Davies and Stacey (1972) examined factors which led to adolescent drinking. Their conclusion was that social and environmental influences, such as having friends who drank, having more pocket money, and attending parties and dances where alcohol was available, were the main factors leading to teenage drinking. A set of items measuring anxiety and stress did not discriminate between drinkers and non-drinkers. This does not, of course, mean that none of the adolescents started drinking as a result of anxiety/stress, but that, if there were any, their numbers were small. On the same theme, Rounsaville et al. (1982) looked at life environment prior to initial drug use in 384 opiate addicts. Only 31% of their sample were found to have experienced at least two traumatic childhood events; 45% of the sample had neither experienced childhood trauma nor were delinquent prior to drug use. Again, although some individuals may have started using drugs in response to stress, this was certainly not the case for most users.

In another study, however, Duncan (1977) examined the incidence of stressful events amongst a group of 31 drug-dependent adolescents and compared it with the norms for junior and high-school children. Increased levels of stressful life events were found for the drug users. A major problem with this study, however, is that many groups, when compared to norms for 2000 unmatched 'controls', might exhibit different scores for any number of reasons due to uncontrolled factors (e.g. social, employment, educational, family situation). Thus the authors conclusion that 'drug use is a stress induced disorder' is a dubious one.

With respect to the onset of smoking, Brunswick and Messeri (1983) carried out a longitudinal study of adolescents. Different predictors of smoking were found for males and females, but poor academic record and certain socioeconomic variables were important predictors of smoking for all. However, the model derived from this study was useful for only a small number of smokers, showing once again that drug users are not a homogeneous group. If stress is an important predictor of smoking, it appears to be so only for a small number of people. In a similar vein, the classic study of young smokers by Bynner (1969) showed that smoking amongst 11–15 year olds was associated with social, economic, educational and attitudinal factors.

It remains now to consider the alternative hypothesis, namely that increased life change or increased stress leads to remission from drug problems. Some support for this is to be found in the literature on spontaneous remission.

Spontaneous Remission

Smart (1976), in a review of the alcohol literature, found that the factors people reported as assisting recovery from alcohol problems included changes in health, employment, marital status and residence—all of which are standard items on life event scales. Thus, increased life stress is reported both by drinkers who have relapsed, as in the previous studies, and by drinkers who are in remission. Saunders and Kershaw (1979) and Tuchfeld (1981) have confirmed Smart's conclusions. Both of these studies involved identifying and interviewing a population of ex-problem drinkers, and examining the reasons which they gave for giving up problem drinking. Broadly similar reasons were given by subjects in the two studies, including major life events, such as marriage, job change, death of a relative, and changes in health. Similarly, an important study by Stimson and Oppenheimer (1982), which followed up 128 heroin users 10 years after they had first registered as addicts with London clinics, found that of the 31% who were subsequently found to be drug free, the majority cited changing personal circumstances, with or without added 'triggers', as the main cause of their remission. The added triggers were often stressful life events, and included such things as death of a friend while in the clinic waiting room. In all the above studies, however, the problems of retrospective data collection and attribution of meaning to events in the past are apparent.

Finally, in relation to tobacco use, Eisinger (1972) found in a prospective study that the ill-health of a friend or relative as a result of smoking was the best predictor of giving up smoking.

The studies of smokers, drinkers and heroin users referred to above give some idea of the complex relationship between stressful events and addiction. Whereas for some individuals stress may be an important trigger in starting use, this explanation is certainly not appropriate for the majority of users. Most people start using drugs as a pleasurable activity, and sociodemographic variables, family and peer group influences are extremely important factors in determining who will and who will not use. On the other hand, stressful events undoubtedly arise in the course of problem use of these substances, sometimes as a consequence of the drug use itself. The impact of any or all of these events may be to increase or maintain consumption, or it may be to reduce consumption and may lead to the person 'coming off' and giving up drug use altogether.

There is no simple explanation for how that varying role of stress operates, and the task for future research is to provide some theoretical insight into how such a mechanism might operate.

Preliminary Results of a Recent Study

In the light of comments made in the introduction, and the specific points made in the review section, it seems appropriate to provide a brief description of some of the methods employed, and results obtained, from a recent investigation carried out by the Addiction Research Group at the University of Strathclyde (O'Doherty and Davies, 1987b). The study involved three groups of substance users, all encountering problems with their use, and a pool of control subjects. The target groups were smokers, drinkers, and users of illicit drugs (principally heroin), and the pool of control subjects was derived so as to provide comparable groups in terms of age, sex, social class and demographic variables. The heroin users and those with alcohol problems were recruited from a variety of sources, including in-patient treatment centres, out-patient clinics and day centres. The smokers were recruited through 'stop smoking' clinics or through newspaper advertisements. All the smokers expressed, if intermittently, a desire to give up smoking. Controls were recruited mainly through contacts of the substance-using groups. All controls identified themselves as non-smokers, non-drug users and non-heavy drinkers.

An attempt was made to tackle some of the methodological problems referred to earlier. In order to minimize the problems associated with retrospective recall, each subject was interviewed repeatedly, at 3-monthly intervals, with up to six interviews per person. At each interview they recalled events over the previous 3 months only. Most subjects were interviewed five times, at which point the recontact rate was about 69% overall. There were 171 subjects involved, including 32 heroin users, 37 smokers and 25 drinkers. Furthermore, at each stage of analysis, each group (e.g. the heroin users, etc.) was compared in terms of the variables being investigated to a matched group of controls drawn from the 'pool' of control subjects, selected so as maximally to resemble the target group.

Each participant in the study was interviewed using a semistructured interview schedule which covered a wide variety of issues. Central topics included an account of the previous week's drug consumption and an account of significant events occurring during the prior 3 months. A rating by the subject of the specific ways in which each reported event was perceived as having an impact, if any, on different areas of his or her life, and whether such events had occurred to the subject personally or to significant others in his or her life, were also included in the interview.

We were interested to use the data obtained to try to find answers to three questions. First, would the life events data enable us to distinguish between the lives of the drug misusers and their group of matched controls? Second, at an individual level, did periods of use and non-use coincide with times when stressful events were occurring or not occurring? Finally, was there any relationship between subjects' *perceptions* of events and periods of lighter or heavier use?

To answer the first of these questions we looked at the illicit drug users, drinkers, smokers, and their control groups individually. A degree of consensus emerged. For the heroin users and the drinkers it was apparent that more events were reported than by the controls. They reported significantly more events happening to themselves; but, paradoxically, they reported fewer events happening to their friends and family (significant others) than did their respective control groups. One final aspect of interest emerged when we looked at subjects' answers to the question as to whether the event(s) reported were unrelated to the addiction, or were an actual consequence of it. It was found that the majority of the events reported were *consequences* of the addiction itself. When we repeated the comparison, taking out these consequential events, the heroin users actually reported fewer events than the controls. A comparable picture emerged for the alcohol misusers. The smokers, on the other hand, presented a similar picture to their control group. Our conclusion on this first point is that our three substance-abusing groups did not experience more stressful life events than did their respective control groups (other than events caused by the addiction itself). Secondly, the fact that both the heroin users and the alcohol misusers reported more events happening to themselves, but fewer events happening to others, implies some sort of selectivity in reporting. Speculatively, it seems possible that problematic alcohol and heroin use develop to the point where less attention is given to aspects of the world not related to the self and the drug. The results are quite clearcut, and there is no other plausible reason why fewer things should happen to the friends and families of drug misusers than to the friends and families of controls.

In our second analysis we examined the hypothesis that, at an individual (within-subjects) level, periods of use and non-use would be related to differing incidence of stressful (or other) life events. Once again, the data produced results which failed to confirm any clear-cut version of the life-events theory. It should be borne in mind that for each of the analyses described, we looked not merely at the number of events which occurred. The analyses were repeated taking into account the type of event (whether it concerned health, social relationships, economic state, legal position, employment status or mood); and similar analysis took place using the 'most serious' events as criteria. The failure to find any link between drug use and events applied across the board, and the data revealed that such events occurred regularly all the time and were just as likely to happen during periods of use as during periods of non-use.

The above findings raised the question as to why subjects' reports that particular events had affected their drug use were so consistently unsupported by the data, and consideration of this issue leads, naturally enough, to the topic of social perception. It could be that although events (of whatever type) are more or less evenly distributed throughout periods of use and non-use, the subject perceives such events as reasons for coming off at particular times, but not at others; and also as reasons for relapsing at some times but not at others. We examined this issue by making use of the data obtained on subjects' perceptions of events, and the impact they were reported as having in different life areas. It was found that although there was, in fact, no difference between times of use and non-use in terms of number or nature of events, the heroin users *perceived* these events as having significantly less impact on social, financial and legal circumstances at times of non-use. For the alcohol users, a nearly identical picture emerged; at times of non-use, events were perceived as having significantly less impact on social and financial affairs.

Thus the only data set to produce support for the life-events theory concerned the perception of events rather than reports of the events themselves. Although subjects reported similar numbers and types of events whether they were using or not, they appeared to interpret these differently at times of non-use. This finding, if it were supported in future studies, would have an impact on the existing dilemmas in this area. Whilst, as we have seen, there is little consistency in the literature with respect to reports of life events and the relationship of these to drug use, the consistency of the phenomena involved might lie at quite a different level. If this is indeed the case, then the pressing question becomes. '*Why* are events interpreted differently at different times?'. It is this issue which is specifically addressed in the next section, where we describe a model which provides a theoretical basis for expecting such changes in social perception to occur.

Before moving on to this new topic, however, there are two peripheral points emerging from the data which deserve special mention. Firstly, the findings described above emerge principally from the alcohol- and heroin-using groups. The smokers in the main failed to produce consistencies of any kind. This is probably because, whilst smoking and heavy smoking have consequences primarily for the individual at the level of health, the nicotine addict is not viewed with the same approbrium as an 'alcoholic' or a 'junkie'; and his or her habit does not have the same legal or social consequences. Secondly, at a purely practical level, our data show that while virtually all the illicit drug users cycled through periods of use and non-use with some regularity, and the alcohol users behaved in a similar if less marked fashion, there were only two of our smokers who provided us with non-use periods. We are inclined to conclude that whilst illicit drug users are giving up all the time (whether they stay off is a different matter), smokers only give up once, and then usually when it is too late.

A PROPOSED MODEL OF THE ADDICTION PROCESS

The intriguing findings from the above study suggest that naturally occurring events have a different impact on an individual at different times, and it now remains to offer some explanation as to why similar events are perceived differently by the same person on different occasions. A speculative theory is outlined below which goes some way towards this; and although the idea requires to be tested rigorously, preliminary analyses suggest it may have some value.

The suggestion is that 'tolerance' (i.e. the change in the effect of a drug with repeated use) is the key to this change in the perception of events. The fact that, with continued use, more of a drug is required to produce the same effect, is well documented. Thus, a regular heroin user may progress to a level of daily use that would prove fatal to an initiate. A similar picture is seen with alcohol. In order to obtain the same effect as with first use, a regular drinker increases the quantity of alcohol consumed. The picture with respect to tobacco is, however, less clear. Undoubtedly tolerance does develop, but possibly over a much longer time span than is the case for either heroin or alcohol.

Although the mechanisms underlying tolerance to a drug can be explained in pharmacological and physiological terms, tolerance is also observed in circumstances in which no drug is involved. For example, people who like to travel may escalate the distances involved to cover more and more exotic places, in order to get the same satisfaction they experienced from more modest excursions at an earlier time. It seems that, even in the absence of drugs, people often want progressively more of what they enjoy. In such circumstances tolerance tends to be explained at a 'psychological' level (despite the fact that the mechanisms underlying tolerance in these situations and in situations where a drug is used can both be explained in the same terms). These common 'psychological' factors are often seriously underestimated in accounts of tolerance to drugs, where the explanation is often given purely in terms of the physiology/pharmacology of drug action. Tolerance thus requires explanation on at least two levels, and cannot adequately be explained at any one level. For the present purposes, we merely invoke the phenomenon of tolerance, without subscribing to any one view of the mechanisms involved.

The central idea of the model is that changes in the perception of events take place as a consequence of changes in tolerance. At an early stage, the 'high' is achieved on a modest amount of drug, with relatively little by way of economic pressure and other 'hassles'. As tolerance develops, this balance changes. More drug is required, costing more money, and involving more 'hassles', but the 'high' remains more or less constant. Eventually, a point is reached where the 'high' gets harder and harder to achieve, despite continuing use of the drug. At this point users often feel that they have reached some sort of plateau, and are using only 'to keep normal' or 'straight'. Avoidance of withdrawal symptoms becomes the main reinforcer of the behaviour as its pleasurable component (i.e. the 'high') is now less frequent. Finally, the absence of this reinforcing 'high', plus the frequent negative consequences associated with a high level of use, now present a very different 'cost-benefit' picture than was the case in the early stages of drug use.

In the context of the above, we can now speculate as to how events might be perceived differently at different times. For instance, a health event such as hospitalization will not be interpreted as a reason for stopping if 'highs' are easily and cheaply achieved. On the other hand, it may be a reason for stopping drug taking if it comes at a time of heavy use and 'hassles', and without the reinforcing effect of the 'high'. Thus, costs and benefits of use are reassessed as the user moves through a 'tolerance cycle'. (The word 'cycle' is taken to imply a process which can repeat many times.) Furthermore, since, after a period of abstinence, tolerance returns to more normal levels, the conditions are created for a new cycle of drug use possibly to commence. Finally, with the achievement of a lower level of tolerance (following a period of abstinence), an event which was previously maintaining abstinence may now be perceived as a reason for relapse.

On the basis of observation, it seems that some individuals may move more quickly through the cycle than others; and also that heroin users seem to cycle more rapidly and frequently than alcohol users and smokers. A further observation is that some drug users (for instance social drinkers) do not cycle through the stages outlined, remaining instead at stages 1 and 2 (see Fig. 15.1). Presumably, individuals whose drug taking has stabilized are able to exercise control over the conditions under which high tolerance is likely to develop.

The model, outlined in Figure 15.1, still requires considerable development; however, it serves as a starting point for the elaboration of a theory of how life events influence the addiction process. It represents an effort to rectify the problem of lack of a theory which, as pointed out in the opening sections of this chapter, creates major problems in this area.

OVERVIEW

Despite the belief in many quarters that stressful life events play an important causal role in the development of drug-related problems, our review of the literature on life events and addiction does not provide clear-cut evidence for this proposition. The evidence for the hypothesis is equivocal, and the picture is clouded by a number of confounding factors. It may be the case that future research, focusing more clearly on problems of retrospective recall and matched control groups, and with a greater degree of theoretical specificity, will provide more satisfactory evidence for the main proposition. In the mean time, the picture remains uncertain. It is also worth bearing in mind that many of the problems

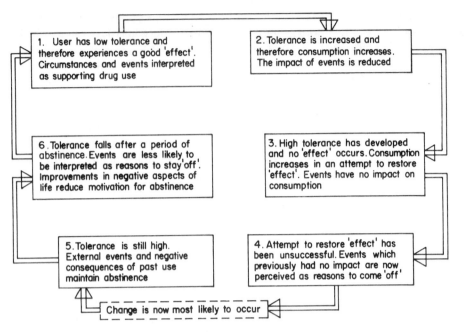

FIG. 15.1   A cyclical model of problem substance use.

thrown up by studies in the area of addiction are also to varying degrees present in the broader life-events and illness literature, and that the specific area of drug use is not uniquely afflicted with these difficulties. It is worth taking note of a quote from Schroeder and Costa (1984) referring to research into life events and illness generally, that 'the life-event paradigm does not employ an appropriate operationalization of stress'.

Our own studies go only part of the way towards solving some of these problems, though we feel they may possibly suggest a few new strategies for the future. The main suggestion for further research, arising from our own work, is that more account needs to be taken of people's own *perceptions* of the things that happen to them. Even the use of independent raters does not overcome the problem of idiosyncratic interpretation, yet it is this individual interpretation of events which seems most likely to support the life-events-and-addiction link. The problem remains as to how one elicits this interpretation without the reintroduction of confounding factors. This is not an easy problem to solve, but the answer, although not a definitive solution, lies somewhere in the realm of prospective design.

Although further research could be carried out on vulnerability factors which undoubtedly account for some individuals' greater susceptibility to stress, possibly leading to increased likelihood of drug use, research in these areas has not proved very productive to date. As outlined in the introduction to this chapter, the search for genetic links, or 'addictive personality types', has been of limited usefulness. Vulnerability factors which have been found to be predictive of drug use are for the most part social and demographic in nature.

It seems, then, that future research might usefully give attention to the individual's personal perception of the costs and benefits of use, if sense is to be made of the frequently cited link between life events and addiction. As Bannister and Fransella (1971) wrote, 'A man does not respond to a stimulus, but to what he perceives that stimulus to be'. This statement is fundamental, but also misleading if we believe that we can isolate *the* perception and use that as our main dependent variable (a procedure implied by consensus ratings of life events, for example) when in fact perception changes according to circumstance, expectations and so forth. There is in fact no single perception that can be tied to an event. The whole point about social perception is that it changes where the event does not.

One of the basic questions arising from this chapter is, 'Can stress cause drug use?'. From the review of the literature and the conclusions of our own study, it seems that the answer is 'sometimes'. On the other hand, the answer to the question 'Is drug use primarily a response to stressful circumstances?', on the basis of the available evidence, appears to be 'No'. This apparent contradiction is explained by the fact that whilst drug users do not comprise a homogeneous group, the majority of them begin and continue using drugs (frequently in a manner which leads eventually to serious problems) because drug use is, amongst other things, pleasurable and self-reinforcing. A number of people use drugs to alleviate stresses in their lives, but there is little justification for generalizing this fact to explain drug use in the general population.

SUMMARY AND CONCLUSIONS

Methodological and conceptual problems abound in studies of life events and addiction. Furthermore, the absence of any strong theoretical model is exceedingly problematic. In our own studies, we have failed to find any differences in the number or type of stressful life events which distinguish users from non-users, with the exception of events which are consequential on the addiction itself. A model is proposed which explains the relationship between life events and addiction as resulting from changes in tolerance which alter the balance of costs and benefits associated with drug use, and thereby influences the way in which life events are interpreted.

REFERENCES

Bannister, D., & Fransella, F. (1971). *Inquiring man: the theory of personal constructs.* Harmondsworth: Penguin.

Billings, A.G., & Moos, R.H. (1983). Psychosocial processes of recovery among alcoholics and their families: Implications for clinicians and programme evaluators. *Addictive Behaviours, 8,* 205–218.

Brunswick, A., & Messeri, P. (1983). Causal factors in onset of adolescents cigarette smoking. In H. Shaffer & B. Stimmel (eds), *The addictive behaviours.* New York: Hawthorn Press.

Bynner, J.M. (1969). The young smoker. London: HMSO.

Davies, J., & Stacey, B. (1972). Teenagers and alcohol. London: HMSO.

Dudley, D.L., Roszell, D.K., & Mules, J.E. (1974). Heroin and alcohol addiction—Quantifiable psychosocial similarities and differences. *Journal of Psychosomatic Research, 18,* 327–335.

Dudley, D.L., Mules, J.E., Roszell, D.K., Glickfeld, G., & Hague, W.H. (1976). Frequency and magnitude distribution of life change in heroin and alcohol addicts. *International Journal of the Addictions, 11*(6), 977–987.

Duncan, D.F. (1977). Life stress as a precurser to adolescent drug dependence. *International Journal of Addictions, 12*(8), 1047–1056.

Edwards, G. (1984). Drinking in longitudinal perspective: Career and natural history. *British Journal of Addiction, 79,* 175–183.

Eisinger, R.A. (1972). Psychological predictors of smoking behaviour change. *Social Science and Medicine, 6,* 137–144.

Gunn, R.C. (1983). Smoking clinic failures and recent life stress. *Addictive Behaviours, 8*(1), 83–87.

Holmes, T.H. & Rahe, R.H. (1967). The Social Readjustment Rating Scale. *Journal of Psychosomatic Research, 11,* 213–218.

Kosten, T.R., Rounsaville, M.D., Herbert, D., & Kleber, M.D. (1986). A 2.5 year follow up of depression, life crisis and treatment effects on abstinence among opioid addicts. *Archives of General Psychiatry, 43,* 733–738.

Kosten, T.R., Rounsaville, B.J., & Kleber, H.D. (1983). Relationship of depression to psychosocial stressors in heroin addicts. *Journal of Nervous and Mental Disorders, 171*(2), 97–104.

Krueger, D.W. (1981). Stressful life events and the return to heroin use. *Human Stress, 7,* 3–8.

Miller, W.R., Hendrick, K.E., & Taylor, C.A. (1983). Addictive behaviour and life problems before and after behavioural treatment of problem drinkers. *Addictive Behaviours, 8,* 403–412.

Moos, R.H., Bromet, E., Tsu, V., & Moos, B. (1979). Family characteristics and the outcome of treatment for alcoholism. *Journal of Studies on Alcohol, 40*(1), 78–88.

Neff, J.A., & Husaini, B.A. (1982). Life events, drinking patterns and symptomatology. *Journal of Studies on Alcohol, 43*(3), 301–318.

O'Doherty, F., & Davies, J. (1987a). Life events and addiction: A critical review. *British Journal of Addiction, 82,* 127–137.

O'Doherty, F., & Davies, J. (1987b). The effect of naturally occurring life events on changes in consumption of alcohol, tobacco and heroin. Unpublished study.

Prochaska, J.D., & Lapsanski, D.V. (1982). Life changes, cessation and maintenance of smoking: A preliminary report. *Psychological Reports, 50,* 609–610.

Reinecker, H., & Zauner, H. (1983). Critical life events as risk factors for alcoholism. *Archiv für Psychiatrie und Nervenkrankheiten 233*(4), 333–346.

Rosenberg, H. (1983). Relapsed versus non-relapsed alcohol abusers: coping skills, life events, and social support. *Addictive Behaviours, 8,* 183–186.

Rounsaville, B.J., Weissman, M.M., Wilber, C.H., & Kleber, H.D. (1982). Pathways to opiate addiction: An evaluation of differing antecedents. *British Journal of Psychiatry, 141,* 437–446.

Royal College of Psychiatrists (1987). *Drug scenes: A report on drugs and drug dependence.* London: Gaskell.

Saunders, W.M., & Kershaw, P.W. (1979). Spontaneous remission from alcoholism: A community study. *British Journal of Addictions, 74,* 251–265.

Schroeder, D.H., & Costa, P.T. (1984). Influence of life event stress on physical illness: Substantive effects or methodological flaws? *Journal of Personality and Social Psychology, 46,* 853–863.

Smart, R.G. (1976). Spontaneous recovery in alcoholics: A review and analysis of the available research. *Drug and Alcohol Dependence, 1,* 277–285.

Stimson, G., & Oppenheimer, E. (1982). *Heroin addiction.* London: Tavistock.

Tuchfeld, B.S. (1981). Spontaneous remission in alcoholics. *Journal of Studies on Alcohol, 42,* 626–641.

KEY WORDS

Life events, addiction, heroin, alcohol, tobacco, stress, consumption, substance use, tolerance, cyclical model.

Handbook of Life Stress, Cognition and Health
Edited by S. Fisher and J. Reason
© 1988 John Wiley & Sons Ltd.

16

Stress and Heart Disease

BRUCE BOMAN
Repatriation General Hospital, Concord, Australia

INTRODUCTION

Psychosocial variables are now recognized as contributing (along with high blood pressure, obesity, lack of exercise, cigarette smoking and high blood cholesterol) to the development of coronary heart disease. A common denominator for many of these psychosocial variables is a significant change to one's personal, social or cultural environment which requires major adjustment and adaptation. Such stresses include rapid economic change, bereavement, migration, upward social mobility, and employment pressures. Individuals whose personalities drive them into a striving, competitive and acquisitive lifestyle have a greater risk of heart disease, while social support and cultural cohesion offer a significant degree of protection against its development.

Clinicians have been impressed for many years by an association between ischaemic heart disease and both stressful life events and a certain personality configuration (Friedman and Rosenman, 1974). In 1910, Sir William Osler described his typical angina case as 'not the delicate, neurotic person but the robust, the vigorous in mind and body, the keen and ambitious man, the indicator of whose engine is always at full speed ahead!'.

Such soundly based clinical impressions have subsequently been bolstered by a substantial amount of research evidence, and it can now be confidently asserted that psychosocial influences constitute (along with smoking, obesity, hypertension, diet, raised serum cholesterol, diabetes and lack of exercise) a risk factor for ischaemic heart disease. While the exact nature of this variable has yet to be refined and its mechanism of action is still unclear, nine main strands can be discerned from the presently available data. These will now be elaborated on in turn.

TYPE A BEHAVIOUR AND ISCHAEMIC HEART DISEASE

Physicians have long noted an association between behavioural styles and coronary artery disease. As already mentioned, Sir William Osler (1910) described the

301

angina patient as one who worked at maximum capacity, incessantly striving for success in commercial, professional or political life. In 1868, Van Dusch observed a relationship between coronary artery disease and persons with excessive work involvement who exhibited a loud and forceful type of speech, and Flanders Dunbar (1947), in her pioneering writings on psychosomatics, gave a description of the personality type likely to develop coronary heart disease as ambitious, overachieving, compulsive and striving after goals.

However, systematic research in this area only began in the 1950s, with the work of Friedman and Rosenman (see review by Matthews, 1982). Starting with observations made in their clinical practice on the similarity in behavioural characteristics of young men with ischaemic heart disease, they went on to define a specific behavioural pattern associated with the development of this disease, which they called Type A.

The Type A behavioural pattern (TABP) comprises a cluster of actions and emotions exhibited by individuals who engage themselves in a chronic struggle to achieve more and more in less and less time, and usually in the face of opposition from people and events in their environment. Consequently, they are performing persistently at near-maximum capacity, have a hyperresponsivity to what they perceive as any challenge to their success, see those around them as competitors, display a generalized hostility and sense of time urgency, and often concentrate on more than one task at a time. Such individuals are preoccupied with themselves and their advancement and have a driving need for control and mastery, which usually leads them to neglect aspects of their life other than their careers (Friedman and Rosenman, 1974).

Friedman and Rosenman have developed a challenging interview known as the Structured Interview (SI) to bring out and assess such qualities. In this, subjects are asked about their habitual responses to situations engendering impatience, hostility and competitiveness, in addition, some of the questions are deliberately presented in a provocative manner, with the assessment of resultant speech patterns and non-verbal behaviours comprising a significant part of the diagnostic process. The Diagnostic Interview places individuals in one of four categories: A1, fully developed Type A behaviour pattern; A2, incompletely developed Type A behaviour; X, an equal representation of Type A and Type B characteristics; and B, the absence of Type A features. It also has the curious propensity of dividing a population (at least a white, middle-class American one) into roughly half Type As and half Type Bs.

A second technique for assessing the TABP is the Jenkin's Activity Survey (JAS), a self-report questionnaire based on a series of discriminant function analyses of a large population administered the SI. Factor analysis of the items has yielded three independent factors: H, or hard-driving competitiveness; S, or speed and impatience; and J, or job involvement (Jenkins et al., 1971). Other self-report measures developed to assess the TABP are the Framingham Type A Scale and the Bortner Scale (Haynes and Feinleib, 1982; Bortner, 1969). While all of these measures possess a reasonable degree of reliability, their degree of correlation is not particularly impressive, with the three self-rating scales concurring with the SI at only between 10% and 25% above chance levels (Matthews, 1982).

As one might anticipate, prevalence studies in both the US and Europe have found that the TABP tends to be concentrated among successful, well-educated, male, white-collar workers occupying higher occupational and socioeconomic positions and dwelling in densely populated and industrialized urban environments (Matthews, 1982).

Numerous studies have now demonstrated an excess of TABP among patients suffering from coronary heart disease (CHD) over non-coronary controls, an association most marked among younger CHD sufferers and in those with symptomatic angina (Matthews, 1982). Cases of myocardial infarction not complicated by angina, and patients with asymptomatic electrocardiographic findings are less likely to manifest Type A behaviors (Haynes and Feinleib, 1982). The most impressive evidence, however, linking the TABP with CHD has been provided by three large-scale prospective studies carried out in California, Framingham and France/Belgium.

The Western Collaborative Group Study involved the follow-up, over a mean time span of 8.5 years, of over 3000 initially healthy males (Rosenman *et al.*, 1975); 257 of these went on to develop CHD, with Type As being twice as likely to get the disorder as Type Bs. When the autopsy findings of those subjects who had died from non-coronary causes were examined, it was found that Type A subjects had a more advanced degree of atherosclerosis in their major coronary vessels.

The Framingham Study followed up for 10 years 750 females and 580 males, who were CHD free at the time of their initial assessment (Haynes and Feinleib, 1982). The TABP emerged as a significant risk factor for the subsequent development of CHD, especially angina-related coronary disease. Type A men in white-collar employment, for example, went on twice as often to develop angina complicating other manifestations of CHD. Among women aged 45 to 64 years of age, Type A behaviour doubled the risk of developing both angina and coronary heart disease overall. However, both Western Collaborative Group and Framingham studies discerned little linkage between TABP and either silent, unrecognized myocardial infarctions or infarctions uncomplicated by angina (Haynes and Feinleib, 1982). Another finding from these two studies was that Type A behaviour amplifies the pathogenic effects of other coronary risk factors (Matthews, 1982).

The French–Belgian Collaborative Study was an 8-year prospective follow-up of some 3000 male factory workers and civil servants, which found that Type A behaviour, as measured by the Bortner Scale, correlated with the development of fatal and non-fatal myocardial infarctions, sudden cardiac deaths, and the total incidence of CHD (French–Belgian Collaborative Group, 1982). In addition, the risk of angina, infarction and sudden death increased in parallel with Bortner Scale scores, and these associations held true independent of age, systolic blood pressure, and smoking.

Hostility (one of the elements comprising the TABP) is, by itself, and independent of TABP, a risk factor for arteriographically documented coronary atherosclerosis. Thus, in a 25-year follow-up study on a large group of medical students, high hostility scores on the Minnesota Multiphase Personality Inventory during medical training correlated with both the development of clinical coronary disease as well as overall mortality (Barefoot *et al.*, 1983). Similarly, in the Western Electric Study, high hostility scores at the time of induction into the research project were predicative of both CHD and mortality rates over the subsequent 20-year follow-up period (Shekelle *et al.*, 1983).

For over 20 years, it has been appreciated that the TABP is associated with a cluster of physiological and biochemical abnormalities, all of which are potentially capable of inducing atheroma formation. The list includes higher secretion rates of catecholamines and ACTH, lower growth hormone levels, enhanced blood clotting and platelet aggregation, greater serum levels of cholesterol, fasting levels of triglycerides, phospholipids and low-density lipoprotein lipids, and lowered alpha to beta lipoprotein cholesterol ratios (Friedman and Rosenman, 1974). The behavioural challenge which particularly leads to excess sympathetic autonomic activity in Type As appears to be one which combines difficulty and a moderate degree of competitiveness with the need for a slow, careful and patient response (Matthews, 1982).

LIFE EVENTS AND CORONARY PATHOLOGY

There is little doubt that acute psychophysiological arousal can trigger a potentially lethal coronary event (Lown *et al.*, 1980). One of the most notable examples of this was John Hunter's sudden death in 1793 soon after a particularly heated board meeting at St George's Hospital in London, and, as a salutary warning to his administrative successors, the couch on which he expired is still kept in the hospital boardroom.

Three mechanisms exist to explain such a phenomenon.

(a) The sympathetic arousal caused by the stressful event can trigger a ventricular arrhythmia in an electrically irritable heart (Lown *et al.*, 1980). This was nicely demonstrated when a group of sufferers from ischaemic heart disease was taken to a football match and their electrocardiograms telemetrically recorded (Rose, 1974). About half of them developed ECG changes during tense moments of the game.

(b) Stresses, especially those involving object loss, have been shown to push vulnerable individuals into congestive cardiac failure and acute pulmonary oedema (Chambers and Reiser, 1953).

(c) Affective states involving depression, helplessness, hopelessness and giving up have been implicated in excessive parasympathetic discharge down the vagal nerve to the heart, with consequent extreme cardiac slowing and even standstill (Engel, 1971). Clinical reports from the Rochester group (Engel, 1971) have provided evidence for this phenomenon, and a prospective study has revealed that an emotional climate of fatigue, apathy, malaise and depression is often a prodrome to myocardial infarction (Falger and Apels, 1982).

While life event research is bedevilled with methodological difficulties, Theorell and Rahe's group have provided impressive evidence showing that individuals who have myocardial infarctions or who die suddenly from cardiac causes have experienced an excess of life events in the weeks and months beforehand, and that there is an association between the severity of the cardiac event and the number of life changes (Theorell, 1982).

Nowadays, many researchers would view these 'first generation' studies as somewhat simplistic in failing to take appropriate cognizance of an individual's unique and personal perception of a life event and the singular emotional impact it has on him as a result of his particular character structure and his previous experiences. Such research is also confounded by a retrospective search after meaning, as the coronary sufferer sifts through the time before the heart attack, searching for its 'cause'. As a result, an event which otherwise might have been seen as mundane and innocuous could be ascribed unwarranted import and significance. On the other hand, events of some significance could be forgotten, inaccurately recalled or glossed over. To get around these problems, recent researchers have included measures of individual impact of life change. For example, Lundberg et al. (1975) found, when using standard life change unit parameters, that there was no difference in life-event scores between myocardial infarct patients and controls. However, when scales were individually developed for each subject, a quite significant difference did emerge.

The natural tendency of people either to forget or to selectively recall life events has been circumvented by asking a group of post-myocardial infarction patients to score events as they happened, and it was found that subjects who subsequently had a fatal coronary event had reported more life changes than survivors (Theorell, 1982). Brown's group at Bedford College, London, has developed a sophisticated and objective technique for eliciting and rating life events and, using this method, an excess of disturbing life events was discerned in the 3 weeks prior to infarction in a group of coronary care patients who had not experienced any preinfarction angina (Connolly, 1976).

A New Zealand study compared the life changes of a group of infarct patients with those of a group of surgical patients and found that the former group had reported approximately two and a half times as many adverse life events as the controls (Bianchi et al., 1978). This study tends to mitigate the 'search for meaning' criticism of life-event work because the surgical patients would have been just as eagerly reviewing their immediate pasts for explanations of their illnesses. Also, the authors, aware of such criticism, incorporated into their paper data on life changes independently gathered from a 'close informant' of each type of patient.

Work has also been done linking life events and the Type A behaviour pattern. Firstly, it seems that Type As, by their very behaviour, engender an excess of life events over Type Bs, that is, the TABP promotes a lifestyle which facilitates exposure to a range of social, personal and occupational stresses, the last mentioned having been shown to be particularly common (Byrne and Rosenman, 1986). Secondly, it seems that it is not so much the number or severity of life changes that engenders distress in Type As, but only those events that are perceived as being out of the individual's control (Glass, 1978).

NEUROTIC SYMPTOMS, CHARACTER STYLES AND CORONARY HEART DISEASE

While the TABP is a cluster of observable behaviours, rather than a reflection of any underlying neuroticism or character style, these two latter variables have also been linked to the risk of developing CHD.

Firstly, it has been demonstrated that the diagnosis of a neurotic disorder is substantially associated with both coronary morbidity and mortality; secondly, that patients with heart disease display an excess of neurotic symptomatology; and thirdly, that a character style associated with the expression or suppression of anger puts a person at greater risk for cardiac morbidity and mortality (Boman, 1982).

Thus mortality surveys of neurotic patients from Birmingham, Scotland, Sweden and New York have all found an increased chance of dying from cardiovascular causes at a rate about twice that expected (see review by Boman, 1982), and in men awaiting coronary angiography, a close relationship exists between scores for neuroticism and the severity of coronary artery pathology detected on their angiograms (Zyzanski *et al.*, 1976). Though burdened by all the difficulties of retrospective research, another way of examining the relationship between neurotic illness and coronary heart disease is to see whether patients suffering from cardiac disorders actually have more symptoms than a healthy control group. It is impossible, of course, to know if the anxiety and depression so described actually pre-date the onset of heart disease or were an emotional response arising from it. There have been a whole cluster of such retrospective studies, using a wide variety of measures of neurotic symptomatology and a disparate collection of experimental groups, which have found that subjects with clinically apparent coronary heart disease have reported an excess of neurotic symptoms in the periods both before and after they fell ill (see review by Boman, 1982). However, the most convincing studies linking neurotic symptoms with coronary heart disease are those prospectively examining which psychosocial variables equate with the later manifestation of heart disorders.

Ostfeld *et al.* conducted a prospective epidemiological study of 1990 initially healthy males, aged between 40 and 45, followed up over a 4.5-year period. Those who went on to develop ischaemic heart disease had complained of more subjective feelings of tension, and, of those who had a myocardial infarction, subjects who had initially scored higher on scales for anxiety and depression were at a greater risk of dying (Lebovits *et al.*, 1967). Paffenbarger's group examined the health records of students who had attended university between 1926 and 1946, and then conducted a follow-up survey in 1962. A high score on an anxiety quotient during college years correlated with non-fatal infarctions and sudden deaths in later life (Thorne *et al.*, 1968). In 1963 an Israeli group commenced a 5-year prospective study of 10 000 male government employees. Measures of anxiety, subjective tension and sleep problems correlated with the later development of coronary heart disease (Groen, 1974). The French–Belgian heart disease project (1982) found that neuroticism was strongly associated with the development of angina, independent of other risk factors. Likewise, those Framingham subjects who went on to develop CHD had initially reported that they habitually suppressed their anger and experienced tension and anxiety (Haynes and Feinleib, 1982).

FAMILY, EMPLOYMENT, LIFESTYLE STRESSES AND CORONARY HEART DISEASE

Before going on to examine this area, it might be useful to see how stress could possibly induce coronary artery atheroma. For example, it was discovered that the serum cholesterol levels of a group of accountants fluctuated during the financial year according to the amount of stress they were under: the highest levels of cholesterol coincided with the time of greatest work pressure (Friedman and Rosenman, 1974); and in a comprehensive literature review, Rosenman and Friedman (1958) pointed out that the predisposing factors for coronary heart disease (increased plasma lipids, intimal damage, altered haemodynamics and accelerated blood clotting) are all stimulated by stress.

In a now quite classical piece of research from 1953, Morris *et al.* looked at the coronary heart disease experience of male London Transport bus drivers and conductors, and showed that the latter had a significantly lower incidence of heart disease, and that in this group, when it did appear, it did so both at a later age and in a less severe form. One of the risk factors suggested for the drivers was the more responsible and stressful nature of their work. Russek and Zohman (1958) observed in young coronary patients that prolonged emotional strain, associated with job responsibility, had almost inevitably preceded their attacks, and in fact those with heart disease could be more readily differentiated from controls by occupational stress levels than by fat intake, obesity, smoking or lack of exercise. In a subsequent survey on 12 000 professional men in fourteen occupational categories, a marked gradient in distribution of heart disease was unassociated with either heredity or diet, but was strikingly related to the relative stressfulness of occupational activity (Russek, 1965). It has also been shown that if job dissatisfaction is measured for various occupational groups, then those reporting most dissatisfaction have the highest rate of coronary heart disease (Sales and House, 1971).

In research associating autopsy findings with work problem, the first-degree relatives of a group of deceased patients were asked whether in the preceding 2 years their dead relative had experienced problems at work; 53% of these cases for whom the question had been answered in the affirmative were found at autopsy to have suffered a fatal myocardial infarction, whereas only 17% of those with few or no work problems were found to have so died (Groen, 1974). In a prospective study (Groen, 1974), workers had been asked whether in the preceding 2 years they had had work problems. Of those who said they had, 13% went on to develop coronary heart disease over the next 5 years; however, only 5% of those who had reported few or no such problems went on to develop the disease. Other prestudy variables which correlated with the development of heart disease were feeling unliked by co-workers, having conflicts with the boss, and feeling that not enough affection was being shown by wives. Theorells' prospective study of 6500 middle-aged males in the Swedish construction industry found a Discord Index measuring dissatisfaction with domestic and working life was predictive of suffering a myocardial infarction during the subsequent 2 years. Work problems had a significantly greater relationship than domestic ones (Theorell and Floderus-Myrhed, 1977). Karasek's group in Sweden (1982) has gone on to explore the kinds of work stresses that may be associated with cardiac pathology, and they have proposed a model which links high work demands with an inability to make decisions, and, in three studies, they have provided substantial evidence to support their hypothesis. The Framingham Study has also demonstrated the significance of lifestyle, employment and interpersonal stresses by showing that in males under 65, ageing worries and daily stress and tension were associated with a greater risk of developing CHD, while for males and females over 65, marital dissatisfaction or disagreements were risk factors. In addition, work overload in males emerged as a factor predictive of CHD (Haynes and Feinleib, 1982).

STRESSES ASSOCIATED WITH TRANSGRESSING SOCIOCULTURAL AND ECONOMIC BOUNDARIES

Crossing barriers of social and economic class and culture produces stresses which also have been shown to be linked with coronary heart disease. In a prospective study of an annually medically examined industrial population, it was discovered that men were at a significantly higher risk of developing coronary heart disease if their social class in childhood was substantially different to the one they now occupied (Shekelle et al., 1969), and in a prospective study of Harvard graduates intergenerational mobility, in regard to father's status, was associated with later sudden cardiac death and non-fatal myocardial infarctions, even when allowance was made for standard coronary risk factors (Gillum and Paffenbarger, 1978). Similarly, among Whitehall civil servants, a changing social gradient, reflected by coming from a background of childhood poverty and deprivation, was linked with excess CHD mortality (Marmot, 1982). The Framingham Study also showed that men undergoing frequent work promotions sustained an increased chance of developing CHD (Haynes and Feinleib, 1982).

The association between the crossing of cultural boundaries and the risk of CHD has been nicely demonstrated by a gradient of increasing CHD rate (especially among young males) for Japanese resident in, respectively, their native land, Hawaii and California, independent of diet, serum cholesterol levels and blood pressure (Marmot, 1982). However, Japanese who maintain their traditional way of life, values and language after their emigration to the US do not have this increased rate, highlighting the part cultural cohesion and support play in protecting against coronary disease (Marmot, 1982).

SOCIAL SUPPORT AND CORONARY HEART DISEASE

It had long been suspected that belonging to a supportive social network and having community ties and resources promote emotional and physical well-being as well as protecting against the onset of psychiatric and organic pathology. However, this has now been partly validated by a series of studies which have shown an inverse relationship between social support and mortality rates, with three of these specifically addressing CHD mortality (Berkman, 1982). The first found that men who were lacking in social ties were over twice as likely to die from CHD as men with many contacts, and that women lacking such ties were over three times more likely to have suffered in fatal coronary event. In the second study, death rates from CHD were higher in those having a lower level of social relationship, with, again, a stronger linkage holding for women. The third study of Japanese–American males found that those with the lowest level of social affiliation had double the risk of developing CHD as those with the highest. Marmot's work on Whitehall civil servants and that on Japanese–Americans has also added to the evidence of the cardiotoxic effect of perceived inadequacies in one's social support network (Marmot, 1982).

Two studies from the 1960s, whose methodology was not as rigorous, are still often quoted as evidence for the buffering effect of a cohesive social support network against life stresses in the development of heart disease. Both examined small and tightly knit ethnic rural communities in Pennsylvania and found that the amount of CHD was substantially less than that found in the surrounding countryside, a fact that could not be accounted for by differences in standard coronary risk factors (Stout et al., 1964; Bruhn et al., 1968). Among workers with NASA, there was little relationship between occupational stress and heart disease risk for men reporting high levels of co-worker support, but among those without support, a significant association was found (Caplan, 1971). One possible underlying mechanism is suggested by the finding that the crisis of retrenchment produces rises in serum cholesterol levels much more often in men who lack emotional support from their wives (Gore, 1978).

Studies of marital status have repeatedly shown that the single, widowed or divorced have higher CHD mortality rates (Berkman, 1982), and that this excess is independent of standard coronary risk factors such as serum cholesterol levels, blood pressure and obesity, as well as social class (Weiss, 1973).

BEREAVEMENT AND CORONARY HEART DISEASE

There is a good deal of evidence showing that mortality rates increase substantially in the months subsequent to a conjugal bereavement, indeed, the death of a close family member triggering a lethal heart attack has been part of our folk lore for generations, with terms such as 'dying from a broken heart' being in common coinage. Thus, in Dr Heberden's Bill classifying the causes of death in London during 1657, 'griefe' figured as the fifth most common cause of death, and Benjamin Rush, one of the signatories of the US Declaration of Independence, wrote in his *Medical inquiries and observations upon diseases of the mind* in 1835: 'dissection of persons who have died of grief show congestion in, and inflammation of the heart, with rupture of its auricles and ventricles'. In Engle's excellent review (1971) of the sociological–demographic literature on the causes of sudden death, he classified them into eight categories, including the threat of losing a close person, the sudden impact of the death of such a person, acute grief and chronic mourning, and the anniversary of the death of an important figure on one's life.

Fitting in with these anecdotal observations, it is now well established that the mortality rate is much higher among widows and widowers than among married persons of the same age (Kraus and Lilienfeld, 1959). Young et al. (1963), for example, have shown that a sharp rise in mortality rate takes place during the first 6 months of widowerhood, and when Parkes et al. (1969) examined the causes on the death certificates, it became apparent that 75% of the increased death rate had been due to heart disease. Indeed, no other disease category showed a statistically significant increase. In a similar piece of research, Talbott *et al.* (1981) looked at 80 women who had died suddenly from heart disease, and, in comparison with a control group, they had more often experienced the death of a significant other within the 6 months preceding their demise. As mentioned above, even the anniversary of the death of a loved one has been shown to bear a relationship to the precipitation of a myocardial infarction (Engel, 1971).

MAJOR STRESSES

In a large controlled study examining the mortality of Australian ex-servicemen who had taken part in the war in Vietnam, they were found to be at greater risk of suffering a fatal coronary event than their comrades who had been in the army at the same time but had held an Australian posting (Fett *et al.*, 1984).

Although anecdotal reports of increased rates of coronary heart disease following liberation of both prisoners-of-war and political prisoners exposed to torture have been published, the main body of research evidence comes from studies conducted on survivors of Japanese and North Korean POW camps by Gilbert Beebe (1975) for the US Veterans' Administration. To grade the severity of stresses involved, Beebe compared POWs with their fellows who had served in the same theatres of war but had not been captured. Apart from one 3-year period, from 1946 to 1965 there had been an annual excess of hospitalizations for cardiovascular disease among the Pacific POWs as compared with the controls. Likewise, among the Korean POWs, every year from 1954 to 1961 demonstrated an excess of such disorders in comparison with their non-captured comrades. Also, there were significant differences between the POWs and controls on their scores on the Cornell Medical Index's cardiovascular system section, and the Japanese POWs were receiving disability pensions for heart disease more often.

What of civilian populations exposed to the rigors, deprivations and dangers of war? Reid (1959) reported that during the German air raids over London, there had been a sharp rise in deaths from myocardial infarction, and a dramatic illustration from more recent history has been civil war in Bangladesh, which led to a 54% increase in cardiovascular deaths among a population of 40 000 tea workers (Mackay, 1974).

Studies from communities stricken by natural disasters, especially flooding, have also shown increased morbidity and mortality rates from non-disaster-related disorders, to which increased cardiovascular death rates have contributed, (Bennett, 1970).

Socioeconomic Influences and CHD

The incidence of coronary heart disease varies widely across cultural and socioeconomic groupings, in general being a disease of affluent and industrialized nations (Marmot, 1982). However, even within countries, it is not randomly distributed, being concentrated in Third World countries among prosperous urban elites, while in developed countries it is a disease of the poorer-educated working classes. Thus in northern India, CHD is more common among the wealthy, and in Puerto Rico among urban dwellers with higher incomes (Marmot, 1982).

Illustrative of the situation in industrialized countries is the study of Whitehall civil servants which found that the risk of men in the lowest grades dying from heart disease was almost four times that of men occupying the highest levels of the public service, and that this association was independent of the standard coronary risk factors (Marmot, 1982). A similar white-collar, managerial/blue-collar worker dichotomy of heart disease risk was also observed in the Western Electric Study (Shekelle *et al.*, 1969). This higher coronary rate for the poorer-educated working classes in industrialized nations has been demonstrated in such geographically divergent countries as the US, Norway, Finland, France, Australia and Japan, with the risk being uniformly in the order of two to three times that of the managerial, professional classes (Marmot, 1982). This state of epidemiological affairs is a relatively recent phenomenon, although as late as the 1930s the higher socioeconomic classes in the West had the greatest risk of developing CHD. Hence, in England and Wales prior to the Second World War, classes I and II were at highest risk of dying from CHD, and the mortality rates for classes IV and V did not cross those for classes I and II until around 1955 (Marmot, 1982).

The picture that emerges from these data is that CHD tends to be a disease of recent affluence, and, consistent with this hypothesis have been the rapidly rising CHD rates in the Soviet Union and Eastern Europe since 1960, coinciding with a substantially improved standard of living in these countries. Over the period 1960 to 1980, Soviet Union CHD mortality rates doubled, paralleling what had happened several decades earlier in the West (Eyer, 1982). Part of the explanation for the uneven distribution of coronary risk rates may be that the newly affluent tend to overindulge in what were formerly unaffordable 'luxuries' like smoking, alcohol and foods rich in fats, and have less cause to exercise, promoting a lifestyle conducive to coronary atheroma, hypertension, hypercholesterolaemia, obesity and mature-onset diabetes (Eyer, 1982). Other variables such as lack of control over one's working environment, reduced levels of social support, the cumulative life cycle experience of belonging to a social class or nation undergoing rapid urbanization and industrialization, and less sophisticated medical care, also probably play contributing parts (Eyer, 1982; Marmot, 1982).

SUMMARY AND CONCLUSIONS

As has been seen, then, a very broad mix of psychological, social and cultural variables have been linked with coronary artery disease, and, taken in conjunction with the fact that many of the standard coronary risk factors like smoking, poor diet, obesity, failure to seek treatment for high blood pressure, lack of exercise and excessive consumption of alcohol also have substantial psychosocial determinants, it becomes apparent that coronary artery disease cannot be properly understood, prevented or treated without the adoption of an aetiological model which encompasses such factors. Of course, caution should be exercised in assuming that just because a variable is associated with coronary heart disease it is necessarily causative. In addition, the mix of psychosociocultural variables so far demonstrated to be linked with coronary artery disease is highly reminiscent of the witches' cauldron in 'Macbeth', and it is most unlikely that, for example, the nine discussed in this chapter are independently linked with heart disease.

Two strands can be teased out, though: variables which trigger off clinically manifest symptoms in a person whose heart is already diseased, and those that contribute to the formation of atheroma over a very prolonged time span. The first situation has been demonstrated in life-event research as well as for bereavement, natural disasters and domestic and employment stresses.

A picture is beginning to emerge, too, of what kind of emotional climate, set off by such events, precedes the coronary event and encompasses helplessness and hopelessness, feelings of no longer coping and being in control, a lack of satisfaction with one's marital, interpersonal and employment lives, loneliness, fatigue, apathy, malaise and depression.

Another explanation, though, is needed for the finding that the presence of certain psychosocial variables can predict the onset of coronary symptoms up to several years in advance. Such a phenomenon exists for the Type A behavioural pattern, individuals who manifest high levels of hostility and neuroticism and the crossing of economic and social–cultural boundaries, especially in the situation in which individuals are trying to 'better' themselves. The common denominator that runs through this second cluster of variables is a high level of arousal accompanying a vulnerability to loss or failure. The former has been shown to be associated with a number of biological changes which are potentially atherogenic, while the latter has been shown to produce significant impairments in functioning of the body's immune system. Much remains to be done, though, before the bridge crossing this wide firth between the biological and behavioural contributions to coronary heart disease can be finally completed.

REFERENCES

Barefoot, J.C., Dahlstrom, W.G., & Williams, R.B. (1983). Hostility, C.H.D. incidence and total mortality: a 25 year follow up study of 255 physicians. *Psychosomatic Medicine*, 45, 59–63.

Beebe, G.W. (1975). Follow up studies of World War II and Korean prisoners. *American Journal of Epidemilogy, 101*, 400–422.

Bennett, G. (1970). Bristol floods 1968. Controlled survey of effects on health of local community disaster. *British Medical Journal, 3*, 454–458.

Berkman, L.F. (1982). Social network analysis and coronary heart disease. *Advances in Cardiology, 29*, 37–49.

Bianchi, G. Fergusson, D., & Walshe, J. (1978). Psychiatric antecedents of myocardial infarction. *Medical Journal of Australia, 1*, 297–300.

Boman, B. (1982). Psychosocial stress and ischaemic heart disease. *Australian and New Zealand Journal of Psychiatry, 16*, 265–278.

Bortner, R.W. (1969). A short rating scale as a potential measure of Pattern A behaviour. *Journal of Chronic Disease, 22*, 87–91.

Bruhn, J.G., Wolf, S., & Lynn, T.L. (1968). Social aspects of coronary heart disease in a Pennsylvania German community. *Social Science and Medicine, 2*, 201–212.

Byrne, D.G. & Rosenman, R.H. (1986). The type A behaviour pattern as a precursor to stressful life-events: a confluence of coronary risks. *British Journal of Medical Psychology, 59*, 75–82.

Caplan, R. (1971). Organizational stress and individual strain: a social psychological study of risk factors in coronary heart disease among administrators, engineers, and scientists. PhD thesis, University of Michigan, Ann Arbor.

Chambers, W.N. & Reiser, M.F. (1953). Emotional stress in the precipitation of congestive heart failure. *Psychosomatic Medicine, 15*, 38–60.

Connolly, J. (1976). Life events before myocardial infarction. *Journal of Human Stress, 2*, 3–17.

Dunbar, F. (1947). The mind and the heart. In *Mind and body: Psychosomatic medicine* (pp. 120–145). New York: Random House.

Engel, G.L. (1971). Sudden and rapid death during psychological stress. Folklore or folk wisdom? *Annals of Internal Medicine, 74*, 771–782.

Eyer, J. (1982). Changing trends in ischaemic heart disease: Relations to cohort experience and economic trends in industrial countries. *Advances in Cardiology, 29*, 50–55.

Falger, P., Appels, A. (1982). Psychological risk factors over the life course of myocardial infarction patients. *Advances in Cardiology, 29*, 132–139.

Fett, M.J., Dunn, M., & Adena, M.A. (1984). *Australian Veterans health studies: The mortality report*. Canberra: AGPS.

French–Belgian Collaborative Group (1982). Ischaemic heart disease and psychological patterns. Prevalence and incidence studies in Belgium and France. *Advances in Cardiology, 29*, 25–31.

Friedman, M., & Rosenman, R. (1974). *Type A behaviour and your heart*. New York: Knopf.

Gillum, R.F., & Paffenbarger, R.S. (1978). Chronic disease in former college students. XVII. Sociocultural mobility as a precursor of coronary heart disease and hypertension. *American Journal of Epidemiology, 108*, 289–298.

Glass, D.C. (1978). Pattern A behaviour and uncontrollable stress. In T.I. Dembroski, S.M. Weiss, J.L. Shields, S.G. Haynes & M. Feinleib (eds), *Coronary prone behaviour*. New York: Springer-Verlag.

Gore, S. (1978). The effect of social support in moderating the health consequences of unemployment. *Journal of Health and Social Behaviour, 19*, 157–165.

Groen, J.J. (1974). Psychosomatic aspects of ischaemic (coronary) heart disease. In O.W. Hill (ed.), *Modern trends in psychosomatic medicine*. London: Butterworths.

Haynes, S.G., & Feinleib, M. (1982). Type A behaviour and the incidence of coronary heart disease in the Framingham Heart Study. *Advances in Cardiology, 29*, 85–95.

Jenkins, C.D., Zyzanski, S.J. & Rosenman, R.H. (1971). Progress towards validation of a computer-scored test for the Type A coronary prone behaviour pattern. *Psychosomatic Medicine, 33*, 193–202.

Karasek, R.A., Theorell, T., Schwartz, T., Pieper, C., & Alfredsson, L. (1982). Job, psychological factors and coronary heart disease. *Advances in Cardiology, 29*, 62–67.

Kraus, A.S., & Lilienfeld, A.M. (1959). Mortality by marital status. *Journal of Chronic Diseases, 10*, 207–211.

Lebovits, B.Z., Shekelle, R.B., Ostfeld, A.M., & Paul, O. (1967). Prospective and retrospective pathological studies of coronary heart disease. *Psychosomatic Medicine, 29*, 265–273.

Lown, B., Desilva, R.A., Reich, P., & Murawski, B.J. (1980). Psychophysiologic factors in sudden cardiac death. *American Journal of Psychiatry, 137*, 1325–1335.

Lundberg, U., Theorell, T., & Lind, E. (1975). Life changes and myocardial infarction: Individual differences in life change scaling. *Journal of Psychosomatic Research, 19*, 27–32.

Mackay, D.M. (1974). The effects of civil war on the health of a rural community in Bangladesh. *Journal of Tropical Medicine and Hygiene, 77*, 120–127.

Marmot, M.G. (1982). Socio-economic and cultural factors in ischaemic heart disease. *Advances in Cardiology, 29*, 68–76.

Matthews, K.A. (1982). Psychological perspectives on the Type A behaviour pattern. *Psychological Bulletin, 91*, 293–323.

Morris, J.N., Heady, J.A., Raffle, P.A.B., Roberts, C.G., & Parks, J.W. (1953). Coronary heart disease and physical activity of work. *Lancet, 2*, 1053–1057, 1111–1120.

Osler, W. (1910). The Lumleian Lectures on angina pectoris. *Lancet, 1*, 839.

Parkes, C.M., Benjamin, B., & Fitzgerald, R.G. (1969). Broken heart: A statistical study of increased mortality among widowers. *British Medical Journal, 1*, 740–743.

Reid, D.D. (1959). Unpublished report in Groen (1974).

Rose, K.D. (1974). The post-coronary patient as a spectator sportsman. In R.S. Eliot (ed.), *Stress and the heart* (pp. 207–218). New York: Futura.

Rosenman, R.H., Brand, R.J., & Jenkins, C.D. (1975). Coronary heart disease in the Western Collaborative Group Study. Final follow-up experience of 8½ years. *Journal of the American Medical Association, 233*, 872–877.

Rosenman, R.H., & Friedman, M. (1958). The possible relationship of occupational stress to clinical coronary heart disease. *California Medicine, 89*, 169–174.

Russek, H.I. (1965). Stress, tobacco and coronary disease in North American professional groups. Survey of 12,000 men in 14 occupation groups. *Journal of the American Medical Association, 192*, 189–194.

Russek, H.I., & Zohman, B.L. (1958). Relative significance of heredity, diet and occupational stress in coronary heart disease of young adults. *American Journal of the Medical Sciences, 235*, 266–275.

Sales, S.M., & House, J. (1971). Job dissatisfaction as a possible risk factor in coronary heart disease. *Journal of Chronic Diseases, 23*, 861–873.

Shekelle, R., Gale, M., & Ostfeld, A. (1983). Hostility, risk of coronary heart disease and mortality. *Psychosomatic Medicine, 45* 109–114.

Shekelle, R.B., Ostfeld, A.M., & Paul, O. (1969). Social status and incidence of coronary heart disease. *Journal of Chronic Diseases, 22*, 381–394.

Stout, C., Morrow, J., Brandt, E.N., & Wolf, S. (1964). Usually low incidence of death from myocardial infarction: Study of an Italian–American community in Pennsylvania. *Journal of the American Medical Association, 188*, 845–849.

Talbott, E., Kuller, L.H., Perper, J., & Murphy, P.A. (1981). Sudden unexpected death in women. Biologic and psychosocial origins. *American Journal of Epidemiology, 114*, 671–682.

Theorell, T.G.T. (1982). Review of research on life events and cardiovascular illness. *Advances in Cardiology, 29*, 140–147.

Theorell, T., & Floderus-Myrhed, B. (1977). Workload and risk of myocardial infarction— a prospective psychosocial analysis. *International Journal of Epidemiology, 6*, 17–21.

Thorne, M.C., Wing, A.L., & Paffenbarger, R.S. (1968). Chronic disease in former college students. VII. Early precursors of non fatal coronary heart disease. *American Journal of Epidemiology, 87*, 520–529.

Van Dusch, T. (1868). *Lehrbuch der Herzkrankheiten*. Leipzig: Whilhelm Engelman.

Weiss, N.S. (1973). Marital status and risk factors for coronary heart disease: The United States health examination survey of adults. *British Journal of Preventive and Social Medicine, 27*, 41–43.

Young, M., Benjamin, B., & Wallis, C. (1963). Mortality of widowers. *Lancet, 2*, 454–456.

Zyzanski, S.J., Jenkins, C.D., Ryan, T.J., Flessas, A., & Everist, M. (1976). Psychological correlates of coronary angiographic findings. *Archives of Internal Medicine, 136*, 1234–1237.

KEY WORDS

Heart disease, cardiovascular disease, coronoary heart disease, ischaemic, heart disease, Type A behavioural pattern, Type B behavioural pattern, neurotic symptoms, family employment, life style stresses, social support, socioeconomic influences, bereavement emotions and behaviour.

Handbook of Life Stress, Cognition and Health
Edited by S. Fisher and J. Reason
© 1988 John Wiley & Sons Ltd.

17

Recent Life Changes and Coronary Heart Disease: 10 Years' Research

RICHARD H. RAHE
University of Nevada School of Medicine

INTRODUCTION

The brain, with its rich interconnections and multiple influences on all organ systems of the body, appears to respond to psychosocial stresses primarily through neurotransmitter and hormonal pathways (Kasl *et al.*, 1968; Rahe *et al.*, 1968; Mason, 1975; Rubin *et al.*, 1969; Schleifer *et al.*, 1983; Barchas *et al.*, 1978). These brain effects are secondarily transmitted to most organ systems of the body. Which of these stress-related alterations are singled out for study depends on the physiological interests of the investigators. For example, studies of coronary heart disease (CHD) have focused on systemic catecholamine levels, blood platelets, serum lipids, and cardiovascular electrophysiology (Dimsdale and Moss, 1980; Wolf *et al.*, 1962; Haft and Fani, 1973; Lown *et al.*, 1973).

To estimate psychosocial stress in a meaningful and standardized fashion, the author helped to devise an instrument formulated from concepts of physiology. Anticipated life stresses, for example, have been shown to lead to physiological arousal very close in time to the life event itself (Ekman and Lundberg, 1971). Imminent job loss, for example, does not cause measurable psychophysiological upheaval until a few weeks, or even a few days, prior to termination (Kasl *et al.*, 1968). A physiological analog of this phenomenon is the pulse rate and blood pressure increases seen in man prior to competing in a sports event; only hours to minutes prior to actual athletic performance are these physiological parameters elevated (Mason *et al.*, 1973). Therefore, our life change questionnaire ignores anticipated life stresses until they are imminent. Conversely, stresses of long standing appear to be accommodated to gradually (Horowitz *et al.*, 1974). In physiological terms, this phenomenon is similar to habituation. Thus, long-term stress, which does not fluctuate in its intensity, may not have great relevance for life change questionnaires. Chronic stress which does fluctuate in its intensity may well have continuing physiological effects (Schaeffer and Baum, 1984). What does seem to have relevance psychophysiologically is *recent* psychosocial change.

Changes in one's steady state of psychosocial adaptation over the recent days, weeks, or several months are what are assessed in our stress measurement instrument.

Systematic evaluation of significant changes in a person's recent life is best performed by interview coupled with a research instrument such as the Recent Life Changes Questionnaire (RLCQ; Rahe and Arthur, 1978; Rahe, 1975). The RLCQ is an expansion of the Schedule of Recent Experience (SRE) questionnaire, designed by the author and Thomas H. Holmes (Rahe et al., 1964). Both instruments sample recent alterations in a person's work, family, social, interpersonal, religious, and financial life. The vast majority of the studies to be reviewed in this chapter used the SRE, with standardized life change intensity values assigned to the life change events. These values, called life change units (LCU), add a dimension of quantification to the recent life change events. For example, the average significance of a death of a spouse is generally rated twice that of marriage (Rahe, 1969; Rahe, 1975). Life change units have dropped from use over the past few years, since in large-scale studies the most frequently reported life change events tend to have very similar (moderately weighted) LCU values. Thus, correlations run between LCUs and a simple counting of life changes events have been as high as 0.9 (Rahe, 1978). Small-scale studies, on the other hand, especially of persons at risk to experience high-value LCU events (such as bereavement), have utilized LCU scoring with good results (DeFaire, 1975).

The importance of constitutional (both genetic and acquired) susceptibility to disease should be mentioned. In coronary heart disease, an overweight, sedentary, cigarette-smoking, hypertensive, middle-aged male is constitutionally more likely to develop signs and symptoms of CHD when under stress than is a slim, young, physically fit female experiencing a similar degree of life stress. Studies of CHD patients' recent life changes and the clinical onset of their disease have contributed, in the main, to our understanding of the timing of illness onset. That is, why does a person who is constitutionally predisposed to CHD develop clinical signs and symptoms of their disease when they do?

In studies of recent life change and disease, four separate steps should be followed to arrive at an adequate understanding of critical methodological issues. These steps are: (1) establish the person's baseline life change estimates; (2) determine the subject's pre-illness, illness, and post-illness life change levels; (3) cross-validate the initial findings; and (4) progress from retrospective studies to prospective investigations. In the material to follow, more than a decade of research was necessary to complete these four steps.

RECENT LIFE CHANGE AND CORONARY HEART DISEASE

Baseline Estimates

Our early work found that it is the rare individual who experiences no recent life changes (Rahe, 1969); even healthy persons showed low to moderate levels of change. However, recently ill persons generally reported moderate to high levels.

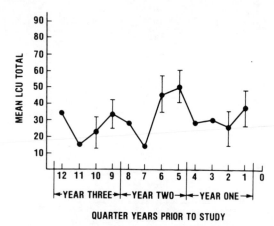

FIG. 17.1   A healthy comparison group. Baseline life change data, by quarter-years, over a 3-year period.

Additionally, those with highest recent life change levels tended to experience major rather than minor illness episodes (Rahe *et al.*, 1967). From this early work, we described a 'normal baseline' of recent life changes for Americans in good health (approximately 150 LCUs per year). In physiological terms, this baseline might be compared to 'background noise' generated by individuals living in an industrialized Western country in the late twentieth century.

Baseline LCU values were seen to vary depending upon the age of the persons studied as well as the culture from which they were drawn. For instance, middle-class, healthy, young adult American males registered one-third greater LCU baselines than did Norwegians with virtually identical demographic characteristics (Rahe *et al.*, 1974a). Older subjects showed lower LCU baselines than did middle-aged individuals (DeFaire, 1975; Rahe, 1969). Baseline LCU estimates also appear to provide information on life changes occurring secondary to societal or economic forces. For example, when we carried out a baseline LCU estimate on healthy, middle-aged males in Stockholm, selected to be a comparison group in the investigation of patients with CHD, we found a small peak of life change occurring in late 1967 (Theorell and Rahe, 1971; Fig. 17.1). A major agricultural reform was enacted that year, with economic ramifications felt across the country. Also, a ruling to change from left-hand to right-hand driving was put into effect in mid-1967. These societal changes may have contributed to the observed peak.

Can subjects remember their recent life changes over the past year or two? Baseline life change estimates can help answer this question. Data can be examined for evidence of a 'forgetting curve'. That is, researchers can look for a fall-off in life change reporting as subjects report over earlier and earlier periods of time. We asked our Swedish subjects to report their recent life changes by quarter-year intervals over the past 3 years. Figure 17.1 shows only modest evidence for subjects forgetting recent life changes 3 years previously, and no evidence of forgetting was seen over the previous 2 years.

In a study of life change before and after recovery from an acute myocardial infarction (MI), 47 Swedish outpatients participated (Rahe and Paasikivi, 1971).

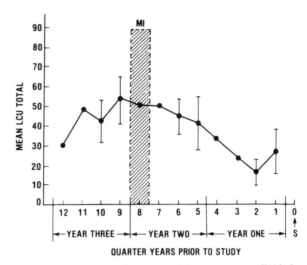

FIG. 17.2   Swedish outpatients who had recovered from a myocardial infarction 2–3 years previously. Quarter-year life changes data prior to and following infarction. (Quarter-year of infarction represented by the stippled bar.)

All subjects had experienced a MI approximately 2 years prior to our study. They were asked to report their life changes over the past 3 years. A summary figure, anchored by the quarter-year of MI, was constructed (Fig. 17.2). Subjects recalled a gradually increasing recent life changes intensity, rising to 50 LCUs for the quarter-year immediately prior to infarct. They also reported a gradual return to an LCU baseline over the 2 years following their infarction. Baseline LCUs appeared to be approximately 25 LCU per quarter-year for this group of men.

A 'forgetting curve' would have shown highest levels of life change over the most recent time intervals, with a decreasing life change level as subjects remembered back into time. In contrast, these men remembered highest levels of life change prior to and shortly following their infarction, which had occurred 1–2 years earlier. They recalled lowest life change levels for their most recent quarter-year intervals. Clearly, in this study, no evidence for a 'forgetting curve' was seen.

Pre-Illness, Illness, and Post-Illness Life Change Levels

Although rarely done, it is critical to compare patients' pre-illness recent life change levels to their own baseline determinations. This was done in the out-patient study outlined above. In further studies, we compared CHD patients' LCU levels over the 6 months prior to the quarter-year of their infarcts, compared to their LCU levels for a chronologically identical time interval 1 year earlier. (As our previous studies did not reveal a 'forgetting curve' over the previous 2 years, this seemed a valid comparison.) As shown in Figure 17.3, when these comparisons were made for 27 Swedish inpatients with an acute myocardial infarction who had experienced *no previous clinical symptoms of heart disease*, the amount of life change reported over the 6 months prior to the quarter-year of their MI was

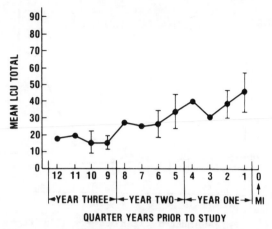

FIG. 17.3 Swedish inpatients, with no prior history for coronary heart disease, recovering from their first myocardial infarction. Quarter-year life changes data reported over the antecedent 3 years.

significantly greater than that given for the chronologically identical 6-month interval 1 year earlier (Theorell and Rahe, 1971). In these patients, a nearly twofold build-up in LCU level was recalled. (In the figures, the quarter-year in which the MI occurred was not counted in order to reduce the risk of including life changes secondary to the onset of the MI itself.)

Clinical episodes of CHD can themselves cause life changes. Recent life change profiles over 2 years prior to MI were gathered in another group of 27 Swedish inpatients, all of whom reported *a previous history of coronary heart disease* (Theorell and Rahe, 1971). No clear LCU build-up was seen in this group (Fig. 17.4). The pre-MI recent life change baselines for these chronically ill persons were found to be elevated, most likely secondary to their chronic illness. Many

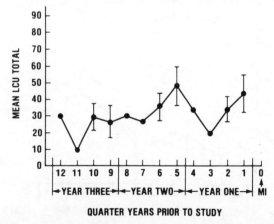

FIG. 17.4 Swedish inpatients, with long-term histories for coronary heart disease, recovering from a myocardial infarction. Quarter-year life changes data reported over the antecedent 3 years.

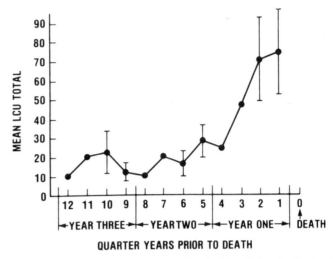

FIG. 17.5   Swedish victims of sudden coronary death. No victims had prior histories for coronary heart disease. Quarter-year life changes data reported over the antecedent 3 years.

stress researchers use hospitalized or clinic patients as 'controls' in their studies. They often discover elevated recent life changes in these 'controls'. True controls must be demographically similar to the patients studied *and* must have been *in good health over the past 3 years*. Otherwise, recent illnesses may well result in enough life changes (both before and following their illness) to elevate their LCU baselines.

Earlier work by the author indicated that recent life change levels are highest in persons experiencing severe illnesses, some of these illnesses even resulting in death (Rahe *et al.*, 1967). Similarly, in our Swedish studies we found that the build-up in life change events reported by next-of-kin of victims of sudden

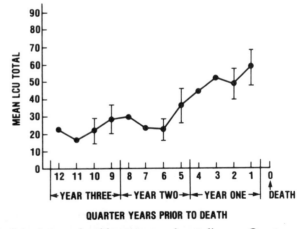

FIG. 17.6   Swedish victims of sudden coronary heart disease. Quarter-year life changes data reported over the antecedent 3 years.

coronary death were higher than those reported by survivors of an acute MI (Rahe and Lind, 1971). Specifically, next-of-kin of 37 Stockholm residents who died suddenly from (autopsy verified) CHD reported a nearly threefold LCU increase over baseline values for the 6 months immediately prior to the quarter-year in which death occurred, compared to the chronologically identical time interval 1 year earlier. This build-up of life changes prior to coronary death was even seen to be statistically significant for those persons *with prior CHD histories* (Figs. 17.5 and 17.6).

Cross-Validation

Our Swedish investigations took on added reliability when they were replicated in much larger groups of persons in Finland. These cross-cultural cross-validation studies consisted of a total population study of 279 residents of Helsinki surviving an MI, and 226 victims of sudden coronary death (Rahe *et al.*, 1973a, 1974b). These were virtually all MI and coronary death victims seen in that capital city over a 6-month period. Findings from these Finnish studies proved to be nearly identical to our earlier Swedish investigations (Figs. 17.7 and 17.8). That is, recent life change build-up for individuals surviving an MI was approximately twofold over baseline values, and the build-up for coronary death victims was seen to be nearly threefold. (Note in Figures 17.7 and 17.8 that an increase in LCU baseline was found once again for patients with prior histories for CHD compared to persons with no CHD histories.)

As a control for possibly inflated LCU reporting by next-of-kin, most of whom were spouses who provided coronary death victims' data, spouses' reports for MI survivors' recent life changes were also collected in these Finnish studies (Rahe *et*

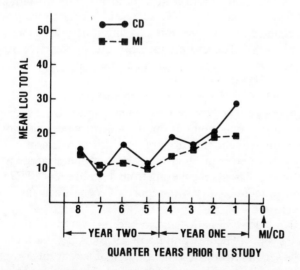

FIG. 17.7 Finnish survivors of an acute myocardial infarction and Finnish victims of sudden coronary death. Both groups had no prior histories for coronary heart disease. Quarter-year life changes data reported over the antecedent 2 years.

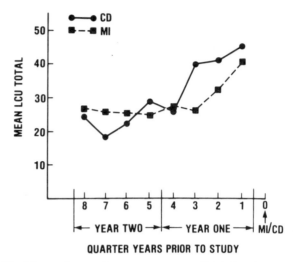

FIG. 17.8   Finnish survivors of an acute myocardial infarction and Finnish victims c sudden coronary death. Both groups had long-standing histories for coronary hea. disease. Quarter-year life changes data reported over the antecedent 2 years.

al., 1973a). When the two sets of spouses' reports were compared, no evidenc was found for LCU inflation on this account.

Retrospective Studies Leading to Prospective Investigations

Major difficulties are encountered in using recent life changes data to predict ne episodes of CHD in populations of healthy persons. First, thousands of person must be followed over a decade or longer in order to observe sufficient numbers c new cases to perform accurate statistical analyses. Second, recent life chang elevations are associated with the onset of many different illnesses, not just CHI (Rahe and Arthur, 1978). Therefore, not only are prospective studies tim consuming and expensive, but recently elevated life change levels predict illnes onset in general, not CHD in particular.

   One way around such obstacles is to predict recurrences of clinical episodes o CHD in samples of persons who have already demonstrated their susceptibility t this disease. For example, one might attempt to identify persons most likely t experience reinfarction, or sudden coronary death, from a group of individua who have recently recovered from their first MI. Another strategy would be t follow closely a group of patients recovering from a MI to see if CHD symptoms and selected CHD risk factors, vary with reported recent life changes. Two suc studies have been carried out.

   In one prospective study, 36 patients who had recovered from their first M were followed over 8 years (Theorell and Rahe, 1975). After this interval, half o them had suffered a second MI or become a victim of an abrupt coronary death the other half remained in good health. The utility of recent life change data i predicting those patients who ultimately suffered CHD recurrences is shown i Figure 17.9. Mean LCU levels were seen to remain quite stable for the 18 patient

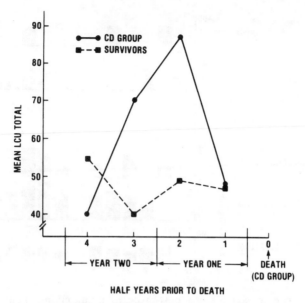

FIG. 17.9 American post-infarction survivors who either remained in good health or became victims of coronary death, or severe reinfarction, over a 4-year period. Half-year life change data, collected prospectively, over the 2 years prior to reinfarction or death. (Reproduced by permission of *Journal of Human Stress*.)

who remained healthy. In contrast, a significant increase in mean LCU level was observed to occur over the year prior to reinfarction, or coronary death, in the afflicted group. Of major interest was the finding that life change build-up was seen to precede, by many months, any physical evidence of incipient cardiac decompensation—such as abnormal ejection fractions as measured by serial ballistocardiography.

The other prospective study followed 21 patients who had recently recovered from their first MI (Theorell *et al.*, 1972). These patients reported to the hospital once a week, over a 2–3 month period. At each clinic visit they completed an RLCQ for life changes which had occurred *during the past week*, and brought with them a 24-hour urine sample collected over the previous day. Urine samples were analyzed for catecholamines. Blood samples were drawn for serum cholesterol determinations. Most patients did well following their MI, but a few developed exacerbations of post-infarction angina pectoris. The overall correlation found between all subjects' weekly LCU levels and their final day urinary epinephrine excretion was seen to be 0.37. This was statistically significant at the 0.05 level.

A case example from the above study is represented in Figure 17.10. A 49-year-old, married foreman of a shop of mechanics reported some work difficulties and personal strains at home over his first week of follow-up. The next week his mother discovered she had breast cancer. Further personal problems occurred during the subject's third follow-up week. The patient's urinary epinephrine excretion was seen to build to a small peak over these first 3 weeks. A second crescendo of life events began during the seventh follow-up week, when

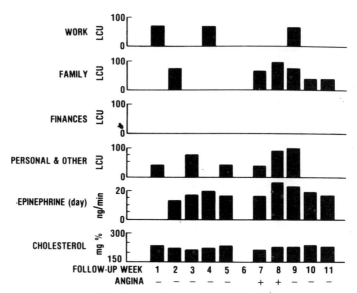

FIG. 17.10   A case example of a post-myocardial infarction patient who was followed every week over the first 3 months after his hospital discharge. Weekly life changes scores were reported. Urinary catecholamine excretion, serum cholesterol level, and the presence or absence of post-infarction angina pectoris were also measured each week over the 3 months.

the patient reported marital difficulties, and a close friend developed an acute MI. During the eighth follow-up week his mother underwent cancer surgery and the patient subsequently missed a good deal of work—leading to difficulties with his boss. Shortly following this second build-up in life change events the patient demonstrated his highest urinary epinephrine excretion. It was also during the seventh and eighth weeks of follow-up that the patient developed his only experience with post-infarction angina. Life changes, catecholamines, and symptoms gradually abated over the final 2 weeks of follow-up. Though not statistically significant, the patient's serum cholesterol concentrations appeared to vary inversely with his recent life changes and his urinary epinephrine excretion.

EMOTIONS AND BEHAVIOR

The notion that certain emotions and behaviors are of potential etiological significance for individuals with CHD was perhaps first mentioned by John Hunter—the 'father of modern surgery' (Peete, 1955). Hunter's observation that his life was at the mercy of anyone who made him angry, illustrated nearly 100 years ago the dysrhythmic potential of hostility for CHD patients. In the early part of this century, Sir William Osler wrote that in his private practice he had a number of Jewish physicians with CHD (angina pectoris), most of whom appeared to be driven by the 'incessant treadmill of practice' (Osler, 1910). He also noted that these men suffered an inordinate amount of worry over life and its vicissitudes (Osler, 1910). Twenty to thirty years later, Dunbar added her observations that a facade of strong independence appeared to be characteristic of CHD patients (Dunbar, 1943).

Not initially aware of this earlier work, Friedman and Rosenman, in the late 1950s, described patients with CHD as exhibiting rapidly spoken and explosive speech, using frequent emphatic gestures, reporting enormous dedication to their work, demonstrating extreme competitiveness and easily elicited hostility, with preoccupations concerning achievement and frequent, self-imposed, time deadlines (Friedman and Rosenman, 1959). Around the same time, Bruhn and Wolf, as well as Van Der Valk and Groen, focused on home problems and life dissatisfactions as key emotional issues of patients with CHD (Bruhn et al., 1968; Van Der Valk and Groen, 1967).

In the late 1960s, the author collaborated in a study of CHD in middle-aged, male, identical twins, in Sweden (Liljefors and Rahe, 1970). From the observations mentioned above, we selected four emotions and behaviors to study: (1) dedication to work; (2) lack of leisure/time-urgency; (3) home problems; and (4) life dissatisfactions. A total population study of all middle-aged male Swedish identical twins between the ages of 45 and 70 was carried out. After a thorough physical exam, CHD in these men was scaled over seven gradations—from no apparent disease to a previously documented myocardial infarction. Of 47 monozygotic twin pairs studied, 32 pairs were found to have at least some degree of discordance in their gradations of CHD. Identical twins discordant for CHD could not be differentiated from one another on the basis of their physical characteristics, such as height, weight, ponderal index, serum cholesterol, glucose metabolism, or even by cigarette-smoking history. However, the twin brother with the more severe CHD could be differentiated from his less afflicted brother by our emotion and behavior measures. The more diseased twin showed a higher degree of overwork, greater time urgency, more home problems, and, in particular, greater life dissatisfactions than did his healthier brother.

In the life change studies presented earlier, Swedish subjects with CHD were also asked to scale themselves on a slightly more expanded group of emotions and behaviors than that used in the twin study (Theorell and Rahe, 1972; Romo et al., 1974). Swedish subjects who had recovered from their first MI were also divided into professional and skilled workers (Theorell and Rahe, 1972). Their answers on the emotion and behaviour questions were compared to those of their matched controls, and prevalence rates for these emotions and behaviors were seen to vary between 10% and 85%. Regardless of socioeconomic status, post-MI patients expressed significantly higher work dissatisfactions, less relaxation, and significantly greater hostility than did controls. The CHD patients also showed significantly higher overtime work than did controls. As a group, the professionals were more satisfied with their work, finances, living conditions, and achievement of life goals than were the skilled workers.

These emotions and behaviors were examined in a cross-cultural study of Swedish, Finnish, and American post-MI subjects (Romo et al., 1974). Their emotions and behavior prevalence rates varied between 20% and 75%. We found that Swedes reported significantly more overtime work than did either Americans or Finns, whereas Americans took their work home at a significantly higher rate than did either of the two Scandinavian samples. Americans claimed to have more time for relaxation during the day than both of the other groups. Finns and Swedes both claimed more work dissatisfaction than did Americans. Time urgency appeared to be significantly more characteristic of Swedes—nearly twice the prevalence reported for Finns or Americans. Finns appeared to be the most dissatisfied with their lives of the three groups; in particular, they reported greatest dissatisfaction with their level of education, their lack of achievement of life goals, and their present level of income. Finn's life dissatisfactions were seen to be at nearly twice the prevalence levels reported by Americans or Swedes.

In summary, certain emotions (hostility, home problems, and life dissatisfactions) and selected behaviors (overwork and time urgency) were found to be variables that significantly differentiated between identical twin pairs discordant for CHD and for patients with CHD compared to healthy controls. However, between 15% and 90% of our post-MI patients did *not* admit to various individual emotions or behaviors. Therefore, CHD emotions and behaviors are far from universal features of patients with this disease. When they did occur, they appeared to be significantly influenced by culture and modestly affected by social class.

REHABILITATION

Rehabilitation should always begin as soon as possible after a patient is admitted to the coronary care unit. More importantly, it should not end at discharge. At the University of California at Los Angeles, we established an educational rehabilitation program for CHD patients, and their spouses, which began the first day or two after hospitalization (Rahe *et al.*, 1975a). We tested patients by questionnaire on their knowledge of their disease and the optimal plans for their rehabilitation. The same questionnaire was given early and late during their hospital stay. The results from the second test were compared to the results from the first to assess what had been learned. Despite the ward staff's conviction that our educational program was extremely effective, no significant learning effect could be demonstrated. In a second study, the author combined in-hospital educational approaches with outpatient treatment over the first few weeks following hospital discharge (Rahe *et al.*, 1973b; 1975b; 1979). Patients completing the combined inpatient and outpatient programs did show a significant learning effect on their questionnaires.

A highly effective use of recent life changes data from CHD patients is in the area of rehabilitation. Recent life changes, along with the individual's reactions to these changes, provide several areas for potential therapeutic intervention. Adjustments to and re-evaluations of recent life change events are facilitated by the group therapy format. The author carried out an experimental program in which group therapy was added to the standard medical outpatient care of patients surviving their first MI (Rahe *et al.*, 1975b; 1979). During these group sessions, recent life changes information, along with key emotions and behaviors were discussed. Lifestyle modifications were suggested: for example, one severely time-urgent patient experimented with taking off his wrist watch for longer and longer portions of the day. This resulted in his learning new behaviors concerning his management of time. His experiences were discussed during the next group session. In a similar vein, recent life change stresses of one patient facilitated group discussions of this topic. Other lifestyle issues discussed were subjects' approaches to their work, their family relationships, and the presence or absence of life satisfactions.

The author's long-term study included a controlled trial, with random assignment of patients to either group therapy plus medical treatment or to medical treatment alone. Forty-four post-MI patients were followed over 3–4 years. In a replication experiment, another seventeen patients were given group therapy plus standard medical treatment. All groups of patients were compared in terms of their past medical histories, demographic characteristics, severity of infarct, and prognosis (Norris Index). (No significant differences were found among any of the groups.) All groups then received identical medical follow-up care, which included counseling regarding diet, information concerning physical exercise, periodic checks on blood pressure and cardiac function, and requisite medicines. Patients receiving group therapy attended six 1.5 hour bi-weekly sessions. The first session was often attended by patients during their second week in the hospital. The remaining sessions were continued over the first 2–3 months following hospital discharge.

Group therapy sessions were roughly as follows. Between four and ten patients comprised a group and were seen as a cadre throughout their sessions. The first session usually dealt with recent life changes over the 6 months prior to their MI as well as an assessment of physical 'risk factors' (e.g. serum cholesterol, hypertension, diabetes, physical inactivity, and cigarette smoking). The focus of this session was: 'Why vulnerable persons (like themselves) develop this disease when they do.' The second session dealth with key emotions and behaviors. These variables were defined to patients as 'psychological risk factors' for CHD. The third session usually focused on problems patients might be having with their attempts to modify physical as well as psychological risk factors. The fourth session frequently centered around home problems—especially family interrelationships concerning diet, sex, and exercise. The final two sessions varied according to the needs of the group. In general, these sessions were geared towards the patients' plans to return to work as well as to strategies to minimize previous life stresses, key emotions, and behaviors.

Follow-up over 3–4 years showed the expected 5% per year reinfarction rate, as well as the expected 3% to 5% per year mortality rate from this disease, *in the control group*. However, no reinfarctions and no coronary deaths were seen in either treatment group over follow-up (Rahe *et al.*, 1979). These intergroup differences were significant at the 0.05 level. In addition, treatment groups achieved a significantly higher return to work percentage (85% and 94%) than did controls (50%). Thus, in terms of crucial medical and social indicators, patients in the group therapy treatment groups fared significantly better than did controls. The control group did no worse, however, than control groups in large, randomly allocated drug studies carried out in the USA (The Pooling Project Research Group, 1978).

Once returned to work, group therapy patients did indicate a significant reduction in the number of hours per week they spent at work, a significant increase in the minutes per day they allowed for lunch, as well as a significant increase in the number of vacation days they took per year (overwork measures). In addition, group therapy patients in the controlled trial reported a significant reduction in their feelings of time urgency compared to control patients. No differences in life satisfaction levels were noted between groups over time and, if anything, controls showed better compliance with physical risk factor modifications (diet, body weight, exercise, and cessation of cigarette smoking) than did either treatment group. Although we felt our achievements in modifying coronary behaviors were important, it seemed these few discrete changes in behavior did not explain all of the variance. The coping advantage these patients achieved from group discussions of their recent life stress, key emotions and behaviors, and CHD management issues seemed immensely important.

SUMMARY AND CONCLUSIONS

Problems have arisen from researchers attempting to use recent life changes data in large-scale predictive studies, hoping to identify those at high risk for near-future CHD (Theorell et al., 1975). What these researchers 'rediscovered' was that high recent life change levels predict illnesses in general, not CHD in particular. In fact, compared to most other disease entities studied by this approach, CHD patients tend to report relatively low recent life changes baselines. Thus, a two- to threefold increase from their low baseline levels does not produce an LCU level grossly divergent from the higher baselines of non-CHD individuals. When these researchers added key emotions and behaviors to their life changes data, their ability to predict persons susceptible to near-future CHD episodes improved (Theorell et al., 1975).

As mentioned in the introduction, the search for physiological correlates of life changes stress and selected emotions and behaviors continues (Theorell et al., 1972; Krantz and Manuk, 1984; Houston, 1983). The sympathetic nervous system, as measured by catecholamine serum levels and excretion rates, is currently thought to be a very important correlate. Further, catecholamines influence a wide variety of cardiovascular functions (e.g. heart rate, rhythm, and blood pressure) as well as lipid mobilization from body stores and platelet agglutination leading to thrombosis (Dimsdale and Moss, 1980; Wolf et al., 1962; Haft and Fani, 1973; Lown et al., 1973). Unless mechanisms linking stress measures with pathophysiology are elucidated, physicians will pay little attention to life stress and illness studies.

It is clear from the perspective of rehabilitation that patients' recent life changes data, along with information regarding selected emotions and behaviors, have added greatly to educational and life restructuring goals needed following a heart attack. Emphasis on physical risk factors alone (diet, smoking, exercise, etc.) tends to ignore psychological and behavioral issues important to disease onset. Also, the chance of compliance goes up if patients are provided with several areas of concentration in their rehabilitation rather than just a few. In our rehabilitation study, patients found it very difficult to modify their smoking and body weight over 3–4 years following MI. They were more successful with exercise, and with the modification of selected emotions (e.g. anger, hostility). They were most successful in their modification of key behaviors (e.g. rushing against time and overwork). Finally, patients' overall feelings of achieved control over their several areas of coronary risk, plus group support in accomplishing this task, gave our patients a distinct, and significant, rehabilitation advantage over our controls.

The author has outlined several of his studies which support the utility of using standardized recent life changes information in helping to understand why persons susceptible to clinical episodes of CHD develop them when they do. A full and meaningful appraisal of such information requires four distinct research steps: baseline life change estimations; pre-illness, illness, and post-illness life change measurements; cross-validation (replication); and retrospective studies leading to prospective investigations. To accomplish the author's series of such studies required extensive collaboration with other specialists for over a decade. Each new study was guided by results of our previous work.

Selected emotions and behaviors were also explored in these studies. Results agreed with the findings of clinicians over the previous 100 years. However, as in our studies of recent life change, individual variability was found to be large. Some commonly assumed characteristic emotions and behaviors of patients with CHD were endorsed at prevalence rates as low as 10%.

Rehabilitation following non-fatal clinical episodes of CHD has been broadened significantly by inclusions of recent life changes data as well as by attention paid to selected emotions and behaviors. Examples of the author's long-term rehabilitation studies using this information in a group therapy format are presented.

REFERENCES

Barchas, J.D., Akil, H., Elliott, G.R., Holman, R.B., & Watson, S.J. (1978). Behavioral neurochemistry: Neurotransmitters and behavioral states. *Science, 200*, 964–973.
Bruhn, J.G., Wolf, S., Lynn, T.N., *et al.* (1968). Social aspects of coronary heart disease in a Pennsylvania German community. *Social Science and Medicine, 2*, 201.
DeFaire, U. (1975). Life change patterns prior to death in ischaemic heart disease: A study of death-discordant twins. *Journal of Psychosomatic Research, 19*, 273–278.
Dimsdale, J.E., & Moss, J. (1980). Short term catecholamine responses to psychological stress. *Psychosomatic Medicine, 42*, 493–497.
Dunbar, F. (1943). *Psychosomatic diagnosis*. New York: Hoeber.
Ekman, G., & Lundberg, U. (1971). Emotional reaction to past and future events as a function of temporal distance. *Acta Psychologica, 35*, 430–441.
Friedman, M., & Rosenman, R.H. (1959). Association of specific overt behavior pattern with blood and cardiovascular findings. *Journal of the American Medical Association, 169*, 1286.
Haft, J., & Fani, K. (1973). Stress and the induction of intravascular platelet aggregation in the heart. *Circulation, 48*, 164–169.
Horowitz, M.J., Schaefer, C., & Cooney, P. (1974). Life event scaling for recency of experience. In E.K.E. Gunderson, R.H. Rahe (eds), *Life stress and illness*. Springfield, Illinois: Charles C Thomas.

Houston, K.B. (1983). Psychophysiological responsivity and the Type A behavior pattern. *Journal of Research into Personality, 17*, 22–39.

Kasl, S., Cobb, S., & Brooks, G.W. (1968). Changes in serum uric acid and cholesterol levels in men undergoing job loss. *Journal of the American Medical Association, 206*, 1500–1507.

Krantz, D.S., Manuk, S.B. (1984). Acute psychophysiologic reactivity and risk of cardiovascular disease: A review and methodologic critique. *Psychology Bulletin, 96*, 435–464.

Liljefors, I., & Rahe, R.H. (1970). An identical twin study of psychosocial factors in coronary heart disease in Sweden. *Psychosomatic Medicine, 32*, 523–542.

Lown, B., Verrier, R., & Corbulan, R. (1973). Psychologic stress and threshold for repetitive ventricular response. *Science, 182*, 834–836.

Mason, J.W. (1975). A historical view of the stress field. *Journal of Human Stress, 1*, 22–36.

Mason, J.W., Hartley, L.H., Kotchen, T.A., Mougey, E.H., Richetts, P.T., & Jones, L.G. (1973). Plasma cortisol and norepinephrine responses in anticipation of muscular exercise. *Psychosomatic Medicine, 35*, 406–414.

Osler, W. (1910). The Humleian lectures on angina pectoris. *Lancet, 1*, 697–702.

Peete, D.C. (1955). *The psychosomatic genesis of coronary heart disease.* Springfield, Illinois: Charles C Thomas.

The Pooling Project Research Group (1978). Relationship of blood pressure, serum cholesterol, smoking habit, relative weight, and ECG abnormalities to incidence of major coronary events. Final report of the pooling project. *Journal of Chronic Diseases, 31*, 201–306.

Rahe, R.H. (1969). Life crisis and health change. In P.R.A. May & R. Whittenborn (eds), *Psychotropic drug response: Advances in prediction*, pp. 92–125. Springfield, Illinois: Charles C Thomas.

Rahe, R.H. (1975). Epidemiological studies of life change and illness. *International Journal of Psychiatry and Medicine, 6*, 133–146.

Rahe, R.H. (1978). Life change measurement clarification. *Psychosomatic Medicine, 40*, 95–98.

Rahe, R.H., & Arthur, R.J. (1978). Life change and illness studies: Past history and future directions. *Journal of Human Stress, 4*, 3–15.

Rahe, R.H., & Lind, E. (1971). Psychosocial factors and sudden cardiac death. *Journal of Psychosomatic Research, 15*, 19–24.

Rahe, R.H., McKean, J.D., & Arthur, R.J. (1967). A longitudinal study of life change and illness patterns. *Journal of Psychosomatic Research, 10*, 355–366.

Rahe, R.H., & Paasikivi, J. (1971). Psychosocial factors and myocardial infarction, II. An outpatient study in Sweden. *Journal of Psychosomatic Research, 15*, 33–39.

Rahe, R.H., Scalzi, C., & Shine, K. (1975a). A teaching evaluation questionnaire for post-myocardial infarction patients. *Heart Lung, 4*, 759–766.

Rahe, R.H., Ward, H.W., & Hayes, V. (1979). Brief group therapy in myocardial infarction rehabilitation: Three to four year follow-up of a controlled trial. *Psychosomatic Medicine, 41*, 229–242.

Rahe, R.H., Meyer, M., Smith, M., Kjaer, G., & Holmes, T.H. (1964). Social stress and illness onset. *Journal of Psychosomatic Research, 8*, 35–44.

Rahe, R.H., Rubin, R.T., Arthur, R.J., & Clark, B.R. (1968). Serum uric acid and cholesterol variability: A comprehensive view of underwater demolition team training. *Journal of the American Medical Association, 206*, 2875–2880.

Rahe, R.H., Bennett, L.K., Romo, M., Siltanen, P., & Arthur, R.J. (1973a). Subjects' recent life changes and coronary heart disease in Finland. *American Journal of Psychology, 130*, 1222–1226.

Rahe, R.H., Tuffli, C.F., Suchor, R.J., & Arthur, R.J. (1973b). Group therapy in the outpatient management of post-myocardial infarction patients. *Psychology in Medicine, 4*, 77–88.

Rahe, R.H., Floistad, I., Bergan, T. et al. (1974a). A model for life changes and illness research: Cross-cultural data from the Norwegian Navy. *Archives of General Psychiatry, 31*, 172–177.

Rahe, R.H., Romo, M., Bennett, L.K., & Siltanen, P. (1974b). Subjects' recent life changes, myocardial infarction, and sudden coronary death. *Archives of Internal Medicine, 133*, 221–228.

Rahe, R.H., O'Neil, T., Hagan, A., & Arthur, R.J. (1975b). Brief group therapy following myocardial infarction: Eighteen month follow-up of a controlled trial. *International Journal of Psychiatry and Medicine, 6*, 349–358.

Romo, M., Siltanen, P., Theorell, T., & Rahe, R.H. (1974). Work behavior, time urgency and life dissatisfactions in subjects with myocardial infarction: A cross-cultural study. *Journal of Psychosomatic Research, 18*, 1–8.

Rubin, R.T., Rahe, R.H., Arthur, R.J., & Clark, B.R. (1969). Adrenal cortical activity changes during underwater demolition team training. *Psychosomatic Medicine, 31*, 553–564.

Schaeffer, M.A., & Baum, A. (1984). Adrenal cortical response to stress at Three Mile Island. *Psychosomatic Medicine, 46*, 227–237.

Schleifer, S.J., Keller, S.E., Camerino, M., Thornton, J.C., & Stein, M. (1983). Suppression of lymphocyte stimulation following bereavement. *Journal of the American Medical Association, 250*, 374–377.

Theorell, T., Lind, E., & Floderus, B. (1975). The relationship of disturbing life changes and emotions in the early development of myocardial infarction and other serious illnesses. *International Journal of Epidemiology, 4*, 281–293.

Theorell, T., & Rahe, R.H. (1971). Psychosocial factors and myocardial infarction. I. An inpatient study in Sweden. *Journal of Psychosomatic Research, 15*, 25–32.

Theorell, T., & Rahe, R.H. (1975). Life change events ballistocardiography, and coronary death. *Journal of Human Stress, 1*, 18–24.

Theorell, T., & Rahe, R.H. (1972). Behavior and life satisfactions characteristics of Swedish subjects with myocardial infarction. *Journal of Chronic Disease, 25*, 139–147.

Theorell, T., Lind, E., Froberg, J. *et al.* (1972). A longitudinal study of 21 subjects with coronary heart disease: Life changes, catecholamine excretion, and related biochemical reactions. *Psychosomatic Medicine, 34*, 505–516.

Van Der Valk, J.M., & Groen, J.J. (1967). Personality structure and conflict situation in patients with myocardial infarction. *Journal of Psychosomatic Research, 11*, 41.

Wolf, S., McCabe, W., Yamamoto, J., Adsett, C., & Schottstaedt, W. (1962). Changes in serum lipids in relation to emotional stress during rigid control of diet and exercise. *Circulation, 26*, 379–387.

KEY WORDS

Recent life changes, life change units, rehabilitation, stress, coping, coronary heart disease, myocardial infarction, sudden death.

Handbook of Life Stress, Cognition and Health
Edited by S. Fisher and J. Reason
© 1988 John Wiley & Sons Ltd.

18

Stress, Disability and Handicap

CHRISTINA KNUSSEN and CLIFF C. CUNNINGHAM
University of Manchester, England

INTRODUCTION

While disability and stress are relatively distinct areas of concern in terms of theory and practice, they have many features in common and are undergoing comparable shifts in orientation. Researchers in both areas have been abandoning simple, univariate, stimulus–response models with assumptions of inevitability of outcome, in favour of transactional, multivariate, mediated models with outcomes that are specific to the situation. Several recent studies capitalize on the congruities between theories of stress and disability, to discuss the effects of disability on the individual, the family and the community (e.g. Crnic *et al.*, 1983). In fact, some of the studies incorporate concepts from other areas, such as Bronfenbrenner's (1979) social system theory (e.g. Dunst *et al.*, 1986; Kazak, 1986); Kelly's (1955) personal construct theory (e.g. Cunningham and Davis, 1985; Schontz, 1969); and Rotter's (1966) theory of locus of control (e.g. Maisto and German, 1981).

The aims of this chapter are to evaluate some current approaches to the study of stress and disability, to draw parallels between the two areas, and to incorporate the concept of disability into a transactional model of stress. We then review examples of recent findings and discuss the insights afforded by some other frameworks.

DISABILITY AND HANDICAP

The World Health Organization (WHO, 1980) has provided clear and useful definitions of the terms impairment, disability and handicap, which have been widely used in the fields of physical and mental (or intellectual) disability (Gokhale, 1984; Heron and Myers, 1983; Mittler and Serpell, 1985).

Impairment is defined as follows: 'In the context of health experience, an impairment is any loss or abnormality of psychological, physiological or anatomical structure or function'. Thus, the loss of a limb and a chromosomal abnormality are both types of impairment.

335

Disability is defined as '. . . any restriction or lack (resulting from an impairment) of ability to perform an activity in the manner or within the range considered normal for a human being.' Thus a limp and a speech impediment are both examples of disability resulting from impairment.

Handicap is defined as '. . . a disadvantage for an individual, resulting from an impairment or a disability, that limits or prevents the fulfilment of a role that is normal (depending on age, sex, and social and cultural factors) for that individual.' Handicap therefore results from the interaction between the person and the social environment: it is a failure to meet the expectations of a particular situation. Using the WHO definitions, it is possible to say that the person with a limp is handicapped in situations which require him or her to walk, run or move without a limp, and the person who has a speech impediment is handicapped in situations which require or demand a certain facility of speech. Although the WHO definitions focus on organic sources of disability, difficulties in aspects such as problem solving can result not only from cognitive impairments, but also from social factors such as the lack of experience or opportunity. Social disadvantages, therefore, may also be seen as possible antecedents of handicaps, in that they prevent 'the fulfilment of a role that is normal . . . for that individual'.

Some disabilities invariably lead to handicap in certain situations; a person who is blind will always be visually handicapped to some extent. The extent, however, will depend upon such things as the context, access to education, and compensatory aids. The mediating roles of personal factors, such as attitudes, values, problem-solving skills and past history, are thus acknowledged. Furthermore, the disability may mark out areas of vulnerability for the individual, although this does not mean that the outcome of disability is always negative. The person with a loss of sight may, for example, develop increased powers of perception. Similarly, many parents state that a child with disabilities increases the quality of family life. Following this line of argument, handicap is a function of behavioural and social responses to disability. It should be defined in terms of the special needs of an individual to function as normally as possible in the environment. Special needs are not aetiological categories of impairment, therefore, but are such things as increased mobility, increased finance, access to an advocate and to a social network.

In this framework, handicap is neither an inevitable nor a permanent consequence of disability; it is dependent upon the transactions and interactions among a whole range of social, cultural and behavioural variables. Recognizing this, the current trend is towards using multivariable approaches to identify the individual, family and environmental factors responsible for, and associated with, successful functioning in society. Such an approach acknowledges the error in making linear and univariate connections between disability, special needs and handicap. It also acknowledges the danger of using impairment (i.e. a pathology) as the dominant model for making sense of handicap. This is likely to result in additional handicap as it implies that there is nothing that can be done to remedy the situation. When this happens the prediction is fulfilled, because nothing is done and consequently the individual or family is deprived of necessary resources. This pathological model becomes pathological in a further sense, by failing to generate the search for solutions to a problem. Thus the reason for defining a handicap in terms of special needs is to identify the resources required to meet those needs. In this sense, handicap is also a consequence of lack of resources, and the degree of handicap experienced within specific situations will be dependent upon the resources available to meet current needs. Handicap is seen as an everchanging outcome dependent upon the transactions among needs, resources and contexts. As such, the framework is characterized by the active search for solutions rather than static explanations of inevitable consequence. This framework is very close to current models of stress.

STRESS AND DISABILITY: THEORY

Stress is increasingly defined as an interaction, transaction or process mediated by other factors (see Fisher, 1986; Johnson, 1986). In this dynamic framework, it complements the changes in the field of disability. The model of stress described by Lazarus and his colleagues (e.g. Folkman, 1984; Folkman and Lazarus, 1985; Lazarus et al., 1985; Lazarus and Folkman, 1984) is increasingly being used by researchers primarily interested in disability; this is because it allows for a wide variety of coping resources and responses, focuses on the response of the individual, and is comprehensive yet adaptable (Friedrich et al., 1985; Silver and Wortman, 1980). Within the Lazarus model, stress is defined as: '. . . a relationship between the person and the environment that is appraised by the person as taxing or exceeding his or her resources and as endangering his or her well-being' (Folkman, 1984; p. 840).

Thus stress is not a stimulus (such as disability), an intrapersonal conflict (such as anxiety), nor a response (such as distress); it is a process which is dynamic, interactive and reactive. The stress process is mediated by two other processes: cognitive appraisal and coping.

Appraisal

Appraisal refers to processes by which the meaning of an event or an encounter is determined. Appraisal is central to the model in that nothing is stressful unless it is appraised as such by an individual. There are two main levels of appraisal. The first, primary appraisal, is concerned with judging whether an event is (a) irrelevant, (b) benign or positive, or (c) negative. If it is negative, it can be concerned with (i) existing harm or loss, such as impairment, disability or other vulnerability, (ii) threat, which is the potential for harm or loss, or (iii) challenge, which is an opportunity for gain, growth or mastery. Primary appraisal is influenced by personal factors, such as beliefs and commitments, and by environmental or situational factors, such as the familiarity of the event, the likelihood of its occurrence and the nature of the possible outcome.

If the event is appraised as stressful, the individual then asks what might be done about it. This is secondary appraisal, and it involves the evaluation of the following coping resources.

a) Physical assets, e.g. health, energy and stamina.
b) Social assets, e.g. social networks, support systems.
c) Psychological assets, e.g. beliefs and values, problem-solving skills, self-esteem and morale.
d) Material assets, e.g. money, equipment, tools.

These coping resources are derived from the personal and environmental variables which are operative at any one time. If such resources are required but insufficient, then they may be viewed as special needs.

Coping

Coping refers to 'cognitive and behavioural efforts to master, reduce, or tolerate the internal and/or external demands that are created by a stressful transaction' (Folkman, 1984; p. 843). It is therefore a process which is independent of whether its outcome is successful or not. Broadly, coping can be focused on the regulation of emotion, or on the management of the problem, but most people will not restrict themselves to one type of coping.

The *outcome,* or effects, of coping will be both immediate and long term. These effects can lead to changes in (a) psychological well-being, (b) somatic health, or (c) social functioning.

The term *encounter* is used by Lazarus *et al.* (1985) to describe the specific occasion when something like an event or feature is appraised. The relationship between the encounter and the outcome corresponds to that between disability and handicap, in that handicap will vary according to personal and environmental factors, and the extent to which resources are available to meet special needs. The concept of a *vulnerability* is particularly useful in this context: a vulnerability is a particular weakness or susceptibility associated with one of the personal or environmental variables. It can result from a previous stressful encounter, or such things as circumstantial and dispositional factors. In this sense, a disability can create vulnerabilities in resources via the personal and environmental variables, dependent upon the situation. Vulnerability can therefore explain why some encounters are more likely to occur than others.

It will be seen that the stress process is dynamic, in that the processes of appraisal and coping influence each other. If the immediate outcome of coping is not successful, reappraisal can initiate a search for new coping strategies from the resources. The long-term outcomes of an encounter can make an impact on coping resources. For example, reactions to a stressful encounter, such as loss of sleep and headaches, can drain physical strength, and become sources of stress in themselves. Congruent with the earlier discussion of disability and handicap, the outcome of a stressful encounter is not always negative; people can gain in self-confidence and self-esteem when they have coped successfully with a stressful situation, thereby increasing their psychological resources. Both frameworks, therefore, avoid the pitfalls of pathological models.

The following example illustrates the ways in which the processes operate. A man who has an amputation of his leg (impairment) may find that he can no longer drive his car (disability), because he cannot operate the clutch with the artificial limb. He finds this stressful (primary appraisal) because he can no longer get to work easily; it hurts his pride to have to depend on others to drive him around; he cannot walk far enough to enable him to use public transport; and his freedom is severely restricted (personal and environmental variables). Without his car, he is handicapped in many situations (outcome). He decides that he wants to change this situation (reappraisal), and notes that his special needs are increased mobility and modifications to the vehicle. He assesses his options (secondary appraisal), and decides that he can afford to have his car adapted, and has the self-confidence to learn to drive again (coping resources). The long-term outcome is increased self-esteem and confidence, and the reduction of various handicaps and vulnerabilities resulting from the disability.

The Role of the Perceiver

One of the attractions of this framework for people in the field of disability is that it highlights the central role of the individual in the process; within the field, there has been a strong movement towards approaches which accept that the views of the individual with disabilities, and of his or her family, concerning their needs and preferences, are paramount, e.g. self-advocacy and consumer partnership models of working with parents (Cunningham and Davis, 1985). In a similar manner, Lazarus et al. (1985) emphasized that stress depends on the appraisal of the relationship between an environmental event and the demands it makes in terms of coping resources: 'there are no environmental stressors without vulnerable people whose agendas and resources influence whether they experience stress, the form it will take, and its short- and long-run outcomes . . . No environmental event can be identified as a stressor independent of its appraisal by the person' (p. 776).

This philosophical congruity is also reflected in clinical models such as Kelly's (1955) personal construct theory, and in various approaches to counselling (e.g. Rogers, 1980). Fundamental to these approaches is that the individual has to interpret and control his or her own processes. For example, it is often assumed by professionals that parents who are told that their child has a condition such as cerebral palsy will suffer greater distress than those told that their child has dyslexia. This judgement fails to take into account the values, hopes, knowledge and aspirations of the parents. It ignores the variability of people's responses to stressful situations (Johnson, 1986). Cunningham and Davis (1985) have described a model, based on Kelly's theory, of the process of adaptation following the disclosure to parents of a diagnosis of disability. The task faced by parents is to construct a framework to understand the 'new child' in relation to the 'label'; to make sense of themselves as parents of such a child, which will involve both an appraisal of their reactions (often very intense and frightening), and their abilities to cope. Inherent in the model is the concept that parental reaction, such as denial, should not be construed as being maladaptive, but instead as signifying that parents are giving themselves the opportunity to explore and reconstrue. In the same way, anxiety, according to Kelly, is an individual's awareness that events are outside the realm of his or her present personal construct system; thus anxiety is a precursor of change, and should not automatically be interpreted as a negative consequence. In other words, anxiety is related to the uncertainty experienced in the encounter, but whether it is experienced as a negative or a positive factor will be determined by the individual's resources. Faerstein (1986) investigated mothers' reactions to the diagnosis of a child's disabilities. She noted that reactions such as self-blame and denial can be positively related to successful coping if they are used to free the individual to focus on mastery of the problem. If the defences are ineffectual, however, anxiety will result.

Fundamental to these approaches is the need to measure the perceptions of the individuals in determining the outcome. Within the framework, one cannot talk about an environmental stressor or a stressful event external to the perceptions of the individual involved. Studies which have concentrated solely on the environmental event or feature have not produced consistent results, as concluded by Zimmerman (1983) in his review of measures of life events. Similarly, Henderson (1978) found that perceptions of adequacy of support were more predictive of positive outcome in patients with mental illness than factual data describing the availability of support. In our recent research, we have found substantial discrepancies between scores on checklists of behaviour difficulties in children with Down's syndrome, and parental perceptions of whether the children had behaviour difficulties. This was particularly apparent in a study which identified two groups of the children who had similar profiles on the checklist of behaviour difficulties (Cunningham, 1986). The mothers of one group perceived that their children were particularly difficult to manage, and the mothers of the second group perceived no management difficulty. The mothers who perceived they had management problems had poorer relationships with their children, expressed less affection for them, were less well adjusted to them, and had higher levels of psychosomatic symptoms, as assessed on the Malaise Inventory (Rutter et al. 1970), than the other mothers. However, the mothers did not differ in terms of demographic and family variables. Without the measures of parental perception there would have been a danger of generalizing about the relationship between behaviour difficulties and measures of negative outcome. Therefore, studies that use disability as an independent variable (i.e. as an environmental stressor) are likely to promote a potentially damaging determinism.

On the other hand, Dohrenwend et al. (1984) and Dohrenwend and Shrout (1985) have argued that if the objective characteristics of events or situations are not recorded, there is no way to determine the contribution of personal and social factors to coping and outcome measures. Measures of appraisal of an event, coping resources, coping strategies and outcome will all correlate highly because they are all measuring the same subjective feelings of 'stress'.

Lazarus et al. (1985) have responded by suggesting that confounding can be reduced by studying the relationships among variables across a series of time points. They also confirm that the focus of study should be the personal and environmental variables which influence appraisal: in other words, determining what it is about the individual and the situation that produces different appraisal and outcomes.

In studying disability and handicap, a useful approach would seem to be the concentrate on the vulnerabilities in personal and environmental variables; this assumes that disabilities can create vulnerabilities. This is not a pathological approach, since vulnerabilities are not inevitably 'stressors', and are not independent of other variables.

The frameworks discussed above imply that studies which rely solely on measuring the univariate relationships between the external event and negative outcome are misleading, especially if they also fail to take the appraisal of the individual into account. Furthermore, many of these studies rely on simplistic statistical analyses which often ignore the intercorrelations among independent variables, and fail to delineate an organizing theoretical framework. The results of such studies, however, can indicate, at a generalized level, gross vulnerabilities which might be associated with disability. This does not mean that the measures themselves are not intrinsically valuable. One such measure is the Malaise Inventory (Rutter *et al.*, 1970). This was adapted from the Cornell Medical Index and designed to assess psychosomatic symptoms associated with emotional disturbance. It consists of 24 'yes/no' items concerning physical or emotional states with an underlying psychological component; the total number of positive responses yields the Malaise score. With a sample of children with Down's syndrome, Cunningham (1986) found that the score of mothers on the Malaise Inventory correlated significantly with reported life events in the past year ($r=0.49$, $p<0.001$). Similar significant correlations were found between Malaise scores and variables such as unemployment, various behaviour problems in the children and a measure of adaptation to the child. Hirst (1983) criticized the Malaise Inventory on the grounds that it lacks a single unifying construct of emotional disturbance. However, it has recently been demonstrated that Hirst's conclusion was due to an inappropriate analysis (Bebbington and Quine, 1987), and that it has satisfactory psychometric properties (McGee *et al.*, 1986). It is thus worth noting that despite its limitations, the Malaise Inventory may be useful as one of a battery of outcome measures. A range of measures is of course essential in determining interrelationships in multivariable frameworks.

In the next section, we review studies which focus on families of children with disabilities, in order to consider methodological issues and highlight features which may put some individuals 'at risk'.

STRESS AND DISABILITY: RESEARCH STUDIES

Byrne and Cunningham (1985) described three current approaches to the study of stress in families which include a child with disabilities. The first is concerned with determining the factors which correlate with outcome measures of stress (e.g. type of disability, health and behaviour problems, demographic variables), the second is related to the practical or material needs of families (e.g. contact with services, financial assistance, respite care), and the third is concerned with factors that facilitate coping and adaptation (e.g. marital relationship, family cohesion, social support networks).

With the first approach, typically the independent variables—demographic, child characteristics, family characteristics—are correlated with a measure of perceived or psychosomatic symptoms such as the Malaise Inventory (Rutter *et al.*, 1970), the Questionnaire on Resources and Stress (Holroyd, 1974), or the Beck Depression Inventory (Beck *et al.*, 1961). Tew and Laurence (1975), for example, correlated a series of child and demographic variables with scores on the Malaise Inventory, and presented these to support their conclusion that parental stress is highest when the child is severely handicapped. However, no attempt was made to determine the unique contributions of each variable by controlling for the effects of other variables.

Beckman (1983) improved on this approach somewhat and reported a series of correlations and intercorrelations among child and family demographic variables and scores on the Questionnaire on Resources and Stress (QRS) (Holroyd, 1974) completed by mothers. The QRS consists of 285 items and 15 scales, yielding three major scale clusters: parent problems, family problems and child problems. It was designed to measure adaptation and coping in families including a child with disabilities. The QRS score used by Beckman was derived from the total number of parent and family problems. She concluded that four of the five child characteristics (caregiving demands, social responsiveness, temperament and repetitive behaviours) were significantly related to QRS scores, but that it was likely that they were all highly intercorrelated. Using the author's reported correlation coefficients in a partial correlation analysis, we found that the effect of the fifth child characteristic (rate of progress) emerged as significantly related to the QRS score, so that the higher the rate of progress, the higher the scores. Furthermore, although the number of caregiving demands was still the best predictor of QRS scores when the effects of other variables were partialled out, two variables (social responsiveness and temperament) had been mediated by the other factors, and were no longer significantly associated with the outcome measure.

Quine and Pahl (1985) focused on the service needs of mothers. This study is strengthened by a more multivariable approach, but it relies on a single outcome measure—the score on the Malaise Inventory. The effects of a series of child and family characteristics on the scores were considered individually and uniquely through a multiple regression analysis. Some of the predictor variables were independent of objective ratings, and some were based on subjective parental reports, such as social isolation, and problems with the child's appearance. An independent measure of behaviour problems emerged as the best predictor of the score on the Malaise Inventory. No differences on scores on the Malaise Inventory were found between mothers of children of different disability groups (such as Down's syndrome and spina bifida). However, there was a significant relationship between such scores and the number of the child's impairments or disabilities. Thus, as predicted by the Lazarus model, there is no clear evidence that diagnostic category of disability can be used to predict the nature and outcome of the stress process. However, in this and other studies, the largest amount of variance related to negative outcome measures is accounted for by unusual caregiving demands related to independent functioning, physical incapacities and behavioural difficulties (e.g. Bristol, 1983; Bradshaw and Lawton, 1978). Caregiving demands are often independent of measures of the child's mental abilities, and the negative consequences are generally associated with the supervisory needs of the child. With quite able children with Down's syndrome, we find that parents are likely to describe their supervisory role as the major demand on resources. Even so, the degree of the parents' vulnerability depends upon personal and environmental variables, and will vary across the life-span. For example, many studies report that disturbance of sleep is found in large numbers of children with intellectual disabilities. Yet we found that parental perceptions of whether or not this constitutes a problem are dependent upon such variables as age of child, family structure, housing arrangements, and the child's health (Cunningham, 1986).

Friedrich et al. (1985) examined the extent to which variations in coping resources predict coping outcome or 'family functioning' in the context of a model derived from that of Lazarus (Crnic et al., 1983). Several aspects of coping resources were measured, including family income, parental education and age, depression, psychological well-being, marital satisfaction, and family relationships. Measures were also taken of aspects of child behaviour and child health. The outcome measure was derived from a version of the Questionnaire on Resources and Stress (Friedrich et al., 1983), representing parent and family problems. Multiple regression procedures were used to determine the unique contributions of these variables to the outcome measures. The variables found to be associated with QRS scores were child medical and behavioural problems, maternal depression, marital happiness, and family relationships. The study was repeated after an interval of 8 months with the same subjects; changes in marital happiness predicted both changes in coping outcome and changes in depression. The strength of this study lies in its clarification of the interrelatedness of the variables, but it is possible that some of the measures of coping resources may not have been the most appropriate for this population. For example, since the parents were mostly well educated with above average incomes, there were probably very few families for whom lack of finance presented a need or vulnerability. More importantly, there is no clear indication of the exact nature of the theoretical framework. The opening statement undermines the authors' alleged faith in the Lazarus model: 'The presence of a chronic disability in a child is a stressor that requires an ongoing coping response by the parents.' (p. 130).

In conclusion, the use of the concept of an 'environmental stressor' (e.g. the aetiological label, unemployment) has not proved useful in explaining variation in outcome measures of the stress process. Rather, variables associated with special needs or demands on resources (e.g. caregiving demands) seem more potent. Such variables are likely to tap vulnerabilities, such as limited time and energy, and to transact with a range of other variables, such as family cohesion, access to support, and parental adjustment to disability. Such variables are easily located in the coping resources of the Lazarus model. Consequently, the model is beginning to be used in support programmes for families with children with disabilities (e.g. Zeitlin et al., 1986), and offers the potential for predicting which variables should be included in studies aimed at tracing the coping strategies of individuals with disabilities and their families. At present, however, the literature cannot be interpreted with any confidence because of the limited range of studies using transactional models with representative samples. Not surprisingly, the literature does indicate that disability can create gross vulnerabilities. Although these are generalizations, they do go some way in answering the key question: which people need which resources at which times? At present, however, there is insufficient detail to indicate the characteristic clusters of variables related to vulnerabilities and coping processes. More research is required based on multivariate approaches. However, this methodology is unlikely to be effective without better theoretical underpinning. This can be seen in the area of social support.

SOCIAL SUPPORT

Social support is one of the main coping resources in the Lazarus model, and has received a lot of attention. It is generally claimed, for example, that social networks are sources of material help, recreation and emotional support, and provide opportunities to try out new ideas (e.g. Dunst *et al.*, 1986). Many studies have reported that parents of children with disabilities, particularly mothers, experience feelings of isolation (e.g. Bradshaw and Lawton, 1978; Quine and Pahl, 1985; Wishart *et al.*, 1981). However, other studies have reported that families of children with disabilities are no more isolated than other families (Kazak, 1987), and that mothers of children with Down's syndrome do not feel that the child restricts them socially (Byrne *et al.*, 1988; Carr, 1975). While this confusion may be due, in part, to a failure to partial out other variables (such as age and family characteristics), there appear to be more serious problems. Barrera (1986) found that definitions of social support tend to be so vague that as a single construct, it is no longer useful; for example, social isolation can include restriction of movement, lack of social contact, and perceived emotional isolation. Barrera suggested that it should be 'broken down' into its various components and that more precise models should be developed to investigate the relationships between aspects of social support and other variables. Alloway and Bebbington (1987) also reported a lack of generally accepted measures of social support. Consequently, only gross conclusions can be drawn from the literature—that, for example, parents of children with disabilities may be vulnerable to feelings of isolation or alienation. In accordance with other studies, Byrne *et al.* (1988) found that most emotional and practical support for mothers of children with Down's syndrome comes from kinship networks, particularly from the husband and from her own female relatives. Support is also gained from other parents of similar children.

Although sparse, research on the friendship patterns of people with major disabilities is less diffuse. Such friendships tend to be restricted in number, and often the individuals with disabilities are spectators rather than direct interactors. Friendship patterns change over the lifespan, but many children with disabilities do not have the opportunities to learn and develop personal and social interactive skills, often because of the nature of the disability and the limited social networks they experience in segregated settings. A long-term consequence of this is that when they eventually enter into adult life, with limitations for employment, they may also have limitations on how they can extend their leisure and social life. The same problem can also be seen in people as they age, or lose employment through disability, who have an increase in leisure time but have a concomitant deterioration of skills. Consequently, this may result in increased vulnerabilities in both groups, associated with isolation or alienation. A major issue related to the use and function of social support variables is that of independence and control. In the next section, we explore this in order to illustrate yet again the usefulness of the interrelating theory of stress and disability.

ASPECTS OF CONTROL

One of the basic beliefs held by most practitioners working with people with disabilities and their families is that people should be helped to achieve as great a degree of independence as possible in order to increase feelings of fulfillment. Independence assumes that people have control over their own lives, and that they make their own choices; however, parents can find it difficult to allow a child with disabilities to do things for him or herself (and to make their own mistakes), and the child may also find it difficult to act independently. Nihira *et al.* (1981) found that self-concept and self-esteem in children with intellectual disabilities were related to the quality of the home environment. In the field of special education, the curricula for people with disabilities are increasingly emphasizing control over the environment with the attendant increase in self-esteem, as opposed to mere rote-training of motor and perceptual skills.

In the field of stress, there have been many good reviews of the concept of control (see Fisher, 1986; Folkman, 1984). We concentrate on the effects of control and of self-blame on adaptation and coping with disability, as developing areas of potential importance.

Kagan (1970) asserted that the degree to which a mother perceives that she has control over the general environment is also related to her perception of the control she has over her children's development. Maisto and German (1981) looked at the relationship between the developmental gain of infants 'at risk' for developmental delay, and the scores of mothers on the Rotter Internal–External Locus of Control Scale (Rotter, 1966). Rotter assumed that the higher the 'internal' score, the greater the perceived control over the environment. However, Brewin and Shapiro (1984) showed that the Rotter I–E Scale measures control over positive outcomes (or achievements or luck) but not control over negative outcomes (failures or misfortunes). The mothers and children in the study were all involved in an intervention programme for at least a year, starting when the children were around 10 months old. Assessments were made during the intervention, and approximately 3 years later. The correlations between 'internality' and developmental gain were not significant during the period of intervention, but 3 years later significant correlations were found between 'internality' and cognitive and language developmental gain. No relationship was found between locus of control and motor developmental gain. It was not possible to determine conclusively the direction of the relationship, i.e. whether the perception of control influenced the development, or vice versa. However, it was suggested that the intervention programme may have temporarily enhanced perception of internality of control, or that locus of control may only emerge as a significant factor when the child is older. Thus, it would appear that the mothers who had low 'internal' scores felt that the rate of their child's development was due to luck or other external sources, and hence they may be less likely to make directed interactions with the child. Some support for this conclusion can also be inferred from a study by McConkey and McEvoy (1984), who investigated the reasons given by mothers of preschool children with intellectual disabilities for not enrolling on a Parental Involvement Course. They report that most of the mothers felt that they were already doing as good a job as possible as parents, and that they did not believe that they could influence the child's development. The mothers were also observed to be less actively involved in play with their children.

Control over negative outcomes is quite a different factor, and may not be a unitary concept. Brewin and Shapiro (1984) noted that control over negative outcomes could mean being able to escape or avoid the outcome, or, alternatively, it could mean being responsible for the outcome. This responsibility could be further divided into faults in character or in behaviour. Janoff-Bulman (1979) also distinguished between self-blame that is 'characterological' (belonging to stable aspects of the person's character, and therefore largely unavoidable) and 'behavioural' (belonging to a person's own modifiable behaviour). Characterological self-blame may be related to depression and lowered self-esteem, while behavioural self-blame may be associated with a belief that negative outcomes can be avoided in the future. Affleck et al. (1985) used these distinctions to investigate the effects of mothers' beliefs about the cause of their infants' developmental delay, irrespective of the actual cause. Over 40% of their sample reported suspected behavioural causes for their child's condition, that was either blaming self or others. All of the cases of self-blame were behavioural rather than characterological, and this self-blame was found to be associated with more positive outcomes (better mood states, fewer caretaking problems, and a better quality of environment for the child) at 9 and 18 months after the birth of the child. Blaming others was related to less favourable outcomes. One would predict that the self-blaming mothers in this study would have achieved high 'internal' scores on the Rotter scale, reflecting a belief in control over positive outcome.

Although it can often be difficult to differentiate between the various aspects of control, it is theoretically important to separate generalized and specific beliefs about control from the use of control as a coping strategy. This helps in understanding why sometimes heightened perceptions of control can be counter-productive, or associated with negative outcomes, depending on coping resources and other beliefs and commitments. For example, a mother who believes that she can influence her disabled child's development may feel guilty if she does this at the expense of attention she is able to give to another child, or if she is repeatedly unable to purchase toys, equipment and items which she believes will help the child.

Similar processes have been indicated in other areas of disability. Bulman and Wortman (1977), for example, found that amongst people suffering severe spinal cord injuries, the best predictors of judged good coping were high levels of self-blame, low blame on others and low perceived avoidability, i.e. those who felt that they could not have avoided the accident but who felt that they were nevertheless to blame. This seemed to be related to the circumstances of the accident. It helped when the person was involved in a customary or usual activity that was enjoyable or associated with leisure. In a similar way, Brewin (1982) distinguished between causal responsibility and culpability as aspects of behavioural self-blame—causal responsibility being the extent to which actions result in a particular outcome, and culpability being the moral evaluation of 'deservingness' of blame. Brewin suggested that Bulman and Wortman's (1977) self-blame was allied to feelings of causal responsibility, and avoidability was allied to culpability: those who felt responsible for the accident ('self-blame') may have coped better than those who felt culpable ('avoidability') because the latter felt the actions which led to the accident had been 'mistakes'. Brewin found that among men who had suffered fairly minor industrial accidents, both causal responsibility and culpability were associated with 'good' coping and positive outcome, and he suggested that the serious and permanent nature of the injuries sustained by Bulman and Wortman's sample may have made culpability particularly difficult to bear. Thus, feelings of control can contribute to both negative and positive outcomes, depending upon personal and environmental variables, and interact with aspects of the situation such as perceived likelihood of recovery.

In conclusion, these studies again suggest that the individual's appraisal of a disability, and the coping resources he or she has at his or her disposal, must form the centre of any discussion of the effects of the disability. Although it would seem that an individual is 'at risk' or vulnerable if appraisal of control does not match reality, this appraisal may facilitate successful coping and adaptation. As has been indicated, there is no reason to believe that the principles and processes involved in adaptation vary across areas of disability as diverse as accidental injury to an adult and the diagnosis of disability in an infant. It would perhaps be worth investigating whether or not it is necessary to blame oneself for past behaviour in order to perceive that one has control over future outcome. Self-blame would seem to be an aid to this process, but perhaps intervention would permit this to be diverted into something more useful. It is certainly an area worthy of more detailed consideration by those investigators interested in describing vulnerabilities and developing preventative interventions.

Although it is generally assumed that beliefs and values about oneself, one's children and disability strongly influence expectations, aspirations and, in turn, behaviour, there has been little systematic effort to delineate either changes in parents' construct system or its effects. Despite this, such constructs appear to be given paramount standing in clinical practice, as indicated by descriptions of parents as 'unaccepting', 'uncaring', 'unrealistic', 'self-blaming' and 'guilt-ridden'—all of which are often used in an accusational and pathological manner. Values and perceptions of children and of intellectual disability and aspirations have also been found to influence adjustment, and to change over time. As a child with disabilities matures, there is some evidence that the parents become more resistant to concepts of normalization and independent living, and to perceive the community as less accepting of the disability (Ferrara, 1979; Suelzle and Keenan, 1981). Clearly, we need a better understanding of how an individual's appraisal of his or her own disability, or that of a family member, changes over the lifespan.

SUMMARY AND CONCLUSIONS

This chapter focuses on the parallels between changing concepts and methods in disability and handicap, and stress. Both areas have moved towards the use of multivariate and transactional models centred on process, and away from univariate approaches that are largely based on the search for associations with negative outcomes. The latter has produced research in danger of generating oversimplified and pathological generalizations. A more positive construction is that disability may, but not inevitably, create vulnerabilities; whether this results in handicap is dependent upon the mediating role of personal and environmental resources. Central to the issue of determining which individuals at which point in their lifespan require which resources, is the perception of the situation by the individual.

This work was prepared whilst the authors were in receipt of funding from the Department of Health and Social Security for the Manchester Down's Syndrome Cohort Study.

REFERENCES

Affleck, G., McGrade, B.J., Allen, D.A., & McQueeny, M. (1985). Mothers' beliefs about behavioral causes for their developmentally disabled infants' condition: What do they signify? *Journal of Pediatric Psychology, 10,* 293–304.

Alloway, R., & Bebbington, P. (1987). The buffer theory of social support—a review of the literature. *Psychological Medicine, 17,* 91–108.

Barrera, M. (1986). Distinctions between social support concepts, measures and models. *American Journal of Community Psychology, 14,* 413–445.

Bebbington, A.C., & Quine, L. (1987). A comment on Hirst's 'Evaluating the Malaise Inventory'. *Social Psychiatry, 22,* 5–7.

Beck, A.T., Ward, C.H., Mendelson, M., Mock, J., & Erbaugh, J. (1961). An inventory for measuring depression. *Archives of General Psychiatry, 4,* 561–571.

Beckman, P.J. (1983). Influence of selected child characteristics on stress in families of handicapped infants. *American Journal of Mental Deficiency, 88,* 150–156.

Bradshaw, J., & Lawton, D. (1978). Tracing the causes of stress in families with handicapped children. *British Journal of Social Work, 8,* 181–192.

Brewin, C.R. (1982). Adaptive aspects of self-blame in coping with accidental injury. In C. Antaki & C.R. Brewin (eds), *Attributions and psychological change* (pp. 119–134). London: Academic Press.

Brewin, C.R., & Shapiro, D.A. (1984). Beyond locus of control: Attribution of responsibility for positive and negative outcomes. *British Journal of Psychology, 75,* 43–49.

Bristol, M.M. (1983). Family resources and successful adaptation to autistic children. In E. Schopler & G. Mesibov (eds), *Families of auutistic children* New York: Plenum Press.

Bronfenbrenner, U. (1979). *The ecology of human development.* Cambridge, Mass.: Harvard University Press.

Bulman, R.J., & Wortman, C.B. (1977). Attributions of blame and coping in the 'real world': Severe accident victims react to their lot. *Journal of Personality and Social Psychology, 35,* 351–363.

Byrne, E.A., & Cunningham, C.C. (1985). The effects of mentally handicapped children on families—a conceptual review. *Journal of Child Psychology and Psychiatry, 26,* 847–864.

Byrne, E.A., Cunningham, C.C., & Sloper, P. (1988). *Families and their children with Down's syndrome: One feature in common.* London: Croom Helm.

Carr, J. (1975). *Young children and Down's syndrome,* IRMMH Monograph 4. London: Butterworths.

Crnic, K.A., Friedrich, W.N., & Greenberg, M.T. (1983). Adaptation of families with mentally retarded children: A model of stress, coping, and family ecology. *American Journal of Mental Deficiency, 88,* 125–138.

Cunningham, C.C. (1986). The effects of early intervention on the occurrence and nature of behaviour problems in children with Down's syndrome. Final Report to DHSS. Hester Adrian Research Centre, University of Manchester.

Cunningham, C.C., & Davis, H. (1985). *Working with parents: Frameworks for collaboration.* Milton Keynes: Open University Press.

Dohrenwend, B.P., & Shrout, P.E. (1985). 'Hassles' in the conceptualization and measurement of life stress variables. *American Psychologist, 40,* 780–785.

Dohrenwend, B.S., Dohrenwend, B.P., Dodson, M., & Shrout, P.E. (1984). Symptoms, hassles, social supports, and life events: Problem of confounded measures. *Journal of Abnormal Psychology, 93,* 222–230.

Dunst, C.J., Trivette, C.M., & Cross, A.H. (1986). Mediating influences of social support: Personal, family and child outcomes. *American Journal of Mental Deficiency, 90,* 403–417.

Faerstein, L.M. (1986). Coping and defense mechanisms of mothers of learning disabled children. *Journal of Learning Disabilities, 19,* 8–11.

Ferrara, D.M., (1979). Attitudes of parents of mentally retarded children towards normalization activities. *American Journal of Mental Deficiency, 84,* 145–151.

Fisher, S. (1986). *Stress and strategy.* London: Lawrence Erlbaum Associates.

Folkman, S. (1984). Personal control and stress and coping processes: A theoretical analysis. *Journal of Personality and Social Psychology, 46,* 839–852.

Folkman, S., & Lazarus, R.S. (1985). If it changes it must be a process: A study of emotion and coping during three stages of a college examination. *Journal of Personality and Social Psychology, 48,* 150–170.

Friedrich, W.N., Greenberg, M.T., & Crnic, K. (1983). A short form of the Questionnaire on Resources and Stress. *American Journal of Mental Deficiency, 88,* 41–48.

Friedrich, W.N., Wilturner, L.T., & Cohen, D.S. (1985). Coping resources and parenting mentally retarded children. *American Journal of Mental Deficiency, 90,* 130–139.

Gokhale, S.D. (1984). The disabled and the third world. In R.C. Nann, D.S. Butt & L. Ladrido-Ignacio (eds), *Mental health, cultural values and social development* (pp. 259–271). Dordrecht, Holland: Reidal.

Henderson, S. (1978). The patient's primary group. *British Journal of Psychiatry, 132,* 74–86.

Heron, A., & Myers, M. (1983). *Intellectual impairment: The battle against handicap.* London: Academic Press.

Hirst, M.A. (1983). Evaluating the Malaise Inventory: An item analysis. *Social Psychiatry, 18,* 181–184.

Holroyd, J. (1974). The Questionnaire on Resources and Stress: An instrument to measure family response to a handicapped family member. *Journal of Community Psychology, 2,* 92–94.

Janoff-Bulman, R. (1979). Characterological versus behavioral self-blame: Inquiries into depression and rape. *Journal of Personality and Social Psychology, 37,* 1798–1809.

Johnson, J. (1986). *Life events as stressors in childhood and adolescence.* London: Sage Publications.

Kagan, J. (1970). On class differences and early development. In V.H. Deneenberg (ed.), *Education of the infant and young child.* New York: Academic Press.

Kazak, A.E. (1986). Families with physically handicapped children: Social ecology and family systems. *Family Process, 25,* 265–281.

Kazak, A.E. (1987). Families with disabled children: Stress and social networks in three samples. *Journal of Abnormal Child Psychology, 15,* 137–146.

Kelly, G. (1955). *The psychology of personal constructs.* New York: Norton.

Lazarus, R.S., & Folkman, S. (1984). *Stress, appraisal, and coping.* New York: Springer.

Lazarus, R.S., DeLongis, A., Folkman, S., & Gruen, R. (1985). Stress and adaptational outcomes: The problem of confounded measures. *American Psychologist, 40,* 770–779.

Maisto, A.A., & German, M.L. (1981). Maternal locus of control and developmental gain demonstrated by high risk infants: A longitudinal analysis. *The Journal of Psychology, 109*, 213–221.

McConkey, R., & McEvoy, J. (1984). Parental Involvement Courses: Contrasts between mothers who enrol and those who do not. In J.M. Berg (ed.), *Perspectives and progress in mental retardation*, Vol. 1. Baltimore: University Park Press.

McGee, R., Williams, S., & Silva, P.A. (1986). An evaluation of the Malaise Inventory. *Journal of Psychosomatic Research, 30*, 147–152.

Mittler, P., & Serpell, R. (1985). Services: An international perspective. In A.M. Clarke, A.D.B. Clark & J.M. Berg (eds), *Mental deficiency: The changing outlook*, 4th edn (pp. 715–787). London: Methuen.

Nihira, K., Mink, I.T., & Meyers, C.E. (1981). Relationship between home environment and school adjustment of TMR children. *American Journal of Mental Deficiency, 86*, 8–15.

Quine, L., & Pahl, J. (1985). Examining the causes of stress in families with severely mentally handicapped children. *British Journal of Social Work, 15*, 501–517.

Rogers, C.R. (1980). *A way of being*. Boston: Houghton Mifflin.

Rotter, J.B. (1966). Generalized expectancies for internal versus external control of reinforcement. *Psychological Monographs: General and Applied, 80* (1, Whole No. 609).

Rutter, M., Tizard, J., & Whitmore, K. (1970). *Education, health and behaviour*. London: Longman.

Shontz, F.C. (1969). *Perceptual and cognitive aspects of body experience*. London: Academic Press.

Silver, R.L., & Wortman, C.B. (1980). Coping with undesirable life events. In J. Garber & M.E.P. Seligman (eds), *Human helplessness: Theory and applications* (pp. 279–375). New York: Academic Press.

Suelzle, M., & Keenan, V. (1981). Changes in family support networks over the life-cycle of mentally retarded persons. *American Journal of Mental Deficiency, 86*, 267–274.

Tew, B., & Laurence, K.M. (1975). Some sources of stress found in mothers of spina bifida children. *British Journal of Preventive Social Medicine, 29*, 27–30.

WHO (World Health Organization) (1980). *International classification of impairments, disabilities and handicaps*. Geneva: WHO.

Wishart, M.C., Bidder, R.T., & Gray, O.P. (1981). Parents' reports of family life with a developmentally delayed child. *Child: care, health and development, 7*, 267–279.

Zeitlin, S., Rosenblatt, W.P., & Williamson, G.G. (1986). Family stress: A coping model for intervention. *B.C. Journal of Special Education, 10*, 231–242.

Zimmerman, M. (1983). Methodological issues in the assessment of life events: A review of issues and research. *Clinical Psychology Review, 3*, 339–370.

KEY WORDS

Stress, disability, handicap, families and disability, coping and disability, adaptation and disability, vulnerability, adjustment to diagnosis, perception of disability, self-blame and disability.

Handbook of Life Stress, Cognition and Health
Edited by S. Fisher and J. Reason
© 1988 John Wiley & Sons Ltd.

19

Anorexia Nervosa

RACHEL BRYANT-WAUGH
The Hospital for Sick Children, Great Ormond Street, London

INTRODUCTION

Current understanding of the aetiology of anorexia nervosa is unsatisfactorily vague. There is no undisputed specific cause, the processes involved in its development remain speculative, and the exact nature of the interaction between psychological and physiological aspects of the disorder is unclear. Because it is not known precisely why individuals develop anorexia nervosa, the potential for a preventative approach is limited. Anorexia nervosa is a serious disorder with an established death rate. It has a tendency to become chronic and is associated with an increasing incidence in Western society. Any attempts to elucidate aetiological mechanisms that might assist prevention must therefore be considered worthwhile. At present, the most that can be achieved in this context is the identification of risk factors, usually on the basis of retrospective enquiry, that may shed some light on vulnerability to anorexia nervosa.

It is now widely accepted that anorexia nervosa can best be regarded as multidetermined and that different causal factors will influence the development of the disorder in each individual (Garfinkel and Garner, 1982). Figure 19.1 provides an overview of some of the main areas of disturbance that have been associated with the development of anorexia nervosa. Almost all the contributory factors identified are not specific to anorexia nervosa, which further supports the notion that a unitary cause is unlikely, and that a more valid approach to understanding its aetiology is in terms of the concept of a combination of stressors operating on a vulnerable individual.

Taking this view, anorexia nervosa can be regarded as a response to an intolerable situation; change—in this case pathological change—is initiated as a means of managing a life situation that the individual is otherwise unable to tolerate. Slade's (1982) view of anorexia nervosa as an attempted adaptive strategy in the face of certain major 'setting' conditions and specific psychosocial stimuli is consistent with this interpretation. If anorexia nervosa is to be regarded as the net result of a particular combination of external stressors and internal

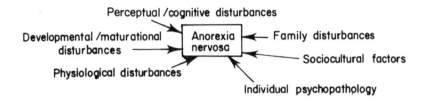

FIG. 19.1   Aetiological models of anorexia nervosa.

characteristics, it is clearly of limited value simply to conclude that the disorder is 'stress related' or 'stress induced'. Such terms are applied to a wide variety of disorders and difficulties and do not adequately convey the complexity of inter-linked antecedent events and conditions that combine to produce the clinical picture of anorexia nervosa. Although the precise nature of the interaction between different combinations of factors in the development of anorexia nervosa is not immediately apparent, there are clear indications in the literature that certain types of stressful events or conditions are identified relatively frequently as precipitating factors in individuals who have an established eating disorder. These are presented in the following sections.

ADOLESCENCE

Pubertal and adolescent conflicts are considered to be of central importance to the development of anorexia nervosa by many authors. In support of this is the fact that the disorder typically occurs in adolescent females soon after puberty. Adolescents of both sexes tend to be acutely aware of their outward appearance, many suffering considerable distress from the normal changes that accompany pubertal physical development. In the light of the common adolescent sense of uncertainty, physical changes may represent a challenge to the sense of self. A recent study of dietary and body shape concerns in a group of British schoolgirls found that whereas less than 4% were overweight, over 40% considered them-selves so, and approximately half wanted to lose weight (Davies and Furnham, 1986). These results are consistent with the impression that in adolescent females, thinness is highly correlated with attractiveness, and dieting to lose weight is associated with becoming more appealing (Halmi et al., 1979). Dieting behaviour and dissatisfaction with body weight appear to be related to some extent to pubertal development, with more developed female adolescents tending to be more dissatisfied about their weight (Tobin-Richards et al., 1983). Crisp (1984) found increasing dissatisfaction with age; within his study, 30% of 12 year olds expressed dissatisfaction, compared to 65% of 16 and 18 year olds. In the 13–15-year group, dissatisfaction with body weight and shape was reported to be greatest in those who were post-menarchal (Crisp, 1984). The heightened 'weight sensitivity' of female adolescents, which is related to physical development and to a cultural preference for slimness in women, results in dieting behaviour being relatively common in this age group. Self-consciousness and uncertainty are associated to an important extent with body development and a sensitivity to fatness (Vandereycken and Meerman, 1984). This sensitivity to fatness has its origins in the physical changes of puberty, and may be triggered at any stage of pubertal development (Crisp, 1983). Dieting may follow chance comments about size or shape, teasing, or observation of friends or family members dieting, all of which have been directly associated with the onset of anorexia nervosa in some individuals (Margo, 1985). It is, however, not clear why some individuals go on to develop the full syndrome of anorexia nervosa whereas others do not (Wakeling, 1985).

During adolescence, with rapid physical growth, individuals of both sexes are confronted with their own sexuality. Sexual development necessitates an altered attitude to self and others, and different role requirements. If these attitudes and requirements are perceived as negative and left unrevised, considerable problems with self-esteem and social functioning may ensue. It has often been suggested that anorexia nervosa represents a rejection of the role and body of a sexually functioning adult female, although this is not always found to be the case (see, for example, Buvat-Herbaut et al., 1983).

Conflicts around the issues of attachment and autonomy are relatively common in adolescence. The smoothness of the transition from the dependence of child-hood to the independence of adulthood will be affected by many factors, both internal and external to the adolescent. Dependency issues and separation difficulties may contribute to the general sense of dissatisfaction with life and low self-esteem experienced by many adolescents (Slade, 1982). In the context of anorexia nervosa, separation conflicts often appear to be manifested in the form of a typically 'model' child showing difficulties in becoming an independent, self-reliant individual (Vandereycken and Meerman, 1984). Halmi et al. (1979) have commented that the peak ages of incidence of anorexia nervosa occur at those times when dependency on the family is most challenged. Adolescents in our society are expected to learn to form qualitatively new types of social interaction—a process that involves taking risks and meeting challenges (Pillay and Crisp, 1977). Individuals who experience difficulty separating from the family, forming new relationships or revising existing ones, may choose to 'opt out' by withdrawing or regressing to the safer arena of childlike relationships. Anorexia nervosa can be viewed as an extreme example of such behaviour, where the regression is both physical and emotional.

The presence of an adolescent results in a period of role revision for all family members. Parents may be reminded of their own adolescent development, or may be faced with unresolved conflicts of their own which they had hitherto successful-ly concealed or forgotten (Crisp, 1977). Close families may be fearful of and feel threatened by the adolescent's emerging sexuality. A marriage that requires the presence of children for its continuation, a precariously adjusted parental rela-tionship and the stability of the family as a unit, may be threatened at this time. Such factors have all been identified in the families of individuals who have developed anorexia nervosa.

There are various interpretations of the mechanisms by which maturational, pubertal and adolescent stress factors are involved in the development of anorexia nervosa. Crisp has described the disorder as a psychobiological regression in response to adolescent and related family turmoil, where maturational conflicts are construed by the adolescent in terms of weight and body shape. He claims that carbohydrate avoidance and weight loss serve to deflect the psychosocial and biological pressures of adolescence, and can be regarded as a dysfunctional 'solution' to the adolescent's crisis. He further suggests that the presence of puppy fat, and the necessary minimum body weight required for menarche to occur, when overlaid on to a background of adolescent psychosocial stress, are important contributory factors to the development of anorexia nervosa (Crisp, 1977; 1980; 1983).

Other authors focus more on the fact that the individual with anorexia nervosa has been ill-prepared as a child for the stresses of adolescence (Bruch, 1973). Excessively close or negative relationships have been identified between individuals with anorexia nervosa and one or both parents, which in some cases have acted as powerful barriers to normal adolescent development (Kellet et al., 1976).

Sex differences in adolescent stresses are often invoked in explanations for the preponderance of female anorectics, males are generally believed to represent 5%–10% of the total anorectic population (Palmer, 1980; Dally et al., 1979), although this figure is believed to be much higher in childhood anorectics (Fosson et al., 1987). It has been suggested that males receive some protection because they tend to reach puberty slightly later than girls (Crisp and Toms, 1972). In addition, changes in the male body are not so extreme as those in females at puberty. Fatness in males is of more limited personal significance and of less sociocultural interest than it is in female adolescents. Crisp (1977) maintains that there are clear sex differences between attitudes to body weight and shape in adolescents. Whereas females usually wish to minimize their shape, often seeing themselves as fat, this is much less common in males. Nevertheless, there are many similarities in the maturational problems identified in both male and female anorectics, problems that are not specific to anorexia nervosa, and in other individuals might either be dealt with effectively or develop into alternative disorders (Crisp and Toms, 1972).

Of course, not all anorectics are adolescents, and although it seems that puberty represents a significant contributory factor in many cases, it is likely that alternative stressors are more important in prepubertal cases, older individuals and some male patients. Jacobs and Isaacs (1986) found a relatively high incidence of major life events and of premorbid emotional and behavioural disturbances in prepubertal patients. They suggest that the post-pubertal group might be subjected to lower levels of stress, until the pressure of entering puberty makes them more vulnerable.

Cases of anorexia nervosa associated with pregnancy and childbirth have also been reported (e.g. Nwaefuna, 1981) and cannot in most instances be directly related to puberty or adolescence. Slade (1977) has identified changes in body image occurring during pregnancy which, coupled with food cravings, may lead to a fear of losing control over weight and eating behaviour (Vandereycken and Meerman, 1984). This in turn may lead to episodes of bingeing or severe food restriction. Post-menopausal women have also been documented as developing anorexia nervosa: Kellet *et al.* (1976) describe the case of a 56-year-old woman who developed the disorder, apparently in relation to the marriages of her daughters.

FAMILY FACTORS

The family approach to the understanding of anorexia nervosa focuses on family background and functioning, the supposition being that certain dysfunctional behaviours or interaction patterns play a role in the aetiology and prognosis of anorexia nervosa in one of the family members (Morgan and Russell, 1975; Yager, 1981; Bryant-Waugh *et al.*, 1987). The suggestion that family-related stress can result in physical or emotional disturbance is not unique to anorexia nervosa, and the importance of families in the development of psychosomatic symptoms has long been recognized (Table 19.1). Clinical observations of families with an anorectic member have led to attempts to identify common characteristics of such families. The characteristics identified vary considerably, and it is certainly not the case that they are present in all families with an anorectic member. Anecdotal observations in the literature are supplemented by a few research papers, such as those by Kalucy *et al.* (1977), Norris and Jones (1979), and Hall (1978).

Minuchin and colleagues have identified a number of characteristics typical of 'anorectic families', namely: enmeshment, overprotectiveness, rigidity, lack of conflict resolution, intense atmosphere with little privacy, and involvement of the anorectic child in unresolved marital or family conflicts (Minuchin *et al.*, 1978). Such families tend to be unable to deal successfully with disagreements, due to their inclination to deny or divert any overt conflict (Liebman *et al.*, 1983). Independence and self-assertiveness may not be encouraged as this could lead to conflict situations and separation from other members of the family (Edwards, 1983).

In the psychoanalytically oriented literature, much importance is attached to

Table 19.1   Family-related stress factors associated with anorexia nervosa

Family move to new neighbourhood
Period spent away from home
Family history of anorexia nervosa/obesity
Parental/sibling dieting
Parental propensity to social avoidance
Close, loyal and mutually dependent family
Family vulnerability to apparently ordinary life events
Family with unusual interest in food, weight and/or shape
Family history of affective disorder or other physical psychiatric disturbances
Parent working in food/fashion industry
Excessive family involvement in caring
Pronounced middle-class value systems
High parental concern and involvement

the mother–daughter relationship, which is regarded as being one in which the needs of the child receive less priority than the mother's notion of what is appropriate or correct. This is held to result in the child entering adolescence with no clear self-concept or sense of self-worth, and with a tendency toward compliant behaviour—Bruch's (1978) 'good girl' who wants to please the family and live up to expectations to the extent that she cannot identify her own needs. Many anorectics describe feeling that they are not good enough or that they are disappointing failures (Vandereycken and Meerman, 1984).

Bruch (1973) further described typical families as those in which expression is not encouraged, the mother is repressed, overprotective and frustrated, and the father somewhat obsessional about health matters. In such families the growth and development of the child tend to be regarded as parental accomplishment (Bruch, 1978). Palazzoli (1974) suggests that parents tend to have an unequal relationship, with the mother being dominant and forceful, and the father passive and emotionally absent. In contrast to this passive, uninvolved father (also reported by other authors, e.g. Sours, 1974; Rowland, 1970), fathers in the families of male anorectic patients have been described as domineering, controlling and rigid, playing a major role in the functioning of the family and often in overt conflict with the anorectic son (Sterling and Sega, 1985).

The identification of marital problems is relatively common in much of the literature on anorexia nervosa. Many authors emphasize the role of parental problems in the development of eating disorders, maintaining that considerable stress is imposed on all family members by a poor marital relationship, which for some individuals may be associated with the onset of anorexia nervosa (e.g. Mazur, 1981). The anorexia nervosa of one member often has a stabilizing effect on dysfunctional family interaction patterns and, in the case of marital difficulties, may serve to keep the family intact.

In times of change or external stress, 'typical' anorectic families have been described as responding poorly—striving to maintain the status quo, attempting to dampen anxiety and conflict, and continuing to use established interaction patterns which may not be appropriate in the altered circumstances (Sours, 1980). Such responses have been identified in the context of normal adolescent development, and may result in a 'chronic state of submerged tension and stress' (Liebman et al., 1983). Features which predispose to difficulties in coping with the stresses imposed by adolescent development appear to be relatively common in anorectic families (Kalucy et al., 1977).

A further common observation is that food plays an important role in these families. This may take the form of the occupational involvement of one of the parents in the food, nutrition or fashion industry (Crisp, 1967; Crisp and Toms, 1972; Sterling and Segal, 1985), or the presence of unusual eating patterns (Dally and Gomez, 1979). In many cases food is used as a form of currency, which is dispensed or withheld according to situations and family values regarding certain foods (Kalucy et al., 1977). The control of weight and the notion of fitness are often highly valued, and equated with a sense of well-being or self-control. Family preoccupation with health and diet is not an uncommon finding. However, Hall et al. (1986) discovered that a history of concern about weight-related matters was at least as common in control families. They conclude that 'weight pathology (defined by Kalucy *et al.* (1977) as deviations in weight, shape, eating behaviour and activity) is not unduly common in the families of anorectic individuals.

The nature of any relationship between a family history of emotional disturbance and the development of anorexia nervosa in another member remains controversial. Many authors have identified a high incidence of psychiatric disorder in relatives of anorectics (Dally, 1969; Morgan and Russell, 1975; Warren, 1968; Winokur *et al.*, 1980), which has been viewed as an indication of a general neurotic morbidity (Crisp and Toms, 1972). It has also been suggested that there is a close relationship between both anorexia nervosa and bulimia, and affective disorder (Cantwell *et al.*, 1977; Yellowlees, 1985). It may be that rather than a genetic vulnerability, the stress caused by living with a relative suffering from mental illness is sufficient to precipitate the onset of an eating disorder. Biederman *et al.* (1985) propose that some individuals who develop anorexia nervosa may have a genetic vulnerability to the development of affective disorder, yet this does not in itself explain why they should initially develop the eating disorder. The nature of the relationship between a family history of emotional disturbance and the development of anorexia nervosa remains unclear, and until more data are available, any conclusions regarding aetiological significance must remain tentative.

It is sometimes all to easy to focus on family-related stress when attempting to explain why an individual has developed an eating disorder. Whilst in most cases there are undoubtedly family factors at play, it must be remembered that anorexia nervosa occurs in a society where dieting, dissatisfaction with size, and over-estimation of body weight are within the cultural norm for adolescent females (Hall, 1978). It is furthermore the case that all of the family stresses identified in the literature may not necessarily have a direct effect on the development of an eating disorder, but a more subtle one, for example by increasing the probability of problems related to adolescent development, which in turn may increase vulnerability to anorexia nervosa. Some of the characteristic family traits identified represent culturally valued characteristics (e.g. emphasis on self-control), and in isolation cannot be viewed as pathological features. Although not specific to anorexia nervosa, such traits may facilitate its development in an individual who regards normal bodily development or functioning as threatening or undesirable. The exercise of self-control may for many be the most obvious way to deal with the perceived threat (Crisp, 1983).

Not all anorectics regard their families as stressful environments; Heron and Leheup (1984) report that many of the patients they interviewed came from close families with apparently few external stresses and with whom they professed to be happy. No doubt the experienced family clinician would identify an element of denial or unresolved conflict. It may be that such 'happy families' offer limited ways of individuating and establishing an identity for someone with an 'anorectic personality' (Heron and Leheup, 1984).

SOCIOCULTURAL FACTORS

In 1939, Ryle suggested that: 'The spread of the slimming fashion, now happily on the wane, and the more emotional lives of the younger generation since the War might have been expected to provide a general increase [in incidence of anorexia nervosa], but these influences may well have been counteracted by the growth of a healthy athleticism among girls and young women and the greater freedom from restraints which they now enjoy.' Since Ryle's comment there have certainly been changes. In particular, the 'slimming fashion' is more popular than ever, placing a great emphasis on the value of slimness in women, which many have associated with heightened weight sensitivity and an increase in incidence of anorexia nervosa (Bruch, 1978; Crisp, 1980; Garner and Garfinkel, 1980). In some cases the social preference for a slim female body shape is so extreme that borderline anorexic shapes may be considered highly attractive (Furnham and Alibhai, 1983). Garner et al. (1980) suggest that the pressure on women to be thin has increased over the past few years, yet in contrast to this, the average weight of females under 30 has risen in the last two decades (Vandereycken and Meerman, 1984).

A major channel for the perpetuation of the 'thin ideal' is undoubtedly the media (Faust, 1983). Dieting and slimming magazines attract growing numbers of readers, fashion models are invariably tall and slim, and there are many books and television programmes promoting the desirability of weight control and a slim body. Recently, the fitness industry has seen an increase in popularity, in particular women's keep fit and exercise classes. Davies and Furnham (1986) have highlighted a recent change in the behaviour of weight-conscious adolescent females which they relate to this increasing interest in fitness. They suggest that younger age groups (12–14 years) are becoming increasingly aware of their weight, and that weight-related concern in all age groups (12–18 years) is directed more towards exercising than to dieting (shades of Ryle's 'growth of a healthy athleticism'?). Thus as well as dieting risks, female adolescents are now increasingly exposing themselves to the risks of over-exercise—a trend encouraged by the fitness industry.

The frequency of preoccupation with body weight appears to be increasing in normal adolescent females (Schwartz et al., 1982), with eating disorders and problems related to weight and body image being relatively frequent in normal adolescent girls (Buvat-Herbaut et al., 1983). Crisp (1983) believes that this preoccupation with fatness, encouraged by the media, and the nearly ubiquitous tendency in female adolescents to diet, form the fundamental basis of anorexia nervosa. Excessive dieting and exercising may seriously interfere with social and academic life and may in extreme cases result in the full syndrome of anorexia nervosa. It remains unclear, however, why some individuals persist in their attempts long after they have reached the cultural ideal. It would appear too simplistic to conceptualize anorexia nervosa on a continuum with weight preoccupation and dieting, as this would mean that every woman conscious of her weight (which the majority are) is at risk of anorexia nervosa (Vandereycken and Meerman, 1984). Garner et al. (1983) have identified essential psychological differences between weight-preoccupied dieters and anorexia nervosa patients, in that the former have an expressed desire for physical attractiveness and social approval, whereas the latter are striving for a sense of psychological organization and self-control.

Many existing hypotheses for the relative rarity of anorexia nervosa in males centre on differences in sociological, cultural or environmental stresses on female and male adolescents (Crisp and Toms, 1972). It is generally held that culturally imposed stresses are greater on females, which serves to increase their vulnerability (Bruch, 1973). Furthermore, several studies have shown that females are more sensitive to the existence of obesity in others, take more notice of this in themselves, and express more concern over dieting and body shape than males (Davies and Furnham, 1986). Yet in males who develop anorexia nervosa, very similar features have been identified to those found in females, including hypersensitivity to weight and shape, and a slim body ideal. Over the last decade or so, there have been a number of feminist interpretations of eating disorders highlighting the difficulty many women have in accepting their own size and shape and relating eating problems to social and cultural factors incorporated in the female sex role (Boskind-Lodahl, 1976; Orbach, 1978). The increase in eating disorders has been associated with repression of feminine nature in our society and the social rejection of fatness in women (Woodman, 1980; Chernin, 1981). Attitudes to the female sex role are conflicting and changing, particularly for girls from middle-class families who might be expected to combine academic achievement and the pursuit of a career with the more traditional roles of wife and mother. Although feminist literature criticizing societal pressures on women to conform to the notion of an 'ideal woman' may have had some effect on adult women, it does not appear to have affected the behaviour of adolescents, who as a group strive to conform to this norm (Davies and Furnham, 1986).

The social class bias in the incidence of anorexia nervosa, with patients coming predominantly from upper- and middle-class families (Crisp, 1980), has been attributed to the stresses imposed by such families on adolescent females. The typical middle-class family orientation of efficiency, achievement and performance, is clearly reflected in the competitiveness and desire for personal improvement often identified in individuals with anorexia nervosa (Kalucy et al., 1977). Upper and middle-class families as a group are 'not renowned for setting limits on the urge to self-improvement' (BMJ, 1978). Garfinkel and Garner (1982) state that a combination of thin body ideal and competitiveness or high performance expectation represents a high risk factor for anorexia nervosa. Such features are likely to be present in individuals from middle-class families characterized by high achievement orientation. Kalucy et al. (1977) suggest that adolescents from lower social class families are more easily able, and inclined, to consolidate their adolescent social roles more quickly, tending to marry earlier and having less unrealistic and ambitious demands placed on them. Alternatively, social class bias may be an indication that middle- and upper-class families are relatively more weight conscious than the rest of the population (Hall, 1978). Obesity is generally thought to be more tolerated in lower social classes, with less direct emphasis being placed on the high cultural value of slimness (Kalucy et al., 1977). In support of these suggestions, Davies and Furnham (1986) found that a group of middle-class females aged 16 were significantly 'more adamant' in their expressed desire to lose weight than a comparable group of lower class girls—many of whom wished to gain weight. Returning finally to Ryle's (1939) welcoming of the 'greater freedom from restraints', this too can be implicated in the increase in incidence of anorexia nervosa. Crisp (1983) notes that the testing out of limits in order to identify them is a characteristic feature of adolescence. He proposes that in our society, institutionalized and moral limits are decreasing and that consequently the internal controls of some adolescents need to become stronger. Thus 'freedom from restraints' may lead some adolescents to apply stricter self-control—one of the most accessible means of which is the reduction of food intake.

INDIVIDUAL/'PERSONALITY' FACTORS

Various authors have attempted to identify what kind of person tends to develop anorexia nervosa—is there a typical 'anorectic personality' or any characteristic emotional and behavioural traits that might indicate which individuals are at risk? Such individual traits can be viewed as being related to general emotional development and the manner in which demands and challenges have been met in the past, the distillation of these factors having some effect on the individual's later response to stress. Hall (1978) suggests that the increased vulnerability of the individual who develops anorexia nervosa may be the result of early life experiences combined with place or role in the family. Bruch (1973) believes that the fear of becoming fat and the refusal to eat, characteristic of anorexia nervosa, are late secondary features to an underlying personality disorder. The 'typical anorectic' identified in the literature is a weight-sensitive, perfectionistic adolescent, who is generally dissatisfied with life and has low self-esteem (Vandereycken and Meerman, 1984). Such an adolescent will commonly be introverted, conscientious and well behaved, and will have had few problems either at home or in school (Bemis, 1978). The more frequently identified premorbid characteristics include the following: neuroticism; social and personal introversion; obsessional features; social and personal anxiety; depression; somatic complaint; perfectionism; independence; having been excessively good or compliant as a child; tendency to see things in black and white terms; lack of assertiveness; avoidance or negative attitude to heterosexual contacts (Crisp et al., 1971; Crisp and Stonehill, 1972; Crisp, 1981; Duddle, 1973; Halmi et al., 1977; Heron and Leheup, 1984; Slade, 1982; Smart et al., 1976; Vandereycken and Meerman, 1984). Similar premorbid traits have been identified in male anorectics, namely obsessionality; considering self unattractive; high success and achievement orientation; overtly conscientious and hard working; rigid in affect (Sterling and Segal, 1985).

It is often very difficult to distinguish premorbid characteristics from those which begin to appear after the onset of the eating disorder—many of the typical traits identified may be secondary to a state of starvation (Bemis, 1978). Considerable variation exists in opinions regarding the existence of 'typical' traits, but how if they do exist, do such characteristics predispose an individual to anorexia nervosa? Crisp (1981) claims that children with a combination of the traits identified are ill-equipped for the stresses imposed by adolescence. Social interaction difficulties may be particularly handicapping during this period. The failure to enter or remain in a significant personal relationship has been found to be relatively common in the history of anorexia nervosa (Slade, 1982). For individuals with high self-performance demands, such a failure can seem particularly devastating. Perfectionistic tendencies result in anything less than idealized being perceived as a failure (Vandereycken and Meerman, 1984). Slade (1982) suggests that anorectics have a general need for control which becomes a need for complete control over or total success in some aspect of their life. Self-control in the form of regulation of food intake and bodily functioning may be one of the few areas that such control or success can be guaranteed. However, in the case of bulimia, the individual is unsuccessful in attempts to achieve self-control, which further contributes to a sense of worthlessness and low self-esteem (Long and Cordle, 1982). In general, slightly different characteristics are identified in bulimic individuals. Casper *et al.* (1980) note that they tend to be more extroverted, admit more frequently to strong appetite, and show greater anxiety, depression, guilt and interpersonal sensitivity than anorectic individuals. They also tend to show a variety of impulsive behaviours, including stealing, alcohol and drug abuse, self-mutilation and suicidal behaviour (Garfinkel *et al.*, 1980; Welbourne and Purgold, 1984).

Not only are behavioural and emotional traits implicated in the development of eating disorders, they are also believed to play a role in response to treatment and in prognosis (Morgan *et al.*, 1983; Goetz *et al.*, 1977). Low self-esteem, high social sensitivity and obsessional features are common in patients whose weight has been newly restored (Pillay and Crisp, 1977). It is common clinical experience that as treatment progresses, patients become self-conscious, depressed, anxious or panicky. Parents may also show an increase in anxiety and depression (Crisp *et al.*, 1974). The resulting inhibited social interaction and heightened sensitivity may represent considerable sources of stress to the recovering anorectic and his or her family. In some cases this may reach a level where progress is hampered and relapse occurs. In terms of prognosis, apprehensiveness, obsessionality, lack of assertion, neuroticism and hysterical symptoms have all been associated with poor outcome (Wakeling, 1985; Bemis, 1978). Again, such findings are by no means uniform, and the relationship of personality characteristics to prognosis remains unclear.

PHYSICAL/ILLNESS FACTORS

Various factors related to physical status and health have been identified as antecedents of anorexia nervosa. Some authors believe that these represent risk factors or predisposing factors due to the stress they impose on a vulnerable individual. Others (e.g. Crisp, 1980) view the role of physiological abnormalities in the eating disorder as entirely secondary. Whether primary or secondary, it is certain that organic factors contribute to the perpetuation and often exacerbation of the emotional and physiological disturbances (Bemis, 1978). A relatively commonly identified physical factor is obesity. Premorbid obesity or a history of weight increase has been associated with the development of anorexia nervosa in both males and females (Margo, 1985; Crisp, 1970; Crisp, 1981; Wakeling, 1985; Sterling and Segal, 1985: Crisp and Toms, 1972). Overweight adolescents may be teased about their size or shape, which can apparently precipitate the onset of anorexia nervosa in a sensitive individual. However, by no means all anorectics are overweight, either at the time of onset or during childhood.

Early puberty (Crisp, 1970) and late age of menarche (Hall *et al.*, 1984) have both been mentioned as predisposing factors or as being related to poor outcome. Again, this may be due to comments or teasing from peers which serve to cause the recipient considerable distress. A further potential stress factor is early cessation of menstruation with weight loss (Katz, 1975; Lupton *et al.*, 1976), or a previous history of amenorrhoea (Wakeling 1985). Amenorrhoea during the anorectic illness has a number of possible explanations. One of these is that it may be a consequence of a stress-induced hypothalamic disorder (Slade, 1982). The possibility that the syndrome of anorexia nervosa is the manifestation of a disturbance in hypothalamic functioning has been explored by many authors (e.g. Greenwood and Johnson, 1975). Abnormal thought patterns, psychosexual disturbances and physiological factors characteristic of anorexia nervosa can all be accounted for using a theory of hypothalamic disorder (Bemis, 1978). However, the role of the hypothalamus in the development and maintenance of anorexia nervosa is not yet clear. At present, the possible interpretations include the following. Starvation or psychological stress causes a disturbance in hypothalamic functioning which leads to the clinical picture of anorexia nervosa; or, there is a primary hypothalamic defect of unknown aetiology that finds expression in the symptoms of anorexia nervosa (Mecklenberg *et al.*, 1974). In some cases, an episode of mild physical illness prior to the onset of the eating disorder appears to be a major precipitating factor (Margo, 1985). It has been suggested that the loss of appetite accompanying such an illness may be in some way appealing to the individual, or may provide the opportunity to embark upon a preplanned diet (Beumont *et al.*, 1978; Dally, 1969). In other individuals, a history of relatively serious physical illness appears to produce a non-specific vulnerability to anorexia nervosa: Patton *et al.* (1986) found a higher rate of severe illness in the history of anorectic individuals than of controls, and suggest that such a history be viewed as a risk factor for anorexia nervosa. These authors found that excessive physical illness earlier in life appears to represent more of a risk factor than acute physical illness as a direct precipitant. Furthermore, of the illnesses experienced by the group studied, there was no significant excess of alimentary versus non-alimentary episodes, and no clear trend for illnesses known to cause appetite loss (Patton *et al.*, 1986).

In attempting to arrive at an explanation for the association between anorexia nervosa and illness episodes, Patton *et al.* (1986) focus on the characteristic dysfunctional family interaction patterns of enmeshment and overprotection (Minuchin *et al.*, 1978). They suggest that such potentially pathological relationships may be triggered by an episode of illness, and in turn provide one of the major setting conditions for the development of anorexia nervosa. In studies of family history, a significant degree of physical illness has been identified in the parents of anorectic patients. Halmi *et al.* (1977) found that gastrointestinal disorders were relatively common, whereas Kalucy *et al.* (1977) noted a high incidence of maternal migraine. Hall (1978) emphasized the extent to which the presence of relatively serious illness in a parent was played down, and the rarity of overt illness orientation in families with an anorectic member. It is possible that emotional difficulties tend to be somatized in anorectics and their families, resulting in relatively high rates of reported illness. Dally (1969) found a high percentage of mothers who were of the opinion that their daughters had suffered from considerable ill-health before the onset of the eating disorder. It is difficult to ascertain to what extent such ill-health may have been psychosomatic.

In conclusion, then, at least in some individuals, previous episodes of physical illness may be related to the development of anorexia nervosa. It is not clear whether such factors are primary precipitants or whether anorectic individuals have some kind of predisposing constitutional vulnerability. This latter suggestion is consistent with the view that psychophysiological disorders probably have a stress-related aetiology (Bemis, 1978).

SCHOOL FACTORS

Many studies have reported that anorectic individuals are of average or above average intelligence and that they tend to show high scholastic achievement (e.g. Smart et al., 1976). Dally and Gomez (1979) found that 53% of a group of anorectics aged 11–14 years were consistently in the top three of their class. Yet school-related factors are not infrequently identified as precipitants of anorexia nervosa. Stress at school has been found to be highly correlated with anorectic behaviour and attitudes, and with poor prognosis in terms of eating behaviour (Wakeling, 1985). Stress and failure experiences related to school, such as pressure to achieve academically, a move to a larger school, exam pressures, and exam failure (real or threatened), represent risk factors for anorexia nervosa, as such experiences have been associated with the development of the eating disorder in some individuals (Vandereycken and Meerman, 1984; Slade, 1982; Margo, 1985). This can be linked to the commonly reported perfectionist tendencies of anorectics, and the stress experienced in attempting to meet high perceived expectations or self-imposed standards. It has furthermore been suggested that the apparent social class bias in anorexia nervosa is not so much due to socioeconomic factors as to educational factors (Lawrence, 1984). Young women who achieve academically face particular conflicts, which in some may contribute towards the onset of anorexia nervosa. Duddle (1973) noted an increase in the disorder in female university students, all of whom did well academically.

Of course, anorexia nervosa is not restricted to those of high levels of intellectual functioning, nor to the students of academically oriented secondary schools or establishments of higher education. Heron and Leheup (1984) identified the disorder across a whole range of social class, intellectual level and type of schooling. In a follow-up study of 50 females, Hall et al. (1984) found that difficulties at school or work in the year prior to the onset of anorexia nervosa were related to good outcome. This may reflect a tendency for such difficulties to be more easily resolved than, for instance, family or personal difficulties. Alternatively, it may be that when onset is triggered by specific external conditions, the disorder is more amenable to treatment, as, for example, with schizophrenia and depression where it has been found that better outcome is related to a specific stressful event and prompt treatment.

SUMMARY AND CONCLUSIONS

The onset of an eating disorder can be linked to a variety of stressful situations and events in the life of an individual. Several theories of stress involve the notion of being driven beyond existing means of coping (Martin, 1981), and anorexia nervosa can be interpreted using such a model: Bemis (1978) states that 'anorectic behaviour is first manifested in response to new situations for which existing skills seem inadequate'. There are two main types of stressor that have been identified as having some effect on mental health, namely, longer term stresses and significant discrete events. The former tend to be related to ongoing life situations, such as unemployment, poor housing, marital problems or other relationship problems. The latter include life events or other events which may include some degree of stress to a particular individual. There are no certain cause-and-effect relationships between the presence of long-term stresses, significant events and mental health, but, as this discussion of anorexia nervosa illustrates, a combination of such stressors increases vulnerability. The question of why specifically anorexia nervosa should develop, rather than any other disorder or difficulty, can perhaps best be answered by attention to the nature of the stressors identified. It may be that specific combinations of antecedent events and circumstances experienced by an individual with perfectionist or obsessional traits and a need for control, determine that anorexia nervosa will be the pathological response of 'choice'. The perfectionist child from a close family with little overt conflict has relatively few ways to develop a sense of autonomy and identity; exaggerated self-control may come to take the place of interaction with others. Inwardly directed control replaces negative feelings of being out of control and socially ineffective (Lawrence, 1979).

It seems probable that sociocultural preferences have contributed to the rise in incidence of anorexia nervosa, yet such preferences do not directly cause eating disorders. Sociocultural factors interact with individual and family characteristics and circumstances to produce varying levels of stress, to which each individual's response will be different.

Gardiner et al. (1983) make a distinction between two types of anorexia nervosa patients: a 'nutritional' group and a 'stress' group. The latter are claimed to develop anorexia nervosa in response to marked stress, lose substantial amounts of weight, but recover relatively rapidly (however, stress remains present in their families). The 'nutritional' group show slow but continuous improvement in weight and eating behaviour, tend to come from middle-class, stable families, and have a later age at onset. It is interesting to note that the 'nutritional' group are reported to resume menses shortly after restoration of weight, whereas the 'stress' group reveal a persistent endocrine disorder after weight gain (Gardiner et al., 1983). Although the terminology applied to the two groups may be misleading—it is difficult to consider the 'nutritional' group stress free—these findings are potentially of interest. They illustrate that unresolved stress, which has probably contributed to the onset of the disorder, may become translated into a persistent physiological disturbance after many of the original symptoms of the eating disorder have disappeared.

In conclusion, anorexia nervosa can be viewed as an extreme form of self-control, exercised as a means of coping with a combination of external and internal stress factors. In bulimia, self-control, although desired is less successfully achieved (Strober, 1980).

It is hoped that the material discussed in this chapter provides some context for understanding stress-related attitudes and behaviour regarding food and weight.

REFERENCES

Bemis, K. (1978). Current approaches to the etiology and treatment of anorexia nervosa. *Psychological Bulletin, 85*, 593–617.

Beumont, P.J.V., Abraham, S.F., Argall, W.J., George, G.C.W., & Glaun, D.E. (1978). The onset of anorexia nervosa. *Australian and New Zealand Journal of Psychiatry, 12*, 145–149.

Biederman, J., Rivinus, T., Kemper, K., Hamilton, D., MacFadyen, J., & Harmatz, J. (1985). Depressive disorders in relatives of anorexia nervosa patients with and without a current episode of nonbipolar major depression. *American Journal of Psychiatry, 142*, 1495–1497.

Boskind-Lodahl, M. (1976). Cinderella's step-sisters: A feminist perspective on anorexia nervosa and bulimia. *Signs: Journal of Women in Culture and Society, 2*, 342–356.

BMJ (1978). Editorial: Anorexia nervosa: Fear of fatness or femininity. *British Medical Journal, 7*, 5.

Bruch, H. (1973). *Eating disorders: Obesity, anorexia nervosa and the person within*. New York: Basic Books.

Bruch, H. (1978). *The golden cage: The enigma of anorexia nervosa*. Cambridge, Mass.: Harvard University Press.

Bryant-Waugh, R., Fosson, A., Kaminski, Z., Knibbs, J., & Lask, B. (1987). Early onset anorexia nervosa—a follow-up study. *Archives of Diseases in Childhood* (in press).

Buvat-Herbaut, M., Hebbinckuys, P., Lemarie, A., & Buvat, J. (1983). Attitudes toward weight, body image, eating, menstruation, pregnancy and sexuality in 81 cases of anorexia compared with 288 normal control girls. *International Journal of Eating Disorders, 2*, 45–59.

Cantwell, D.P., Sturzenberger, S., Burrough, J., Salkin, B., & Green, J. (1977). Anorexia nervosa: An affective disorder? *Archives of General Psychiatry, 34*, 1087–1093.

Casper, R.C., Eckert, E.D., Halmi, K.A., Goldberg, S.C., & Davis, J.M. (1980). Bulimia. Its incidence and clinical importance in patients with anorexia nervosa. *Archives of General Psychiatry, 37*, 1030–1035.

Chernin, K. (1981). *Womanize: The tyranny of slenderness*. London: The Womens Press.

Crisp, A.H. (1967). Anorexia nervosa. *Hospital Medicine*, May, 713–718.

Crisp, A.H. (1970). Anorexia nervosa: 'feeding disorder', 'nervous malnutrition' or 'weight phobia'. *World Review of Nutrition and Diet, 12*, 452–504.

Crisp, A.H. (1977). Some psychobiological aspects of adolescent growth and their relevance for the fat/thin syndrome (anorexia nervosa). *International Journal of Obesity, 1*, 231–238.

Crisp, A.H. (1980). *Anorexia nervosa: Let me be*. London: Academic Press.

Crisp, A.H. (1981). Nutritional disorders and the psychiatric state. In H.M. Van Praag, M.H. Lader & O.J. Rafaelsen *et al.*, (eds), *Handbook of biological psychiatry*, Part IV (pp. 653–683). Marcel Dekker.

366 RACHEL BRYANT-WAUGH

Crisp, A.H. (1983). Anorexia nervosa: Regular review. *British Medical Journal, 287*, 855–858.

Crisp, A.H. (1984). Psychopathology of anorexia nervosa. In A.J. Stunkard & E. Stellar (eds), *Eating and its disorders*. New York: Raven Press.

Crisp, A.H., Harding, B., & McGuinness, B. (1974). Anorexia nervosa: Psychoneurotic characteristics of parents: Relationship to prognosis. *Journal of Psychosomatic Research, 18*, 167–173.

Crisp, A.H., & Stonehill, E. (1972). Some psychological characteristics of patients with anorexia nervosa before and after treatment. Paper read at IXth European Psychosomatic Conference, Vienna.

Crisp, A.H., Stonehill, E., & Fenton, G.W. (1971). The relationship between sleep, nutrition and mood: A study of patients with anorexia nervosa. *Postgraduate Medical Journal, 47*, 207–213.

Crisp, A.H., & Toms, D.A. (1972). Primary anorexia nervosa or weight phobia in the male: Report on 13 cases. *British Medical Journal, 1*, 334–338.

Dally, P.J. (1969). *Anorexia nervosa*. London: Heinemann.

Dally, P.J., & Gomez, J. (1979). *Anorexia nervosa*. London: Heinemann.

Dally, P.J., Gomez, J., & Isaacs, S. (1979). *Anorexia nervosa*. London: Heinemann.

Davies, E., & Furnham, A. (1986). The dieting and body shape concerns of adolescent females. *Journal of Child Psychology and Psychiatry, 27*, 417–428.

Duddle, M. (1973). An increase in anorexia nervosa in a university population. *British Journal of Psychiatry, 123*, 711–712.

Edwards, G. (1983). The making of anorexia nervosa. *Changes, 2*(i), 17–20.

Faust, M.S. (1983). Alternative constructions of adolescent growth. In J. Brooks-Gunn & A.C. Peterson (eds), *Girls at puberty: Biological and psychosocial perspectives*. New York: Plenum Press.

Fosson, A., Bryant-Waugh, R., Knibbs, J., & Lask, B. (1987). Early onset anorexia nervosa—a description of 48 patients. *Archives of Diseases in Childhood, 62*, 114–118.

Furnham, A., & Alibhai, N. (1983). Cross cultural differences in the perception of female body shapes. *Psychological Medicine, 13*, 829–837.

Gardiner, R.J., Martin, F., & Jukier, L. (1983). Anorexia nervosa: Endocrine studies of two distinct clinical subgroups. In P. Darby, P. Garfunkel, D. Garner & D. Coscina (eds), *Anorexia nervosa: Recent developments in research*. New York: Alan R Liss.

Garfinkel, P.E., & Garner, D.M. (1982). *Anorexia nervosa: A multidimensional perspective*. New York: Brunner Mazel.

Garfinkel, P.E., Moldofsky, H., & Garner, D.M. (1980). The heterogeneity of anorexia nervosa: Bulimia as a distinct subgroup. *Archives of General Psychiatry, 37*, 1036–1040.

Garner, D.M., & Garfinkel, P.E. (1980). Sociocultural factors in the development of anorexia nervosa. *Psychological Medicine, 10*, 647–656.

Garner, D.M., Olmsted, M.P., & Garfinkel, P.E. (1983). Does anorexia nervosa occur on a continuum? Differences between weight preoccupied women and anorexia nervosa. *International Journal of Eating Disorders, 2*(4), 11–20.

Garner, D.M., & Garfinkel, P.E. Schwartz, D., & Thompson, M. (1980). Cultural expectations of thinness in women. *Psychological Reports, 47*, 483–491.

Goetz, P.L., Succop, R.A., Reinhart, J.B., & Miller, A. (1977). Anorexia nervosa in children: a follow-up study. *American Journal of Orthopsychiatry, 47*, 597–603.

Greenwood, M.R.C., & Johnson, P. (1975). Behavioural correlates of the obese condition. In M Winick (ed.), *Childhood obesity*. New York: John Wiley & Sons.

Hall, A. (1978). Family structure and relationships of 50 female anorexia nervosa patients. *Australian and New Zealand Journal of Psychiatry, 12*, 263–268.

Hall, A., Slim, E., Hawker, F., & Salmond, C. (1984). Anorexia nervosa: Longterm outcome in 50 female patients. *British Journal of Psychiatry, 145*, 407–413.

Hall, A., Leibrich, J., Walkey, F., & Welch, G. (1986). Investigations of 'weight pathology' of 58 mothers of anorexia nervosa patients and 204 mothers of schoolgirls. *Psychological Medicine, 16*, 71–76.

Halmi, K.A., Goldberg, S.C., Eckert, E., Casper, R., & Davis, J. (1977). Pretreatment evaluation in anorexia nervosa. In R.A. Vigersky (ed), *Anorexia nervosa*. New York: Raven Press.

Halmi, K.A., Casper, R., Eckert, E., Goldberg, S., & Davis, J. (1979). Unique features associated with age of onset of anorexia nervosa. *Psychiatry Research, 1*, 209–215.

Heron, J.M., & Leheup, R.F. (1984). Happy families. *British Journal of Psychiatry, 145*, 136–138.

Jacobs, B., & Isaacs, S. (1986). Pre-pubertal anorexia nervosa: a retrospective controlled study. *Journal of Child Psychology and Psychiatry, 27*, 237–250.

Kalucy, R.S., Crisp, A.H., & Harding, B. (1977). A study of 56 families with anorexia nervosa. *British Journal of Medical Psychology, 50*, 381–395.

Katz, J.L. (1975). Psychoendocrine considerations in anorexia nervosa. In E.J. Sacher (ed.), *Topics in psychoendocrinology*. New York: Grune and Stratton.

Kellet, J., Trimble, M., & Thorley, A. (1976). Anorexia nervosa after the menopause. *British Journal of Psychiatry, 128*, 555–558.

Lawrence, M. (1979). Anorexia nervosa—the control paradox. *Women's Studies International Quarterly, 2*, 93–101.

Lawrence, M. (1984). Anorexia nervosa: An 'update'. *Association for Child Psychiatry and Psychology Newsletter* (July).

Liebman, R., Sargent, J., & Silver, M. (1983). A family systems orientation to the treatment of anorexia nervosa. *Journal of the American Academy of Child Psychiatry, 22*, 128–133.

Long, C.G., & Cordle, C.J. (1982). Psychological treatment of binge eating and self-induced vomiting. *British Journal of Medical Psychology, 55*, 139–145.

Lupton, M., Simon, L., Barry, V., & Klawans, H. (1976). Biological aspects of anorexia nervosa. *Life Sciences, 18*, 1341.

Margo, J.L. (1985). Anorexia nervosa in adolescents. *British Journal of Medical Psychology, 58*, 193–195.

Martin, I. (1981). Biological bases of behaviour. In D. Griffiths (ed.), *Psychology and medicine*. London: The British Psychological Society and Macmillan.

Mazur, D.C. (1981). A starving family: An interactional view of anorexia nervosa. In E. Howell & M. Bayes (eds), *Women and mental health*. New York: Basic Books.

Mecklenberg, R.S., Loriaux, D.L., Thompson, R.H., Andersen, A.E., & Lipsett, M.B. (1974). Hypothalamic dysfunction in patients with anorexia nervosa. *Medicine, 53*, 147–159.

Minuchin, S., Rosman, B., & Baker, L. (1978). *Psychosomatic families: Anorexia nervosa in context*. Cambridge, Mass.: Harvard University Press.

Morgan, H.G., Purgold, J., & Welbourne, J. (1983). Management and outcome in anorexia nervosa. A standardised prognostic study. *British Journal of Psychiatry, 143*, 282–287.

Morgan, H.G., & Russell, G.F.M. (1975). Value of family background and clinical features as predictors of long-term outcome in anorexia nervosa: four year follow-up study of 41 patients. *Psychological Medicine, 5*, 355–371.

Norris, D.L., & Jones, E. (1979). Anorexia nervosa—A clinical study of 10 patients and their family systems. *Journal of Adolescence, 2*, 101–111.

Nwaefuna, A. (1981). Anorexia nervosa in a developing country. *British Journal of Psychiatry, 138*, 270.

Orbach, S. (1978). *Fat is a feminist issue*. London: Hamlyn.

Palazzoli, M.S. (1974). *Self-starvation. From the intrapsychic to the transpersonal approach to anorexia nervosa*. London: Chaucer, Human Context Books.

Palmer, R.L. (1980). *Anorexia nervosa: A guide for sufferers and their families*. Harmondsworth: Penguin.

Patton, G.C., Wood, K. & Johnson-Sabine, E. (1986). Physical illness. A risk factor in anorexia nervosa. *British Journal of Psychiatry, 149*, 756–759.

Pillay, M., & Crisp, A.H. (1977). Some psychological characteristics of patients with anorexia nervosa whose weight has been newly restored. *British Journal of Medical Psychology, 50*, 381–395.

Rowland, C.V. (1970). Anorexia nervosa: A survey of the literature and review of 30 cases. In C.V. Rowland (ed.), *Anorexia and obesity—international psychiatry clinics*, Vol.7. Boston: Little Brown.

Ryle, J.A. (1939). Discussion on anorexia nervosa. *Proceedings of the Royal Society of Medicine, 32*, 735–737.

Schwartz, D.M., Thompson, M.G., & Johnson, C.L. (1982). Anorexia nervosa and bulimia: The sociocultural context. *International Journal of Eating Disorders, 1*(3), 20–26.

Slade, P.D. (1977). Awareness of body dimensions during pregnancy. An analogue study. *Psychological Medicine, 7*, 245–252.

Slade, P.D. (1982). Towards a functional analysis of anorexia nervosa and bulimia nervosa. *British Journal of Clinical Psychology, 21*, 167–179.

Smart, D.E., Beumont, P.J.V., & George, G.C.W. (1976). Some personality characteristics of patients with anorexia nervosa. *British Journal of Psychiatry, 128*, 57–60.

Sours, J.A. (1974). The anorexia nervosa syndrome. *International Journal of Psychoanalysis, 55*, 567–572.

Sours, J.A. (1980). *Starving to death in a sea of objects*. New York: J. Aronson.

Sterling, J.W., & Segal, J.D. (1985). Anorexia nervosa in males: A critical review. *International Journal of Eating Disorders, 4*, 559–572.

Strober, M. (1980). Personality and symptomatological features in young, nonchronic anorexia nervosa patients. *Journal of Psychosomatic Research, 24*, 353–359.

Tobin-Richards, M.H., Boxer, A.H., & Peterson, A.C. (1983). The psychological significance of pubertal change. In J. Brookes-Gunn & A.C. Peterson (eds), *Girls at puberty: Biological and psychosocial perspectives*. New York: Plenum Press.

Vandereycken, W., & Meerman, R. (1984). Anorexia nervosa: Is prevention possible. *International Journal of Psychiatry in Medicine, 14*(3), 191–205.

Wakeling, A. (1985). Risk factors in anorexia nervosa. Paper presented at The Royal College of Psychiatrists, London, November 1985.

Warren, W. (1968). A study of anorexia nervosa in young girls. *Journal of Child Psychology and Psychiatry, 9*, 27–40.

Welbourne, J., & Purgold, J. (1984). *The eating sickness*. Brighton: Harvester Press.

Winokur, A., March, V., & Mendels, J. (1980). Primary affective disorder in relatives of patients with anorexia nervosa. *American Journal of Psychiatry, 137*, 695–698.

Woodman, M. (1980). *The owl was a baker's daughter: Obesity, anorexia and the repressed feminine*. Canada: Inner City Publ.

Yager, J. (1981). Anorexia nervosa and the family. In M. Lansky (ed.), *Family therapy and major psychopathology*. New York: Grune and Stratton.

Yellowlees, A.J. (1985). Anorexia and bulimia in anorexia nervosa: A study of psychosocial functioning and associated psychiatric symptomatology. *British Journal of Psychiatry, 146*, 648–652.

KEY WORDS

Anorexia nervosa, aetiology, risk factors, precipitating factors, adolescence, puberty, dieting, weight sensitivity, sexuality, self-esteem, separation difficulties, regression, family factors, menarche, pregnancy, bingeing/bulimia, family characteristics, marital problems, weight pathology, family psychiatric history, affective disorder, personality characteristics, sociocultural factors, fitness, self-control, feminist interpretations, middle-class characteristics, obesity, perfectionism, impulsive behaviours, illness episides, amenorrhoea, hypothalamic disorder, appetite loss, illness orientation, school factors, long-term stress, life events.

Handbook of Life Stress, Cognition and Health
Edited by S. Fisher and J. Reason
© 1988 John Wiley & Sons Ltd.

20

Personality, Life Stress and Cancerous Disease

CARY L. COOPER
University of Manchester Institute of Science and Technology, England

INTRODUCTION

While research into coronary heart disease and stress has been growing, developing and bearing valuable information (Glass, 1977; Haynes *et al.*, 1980; Cooper, 1983), the same cannot be said of other potentially stress-related illnesses, particularly cancer. Although psychological research work has been conducted in the field of cancer, it has not been as systematic or as unequivocal as in the field of cardiovascular disease. Much of this research has been published in disparate journals and tends to be retrospective in design. Nevertheless, there is a wide body of seminal knowledge available, and in order for us to make progress, it is essential to bring it together to see 'where we are' and 'where we should be going' (Cooper, 1988). The purpose of this chapter is to review the existing research work on the effect of personality and adverse life events in the etiology of cancer. This will also help us to highlight some of the methodological weaknesses of the current research and suggest future developments.

THE RELATIONSHIP OF PSYCHOLOGICAL FACTORS TO CANCER

It was in the late 19th century that attention was first drawn to the possible link of stress and cancer by Paget (1870), who observed that 'the cases are so frequent in which deep anxiety, defended hope and disappointment are quickly followed by the growth and increase of cancer, that we can hardly doubt that mental depression is a weighty addition to the other influences favouring the development of the cancerous constitution.' Herbert Snow (1893), in his acclaimed book *Cancer and the cancer process*, noted that 'We are logically impelled to inquire if the great majority of cases of cancer may now own a neurotic origin? . . . We find

Some of the material used in this chapter was published by the author in the *Journal of Human Stress*.

that the number of instances in which malignant disease of the breast and uterus follows immediately antecedent emotion of a depressing character is too large to be set down to chance, or to that general liability to the buffets of ill fortune which cancer patients, in their passage through life, share with most other people not so afflicted.' Throughout the early part of the 20th century, further suggestions have been made about the relationship between psychosocial factors and cancer, culminating in a book by Evans (1926), *A psychological study of cancer*, in which she suggested that one of the leading causes of cancer was the loss of a love object or an important emotional relationship. Her analysis of cancer patients led her to believe that some people experiencing grief directed their psychic energy inward, against their own natural body defenses.

There have been a number of explanations of just how stress may cause disease. Foque (1931), for example, believed that there was a multiplicity of secondary causes for cancer, such as x-rays, chemicals and viruses. However, in this view, the cells had to be in a receptive state before the cancerous process could start. He believed in 'the role of sad emotions as activators and secondary causes in the activation of human cancers'. These, he added, 'through the instrumentality of the nervous system's effect on metabolism, act on the endocrine balances of the body in such a way that the cell is put into a state where it is sensitive and receptive to the carcinogen'.

Fox (1978), however, suggested that there are two primary cancer-causing mechanisms: (a) 'carcinogenesis, the production of cancer by an agent or mechanism overcoming existing resistance of the body', and (b) 'lowered resistance to cancer, which permits a potential carcinogen normally insufficient to produce cancer to do so' (e.g. weakened emotional state). This latter mechanism involves the immunosuppression system of the body, with an 'immune deficient' individual at risk of one form of cancer or another depending on the vulnerability of particular organs.

Selye (1979), on the other hand, suggested that all organisms go through a 'general adaptation syndrome', which passes through three stages.

1) Alarm reaction, which is comprised of a shock phase ('the initial and immediate reaction to a noxious agent') and a countershock phase ('a mobilization of defenses phase in which the adrenal cortex becomes further enlarged and secretes more corticoid hormones').
2) Stage of resistance, which involves adapting to the stressor stimulus, but decreasing one's ability to cope with subsequent stimuli.
3) Stage of exhaustion, which follows a period of prolonged and severe adaption.

He goes on to say that the hormonal attack (particularly adrenocorticotrophic hormone, ACTH) on the body is the ultimate cancer-producing weapon if it is activated at a frequent, continuous and high level.

Selye (1979) believes that stress plays some role in the development of all diseases: 'these effects may be curative (as illustrated by various forms of externally-induced stress such as shock therapy, physical therapy, and occupational therapy) or damaging, depending on whether the biochemical reactions characteristic of stress (e.g. stress hormones or nervous reactions to stress) combat or accentuate the trouble.'

Although the exact bodily and psychological mechanisms are still not entirely clear, the evidence is mounting that there is some link between psychosocial/ personality factors and certain forms of cancer, even though the methodological weaknesses in the existing research leave something to be desired.

Most of the research in this field can be subdivided into two categories: those studies which focus on the relationship between various psychometric predispositions and cancer, and those which examine the emotional history or adverse life event and the pathogenesis of cancer.

Whereas Fox (1978) and Selye (1979) emphasize the physiological or bodily reactions and processes of stress; Haney (1977), Kissen (1969) and others have concentrated on the psychological processes that may lead to cancer. Kissen has argued that adverse life events and loss of a love object can lead to cancer by the psychological mechanisms of 'despair, depression and hopelessness'. He suggests that 'adverse life situations in an individual with poor emotional outlets, and therefore, with diminished ability to effectively sublimate or dissipate an emotional situation, are likely to result in such affects as depression, despair and hopelessness. It is also possible that adverse life situations may directly precipitate such effects whatever the personality, but it must be conceded that their manifestation is more likely in those with poor emotional outlets.' Haney (1977) argues that personality predispositions may not be directly linked to cancer, but will help to determine 'the psychic and somatic insults to which the individual will be exposed and the meaning these exposures will have for the individual'. There is likely to be a psychocarcinogenic process in operation, which works in such a way that the stressor and bodily predispositions interact and co-vary in the direction of an ultimate carcinoma, one feeding the other.

PERSONALITY PREDISPOSITIONS AND CANCER

Bacon et al. (1952) provided one of the earliest suggestions of a cancer personality. They investigated 40 women with cancer of the breast, and constructed detailed psychoanalytic case histories of each of them. They concluded that these patients had six important behavioral characteristics:

1) a masochistic character structure,
2) inhibited sexuality,
3) inhibited motherhood,
4) inability to discharge or deal appropriately with anger, aggressiveness or hostility, covered over by a facade of pleasantness,
5) an unresolved hostile conflict with the mother handled through denial and unrealistic sacrifice, and
6) delay in securing treatment.

Bacon and her colleagues were inclined to believe that there might be a connection between the psyche and cancer, and that 'it is possible for emotional forces at times to provide a catalyst for the cancer reaction'. LeShan (1959) was one of the first to suggest that cancer may result from the loss of a loved one or some significant other, particularly in persons who are prone to feelings of hopelessness, depression, low self-esteem and introjection. Many of the early researchers in this field have observed that malignancies seem to be associated with what Kissen (1963) and others (Dattore *et al.*, 1980) have termed 'general emotional inhibition, denial and repression'.

LeShan and Worthington (1955) did some of the early work in this field, by comparing 152 cancer patients and 125 patients with other or no illness, using a projective test developed by Worthington. The cancer group differed from the control in the following ways: (a) they had difficulty expressing hostile feelings, (b) they suffered the loss of a 'dear one' prior to diagnosis, and (c) they showed greater potential anxiety about the death of a parent.

Kissen (1963) carried out a study among 335 patients, of whom 161 had been diagnosed as having lung cancer, while others had some other less severe illness. He instrumented a childhood behavior disorder questionnaire and the Maudsley Personality Inventory, and found that the cancer patients suffered from 'a diminished outlet for emotional discharge', both in their childhood experiences and in their present adult lives. Booth's (1963) Rorschach work on 93 lung cancer patients and 82 tubercular patients revealed similar patterns among the cancer patients. He found that cancer patients responded very differently to the inkblots than did tubercular patients, emphasizing emotional repression, the inward direction of anger, and vulnerability to emotional loss.

Studies in the late 1960s and early 1970s used more sophisticated psychometric measures, but still suffered from inadequate or non-representative sampling and inappropriate comparison groups. They nevertheless came up with similar findings to the early work. Pauli and Schmid (1972) carried out an investigation among 57 patients with histologically verified breast cancer and compared them to a group of 34 women with benign disorders of the reproductive organs, using the Minnesota Multiphase Personality Inventory (MMPI). They found that the patients with mastocarcinoma were significantly different on measures of depression, hypochondriasis, and paranoia. Grissom *et al.* (1975) compared healthy subjects and patients with bronchial carcinoma and found that their cancer patients had significantly lower 'personal integration' scores on the Tennessee Self-Concept scales. Individuals with this pattern of behavior frequently direct their frustration, anger and failure inward, and are vulnerable to the loss of an important relationship.

There have been a great number of studies which have explored the psychometric differences between cancer patients and other patients or normals, but they all suffer from being retrospective. The major problem with these investigations stems from the nature of the primary sample, which is usually made up of diagnosed cancer patients. It is extremely difficult in these circumstances to disentangle the interrelationship between cancer and personality. There is enough evidence available to suggest that the awareness of having cancer can alter various personality measures (Craig and Abeloff, 1974), which could make methodological nonsense of existing findings. Prospective work in this field is now underway in the US. Paffenbarger (1977), for example, is engaged in a long-term cohort study of over 35 000 former Harvard students and 16 500 University of Pennsylvania students (of both sexes), on whom physiological and psychological data have been accumulating over a large number of years.

In the meantime, there are a number of premorbid personality studies already available to test some of Kissen's (1963) theories that repression is the fundamental personality mechanism in cancer pathogenesis, particularly in people who have suffered the loss of a love object. To this end, Dattore *et al.* (1980) carried out a very well-designed study of 200 patients (75 cancer and 125 non-cancer patients), on whom premorbid MMPI personality data were available through Veterans' Administration Hospital records. Extensive screening of records was involved to ensure comparable samples. They found that the two groups were significantly different on three scales: repression, depression, and denial of hysteria. Their findings on repression were in the direction of earlier studies, that cancer patients showed significantly higher scores. Their results on depression were unexpected but understandable: they found that cancer patients had significantly lower depression scores than controls. They argued, 'since depression represents such a threatening emotion to the cancer patient, one would expect to see relatively little acknowledgement of depression by subjects in the cancer group'. In addition, they found that cancer patients scored lower on the denial of hysteria measure, which they interpreted as indicating that they were more *insightful* and *introceptive* than non-cancer patients, which is also consistent with earlier theoretical speculations.

Other research has shown the opposite, namely, that extraverts are more prone to cancer. Hagnell (1966) carried out an epidemiological survey of 2550 Swedish women over a 10-year period. It was found that a significantly higher proportion of women who had developed cancer had been originally rated as having a 'substable' personality. This classification of personality types, developed by a Swede, Sjobring (1963), utilizes four dimensions: (a) a capacity factor, (b) a stability factor, (c) a solidity factor, and (d) a validity factor. The 'substable' personality is described as 'warm, hearty, concrete, heavy, industrious, interested in people, social, tending to personal interrelations and inhibition'. Hagnell's findings did not support earlier or subsequent research observations, as his results showed that cancer patients were 'substable' more often than one might expect. 'Substability' in Sjobring's system has traits in common with Eysenck's classification of 'extraversion', which refers to the outgoing, uninhibited social proclivities of a person. Thus, Coppen and Metcalfe (1963), prompted by Hagnell's findings, carried out a survey on 47 women with cancer, using the Maudsley Personal Inventory, which assesses extraversion. They concluded that women who develop breast cancer do have significantly higher extraversion scores, and that this is a 'constitutionally determined' characteristic of these patients rather than a 'temporary reaction' to their illness. This finding confirms Hagnell's result, but does not agree with Kissen's hypothesis that cancer is associated with individuals who have 'poor emotional outlets' and repress their feelings.

In addition, a great deal of recent work has been carried out on the link between clinical depression and cancer. Bieliauskas and Garron (1982) provide an excellent review of most of this research. Many early studies have indicated, mostly retrospectively, that cancer patients tend to suffer from some form of psychological depression (Levine *et al.*, 1978). Probably the best designed prospective study in the field is by Shekelle and his colleagues, (Shekelle *et al.*, 1981), who conducted an epidemiological investigation of 2020 men in whom clinically assessed depression had been measured by the MMPI some 17 years before the mortality records had been examined. For those males who had scored at the top end of the depression scale, there was twice the incidence of deaths due to cancer than for those who did not score at the high end of the depression continuum. The data indicate that the risk was prevalent during the whole 17-year period but was most prominent between 12 and 17 years. Bieliauskas and Garron (1982) indicate that: 'because of the prospective nature, the long period, the use of quantitative measures, attention to their risk factors, and the large number of subjects, this study provides significant evidence of prospective increases in risk of cancer death with increased depression.'

Nevertheless, there were a number of methodological weaknesses. First, the MMPI absolute depression scores for the cancer deaths were not in the pathological range, only linearly more depressive than for the non-cancer deaths. Second, we only have a 'one point of time' measurement of depression (i.e. 17 years ago) and do not have information about the change that may have taken place in the psychological state of the individuals assessed.

While all the results point in a similar direction, with the exception of the few mentioned above, the methodological weaknesses here are very great indeed. Most of these studies suffer from inappropriate samples, uncoordinated and unreliable measuring instruments, inadequate comparison groups, retrospective as opposed to prospective data gathering, and a disregard for fitting the research work into any kind of conceptual or theoretical framework. The issue of an appropriate control group is particularly important, and the difficulties of interpretation in this respect were highlighted in a recent study by Watson and Schuld (1977). They took a sample of cancer patients and matched control groups and found no significant differences on any of the MMPI scales between the two. Although the data were collected on a premorbid basis (i.e. well before any clinical diagnosis of cancer), the sample was comprised of individuals for whom psychopathology had been diagnosed (i.e. they were psychiatric patients). In addition, the malignancy group contained a large proportion of people with alcohol-related problems, six times as many as in the control group (Kellerman, 1977). These kinds of studies create a great deal of confusion in the cancer field and could be controlled by more careful research designs. As Perrin and Pierce (1959) suggest, ideally each study of cancer and personality should contain two control groups, one of subjects who have some chronic, non-cancerous disease sufficient to cause them anxiety about their health, and the other a comparison group of 'healthy' subjects.

LIFE EVENTS AND CANCER

A second category of studies in this field has focused on recent stressful life events and the onset of cancer. Indeed, in LeShan's (1959) early review of 75 studies on psychological factors in the development of malignant disease, he concluded that 'the most consistently reported, relevant psychological factor has been the loss of a major emotional relationship prior to the first-noted symptoms of neoplasm.'

He later developed hypotheses about mortality rates. He predicted that cancer mortality rates should be highest for widowed, next highest for divorced, and lowest for married and then single persons, if the theory of loss of emotional relationships was valid. He analysed epidemiological data from a number of studies and found that some of the data were consistent with this hypothesis.

Muslin *et al.* (1966) carried out an investigation of 165 women who were about to have a breast biopsy. The women were interviewed and given a life events questionnaire prior to diagnosis, and in the end the authors were able to produce 37 matched pairs of malignant and benign subjects, in three different groups of events (i.e. early, recent, and both early and recent). For the recent and combined groups, they found more benign them malignant patients reporting 'losses', but with little statistical significance among the three groups.

Schmale and Iker (1966) explored the same phenomenon among a group of women who were reporting for a cone biopsy as a result of a positive Pap test. They were given psychological tests and interviewed prior to diagnosis, and none of the subjects had any gross abnormality that would lead the physician to suspect cervical cancer. On the basis of high life events scores 6 months prior to the first positive Pap smear, the authors then predicted which women would ultimately be diagnosed as having cervical cancer. It was found that there was a significantly high level of accuracy in their judgments, based solely on life events immediately preceding the first tests.

On the other hand, Schonfield (1975), who interviewed 112 Israeli women on the day before biopsy of a breast lump, found no evidence that stressful life events, particularly losses, precede the onset of cancer. Data from this study show that patients who were subsequently found to have benign tumors of the breast had higher scores (more stress) on Holmes and Rahe's Social Readjustment Rating Scale (SRRS) than those who had malignancies. However, he found that patients who were subsequently found to have malignant tumors had higher cover anxiety and MMPI lie scale scores. This could possibly be the result of the physician unconsciously transmitting to them his own anxiety about their breast lumps.

In addition, Snell and Graham (1971), in their study of 352 breast cancer patients and 670 patients with other types of cancer and non-neoplasmic diseases, could find no difference between these two groups in the experiencing of a single event or a cumulative number of events by themselves or by members of their families. They pointed out the shortcomings of their methodology, and also suggested that there may be events of a different type (not studied by them) which may be related to the development of cancer of the breast.

In recent years a good deal of sustained work has been carried out by Greer and his colleagues (Greer and Morris, 1975; Greer, 1979). In a study on premorbid breast cancer, Greer (1979) studied 160 women admitted to hospital for a breast tumour biopsy. A breast tumour was defined as being 'a tumour with or without palpable auxiliary nodes, with no deep attachment and no distant metastases: 'that is, women with either very early breast cancer which is operable or women with some breast disease which is benign'. These patients were interviewed on the day prior to the biopsy and detailed information was collected on stressful life events (e.g. events which caused them severe and prolonged emotional distress). These events were verified by husbands or close relatives. Additional psychometric data were also collected on depression, hostility, extraversion/neuroticism and other social and psychiatric states. After the operation, 69 of the women were found to have breast cancer, and 91 a benign breast disease. The cancer and controls (i.e. benign group) were matched in most respects (e.g. social class, marital state, etc.), except that the cancer patients were significantly older.

No significant differences were found in respect to the occurrence of stressful life events, including loss of a loved person, or depression, or denial as the characteristic response to life stresses. Although an effort was made to design the research in a way that would minimize the effects of diagnosed cancer on personality and the recall of life events, the author admits himself that 'we had no control over what surgeons told patients before admission'. In addition, he was unable to control for the fear of having an operation which could result in the removal of a breast and the diagnosis of breast cancer. Furthermore, those in the cancer group were significantly older, which could have biased the results. But most important of all, since breast cancer may take several years to develop, and the stressful life events responsible may take place years before that, there is a strong potential 'memory falsification' problem. What is really needed, as Greer himself suggests, are large scale prospective studies with more sophisticated control groups.

In an effort to meet these objectives, Cooper et al. (1986) carried out a large-scale, prospective study on 2163 patients attending breast screening clinics. The Cooper, Cooper and Cheang Life Events Scale was used, which included 42 items (generated from a pilot sample of British females) and 10-point Likert-type scales on the degree of the stressfulness of the event. These women were subsequently diagnosed as having cancer, a cyst, benign breast disease and normal breasts. A well-woman control was also used. It was found that the cancer group had experienced significantly more loss- or illness-related events, perceived life events generally as more stressful, used fewer and poorer coping skills and were significantly lower on Type A behaviour (e.g. less assertive, directed emotions inward).

There have been other studies which have explored traumatic life events and cancer, without using the SRRS. For example, Smith and Sebastian (1976) examined the emotional history of 44 cancer patients and 44 patients with physical abnormalities which were non-cancerous. Structured interviews were carried out to try to identify the frequency, intensity, and duration of emotional states in each person's life, which involved questions about family life, childhood, social and sexual life, career, religion, etc. Their approach was far more open-ended than the traditional life events research just reviewed, in that they relied on interview responses to the following. 'I am going to ask you to remember events that have occurred in your life which have made you feel very concerned, emotional, stressed and so forth. I will ask you to relate the kind of events that provoked emotional feelings in you, the data of the event and the intensity and duration of the events and emotional conditions. We will begin with early childhood and end up with questions about your present life situation.' Critical incidents were then recorded, and rated as high, medium or low, and the intensity and duration of the emotional events for each person were rated on a 15-point scale. It was found that there were significantly more frequent and intense emotional events prior to diagnosis among cancer patients than among the comparison groups.

Another interesting study along these lines was undertaken by Witzel (1970) of 150 cancer patients and 150 patients with other serious diseases. He took personal histories of past illnesses and found that non-cancer patients had a significantly larger number of reported incidents of medical problems throughout their lives than cancer patients. They reported being out-patients three times more often than cancer patients, being in a hospital bed three times more often, having temperatures in excess of 38.5°C seven times more often, and experiencing twice as many minor illnesses and operations. The authors contend that this does not necessarily contradict the other research on adverse life events, because these critical medical incidents may signal the disease process itself. As Fox (1978) has suggested, 'developing cancer had mobilised the immune response, which is capable of fighting many diseases, and which, because of its aroused status, could do so more successfully than that of non-cancer patients'.

Some other research in this area is being undertaken which attempts to predict cancer from psychosocial factors. One such study was carried out by Horne and Picard (1980) among lung cancer patients, who were selected on the basis of the 'presence of an undiagnosed, subacute or chronic lung lesion visible on previous roentgenographic examination'. The patients were then interviewed extensively on a variety of psychosocial factors: childhood stability, job stability, marriage stability, lack of plans for the future, and recent significant loss. A composite score was devised for each patient on the basis of these five life areas. The patient's clinical pathology from 15 to 38 months after the psychosocial interview was determined, to see if predictions could be made from the life events to the diagnosis. The composite score was predictive in 80% of the patients with benign lung disease and in 61% of lung cancer patients. In fact, the predictive power of the psychosocial factors was as good as information on smoking history.

As we have seen, a great deal of research in the stress field has been conducted using life event methodology, much of which has stemmed from the Holmes and Rahe Social Readjustment Rating Scale, and others that followed it have, in the main, utilized weightings for each life event, generated either on a large general population sample or on a smaller but more representative sample of a larger group to be studied.

There are several methodological problems with the SRRS and other similar life event scales that include generic weightings, which may bias or distort research results in the field of stress. First, these scales list a number of events which may be symptoms or consequences of illness rather than critical incidents (e.g. change in number of marital arguments, fired from work, sexual difficulties, etc). Second, the illness itself may impede or prevent the patient from accurately recalling past events (particularly not very important ones), as Napier *et al.* (1972) have found. But, by far the most important methodological weakness of these scales lies in the fact that individual perceptions of the events are not taken into

Table 20.1 Comparison of common items on the Cooper, Cooper and Cheang Life Events Scale and the Social Readjustment Rating Scale (SRRS). (Source: Cooper *et al.*, 1985)

Life event	Percentage experiencing life event over last 2 years		Mean score of ratings		
	Control group	Cancer patients	SRRS	Control group	Cancer patients
Moved house	32	15	2.00	4.29	3.57
Major house renovation	25	13	2.50	4.37	4.40
Got married	6	2	5.00	3.38	1.00
Divorce	1	6	7.30	3.80	7.33
Child started school/ nursery	14	8	2.60	2.70	5.33
Change in nature of work	21	9	3.60	4.01	5.25
Changed job	14	9	2.90	4.30	5.40
Made redundant	3	8	4.70	6.30	8.67
Retired	2	21	4.50	5.00	7.30
Increased/new bank loan	25	11	3.10	3.63	4.50
Financial difficulty	16	13	3.80	5.16	5.50
Death of husband	2	8	10.00	10.00	9.75
Death of a close friend	6	43	6.30	7.46	9.62
Serious illness of yourself	3	8	5.30	5.46	9.25
Pregnancy	5	6	4.00	4.71	9.33
Birth of baby	4	2	3.90	4.93	9.00
Family member left home	12	13	2.90	4.91	3.83
Difficult relationship with parents	11	2	2.90	5.36	5.00

Well-woman group ($n = 418$); breast cancer patients ($n = 53$).

account. Each event of the SRRS may have differential meaning for each subject, yet they are rigidly enumerated in scoring. Cooper *et al.* (1985) carried at a pilot prospective study on 53 women who had attended a breast-screening clinic (at which time we tested them) and later were diagnosed as having breast carcinoma. They also obtained control data on 418 'well women' attending annual medical examinations. They then compared the perceptual life events ratings of the controls and cancer patients against the weighted items in the SRRS, for those 18 life events that were common to the SRRS and the Cooper, Cooper and Cheang Life Events Scale (which included 42 items and was generated for a UK female sample; Table 20.1).

Several points can be made about Table 20.1, which raises questions about the validity of using standardized weighted life event scales. First, it can be seen that the SRRS weights for the various life events were substantially different from the perceptions of the well-women control group. This could reflect cultural differences between the United States (where the weightings for the SRRS were devised) and England, and/or differences between male and female subjects (since the SRRS were generated on a general population of men and women). It is interesting to note, for instance, that events to do with 'the family' (e.g. family member left home, difficult relationship with parents, birth of baby, etc.) are more highly rated in England and/or among a female population than among the American general population. Second, it can be seen that there are also substantial differences between the cancer patients' perceptions of these events (remembering that these perceptions were generated on the first visit to the breast-screening clinic and well in advance of any diagnosis of cancer) and the 'well-women' controls. Thus, if controls had roughly the same proportion of life events as the cancer group, no significant difference would be found between them using standardized weightings, even though the cancer patients may perceive the event as nearly twice as stressful as the controls on SRRS weightings (e.g. changed job). Indeed, we found that of the 42 items in the Cooper, Cooper and Cheang Life Events Scale, cancer patients perceived themselves to be significantly more stressed than controls on 29 of them.

Finally, in generating life events that would be relevant to an English female sample, we carried out extensive in-depth interviews with over 200 women and found a number of life events that were very important to include, but which did not appear on many of the standardized scales. In many cases these items were a significant event for between 25% and 35% of the sample of controls and cancer patients (e.g. death of family member, illness of close family member, increased nursing responsibilities for elderly parents/family members, separation (temporary) of loved ones, etc.). On balance, therefore, it is difficult to justify a culture-specific life event scale with standardized weightings in the field of stress research. What is needed are life event scales designed on a sample of the population on which a larger study will be undertaken, utilizing Likert-type rating scales by the subject or patient concerned.

SUMMARY AND CONCLUSIONS

This chapter attempts to review the research linking personality factors and adverse life events to the cancer process. Much of this research is retrospective, with poor control groups and small samples, but recent investigations are improving in these regards. On balance, the existing research seems to indicate that emotionally inhibited individuals who have experienced significant loss-related events (e.g. death of parent or spouse) are 'at risk' to the cancer process.

The area of stressful life events and the pathogenesis of cancer is, therefore, a potentially fruitful field of future research and must be seriously considered. At the very least, adverse life events must act as an intervening, if not primary, source of illness behavior. As Haney (1977) has recently suggested, 'adverse life events may produce situations and circumstances which heighten the individual's belief in his susceptibility, or increase the perceived threat. Adverse life events may exacerbate existing and often otherwise well-tolerated symptoms and reduce the individual's tendency to deny them or delay help-seeking.'

REFERENCES

Bacon, C.L., Rennecker, R., & and Kutler, M. (1952). Psychosomatic survey of cancer of the breast. *Psychosomatic Medicine, 4*, 453–460.

Bieliauskas, L.A., & Garron, D.C. (1982). Psychological depression and cancer. *General Hospital Psychiatry, 4*, 56.

Booth, G. (1964). Cancer and culture: Psychological disposition and environment (A Rorschach Study). Unpublished.

Cooper, C.L. (1988) *Stress and breast cancer.* Chichester: Wiley.

Cooper, C.L., Cooper, R.D. & Faragher, E.B. (1985). Stress and life event methodology. *Stress Medicine, 1*, 287–289.

Cooper, C.L., Cooper, R.D. & Faragher, E.B. (1986). A prospective study of the relationship between breast cancer and life events, Type A behavior, social support and coping skills. *Stress Medicine, 2*, 271–279.

Coppen, A.J., & Metcalfe, M. (1963). Cancer and extraversion. *British Medical Journal,* 18–19.

Craig, T.J., & Abeloff, M.D. (1974). Psychiatric symptomatology among hospitalized cancer patients. *American Journal of Psychiatry, 131*, 1323–1327.

Dattore, P., Shontz, F. & Coyne, L. (1980). Premorbid personality differentiation of cancer and non-cancer groups. *Journal of Consulting and Clinical Psychology, 48*(3), 388–394.

Evans, E.A. (1926). *Psychological study of cancer.* New York: Dodd-Mead.

Foque, E. (1931). Le probleme au cancer dans les aspects psychiques. *Hospital Gazette (Paris), 104*, 827.

Fox, B.H. (1978). Premorbid psychological factors as related to cancer incidence. *Journal of Behavioral Medicine, 1*(1), 45–133.

Glass, D. (1977). *Behavior patterns, stress and coronary disease.* New Jersey: LEA.

Greer, S. (1979). Psychological enquiry: A contribution to cancer research. *Journal of Psychology and Medicine, 9*, 81–89.

Greer, S., & Morris, T. (1975). Psychological attributes of women who develop breast cancer: A controlled study. *Journal of Psychosomatic Research, 19*, 147–153.

Grissom, J., Weiner, B., & Weiner, E. (1975). Psychological correlates of cancer. *Journal of Consulting and Clinical Psychology, 43*, 113.

Hagnell, O. (1966). The premorbid personality of persons who develop cancer in a total population investigated in 1947 and 1957. In *Psycho-physiological aspects of cancer. Annals of the New York Academy of Science, 846*.

Haney, C.A. (1977), Illness behaviour and psychosocial correlates of cancer. *Journal of Social Science and Medicine, 11*(4), 223–228.

Haynes, S., Feinleib, M., & Kannel, U. (1980). The relationship of psychological factors to coronary heart disease in the Framingham Study. *American Journal of Epidemiology, 111*(1), 37–58.

Holmes, T.H., & Rahe, R.H. (1967). The Social Readjustment Rating Scale. *Journal of Psychosomatic Medicine, 11*, 213–218.

Horne, R.L., & Picard, R.S. (1980). Psychosocial risk factors for lung cancer. *Psychosomatic Medicine, 41*, 503–514.

Kellerman, J. (1978). A note on psychosomatic factors. *Journal of Consulting and Clinical Psychology, 46*, 1422–1523.

Kissen, D. (1963). Personality characteristics in males conducive to lung cancer. *British Journal of Medical Psychology, 36*, 27–36.

Kissen, D. (1969). The present status of psychosomatic cancer research. *Geriatrics, 24*, 129.

LeShan, L. (1959). Psychological states as factors in the development of malignant disease: A critical review. *Journal of the National Cancer Institute, 22*, 1–18.

LeShan, L. (1966). An emotional life-history pattern associated with neoplastic disease. *Annals of the New York Academy of Science, 125*, 780–793.

LeShan, L., & Worthington, R.E. (1955). Some psychological correlates of neoplastic disease: Preliminary report. *Journal of Clinical and Experimental Psychopathology, 16,* 281.

Levine, P.M., Silberfarb, P.M., & Lipowski, A.J. (1978). Mental disorders in cancer patients: A study of 100 psychiatric referrals. *Cancer, 42,* 1385–1391.

Muslin, H.L., Gyarfas, K. & Pieper, W.J. (1966). Separation experience and cancer of the breast. *Annals of the New York Academy of Science, 125,* 802–806.

Napier, J.A., Metzner, H., & Johnson, B.C. (1972). Limitations of morbidity and mortality data obtained from family histories. A report from the Tecumseh studies. *American Journal of Public Health, 62,* 30–35.

Paffenbarger, R.S. (1977). Psychosocial factors in students predictive of cancer. Grant No. IR01 CA 225 74–01, National Cancer Institute, Bethesda, Md.

Paget, J. (1870). *Surgical pathology.* London: Longmans Green.

Pauli, H., & Schmid, V. (1972). Psychosomatic aspects in the clinical manifestation of mastocarcinoma. *Journal of Psychotherapy and Medical Psychology, 22*(2).

Perrin, G.M., & Pierce, I.R. (1959). Psychosomatic aspects of cancer: A review. *Psychosomatic Medicine, 5,* 397–421.

Schmale, A.H., & Iker, H.P. (1966). The affect of hopelessness and the development of cancer. *Journal of Psychosomatic Medicine, 28,* 714–721.

Schonfield, J. (1975). Psychological and life-experience differences between Israeli women with benign and cancerous breast lesions. *Journal of Psychosomatic Research, 19,* 229.

Selye, H. (1979). Correlating stress and cancer. *American Journal of Proctology, Gastro-enterology, Colon and Rectal Surgery, 30*(4), 18–28.

Shekelle, R.B., Raynor, W.J., Ostefeld, A.M. *et al.* (1981). Psychological depression and 17-year risk and death from cancer. *Psychosomatic Medicine, 43,* 117–125.

Sjobring, H. (1963). *La personalite, structure et developpement.* Paris: Doin.

Smith, W.R., & Sebastian, H. (1976). Emotional history and pathogenesis of cancer. *Journal of Clinical Psychology, 32*(4), 63–66.

Snell, L., & Graham, S. (1971). Social trauma as related to cancer of the breast. *British Journal of Cancer, 25*(4), 721.

Snow, H. (1893). *Cancer and the cancer process.* London: Churchill.

Watson, C., & Schuld, D. (1977). Psychosomatic factors in the etiology of neoplasms. *Journal of Consulting and Clinical Psychology, 45*(3), 455–461.

Witzel, L. (1970). Anamnese and Zweiterkrankungen bei Patienten mit bosartigen Neubildungen. (Medical histories of patients with malignant tumors compared with patients with other diseases.) *Medizinische Klinik, 65,* 876–879.

KEY WORDS

Personality predispositions to cancer, life stress, carcinogenesis, lowered resistance to cancer, poor emotional outlet, lowered self-esteem, emotional inhibition, depression, adverse life events, lack of social support, loss of significant other, emotional history, life event methodology.

21

Stress and Diabetes

CLARE BRADLEY
University of Sheffield, England

INTRODUCTION

In the 1980s, there has been a surge of interest in stress and diabetes. It is commonly believed that stress can both precipitate diabetes onset and disrupt diabetes control. Growing evidence suggesting a causal association between chronic hyperglycaemia and subsequent complications of diabetes has motivated research into stress and other factors believed to affect diabetes control.

Stress research in general, and particularly life events research, has been accused of mindless empiricism in failing to consider mechanisms linking life events and illness outcome (Waterhouse, 1984). In diabetes-related stress research, models and mechanisms have been described (e.g. Tarnow and Silverman, 1981–2; Evans, 1985), though the models are unable to accommodate many of the data being produced. A second form of mindlessness noted by Waterhouse (1984) and common in diabetes research is the failure to appreciate and allow for individual variability in the appraisal of stress and failure to consider individual differences in responses to stress. Individual differences all too often ignored also include basic parameters concerning the nature of the subjects' diabetes and their treatment regimens. Some researchers in this field are, however, now recognizing the importance of differences between diabetic individuals responding to apparently similar stressors (Carter *et al.*, 1985; Stabler *et al.*, 1986) or exposed to the same stress management programme (Bradley, 1985), and there is greater recognition of differences between individuals in response to the diabetes itself (e.g. Johnson, 1980; Kosub and Cerreto, 1981).

THE PATHOPHYSIOLOGY OF DIABETES MELLITUS

It is now becoming clear that diabetes mellitus is not a single disorder but is a collection of several disorders with different underlying causes and with multiple

Preparation of this chapter was supported by NIH grant number AM28196 to the author.

hormonal abnormalities. All forms of diabetes mellitus are characterized by disordered carbohydrate metabolism with hyperglycaemia. Diabetes results from a deficiency of insulin function; either the beta cells of the pancreas produce insufficient insulin or the insulin produced may not be used effectively. Relative insufficiency of insulin may be due to hypersecretion or hyperactivity of insulin antagonists such as glucagon from the alpha cells of the pancreas, pituitary, adrenomedullary, or thyroid hormones.

The World Health Organization (1985) estimated that 2%–5% of the UK population and 5%–10% in the USA have some form of diabetes. Estimated prevalence rates elsewhere in the world vary from zero in the highland population of Papua New Guinea to 25% among the Pima Indians and Nauruans.

Insulin from beta cells of the pancreas promotes the uptake of glucose from the blood by the body cells. Without insulin, glucose metabolism and storage are inadequate and glucose accumulates in the blood. When the glucose reaches a sufficiently high level (approximately 10 mmol/l) it spills over into the urine and the volume of urine may increase considerably, causing dehydration. Thus thirst is a common symptom of untreated diabetes. Fat may be used as a metabolic substrate but complete metabolism of fat requires the presence of substances produced during the combustion of glucose. Thus, in the absence of glucose metabolism, fat combustion is incomplete, toxic intermediate metabolites (ketone bodies) are produced which accumulate in the blood. If ketone bodies collect in sufficient amounts, they cause acidosis and eventually coma, which may be fatal. This form of coma associated with untreated diabetes is the high blood glucose, or hyperglycaemic, coma. With insulin-treated diabetes, hypoglycaemic coma is more of a risk. Hypoglycaemia may occur if insulin is not balanced with sufficient carbohydrate intake or if unusual amounts of exercise are not compensated for by increased carbohydrate allowance or reduced insulin dosage. Recovery is rapid if glucose is given orally or intravenously or when the hormone, glucagon, is injected intramuscularly.

Some 85% of people with diabetes do not require insulin to manage their disorder. They have some effective endogenous insulin and some homeostatic control of their blood glucose. There is only a small risk of ketoacidosis and hyperglycaemic coma in people with this form of non-insulin-dependent diabetes (NIDD). In overweight people with NIDD, it is often possible to reduce carbohydrate intake to within a range in which endogenous insulin can cope. In such cases the diabetes can be managed by diet alone. In cases of people with NIDD who are not overweight, there is likely to be insufficient utilization of carbohydrates. Sulphonylureas (hypoglycaemic agents in tablet form) may be used to stimulate insulin secretion or to increase insulin effectiveness (see Lebovitz (1985) for review).

THE CLASSIFICATION OF DIABETES

There is currently active debate over how best to categorize the various types of diabetes which can be identified. The terms used are important for stress researchers to understand as stress responses would be expected to differ between subjects with different kinds of diabetes.

At one time diabetes was classified according to age at the time of diagnosis into 'juvenile-onset' or 'maturity-onset' diabetes. However, although all juvenile-onset patients would be dependent on insulin, the maturity-onset patients form a heterogeneous group including patients treated by diet alone, diet and tablets, and diet and insulin. In the interests of greater precision, diabetes was often described in terms of treatment prescribed. By the beginning of the 1980s a new terminology was being recommended which was intended to reflect different pathogenic mechanisms underlying the diabetes. A distinction between 'type I' and 'type II' diabetes was made on the basis of certain immunological phenomena and genetic markers. However, the methods for measuring these immunological and genetic characteristics are not commonly available. In practice the terms type I and type II have tended to be used synonymously with the labels insulin-dependent diabetes (IDD) and NIDD which refer to clinically descriptive sub-classes where the distinction is based on the patients' dependence for survival on exogenous insulin. Some patients are not easily classified as having IDD or NIDD. The term IDD is sometimes used to refer to anyone who uses insulin in treating their diabetes. A proportion of such patients, however, will have substantial amounts of effective endogenous insulin but have found it impossible to achieve good glycaemic control using other forms of therapy alone. Thus 'insulin treated' is not the same as 'insulin dependent' and this distinction is of particular importance to stress researchers investigating the effects of stress on diabetes control. Only truly IDD patients can be expected to have a complete absence of endogenous insulin and hence to have a lack of homeostatic control over any stress-related changes in blood glucose. Unless precise terminology is used in research reports, the reader may be misled about insulin availability in the subjects studied. C-peptide measures of endogenous insulin availability or details of clinical criteria which may be used in the absence of C-peptide measures (Welborn et al., 1983) are needed to establish the nature of the subject samples studied in psychophysiological research on stress and diabetes control.

COMPLICATIONS OF DIABETES

Both IDD and NIDD are associated with a widespread pattern of tissue damage. Complications may precede diagnosis in older people with NID diabetes and the complications increase with duration of both ID and NID diabetes. It is unusual for people to be complication free after 20 years of diabetes.

Hypertension and hyperlipidaemia are more common among diabetic than among non-diabetic individuals and may contribute to the increased risk of coronary heart disease, cerebral vascular accidents and peripheral vascular disease in the diabetic population. The specific microvascular complications of diabetes include retinopathy, nephropathy and some aspects of neuropathy. There is now substantial evidence (Pirart, 1978; Tchobroutsky, 1978) to suggest that chronic hyperglycaemia associated with poor control of diabetes is one of the major factors responsible for the microvascular (though not the macrovascular) complications of diabetes. Attempts to avoid the microvascular complications are directed mainly at improving blood glucose control.

VARIABILITY OF GLYCAEMIC CONTROL

Variability of glycaemic control would be expected to be greatest for ID patients who have little if any endogenous insulin and least for people with obesity-related NIDD who have normal insulin production and homeostatic control of blood glucose. In IDD, any change in insulin requirements due to unexpected exercise, intercurrent illness, or other factors not anticipated by a well-judged adjustment to insulin dose, will be reflected in deviations of blood glucose levels.

A small proportion of individuals with IDD experience extreme swings of glycaemic control, occasionally with recurrent hypoglycaemic coma, but more often with frequent episodes of ketoacidosis and hyperglycaemic coma. This kind of extreme lability is often called 'brittle diabetes' (Tattersall, 1977) and accounts for a high proportion of emergency admissions in a small number of patients. The cause of brittle diabetes is the subject of much debate (e.g. Pickup *et al.*, 1983; Gill *et al.*, 1985). It is possible that, in some individuals, brittle diabetes is caused by overreactivity to stress. However, most of the studies of stress and diabetes control have ignored individual differences in response to stress, though the little evidence available suggests that such differences are considerable. Before considering these studies, however, the role of stress in the onset of diabetes will be considered and, first, attention will be given to the notion of diabetes as a stressor.

DIABETES AS A STRESSOR

Undoubtedly the onset of diabetes is a stressful experience for many individuals. Although much of the stress and coping literature may be of relevance to helping people with newly diagnosed diabetes, there is little evidence that research on the impact of diabetes has been influenced by this literature. Bradley and Marteau (1986) reviewed recent studies investigating the impact of diabetes on families and found little of direct relevance to health professionals attempting to help patients to cope with diabetes onset. A problem with much of this research has been that the meaning of the diabetes to the individual families has not been considered when investigating families' response to diabetes.

The dangers of assuming that diabetes has uniform implications for all those who have the disorder can be well illustrated with reference to a study by Felton *et al.* (1984). Felton and colleagues chose to study people with one of a number of chronic diseases selected to represent a dimension of controllability. Diabetes was viewed, by the authors, as offering intermediate control between certain forms of cancer and rheumatoid arthritis at the uncontrollable extreme and hypertension at the other extreme. There was no recognition that the degree of actual control possible will vary within diagnostic categories. Certainly, within the category of diabetes, controllability of the disorder would vary widely with the type of diabetes and the treatment regimen followed. It is apparent from research using a recently developed diabetes-specific measure of perceived control that individuals also differ considerably in their perceptions of control of diabetes (Bradley *et al.*, 1984). Furthermore, this measure has proved useful in predicting both choice and efficacy of different forms of treatment (Bradley *et al.*, 1987) and the occurrence of diabetic ketoacidosis (Bradley *et al.*, 1986). It would not be surprising if this measure was also a useful predictor of coping strategies adopted in managing diabetes, but such relationships have yet to be investigated.

Many of the problems in Felton *et al.*'s study could be overcome by studying diagnostic groups separately. If the sample were limited to those with a particular kind of diabetes, differences in diabetes-specific perceived control could be measured and the relationships between perceived control and coping strategies, psychological and physiological adjustment could be investigated. Measures of adjustment could be selected that were known to be appropriate for people with diabetes (but might not have been appropriate for other subject groups), and the coping strategies considered could include those specific to diabetes.

By sharpening up the measurement instruments used, future studies could more precisely test hypotheses derived from the literature on stress and coping. Furthermore, cognitions and coping strategies predictive of positive physiological and psychological adjustment might be identified which would be useful in educating and counselling people with diabetes.

STRESS AND DIABETES ONSET

It is generally accepted that a wide range of environmental factors together with some degree of genetic predisposition are the cause of most forms of diabetes mellitus (Lebovitz, 1984). NIDD appears to have a strong genetic factor, with a 95% to 100% concordance rate in identical twins. However, the nature of the genetic abnormalities associated with insulin resistance and alterations in beta cell function of NIDD are unknown (Lebovitz, 1984).

There is evidence to suggest that IDD (but not NIDD) is an autoimmune disease which arises in susceptible individuals exposed to environmentally triggering events. The genetic contribution of IDD is no more than 50% since this is the maximum estimate of concordance in identical twins with IDD (Bottazzo *et al.*, 1985). The environmental contributions to the aetiology of IDD remain to be identified. Hypothesized events leading up to the clinical manifestation of IDD have been described by Lebovitz (1984). The first postulated step involves some toxic or infectious insult to the beta cells of a genetically susceptible individual. This insult leads to an immunological process that results in circulating antibodies to various components of islet cells. Chronic destruction of beta cells may be caused by one or more of these antibodies. When sufficient beta cells are destroyed, insulin secretion will be reduced to a point where hyperglycaemia and eventually ketoacidosis follow.

The literature on psychoimmunology (reviewed by Solomon *et al.*, 1985) suggests various ways in which psychological stress may be implicated in the initial stage of development of IDD hypothesized above. Stress-related changes in immune function may increase the likelihood of viral or bacterial disease, which may provide the initial insult to the beta cells. The Barts Windsor prospective family study showed that islet cell antibodies preceded the development of overt diabetes by at least 3 years (Gorsuch *et al.*, 1981). Thus any effects of stress on immunocompetence leading to damage to pancreatic beta cells may have occurred long before onset of symptomatic diabetes.

A second mechanism whereby stress may be implicated in diabetes onset may operate around the time when diabetes becomes symptomatic. Stress-related counterregulatory hormone activity may aggravate the metabolic disturbance that has already developed. Indeed, if the already elevated blood glucose levels increase to beyond the renal threshold, dehydration associated with glycosuria may then produce the first symptoms of overt diabetes. The many anecdotal accounts and descriptive reports of life stresses contiguous with symptomatic IDD onset probably reflect this second mechanism.

Some retrospective studies of life events and di· betes onset have used designs prone to recall bias (e.g. Kisch, 1985), such that ρatterns of life events reported may reflect attempts to find an explanation for diabetes onset rather than a difference in events actually encountered. Other studies have avoided any problem of recall bias. Clayer and colleagues (1985) followed up 1526 victims who survived the 1983 bushfires in South Australia. The prevalence of a number of disorders, including diabetes, was significantly increased 12 months after the bushfires. Another study (Robinson and Fuller, 1985) made efforts to reduce recall bias and to estimate the influence of stressful life events on diabetes onset independently of any influence of individual differences in response to such events by employing Brown and Harris' Life Events and Difficulties Schedule. This study investigated thirteen ID diabetic/sibling pairs and neighbourhood controls involved in the Barts Windsor prospective family study. While the parent study was prospective, the offspring was retrospective in design: 77% of the diabetic subjects reported one or more severe life events in the 3 years prior to diagnosis, compared with 39% of siblings and 15% of age- and sex-matched neighbourhood controls. The authors concluded that stressful life events may be triggering factors involved in the aetiology of ID diabetes. This particular study restricted the period over which life events were recalled to 3 years. All diabetic subjects in the study would, therefore, have been expected to have had islet cell antibodies during this entire period. Thus the stresses identified in this study, and in the studies by Clayer *et al.* and Kisch described above, were probably not causally implicated in beta cell damage but more likely simply speeded up the manifestation of diabetes which would have become apparent eventually even in the absence of stress.

Early work which documented retrospectively an increased incidence of stressful experiences among an ID diabetic sample compared with non-diabetic comparison samples (e.g. Stein and Charles, 1975) have been viewed doubtfully by several reviewers (e.g. Fisher *et al.*, 1982; and Johnson, 1980) on account of the length of the period considered prior to symptomatology. Some of the stressful events in Stein and Charles' study were reported to have occurred as much as 10 years before onset of symptomatic diabetes. However, the recent evidence, reviewed above, suggests that many years may elapse between the actions of possibly stress-related causal agents initiating cell damage and the appearance of symptomatic diabetes. It would seem that, after all, it is not unreasonable to consider life events experienced over longer time periods when exploring the role of stress in the aetiology of ID diabetes.

THE EFFECTS OF STRESS ON DIABETES CONTROL

Life Events Research

Studies of life events and diabetes control have produced reasonably consistent results suggesting increased life events are associated with higher levels of blood glucose. Prior to the 1980s, studies were hampered by the lack of convenient measures of glycaemic control. Nevertheless, two studies (Grant et al., 1974; Bradley, 1979) suggested that Holmes and Rahe-type life event measures were associated with disturbances of diabetes measured by a variety of indices.

A number of recent studies followed the development of long-term measures of glycaemic control. Glycosylated haemoglobin (GHb) and the related measures of haemoglobin A1 (HbA1) and haemoglobin AIC (HbAIC) reflect average blood glucose levels over the previous 6 to 8 weeks. These measures are far from perfect, and it is important that their limitations be recognized. In particular, they do not reflect blood glucose variation, only mean blood glucose. Nevertheless, GHb and related measures appeared to offer convenient alternatives to the single blood glucose and urine glucose measures which until recently were the only measures of glycaemic control readily available.

Recent studies have investigated relationships between HbA1 or HbA1C measures of glycaemic control and measures of perceived stress or impact of life events (Linn et al., 1983; Jacobson et al., 1985). One study by Cox et al. (1984) related HbA1 to the number of reported 'Hassles and Uplifts' elicited by Kanner et al.'s (1981) instrument to measure day-to-day stressful events. These studies indicated that life stress, measured in various ways, was associated with increased HbA1 levels. It has usually been presumed that life stress causes increased HbA1 in the simple manner shown in Figure 21.1.

$\uparrow$ life stress $\longrightarrow$ $\uparrow$ HbA1

FIG. 21.1. A unidirectional causal model of the relationship between life stress and diabetes control.

Where studies of life events and diabetes control have compared subgroups of patients, subgroups with stronger associations between life events and HbA1 also reported more life events. Linn et al. (1983) compared Type I and Type II men and found that Type I men reported more life events as well as demonstrating a stronger association between perceived stress associated with life events and HbA1. Comparable findings were reported by Bradley (1979). Jacobson et al. (1985) found that a subgroup of patients with recent onset proliferative retinopathy reported more life events and a stronger life events/HbA1C association than subgroups of patients with long-standing retinopathy or no retinopathy of this kind. The greater number of life events in those who had stronger associations between life events and HbA1 could be explained in a number of ways. A perceptual bias may lead people who experience greater disturbance in association with life events to be more likely to note the occurrence of life events. Thus it could be that the subgroups did not differ in the number of life events actually encountered, only in their perceptions of this number. However, if we assume that differences in the number of life events reported do reflect differences in the number encountered, and if we also assume that the association between life events and glycaemic control is a causal one, then the data may be economically encompassed by the model described in Figure 21.2, where the causal link works both ways: life events disrupt glycaemic control which in turn leads to more life events.

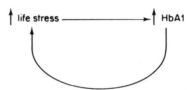

FIG. 21.2. A simple two-way causal model of relationships between life stress and diabetes control.

There are two kinds of mechanism which may account for life events causing raised blood glucose levels. The mechanisms by which counterregulatory hormones (CRHs) may mediate stress-related increases in blood glucose levels are well understood (Tarnow and Silverman, 1981–2; Evans, 1985). However, behavioural mediation of stress-related glycaemic fluctuations is also probable (e.g. Barglow et al., 1984; Cox et al., 1986).

Two of the above studies (Linn et al., 1983; Cox et al., 1984) concluded that the most obvious kind of behavioural influence, compliance with treatment recommendations, did not mediate the relationship between glycaemic control and life stress. However, the measures of compliance used were self-reports of the level of compliance over each study period as a whole. These ratings would not reflect any variability in compliance. Even a conscientious follower of their treatment regimen may well cut corners or temporarily abandon their diet during periods of stress. Such temporary aberrations might not be reflected in the patients' general ratings of compliance, but it is this kind of fluctuation which is interesting in the context of delineating the mechanism whereby stress is associated with poorer glycaemic control. The possibility of behavioural mediation of the relationship between life stress and glycaemic control cannot be excluded on the basis of studies conducted to date.

There are various possible mechanisms whereby poor glycaemic control may cause life events to occur or increase the impact of life events in ID patients. There is growing evidence that cognitive functioning may be impaired with hyperglycaemia (Holmes et al., 1983; Holmes, 1987). Subjective symptoms, both physical symptoms (Cox et al., 1983) and mood symptoms (Moses and Bradley, 1985), have been shown to vary with blood glucose levels. The experience of the hyperglycaemic state by some individuals as arousing, stressful or fatiguing may prime those individuals to note more life events or, indeed, to create more life events. Extremes of hypoglycaemia have also been shown to cause impaired cognitive function (Holmes et al., 1983; Holmes, 1987) and aversive physical symptoms and moods (Gonder-Frederick et al., 1986). Hypoglycaemic episodes can directly cause falls and accidents. Recurrent hypoglycaemic episodes may cause life events by undermining the confidence of the individual and the confidence of employers and others in the individual's reliability. Whatever the psychological impact of hypoglycaemic episodes, the metabolic impact on HbA1 levels will be trivial. In research relating life events to levels of HbA1, only relationships between long-lasting hyperglycaemia and life events will be apparent. Given the transitory nature of hypoglycaemic episodes and the limitations of HbA1 and similar measures of long-term glycaemic control, any associations between life stress and low blood glucose levels will go unnoticed in such research.

Few studies have provided data on individual differences rather than subgroup differences. However, available data point to considerable interindividual variation in the associations between metabolic control and life events experienced (Grant *et al.*, 1974). Cox and colleagues (1984) asked 35 ID patients who had monitored their blood glucose levels for 12 months about their perceptions of how various stress-related states affected their blood glucose levels. Although for most of the negative affects described, the majority of patients reported that their blood glucose levels would be raised, some reported lowered blood glucose, and a substantial number of patients reported no change in their blood glucose. If such differences were reflected in variable responses to life events, then the moderate overall relationship between life events and metabolic control observed masks far more dramatic glycaemic fluctuations among a more reactive subgroup which would include individuals with brittle diabetes.

Figure 21.3 offers a model which acknowledges the possibilities of individual differences in glycaemic response to life events and takes account of the data which suggest that subgroups of individuals not only demonstrate stronger associations between life events and glycaemic control but also report more life

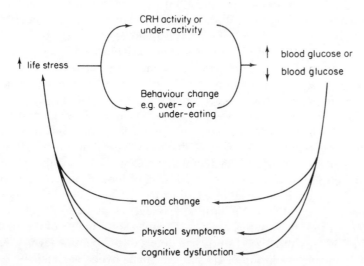

FIG. 21.3.   An elaborated two-way causal model of relationships between life stress and diabetes control.

events. Since CRH activity would be likely to be more disruptive in people who have no endogenous insulin secretion, the model has no difficulty in accounting for differences between subgroups of patients likely to reflect the degree of homeostatic control.

In summary, therefore, life events research using HbA1, or similar measures of long-term glycaemic control, is likely to give a very oversimplified view of the relationship between stress and diabetes control. Mechanisms have been identified which may combine to cause life events to disrupt glycaemic control (CRH activity or inappropriate deviation from usual treatment regimen at times of stress) or to cause poor glycaemic control to increase the frequency or impact of life events (impairments to cognitive function, altered mood states). What few data there are on individual differences suggest that life stress is not infrequently associated with decreased blood glucose levels, though any such associations are obscured by the use of HbA1 measures of long-term glycaemic control.

Studies of the effects of acute stress on diabetes control have produced inconsistent and apparently contradictory findings both between the studies themselves and in comparison with life events research. The use of blood glucose as the measure of glycaemic control in studies of acute stress allows for hypoglycaemic effects of stress to be observed in a way that HbA1 measures used in life events research do not. Thus the range of measurable responses increases. In the section below it is argued that there is a need for greater attention to individual differences in response to acute stress.

Acute Stress and Diabetes Control

Reviews of the early literature (Watts, 1980; Fisher *et al.*, 1982; Bradley, 1982; Barglow *et al.*, 1984) concluded that the stressors used in the early studies had destabilizing effects on diabetes control but that the direction of blood glucose change was not consistent. The studies considered by these reviewers have been criticized by them and others (notably Lustman *et al.*, 1981) on a variety of methodological and conceptual grounds. The variability of findings concerning the direction and extent of blood glucose change associated with various forms of psychological stress have stimulated doubts about the potency of stressors used, the heterogeneity of subjects (both in terms of type of diabetes and degree of glycaemic control), and the adequacy of experimental design and statistical analyses. While such criticisms have been appropriate, the possibility that some of the variability in the findings may be due to individual differences in response to stress has been overlooked. A few more recent studies, while dealing with many of the criticisms of the earlier studies, have looked only for group differences, ignoring individual variability (Edwards and Yates, 1985; Naliboff *et al.*, 1985; Kemmer *et al.*, 1986). Naliboff and colleagues studied subjects with NID diabetes. The other two studies were of ID subjects (though 3 of the 10 diabetic subjects in Edwards and Yates' study had detectable C-peptide levels). Kemmer *et al.*'s study included a group of ID subjects made hyperglycaemic by omission of insulin injections. Stressors included a digit-symbol substitution task, mental arithmetic and public speaking. In none of the three studies did any of the stressors used affect blood glucose levels in any of the groups. Two of the studies showed that self-reports of stress experienced increased significantly with the experimental tasks (Edwards and Yates, 1985; Kemmer et al., 1986). Despite this and despite the evidence for increases in physiological and catecholamine measures of stress in two of the studies (Naliboff et al., 1985; Kemmer et al., 1986) and cortisol increases with one form of stress in one study (Kemmer et al., 1986), no effects of stress on blood glucose levels were observed. Kemmer et al. cited Berk et al. (1985) in suggesting that plasma adrenaline must rise by at least 150–200 pg/ml to cause a clinically relevant increase in hepatic glucose production, and pointed out that the mean increase in their own study barely reached these levels in any of the groups. Mean increases in Naliboff et al.'s groups were even less. No data were provided on individual differences and there is a real possibility that the mean levels reported are misleading. Naliboff and colleagues noted large variability in the levels of catecholamines in their NID subjects, but this was only mentioned in explanation of the lack of significance for the apparently different catecholamine levels in diabetic and non-diabetic comparison groups.

Naliboff and colleagues went on to look for evidence of diabetic autonomic neuropathy which might cause decreased responsiveness in terms of both physiological and metabolic measures. Unfortunately, only group data were presented. The subjects as a group were said to have 'mild autonomic neuropathy' but it is unlikely that the label applied equally to the various members of the group. It would have been more informative to have related the degree of autonomic neuropathy present in an individual subject to that subject's responses to the stressful tasks. This was not done.

It seems that in their very thorough efforts to meet the criticisms levelled at earlier studies, these later studies have overlooked the possibility that individual differences in response to stress might be real and interesting and not a reflection of methodological inadequacies. None of the three studies has addressed the individual differences in their data.

There is some evidence from recent work of individual differences in responses to stress of the kind observed in the early, classic work of Hinkle and Wolf (e.g. Hinkle and Wolf, 1952). Carter and colleagues reported some preliminary data (Carter et al., 1985) indicating that blood glucose change in response to the stress of mental arithmetic was idiosyncratic across subjects but significantly reliable across a 12-week period. Furthermore, the extent of the absolute change in blood glucose was significantly related to the pre-stress level of blood glucose. Further investigations are required to identify the characteristics of stress-responsive individuals and those of individuals with different kinds of blood glucose response.

One obvious candidate for a measure which may differentiate stress-responsive diabetic subjects from those whose blood glucose levels remain stable is a measure of Type A behaviour indicative of competitive drive for achievement, impatience and aggression. There is some evidence from a study by Stabler et al. (1986) that young IDD subjects classified as Type A in behaviour pattern differed from those classified as Type B in their blood glucose responses to 10 minutes of a challenging video game. All but one of the 6 Type A subjects showed increased blood glucose in response to the stress, whereas all but one of the Type B subjects showed a decrease. Stabler and colleagues' study thus lends support to the findings of Carter *et al.* suggesting that individuals with IDD differ in their glycaemic responses to stress. Furthermore, Stabler *et al.* showed that the direction of blood glucose change was related to ratings of Type A behaviour.

The evidence for individual variability in glycaemic response to stress supports the view that a simple model of life stress leading to increased blood glucose levels is inadequate. It is likely that individual differences in the nature and extent of glycaemic response to life stress, comparable to the differences observed in patients under acute laboratory stress, would be observed if the methodology used allowed such differences to be detected.

The simple model of life stress causing raised blood glucose levels inspired much of the use of stress management training as an aid to diabetes control. The results of studies, reviewed below, evaluating the effects of stress management techniques on diabetes control, lend further evidence for the idiosyncratic nature of glycaemic responses to stress in diabetic subjects.

STRESS MANAGEMENT AND DIABETES CONTROL

There is growing evidence to suggest that stress management techniques may be valuable aids to diabetes management for some individuals, while being unhelpful or even damaging to diabetes control for others. Two of the earliest case reports illustrated these two extremes in ID individuals. Fowler *et al.* (1976) and Seeburg and DeBoer (1980) reported that insulin requirements were reduced by relaxation training with electromyographic (EMG) biofeedback. In Seeburg and DeBoer's study, training was terminated when the diabetes became unstable and hypoglycaemic symptoms were troublesome. Unlike the subject of the previous case report by Fowler *et al.*, this subject's diabetes was previously well controlled and no stress-related metabolic disturbances were experienced. It was not clear why relaxation training was thought to be appropriate in such a case.

Surwit and Feinglos (1983) investigated the effects of progressive relaxation training on 12 patients with type II diabetes who were selected because they reported experiencing stress-related fluctuations in diabetes control. Three-hour glucose tolerance tests and intravenous insulin tolerance tests were carried out before and after 5 days hospitalization during which six subjects received relaxation training. The glucose tolerance of the relaxation group was significantly improved and there was no associated change in insulin sensitivity or glucose-stimulated insulin secretory activity; findings which led the authors to suggest that the increases in glucose tolerance were mediated by hepatic mechanisms. In a subsequent letter, Surwit and Feinglos (1984) reported that improvements in glucose tolerance in the relaxation group were associated with decreases in plasma cortisol levels. Plasma levels of catecholamines were reported to have been within normal limits in all subjects and did not change with relaxation. Individual data presented in the original report (Surwit and Feinglos, 1983) suggested that individual differences in response to relaxation in this carefully controlled study of selected patients with NIDD were minimal.

The same authors conducted a comparable study of patients with poorly controlled type I diabetes who reported stress-induced hyperglycaemia (Feinglos *et al.*, 1987) and found no significant differences between relaxation and control groups in glucose tolerance, GHb levels or insulin requirements after 6 weeks practising relaxation at home. The groups did not differ in changes in plasma catecholamines or cortisol levels during the study period. The authors considered various possible explanations for the lack of effect of relaxation on this group of type I patients when significant positive effects had previously been noted for type II patients. They suggested that stress might play a greater role in disturbing control of type II diabetes since endogenous insulin secretion (which will not occur in type I diabetes) is likely to be inhibited by stress in type II individuals, which may add to any problem of raised blood glucose levels due to catecholamine and cortisol effects which would be expected to occur in both type I and type II patients. Secondly, the authors suggested that the patient population with type I diabetes may be heterogeneous in terms of glucose response to stress. They also pointed out that type I subjects tend to show more baseline variability in glycaemic control, which may influence stress response. Unfortunately the authors did not provide any information about the variability of the individual type I subjects. They suggested that future investigations of various means of stress reduction with type I patients should study subjects who have demonstrated hyperglycaemic responses to stress, and that attempts should be made to stabilize the baseline blood glucose of subjects beforehand for better evaluation of stress-related fluctuations and the effects of stress management.

One study in which blood glucose control was stabilized prior to relaxation training was reported by Landis and colleagues (1985). From the HbA1 levels, it appeared that there was little room for further improvement in glycaemic control with relaxation training. Indeed, given that such tight control was possible without relaxation training, it could be argued that stress could not be having much of a disruptive influence on the diabetes control of these individuals. Though it is possible that relaxation training might enable subjects to achieve the same degree of diabetes control more easily, with less juggling of insulin dose, carbohydrate intake and other variables, the data provided indicated that insulin dose, HbA1 levels and average blood glucose levels decreased for some patients and increased for others. However, variability of blood glucose (as indicated by daily range of blood glucose) decreased for four of the five patients studied and remained constant for the fifth patient.

Other recent reports of the use of relaxation in the management of ID diabetes include detailed case reports (Rosenbaum, 1983) and a small-scale study of four subjects by Lammers *et al.* (1984). Considerable variation in response to relaxation treatment was apparent both within and between studies. What little information is available on individual differences suggests that relaxation training was least useful for those subjects whose glycaemic control was good to start with (Landis *et al.*, 1985; Lammers *et al.*, 1984) and was most useful when used by subjects who not only had poor control of diabetes but also felt that stress was a factor in disrupting their control (Lammers *et al.*, 1984).

An extensive study of relaxation techniques to improve control of insulin-requiring diabetes has recently been completed in Sheffield (Bradley *et al.*, 1985). Attempts were made to recruit patients in poor glycaemic control who felt that stress was a factor which affected their blood glucose levels. Thirty-two patients were studied in a baseline, treatment, follow-up design. Treatment involved one of two forms of relaxation training for two of three groups, the third group acting as controls. Measures of glycaemic control improved significantly from baseline to follow-up in all three groups. Differences between the groups did not reach significance. However, within-group differences were considerable: of 22 subjects who received relaxation training, 11 showed clinically significant improvements in glycaemic control. Preliminary analyses suggest that the 11 subjects who benefited from relaxation, differed from the 11 who did not on a number of variables. Those who benefited had poorer glycaemic control at baseline, and higher ratings of stress experienced on an English translation of Kanner *et al.*'s (1981) Hassles and Uplifts scale. These findings suggest that the patients who benefited from relaxation in terms of their glycaemic control were those the recruitment procedure attempted to select. Measures of health beliefs and perceptions of control of diabetes (Bradley *et al.*, 1984) were also obtained and their value in predicting treatment efficacy will be examined. It is plausible that relaxation training, in offering a means of control over psychophysiological reactions which might otherwise disrupt glycaemic control, will be of most use to those people who initially feel least personal control over their diabetes.

There is enormous scope for systematic investigation of the mediating role of cognitive factors in evaluations of stress management techniques as aids to diabetes management. Indeed, cognitive factors have been given scant consideration in research throughout the whole area of stress and diabetes, even though cognitions and beliefs about diabetes are generally considered to be factors important in determining the quality of diabetes care. Recent developments of reliable, diabetes-specific measures of health beliefs (Given *et al.*, 1983; Bradley *et al.*, 1984) and perceived control (Bradley *et al.*, 1984) may encourage wider consideration of individual differences in beliefs and cognitions in the context of research into diabetes and stress.

Mechanisms Whereby Stress Management may Affect Diabetes Control

It has usually been assumed that stress-related sympathetic nervous system activity disrupts diabetes control via mobilization of counterregulatory hormones and that stress management interventions serve to promote parasympathetic nervous system activity thereby counteracting the effects of stress. The evidence presented above suggests that individuals differ in the extent to which stress management techniques are beneficial. Adverse consequences of relaxation training experienced by a minority of individuals (e.g. Seeburg and DeBoer, 1980) may be due to inappropriate promotion of parasympathetic nervous system activity in circumstances where there is no stress-induced sympathetic nervous system activity to counteract. However, positive benefits of relaxation are seen more often than negative, even among IDD subjects with good glycaemic control prior to relaxation training (Landis *et al.*, 1985). One mechanism by which relaxation techniques may be beneficial to glycaemic control is by reducing mood swings which in turn may reduce variability in skin blood flow and hence decrease variability in the absorption rates of subcutaneously injected insulin. There has been considerable interest in the role of skin blood flow and insulin absorption in accounting for within-subject variation in glycaemic control, but the effects of stress and stress management on these parameters have yet to be investigated. A further mechanism by which stress management techniques may improve glycaemic control is via behavioural mediation, perhaps by minimizing disruptive behaviour change associated with periods of life stress. Stress management interventions may break the vicious circle described in Figures 21.2 and 21.3 at the point where life events cause blood glucose change either by moderating CRH activity or by minimizing behavioural reactions to life events. The vicious circle may also be broken at the point where glycaemic disturbance increases the number of life events if the individual uses relaxation to cope with dysphoric moods associated with elevated blood glucose levels.

Thus a number of possible mechanisms can be identified by which stress management may influence diabetes control. Most of the mechanisms postulated would act to improve glycaemic control, though there is a risk of hypoglycaemia due to inappropriate suppression of CRH action or perhaps due to relaxation-induced increase in skin blood flow causing more rapid insulin absorption. Given the present state of knowledge, caution is needed when stress management techniques are used by diabetic individuals; relaxation practice should be avoided when blood glucose is in the low normal range (4 mmol/l or below), and treatment for hypoglycaemia should be readily available.

SUMMARY AND CONCLUSIONS

Few researchers have viewed diabetes as a stressor and approached the study of diabetes from the perspectives offered by the stress and coping literature. Where such a perspective has stimulated research, the unrealistic view of diabetes as a single disease entity with universal demands and consequences has undermined the work. Understanding of the nature of diabetes and its treatment is necessary for understanding the implications of existing research and provides a sound basis for future research.

It seems clear that stress can trigger onset of diabetic symptoms. There is a theoretical possibility that stress may also play a causal role in the initial damage to pancreatic islet cells, though evidence for such a role is thin.

It is becoming clear that individuals with diabetes differ in their response to stress and stress management. Researchers are beginning to appreciate the need to evaluate the effects of stress and the efficacy of therapeutic interventions on individuals rather than heterogeneous groups. It is argued that the apparent consistency of findings from life events studies indicating that HbA1 levels increase with life stress may be due, in part, to measurement artifacts, and that the lack of significant effects of laboratory stress on groups of diabetic subjects masks considerable individual variation in response to stress. By focusing attention on individual differences and working within a more complex model of relationships between stress and diabetes control, we can begin to identify individuals for whom stress management is indicated as a useful addition to their diabetes treatment regimen.

REFERENCES

Barglow, P., Hatcher, R., Edidin, D.V., & Sloan-Rossiter, D. (1984). Stress and metabolic control in diabetes: psychosomatic evidence and evaluation of methods. *Psychosomatic Medicine, 46,* 127–144.

Berk, M.A., Clutter, W.E., Skor, D. *et al.* (1985). Enhanced glycaemic responsiveness to epinephrine in insulin-dependent diabetes mellitus is a result of the inability to secrete insulin: augmented insulin secretion normally limits the glycaemic but not the lipolytic or ketogenic, response to epinephrine in humans. *Journal of Clinical Investigation, 75,* 1842–1851.

Bottazzo, G.F., Rujol-Borrell, R., & Gale, E. (1985). Etiology of diabetes: the role of autoimmune mechanisms. In K.G.M.M. Alberti & L.P. Krall (eds), *The diabetes annual vol. 1.* (pp. 16–52). Amsterdam: Elsevier Science.

Bradley, C. (1979). Life events and the control of diabetes mellitus. *Journal of Psychosomatic Research, 23,* 159–162.

Bradley, C. (1982). Psychophysiological aspects of the management of diabetes mellitus. *International Journal of Mental Health, 11,* 117–132.

Bradley, C. (1985). Psychological aspects of diabetes. In K.G.M.M. Alberti & L.P. Krall (eds), *The diabetes annual.* vol. 1 (pp. 374–387). Amsterdam: Elsevier Science.

Bradley, C., & Marteau, T.M. (1986). Towards an integration of psychological and medical perspectives of diabetes management. In K.G.M.M. Alberti and L.P. Krall (eds), *The diabetes annual* vol. 2 (pp. 374–387). Amsterdam: Elsevier Science.

Bradley, C., Brewin, C.R., Gamsu, D.S., & Moses, J.L. (1984). Development of scales to measure perceived control of diabetes mellitus and diabetes related health beliefs. *Diabetic Medicine, 1,* 213–218.

Bradley, C., Moses, J.L, Gamsu, D.S., Knight, G., & Ward, J.D. (1985). The effects of relaxation on metabolic control of Type I diabetes: a matched controlled study. *Diabetes, 34,* 17A.

Bradley, C., Gamsu, D.S., Knight, G., Boulton, A.J.M., & Ward, J.D. (1986). Predicting risk of diabetic ketoacidosis in patients using continuous subcutaneous insulin infusion. *British Medical Journal, 293,* 242–243.

Bradley, C., Gamsu, D.S., Moses, J.L., Knight, G., Boulton, A.J.M., Drury, J., & Ward, J.D. (1987). The use of diabetes-specific perceived control and health belief measures to predict treatment choice and efficacy in a feasibility study of continuous subcutaneous insulin infusion pumps. *Psychology and Health, 1,* 123–132.

Carter, W.R., Gonder-Frederick, L.A., Cox, D.J., Clark, W.L. & Scott, D. (1985). Effect of stress on blood glucose in IDDM. *Diabetes Care, 8,* 411–412.

Clayer, J.P., Bookless-Pratz, C., & Harris, R.L. (1985). Some health consequences of a natural disaster. *The Medical Journal of Australia, 143,* 182–184.

Cox, D.J., Gonder-Frederick, L.A., Pohl, S., & Pennebaker, J.W. (1983). Reliability of symptom blood glucose relationships among insulin dependent adult diabetics. *Psychosomatic Medicine, 45,* 357–360.

Cox, D.J., Taylor, A.G., Nowacek, G., Holley-Wilcox, P., Pohl, S.L., & Guthrow, E. (1984). The relationship between psychological stress and insulin-dependent diabetic blood glucose control: preliminary investigations. *Health Psychology, 3,* 63–75.

Cox, D.J., Gonder-Frederick, L., Pohl, S. & Pennebaker, J.W. (1986). Diabetes. In K.A. Holroyd & T.L. Creer (eds), *Self-management of chronic disease,* pp. 305–346. New York: Academic Press.

Edwards, C., & Yates, A.J. (1985). The effects of cognitive task demand on subjective stress and blood glucose levels in diabetics and non-diabetics. *Journal of Psychosomatic Research, 29,* 59–69.

Evans, M.B. (1985). Emotional stress and diabetic control: a postulated model for the effect of emotional distress upon intermediary metabolism in the diabetic. *Biofeedback and Self-Regulation, 10,* 241–254.

Feinglos, M.N., Hastedt, P., & Surwit, R.S. (1987). Effects of relaxation therapy on patients with Type I diabetes mellitus. *Diabetes Care, 10,* 72–75.

Felton, B.J., Revenson, T.A., & Hinrichsen, G.A. (1984). Stress and coping in the explanation of psychological adjustment among chronically ill adults. *Social Science and Medicine, 18,* 889–898.

Fisher, E.B. Jr., Delamater, A.M., Bertelson, A.D., & Kirkley, B.G. (1982). Psychological factors in diabetes and its treatment. *Journal of Consulting and Clinical Psychology, 50,* 993–1003.

Fowler, J.E., Budzynski, T.H., & VandenBergh, R.L. (1976). Effects of an EMG biofeedback relaxation program on the control of diabetes: a case study. *Biofeedback and Self-Regulation, 1,* 105–112.

Gill, G.V., Walford, S. & Alberti, K.G.M.M. (1985). Brittle diabetes—present concepts. *Diabetologia, 28,* 579–589.

Given, C.W., Given, B.A., Gallin, R.S. & Condon, J.W. (1983). Development of scales to measure beliefs of diabetic patients. *Research in Nursing and Health, 6,* 127–141.

Gonder-Frederick, L.A., Cox, D.J., Bobbitt, S.A., & Pennebaker, J.W. (1986). Blood glucose symptom beliefs of diabetic patients: accuracy and implications. *Health Psychology, 5,* 327–341.

Gorsuch, A.N., Spencer, K.M., Lister, J., McNally, J.M., Dean, B.M., Bottazzo, G.F., Cudworth, A.G. (1981). The natural history of Type 1 (insulin dependent) diabetes mellitus: evidence for a long pre-diabetic period. *Lancet ii,* 1363–1365.

Grant, I., Kyle, G.C., Teichman, A., & Mendels, J. (1974). Recent life events and diabetes in adults. *Psychosomatic Medicine, 36,* 121–128.

Hinkle, L.E. & Wolf, S. (1952). Importance of life stress in the course and management of diabetes mellitus. *Journal of the American Medical Association, 148,* 513–520.

Holmes, C.S. (1987). Cognitive functioning and diabetes: broadening the paradigm for behavioural and health psychology? *Diabetes Care, 10,* 135–136.

Holmes, T.H. & Rahe, R.H. (1967). The social readjustment rating scale. *Journal of Psychosomatic Research, 11,* 213–218.

Holmes, C.S., Hayford, J.T., Gonzalez, J.L., & Weydert, J.A. (1983). A survey of cognitive functioning at different glucose levels in diabetic persons. *Diabetes Care, 6,* 180–185.

Jacobson, A.M., Rand, L.I., & Hauser, S.T. (1985). Psychologic stress and glycaemic control: a comparison of patients with and without proliferative retinopathy. *Psychosomatic Medicine, 47,* 372–381.

Johnson, S.B. (1980). Psychosocial factors in juvenile diabetes: a review. *Journal of Behavioral Medicine, 3,* 95–116.

Kanner, A.D., Coyne, J.C., Schaefer, C., & Lazarus, R.S. (1981). Comparison of two modes of stress measurement: daily hassles and uplifts versus major life events. *Journal of Behavioural Medicine, 4,* 1–39.

Kemmer, F.W., Bisping, R., Steingruber, H.J., Baar, H., Hardtmann, F., Schlaghhecke, R., & Berger, M. (1986). Psychological stress and metabolic control in patients with type I diabetes mellitus. *New England Journal of Medicine, 314,* 1078–1084.

Kisch, E.S. (1985). Stressful life events and the onset of diabetes mellitus. *Israel Journal of Medical Sciences, 21,* 356–358.

Kosub, S.M., & Cerreto, M.C. (1981). Juvenile diabetes: current trends in psychosocial research. *Social Work in Health Care, 6,* 91–101.

Lammers, C.A., Naliboff, B.D., & Straatmeyer, A.J. (1984). The effects of progressive relaxation on stress and diabetic control. *Behavior Research and Therapy, 22,* 641–650.

Landis, B., Jovanovic, L., Landis, E., Peterson, C.M., Groshen, S., Johnson, K., & Miller, N.E. (1985). Effects of stress reduction on daily glucose range in previously stabilised insulin-dependent diabetic patients. *Diabetes Care, 8,* 624–626.

Lebovitz, H.E. (1984). Etiology and pathogenesis of diabetes mellitus. *Pediatric Clinics of North America, 31,* 521–530.

Lebovitz, H.E. (1985) Oral hypoglycaemic agents. In K.G.M.M. Alberti & L.P. Krall (Eds), *The diabetes annual,* vol. 1 (pp. 93–110). Amsterdam: Elsevier Science.

Linn, M.W., Linn, B.S., Skyler, J.S., & Jensen, J. (1983). Stress and immune function in diabetes mellitus. *Clinical Immunology and Immunopathology, 27,* 223–233.

Lustman, P., Carney, R., & Amado, H. (1981). Acute stress and metabolism in diabetes. *Diabetes Care, 4,* 658–659.

Moses, J.L., & Bradley, C. (1985). Accuracy of subjective blood glucose estimation by patients with insulin-dependent diabetes. *Biofeedback and Self-Regulation, 10,* 301–314.

Naliboff, B.D., Cohen, M.J., & Sowers, J.D. (1985). Physiological and metabolic responses to brief stress in non-insulin dependent diabetic and control subjects. *Journal of Psychosomatic Research, 29,* 367–374.

Pickup, J., Williams, G., Johns, P., & Keen, H. (1983). Clinical features of brittle diabetic patients unresponsive to optimized subcutaneous insulin therapy (continuous subcutaneous insulin infusion). *Diabetes Care, 6,* 279–284.

Pirart, J. (1978). Diabetes mellitus and its degenerative complications: a prospective study of 4,400 patients observed between 1947 and 1973. *Diabetes Care, 1,* 168–188.

Robinson, N., & Fuller, J.H. (1985). Role of life events and difficulties in the onset of diabetes mellitus. *Journal of Psychosomatic Research, 29,* 583–591.

Rosenbaum, L. (1983). Biofeedback-assisted stress management for insulin-treated diabetes mellitus. *Biofeedback and Self-Regulation, 8,* 519–532.

Seeburg, K.N. & DeBoer, K.F. (1980). Effects of EMG biofeedback on diabetes. *Biofeedback and Self-Regulation, 5,* 289–293.

Solomon, G.F., Amkraut, A.A., & Rubin, R.T. (1985). Stress, hormones, neuroregulation and immunity. In S.R. Burchfield (ed.), *Stress: Psychological and Physiological interactions* (pp. 207–221). Washington: Hemisphere.

Stabler, B., Morris, M.A., Litton, J., Feinglos, M.N., & Surwit, R.S. (1986). Differential glycemic response to stress in Type A and Type B individuals with IDDM. *Diabetes Care, 9,* 550–551.

Stein, S.P., & Charles, E.S. (1975), Emotional factors in juvenile diabetes mellitus: a study of early life experience of 8 diabetic children. *Psychosomatic Medicine, 37,* 237–244.

Surwit, R.S., & Feinglos, M.N. (1983). The effects of relaxation on glucose tolerance in non-insulin-dependent diabetes. *Diabetes Care, 6,* 176–179.

Surwit, R.S., & Feinglos, M.N. (1984). Relaxation-induced improvement in glucose tolerance is associated with decreased plasma cortisol. *Diabetes Care, 7,* 203–204.

Tarnow, J.D., & Silverman, S.W. (1981–2). The psychophysiologic aspects of stress in juvenile diabetes mellitus. *International Journal of Psychiatry in Medicine, 11,* 25–44.

Tattersall, R. (1977). Brittle diabetes. *Clinical Endocrinology and Metabolism, 6,* 403–419.

Tchobroutsky, G. (1978). Relation of diabetic control to development of microvascular complications. *Diabetologia, 15,* 143–152.

Waterhouse, I.K. (1984). Presidential address: perspectives on stress, coping and vulnerability. *Australian Psychologist, 19*(2), 115–133.

Watts, F.N. (1980). Behavioural aspects of the management of diabetes mellitus: education, self-care and metabolic control. *Behaviour Research and Therapy, 18,* 171–180.

Welborn, T.A., Garcia-Webb, P., Bonser, A., McCann, V., & Constable, I. (1983). Clinical criteria that reflect C-peptide status in idiopathic diabetes. *Diabetes Care, 6,* 315–316.

World Health Organisation Study Group (1985). *Diabetes mellitus.* Technical Report Series, No. 727. Geneva: World Health Organisation.

KEY WORDS

Diabetes mellitus, stress, stress management, relaxation training, psychological, life events, brittle diabetes, aetiology, psychoimmunology, locus of control, perceived control, health beliefs, type A behaviour, individual differences, counterregulatory hormones, autonomic neuropathy, glycaemic control, blood glucose levels, glycosylated haemoglobin.

Section III: Cognitive Factors which Influence Stress and Health

Handbook of Life Stress, Cognition and Health
Edited by S. Fisher and J. Reason
© 1988 John Wiley & Sons Ltd.

22

Stress and Cognitive Failure

JAMES REASON
University of Manchester, England

INTRODUCTION

On the face of it, the term 'cognitive failure' could embrace all the possible varieties of human fallibility. But since the early 1980s, it has taken on a rather specific meaning. Due largely to the work of Broadbent and his collaborators (Broadbent *et al.*, 1982; 1986), the term has come to be restricted to the commonplace and usually inconsequential failures of perception, memory and motor function that punctuate the everyday activities of all human beings, regardless of age, sex, historical period or cultural background (see Reason and Mycielska, 1982). If, as has been suggested (Reason, 1977; Norman, 1981), the failure of planned actions to achieve their desired outcome may be meaningfully divided into two major classes, *planning failures* (mistakes) and *execution failures* (slips and lapses), then the term 'cognitive failure' refers to the latter rather than to the former, and this is how it will be used in the present chapter.

Although this restricted definition of cognitive failure coincides conveniently with one-half of the planning–execution distinction, it was shaped more by practical than by theoretical considerations. The natural history investigation of everyday cognitive failures has, of necessity, relied extensively upon self-report techniques, involving diaries, questionnaires and daily rating scales. For these to be of any value, it is necessary that errors should be readily detectable by their perpetrators. Whereas inadequate plans, false diagnoses and the like may go unrealized for long periods, deviations from current intention, arising either from attentional slips or memory lapses, are usually recognized as such immediately, or shortly after, they have been committed. Indeed, it has been suggested that one of the principal functions of consciousness is to detect and recover actions-not-as-planned (Mandler, 1975, 1985), though this facility is tuned more to detecting one's own slips than those of others. For example, due to a mix-up in the studio, West Germany's ARD TV network inadvertently broadcast Chancellor Helmut Kohl's 1986 new year message instead of the 1987 message. Most of the 6.86 million viewers did not realize it was the wrong speech until they were wished 'a peaceful 1986'. The Chancellor's spokeswoman was only alerted to the error when she realized 'he didn't have the same suit on'. The Chancellor, however, knew immediately, and '. . . his reaction was correspondingly harsh' (*Guardian,* January 2nd, 1987).

EXTREME STRESS AND REAL-LIFE FAILURES: A BRIEF OVERVIEW

There can be little doubt that extreme stress enhances the probability of cognitive failure. All disciplined armies have based their training of recruits upon the assumption that the rigours of real combat can reduce humans to mindless automata. As a consequence, soldiers have been repeatedly drilled not only in the mechanics of handling their weapons (the numbered sabre 'cuts' of cavalrymen, the elaborate loading sequence for 17th century musketeers, etc.), but also in contingent problem-solving routines, such as the 'immediate actions' required to clear a blocked machine-gun. But even 'second nature' behaviours can crumble in the face of imminent destruction. The American Civil War yielded some poignant instances of cognitive failure. After Gettysburg, over 200 of the muzzle-loading rifles picked up from the battlefield had been loaded five or more times without being fired. One had been loaded 21 times and never fired (Baddeley, 1972). Following the engagement at Kennesaw Mountain, during the battle for Atlanta, tree trunks in front of defensive works were found to be bristling with ramrods, fired off prematurely during the loading sequence by troops under attack.

The greater part of the psychological literature on high levels of stress relates to artificial situations in which the subjects were well aware that real catastrophe would not result from their errors (see Harris *et al.,* 1956; Klier and Linskey, 1960; Robbins *et al.,* 1961; Bell, 1980). Most of the work involving genuine stressors and real consequences deals with the performance of military personnel under combat stress (Grinker and Spiegel, 1963; Marshall, 1978). Marshall, interviewing Second World War combat veterans, found that, on average, not more than 15% of the men questioned had actually fired at the enemy during an engagement. In the best units, only one-quarter of the soldiers used their available firepower, though most of the actions had occurred in conditions where it would have been possible for at least 80% of the troops to have used their weapons in earnest; this indicates around 30% net effectiveness.

Not all panic-induced failures have adverse consequences. During the abortive attack on German shipping at Wilhelmshaven in December 1939, an RAF Wellington bomber came under close and persistent attack by an enemy fighter. The co-pilot, meaning to jettison his bombs prematurely, pulled the flap lever instead of the bomb-door lever, putting down full flap. The Wellington shot upwards, stalled, and then plunged earthwards. The pilot of the attacking Messerschmitt was so taken aback by this unexpected manoeuvre that he lost contact. The English pilot eventually recovered control and the Wellington returned home safely. Most of the other bombers fell prey to the German fighters (Hastings, 1981).

Ronan (1953) interviewed aircrews who had survived in-flight emergencies in B-50 bombers. He was especially interested in critical incidents, actions having

either desirable or unwanted consequences. In data obtained from 153 experienced aircraft commanders (with an average of 2971 flying hours), it was found
that 360 (15%) of 2450 critical incidents involved actions that either failed to
improve or actually exacerbated the situation. This almost certainly underestimated the true failure rate since non-survivors could not be interviewed.

Using data from Ronan and from other investigations involving convincing
simulations of real danger (Berkun et al., 1962; Berkun, 1964), Swain and
Guttmann (1980) sought to establish the error probability of nuclear power plant
(NPP) operators during a serious emergency (i.e. a large loss of coolant accident).
They produced a predicted performance curve in which the human error probability (HEP) was assessed to begin at 1.0 immediately after the occurrence, falling to
0.9 5 minutes later, and to 0.1 after 30 minutes. However, if the highly stressful
conditions persisted throughout the initial half-hour and continued thereafter,
they estimated that the HEP curve would level out at around 0.25 after 30
minutes. They also applied the doubling rule: 'This theory holds that, given an
initial error has been made and perceived as such or that an initial action has failed
to have its intended corrective effect, the error probability for each succeeding
corrective action doubles' (Swain and Guttmann, 1980, pp. 17–21).

Such quantitative estimates are hard to reconcile with the subsequent reality of
NPP emergencies, partly because major incidents are still mercifully too few to
make a proper assessment, and partly because these predictions fail to take proper
account of the *kinds* of errors that are actually committed. To date, there have
been around seven psychologically well-documented NPP emergencies, ranging
from that at Three-Mile Island in 1979 to Chernobyl in 1986 (see Reason, 1986;
1987a; 1987b). These case studies do indeed reveal a reasonably high incidence of
cognitive failures; but most of them were neither as serious in their consequences
nor so plentiful as the simple omission errors made by maintenance personnel in
the course of normal working (INPO, 1985). By the same token, some of the more
disastrous operator errors were not in the least stress related. Thus, the operators
at Chernobyl-4 committed their six major safety violations before they became
aware (in the last minute prior to the explosion) that the reactor was in a highly
dangerous condition (Nature, 1986).

STRESS IS NOT A NECESSARY CONDITION
FOR COGNITIVE FAILURE

This brief review of 'ecologically valid' studies suggests that while high levels of
stress can, and often do, increase the likelihood of cognitive failure, they are not a
necessary condition for its occurrence. This conclusion is further endorsed by an
'extended diary' investigation of the conditions prevailing when absented-minded
slips and lapses were detected during the course of routine daily activities (Reason
and Mycielska, 1982; Reason, 1984).

Sixty-three university students used diaries to record their slips and lapses over
a continuous period of 7 days. In addition to noting down the details of these
cognitive failures, they were also required to complete a set of standardized
ratings for each slip or lapse, as soon as possible after its occurrence. Factors

Table 22.1   Ratings concerning the mental, physical and environmental factors prevailing at the time the cognitive failure occurred. The figures in the body of the table show the per cent cognitive failures (n = 192) associated with each rating scale value for each factor

	(Not at all) 1	2	3	4	5	6	7 (Very)
Preoccupied?	6.4	10.1	9.5	12.6	20.1	27.0	14.3
Distracted by surroundings?	2.6	10.0	15.2	6.7	7.9	20.9	36.7
Feeling upset/worried?	52.9	21.9	6.9	5.8	7.9	3.7	1.1
Feeling emotional/excited?	42.3	22.2	5.3	10.1	11.1	5.8	3.2
Feeling tired/sleepy?	15.3	20.1	9.5	16.4	15.9	13.8	9.0
Feeling unwell?	50.0	22.9	6.4	5.8	9.6	3.7	1.6
Feeling rushed?	30.7	16.4	8.5	7.4	13.8	16.4	6.8
Bothered by surroundings?	48.2	26.7	7.3	8.9	3.1	4.7	1.1
Surroundings familiar?	1.1	0	2.6	1.6	3.1	11.5	80.1

investigated included: (a) the nature of the intended actions; (b) the nature of the erroneous actions; (c) the relationship, if any, between the intended actions and some other activity; (d) the mental and physical state at the time of the slip; and (e) the environmental circumstances. The study 'netted' a total of 192 slips, an average of three per person. (This is likely to be a considerable underestimate, since diarists tend only to record the more notable slips.) The results relating to the effects of possible stressors are shown in Table 22.1.

These and other diary data provide a relatively consistent picture of the circumstances associated with everyday cognitive failures. When the slip occurred, the diarists were carrying out some highly automatized task in extremely familiar surroundings. They were also either preoccupied by some inner concern or distracted by something happening within their immediate vicinity. But they were not feeling particularly upset, emotional or unwell. Responses to the fatigue and time pressure questions, however, did suggest that these factors were influential on some occasions but not on others. Potentially bothersome environmental factors (e.g. temperature, noise, poor illumination, etc.) were not rated as contributing at all significantly to the cognitive failure.

PRONENESS TO COGNITIVE FAILURE: A STABLE DISPOSITION

Since the mid-1970s, a substantial number of questionnaires, designed to obtain a subjective estimate of an individual's proneness to various kinds of cognitive failure, have been administered by different research groups to a wide range of people. This work has been reviewed by Herrmann (1982; 1984), Martin and Jones (1984), and by Morris (1984). Considering the diversity of both the measures and the samples investigated, the findings are remarkably consistent. Those of relevance to the present discussion are summarized below.

1. Responses to these questionnaires reveal wide and consistent individual differences in proneness to minor cognitive failures. Split-half and test-retest reliabilities (over several months) usually lie between 0.7 and 0.8, but are sometimes higher (see Herrmann, 1982; Broadbent et al., 1986). These retest reliabilities indicate that approximately 50% of the variance is the same from one

testing occasion to the next. Of course, it also suggests that a substantial proportion of the variance could also be due to local 'state' factors. Even though these questionnaires require a retrospective assessment over several previous months, it is likely that the responses will be coloured to some degree by the prevailing conditions.

2. Significant correlations have been obtained between self-ratings, as measured by the Cognitive Failures Questionnaire, and ratings of the respondent's level of absent-mindedness made by their spouse. Thus, people's opinions of their own error proneness tend to coincide with the views of those having the opportunity to observe their actual behaviour.

3. Questionnaire items are almost invariably positively correlated one with another. Thus, individuals who acknowledge themselves to be markedly prone to memory lapses also report a relatively high rate of action slips, and conversely. This suggests that susceptibility to these minor failures is governed by some global factor that operates beyond the level of the specific cognitive activities in which these errors reveal themselves. This conclusion is further endorsed by the finding that the total scores obtained from questionnaires focusing upon somewhat different aspects of cognitive function intercorrelate positively and significantly.

4. Few relationships of any importance have yet been found between these error proneness questionnaires and standard measures of intelligence, extraversion–introversion and the like. In short, these cognitive failures questionnaires appear to be tapping something not readily assessed by existing psychometric instruments.

COGNITIVE FAILURE AND VULNERABILITY TO STRESS

One of the most interesting findings to emerge from questionnaire studies of error proneness is the relationship between a characteristically high level of minor cognitive failures, assessed retrospectively over a period of months, and the number and degree of self-reported psychiatric symptoms, experienced during or immediately following a period of stress. This stress-moderated relationship has now been obtained with a variety of samples, subjected to different stresses, and using different measures of error proneness and symptomatology. In general, these findings provide support for Broadbent's stress-vulnerability hypothesis: namely, that high cognitive failures scores are related to increased vulnerability to externally imposed stress (Broadbent et al., 1982). The evidence is summarized below.

Student Nurses on High-Stress Wards

The first statement of this relationship was made by Broadbent and his co-workers (Broadbent et al., 1982). They reported a study by Parkes in which she administered the Cognitive Failures Questionnaire (CFQ) to 101 student nurses just prior to a 6-week period of medical ward training. The CFQ is a 25-item questionnaire that asks about the frequency of 25 everyday breakdowns of performance during the last 6 months. For the 48 nurses who had spent their time on high-stress wards, Parkes found a highly significant tau (0.46) between CFQ score (covering the 6 months prior to the ward duty) and the score obtained subsequently from the Middlesex Hospital Questionnaire (which calls for self-reports of minor psychiatric symptoms). In the case of the 53 nurses who had served on low-stress wards, no such relationship was found (tau = 0.087).

Undergraduates Just Prior to a Major Examination

Gillian Kane (Kane, 1987), a research student at the University of Manchester, gave the Short Inventory of Mental Lapses* (SIML; Reason and Lucas, 1984) and the General Health Questionnaire (GHQ; Goldberg, 1972) to various groups of sixth-form and university students before (n=245) and just after (n=173) sitting a major examination. The sample was divided into stressed and non-stressed groups on the basis of their GHQ scores. Positive and significant correlations were obtained between psychiatric symptomatology and typical levels of cognitive failure (rated over the preceding 12 months) in the former, but not in the latter group, on both testing occasions.

Women Treated Surgically for Breast Cancer

In a 3-year study (Lucas et al., 1985; Lucas, 1986), 100 women were interviewed either during an out-patient clinic just prior to breast surgery, or on the ward shortly after the operation. Sixty-seven of the patients were found to have breast cancer, and 33 had benign breast disease. Sixty of the patients with breast cancer and 29 with benign disorders were interviewed a second time approximately 4 months after surgery.

Both sets of interviews included the administration of a shortened version of the Brown–Birley Life Events Schedule (Brown and Harris, 1978); the Standardised Social Interview (Clare and Cairns, 1978); a shortened version of the Present State Examination (Wing et al., 1974); and the Short Inventory of Mental Lapses (Reason and Lucas, 1982).

Findings at First Interview

SIML scores correlated significantly with the number of psychiatric symptoms reported at the time of the first interview (0.395; p<0.01). There was a significant point-biserial correlation between the presence of depression at first interview and the SIML score. Subjects who reported feeling depressed had higher mean SIML scores (2.20; S.D.=0.613) than those who did not (1.89; S.D.=0.441). However, the point-biserial correlation between SIML score and the presence of

---

* The SIML is a fifteen-item questionnaire comprising twelve frequently occurring slips and lapses (see Reason, 1984d), together with three further items relating to mind-dwelling, concentration and paying attention. Like the CFQ, it asks the respondent to rate approximately how often each slip or lapse has been experienced, but over the past year rather than 6 months. Correlations between the CFQ and SIML have been found to be of the order of 0.6 to 0.7 on several occasions (Reason and Lucas, 1984). The GHQ, as used here, was a 28-item psychiatric self-report instrument designed to assess the degree of 'caseness' in a non-hospitalized population. Like the MHQ, it inquires about the presence of minor psychiatric signs and symptoms.

nervous tension at first interview was effectively zero (-0.024). There was no correlation between the SIML score and the number of negative life events occurring in the year prior to surgery (0.071). In addition to supporting the results of Broadbent and his co-workers, these findings highlight the relationship between general 'absent-mindedness' and symptoms of depression.

Findings at Second Interview

Analyses of the data obtained approximately 4 months after surgery focused upon assessing the reliability of possible predictors of psychiatric morbidity. When the number of psychiatric symptoms yielded by the Present State Examination was used as the dependent measure of morbidity, nine factors accounted for over 35% of variance in a multiple regression analysis (F [9.50]=3.08; p=0.0051). Using the method of elimination, the following ranking of predictors was obtained (figures in parentheses indicate the percentage reduction in the R-squared value when that particular factor is removed from the regression analysis): upset by scar (24.2), absent-mindedness (18.6), radiotherapy (14.9), pain in scar (8.0), no confiding tie (7.9), previous psychiatric problems (1.6), children under 14 (0.7), mastectomy (0.5), difficulty in moving arm (0.3). The test–retest reliability of the SIML scores between the first and second interviews was 0.69. This result accords with earlier findings. A marked degree of absent-mindedness (during the 12-month period prior to the second interview) was a better predictor of the presence of psychiatric symptoms following a period of great stress than a number of more obviously relevant medical and social factors.

The Dundee Student Homesickness Studies

Fisher and Hood (1987) found reported homesickness in 61 (31%) of a group of 196 residential university students. The homesick students had significantly higher mean scores on both the MHQ and the CFQ than those not homesick. Within the total sample, women undergraduates produced higher ratings of the stress associated with moving away from home than the men, and gave significantly higher scores on both the MHQ and the CFQ. The levels of homesickness, however, did not differ significantly between the sexes.

In another study (Fisher *et al.*, 1985), 100 students were investigated during the first 5 weeks of their first term at university. Sixty reported homesickness. The homesick students again produced higher CFQ scores than the non-homesick students, and the CFQ correlated significantly with the frequency of homesickness episodes.

While the Dundee findings considered so far are reasonably consistent with the stress-vulnerability hypothesis, the results of a further study (Fisher *et al.*, 1987) are more ambiguous. Students were administered the CFQ and the MHQ on two separate occasions, 2 months before and 5 weeks after taking up university residential accommodation for the first time. Cognitive failure and depression levels were raised in all subjects *after* the move to university. This result was taken by the authors as indicating that increased symptomatology and raised levels of absent-mindedness are both *consequences* of the stressful relocation. But other interpretations of these data are possible.

Both the timing of the testing sessions and the magnitude of the CFQ/MHQ correlations on both occasions strongly suggest that subjects were stressed *both* before *and* after their move to university (the 'before' session retrospectively embracing major examinations). If this were the case, then these data would not provide adequate grounds for rejecting the stress-vulnerability hypothesis.

WHAT DO COGNITIVE FAILURES QUESTIONNAIRES MEASURE?

The evidence so far reviewed in this chapter suggests three conclusions. First, self-reported liability to minor cognitive failures is a relatively stable and enduring characteristic of the individual. Second, responses to cognitive failures question-naires appear to reflect the operation of some global factor which exerts its influence across a wide variety of cognitive activities. Third, whatever governs this general proneness to everyday slips and lapses also contributes to stress vulner-ability. So what is it that determines the way people answer questions about how often they experience various trivial slips and lapses during the course of everyday life?

1. It is relatively independent of the precise form of the question. As noted earlier, the total scores from various types of cognitive failures questionnaire, employing different question forms and focusing upon different aspects of cogni-tive function, correlate positively and usually significantly one with another (Broadbent *et al.*, 1982; Reason, 1984). All have substantial general factors accounting for a large proportion of the total variance. One possible interpreta-tion of these findings is that the frequency of occurrence estimates given for all items is coloured by the respondents' global impressions of their general 'scatti-ness', and that '. . . these broadly-based metacognitive beliefs are reasonably accurate reflections of the characteristic efficiency with which they manage their cognitive affairs' (Reason, 1984, p. 13).

2. It is not easily discriminated by laboratory measures. However these subjec-tive impressions are derived, they do not readily submit to laboratory analysis. Several studies have tried and failed to find established laboratory measures that discriminate between high and low scorers on cognitive failures questionnaires (Broadbent *et al.*, 1982; Herrmann, 1982; Morris, 1984; Martin and Jones, 1984). However, most of these tests were designed to assess the efficiency of very specific cognitive operations in relatively artificial conditions, whereas self-report instru-ments are tapping the characteristic way in which people deal with the less well-defined and more varied informational demands of everyday life. An ob-vious difference between the laboratory and everyday life is that, in the former, subjects are usually told where to direct their attention. In life, on the other hand, people are faced with the far more complex task of deciding not only where to look at any given moment, but also which of the available sources of information are relevant to the task at hand.

3. It has something to do with attentional deployment. The closer laboratory conditions approximate to the multiple attentional demands of daily life, the more

successful they are in discriminating high and low questionnaire scorers. Among the few studies to achieve positive results are those which have employed *distributed attention* tasks (Wakeford *et al.*, 1980; Harris and Wilkins, 1982; Martin and Jones, 1983, 1984). Here, subjects are required to perform two or more activities concurrently. A general finding is that whereas no differences are found in the performance of each task in isolation, high scorers on the CFQ do worse than low scorers when more than one task is attempted simultaneously. A reasonable inference from these results is that everyday error proneness is bound up with the way in which people typically deploy their limited attentional resources in relation to competing demands. It also accords with the diary study conclusion that some attentional 'capture' is a necessary condition for the natural occurrence of slips and lapses (Reason and Mycielska, 1982).

4. It relates to the selection of coping strategies. Kane (1987) divided her students into high and low error groups on the basis of their pre-examination SIML scores. The Ways of Coping Checklist (Folkman and Lazarus, 1985) revealed reliable differences in the kinds of coping devices employed by these groups. High-error individuals reported a greater use of strategies requiring the exertion of mental effort to deal with or suppress emotions (e.g. displacement, spiritual coping, self-directed coping, confrontive coping, etc.). Those less error prone tended to favour more active, task-related coping measures (e.g. seeking support from others). These data suggest that high-error individuals employ coping strategies that make greater demands upon limited cognitive resources.

In a study of 141 nurses, Parkes (cited by Broadbent *et al.*, 1986) examined the way in which high-CFQ nurses (+1 S.D. from the mean) and low-CFQ nurses (−1 S.D. from the mean) employed active or passive coping strategies in two kinds of situation: (a) when the stress was perceived as being controllable, and (b) where it must be accepted. In the former circumstance (i.e. where the stress level could be modified through action), there was a substantial difference in the degree to which these two groups of nurses used active coping strategies; but in those situations where the stresses had to be accepted, both groups employed active coping strategies to much the same degree. The general conclusion was that low-CFQ nurses used more direct or active means of coping with stress, but only when they perceived the situation as being to some degree controllable. High-CFQ nurses tended to respond to these potentially controllable circumstances with more passive and less directed coping measures.

In short, high-CFQ individuals seem less able to adapt their coping strategies to the discretionary aspects of the situation. Either they are less sensitive to its controllable potential, or they are less flexible in the deployment of their repertoire of coping devices. The latter possibility seems more in tune with the arguments presented above, and receives some support from a recent laboratory study (Broadbent *et al.*, 1986).

Taken together, these various lines of research go some way to explaining why it is that more absent-minded people show greater vulnerability to stress. It is not so much that stress induces a high rate of cognitive failure (though that may indeed be the case). Rather, it would appear that a certain style of cognitive resource-management can lead to *both* absent-mindedness *and* to the inappropriate matching of coping strategies to stressful situations. Whether this cognitive management style has a relatively fixed constitutional basis, or whether it is amenable to corrective training, is an important issue requiring urgent investigation.

COGNITIVE FAILURES AND PSYCHIATRIC SYMPTOMATOLOGY

In the studies considered above, it was shown that stressors moderate the relationship between cognitive failures and psychiatric symptomatology, making it more apparent in high rather than low stress situations. Nevertheless, positive and significant correlations have been found repeatedly between the CFQ and MHQ in groups where the level of stress was not measured or manipulated (Broadbent et al., 1982). As is well known, anxious and depressed people experience a higher rate of cognitive failures than those not so afflicted (Beck et al., 1979). It is therefore important to distinguish between externally imposed stresses (of the kind discussed in the previous section), and the more chronic or 'resident' forms associated with psychiatric illness. The discussion so far has dealt primarily with the former. We will now look briefly at the cognitive effects of 'intrinsic stresses' that some people carry with them from one situation to another.

Psychiatric illnesses of many kinds (and especially those in which the symptoms of anxiety and depression are prominent) are associated with attentional inflexibility. This is usually described by patients as a failure of concentration (Goldberg, 1972; Horowitz, 1979), stemming in large part from an inability to divert the mind from brooding upon some painful or threatening topic. Mental life comes to be dominated by these intrusive ruminations. Or, to put it another way, they 'capture' the limited attentional resource for lengthy periods, leaving little or no reserves to deal with other than the most clamorous external demands. These are just the conditions for inducing actions to slip or memories to lapse. Indeed, as M. Eysenck (1982; 1984) has pointed out, the presence of these intrusive ruminations places the anxious or depressed person in an unbalanced divided-attention predicament, even when performing a single task. Task-irrelevant ruminations gain privileged access to the restricted conscious 'workspace', hindering or preventing the processing of task-relevant data. Small wonder, therefore, that such people are more error prone.

STRESS AND 'CUSTODIAL' ATTENTION

Under normal circumstances, people appear to hold in reserve a part of their limited attentional resource to guard against the occurrence of errors having unacceptable consequences. In everyday language, this custodial role of attention is often referred to as 'taking care'. In crossing a road, we 'take care' to watch out for oncoming traffic. On departing for a holiday, we 'take care' to ensure that the gas is turned off. Before leaving for the airport, we 'take care' that we have our passport, ticket and money, and so on. But when assailed by negative life events, this reserve of 'custodial' attention tends to be used up elsewhere, and we are at risk of making dangerous errors. Support for such a view is derived from a questionnaire study of absent-mindedness in shops together with an analysis of letters written by 67 people believing themselves to be wrongly accused of shop-lifting (Reason and Lucas, 1984). It is also consistent with laboratory studies involving the controlled elicitation of speech errors (Baars *et al.*, 1975; Baars, 1980).

The study of absent-mindedness in shops (Reason and Lucas, 1984) revealed that while people are generally 'present-minded' in regard to certain kinds of 'risky' shopping behaviour under normal circumstances (e.g. transferring goods from the shelf to something other than the standard trolley or basket), this self-directed vigilance is markedly reduced in periods of extreme life stress (as evidenced by the letters of the accused sample). During exceptionally troubled times, there appear to be little or no cognitive resources available to sustain this custodial reserve. In addition, the chances of such 'risky' absent-minded errors slipping by unnoticed are increased by environments, like supermarkets, specifically designed to elicit 'taking' actions. These actions, when performed in a distracted or preoccupied state, are readily linked to habitual and ill-advised 'placing' routines (i.e. putting the article in a pocket, purse, bag, etc.). It is then relatively easy to forget to declare the item at the checkout. Significantly, the goods involved in these arrests were trivial in cost, and, in some cases, neither wanted nor usable by the accused person (e.g. refills for articles not possessed, etc.).

MOOD STATES AND DAILY ERROR RATINGS

While there is now considerable evidence to support the idea that individual error proneness is determined by some relatively stable, trait-like factor, it is also true that error rates show state-related variations. One attempt to gauge the extent of these 'local' fluctuations has involved the combination of (a) an initial 'baseline' assessment of previous error liability (i.e. SIML), and (b) daily ratings of the degree to which each slip or lapse is seen as occurring more or less frequently than this 'typical' value.

Lucas *et al.* (1985) used this technique to investigate the relationship between daily error rates and mood, over repeated 5-day periods, in 60 women (41 with breast cancer and 19 with benign disease) undergoing investigation and treatment at the University Hospital of South Manchester. The subjects were asked to judge whether each of the 15 errors present in the SIML had occurred more or less often than usual—where 'usual' meant the typical rates indicated by their SIML responses. They were also required to complete scales indicating their predominant mood state on each of the assessed days. These judgements concerned feelings of being tense and stressed, being tired, worried, cheerful and being in control. The analysis was performed on a total of 651 days of combined mood and error ratings, obtained from eight groups of patients for three test periods: just before or just after surgery, and at 3 and 12 months later.

During the initial period, an average (over all groups) of 36.6% of the days were rated as ones in which it was difficult to stop worrying. This proportion fell to 11.7% during the 3-month postoperative test period, and rose slightly to 14.1%

Table 22.2   Rank order correlations between daily error changes and mood

Groups	Number of days	Mood ratings Tense	Tired	Worried	Cheerful	In control
First test period						
Cancer Ss	117	0.41[b]	0.18	0.45[b]	−0.35[b]	−0.24[b]
Benign Ss	72	0.39[b]	0.38[b]	0.25[a]	−0.22	−0.01
Postop.	48	0.31[a]	0.23	0.46[b]	−0.32[a]	−0.63[b]
Second test period (3 months post-surgery)						
Mastectomy Ss	108	0.34[b]	0.21[a]	0.13	−0.18	−0.21[a]
WLS Ss (1)	77	0.27[a]	0.51[b]	0.27	0.15	−0.27[a]
Benign Ss	68	0.24[a]	0.05	−0.04	−0.12	−0.04
Third test period (12 months post-surgery)						
Mastectomy Ss	77	0.35[b]	0.21	0.54[b]	−0.11	−0.15
WLS Ss	42	0.49[b]	0.47[b]	0.58[b]	−0.37[a]	−0.52[b]

during the 1-year postoperative period. Levels of experienced tension and stress also declined for all groups over the three testing periods.

All groups reported increases in daily error rates. These varied from approximately 20% of days (in which total net error rates were 'more than usual') in the highly stressed patients awaiting admission for biopsy, to under 7% in those who had just returned home after surgery. Different error types varied in the extent to which they were reported as increasing. Those most sensitive to stress were mind-dwelling, difficulty in concentration, and 'attending but not taking in'. Other SIML items, including memory lapses and slips of action, were also reported as increasing by between 7% and 20% during the very stressful preoperative period.

Further evidence of state-related variations in cognitive failure rates was obtained from correlations between daily 'net error change scores' and the corresponding mood ratings. These are shown in Table 22.2.

The relationships show a clear pattern. For most groups over most test periods, days in which a negative and mood state predominated were associated with increased error rates, and conversely. Comparable correlations between daily cognitive failure rates and mood were found by Kane (1987), using identical measuring instruments, but with pre- and post-examination students. It is clear, therefore, that self-report measures of error proneness are responsive to state-dependent variations when the assessment is restricted to a recent, brief and well-defined time period. Moreover, these daily ratings support the idea of a causal relationship between stress and cognitive failure.

RECONCILING STATE AND TRAIT: COGNITIVE UNDER-SPECIFICATION

Throughout this chapter, we have been considering two apparently contradictory hemes. The evidence from both naturalistic studies and those employing daily ratings indicates that stress promotes cognitive failures. Yet, we have also discussed a number of varied investigations which support Broadbent's hypothesis that characteristically high levels of absent-mindedness are associated with an enhanced vulnerability to the adverse effects of stress. Some investigators (Fisher et al., 1985; Kane, 1987) have presented these as either/or possibilities: either stress causes cognitive failure, or a marked tendency towards absent-mindedness leads to greater stress effects. In this concluding section, it is argued that both alternatives can co-exist within the same theoretical framework.

Let us first consider how cognitive failures arise in people who are neither excessively absent-minded, nor operating in conditions that are especially stressful. Naturalistic observations show that there are three conditions which promote slips and lapses: (a) the performance of some routinized activity in familiar surroundings; (b) an intended or necessary departure from past practice, due to altered goals or modified circumstances; and (c) when attention is claimed by something other than the job in hand, either some internal preoccupation or an external distraction. Moreover, a large proportion of the resulting errors take highly predictable forms: *strong habit intrusions* (e.g. 'Intending to lose weight, I decided to avoid sugar on my cereal; but when I got to the breakfast table, I found myself sprinkling it on as usual.'), or *strong habit exclusions* (e.g. 'I intended to drive home via the fish shop, but went the usual way and arrived back fishless.').

Observations such as these permit three general inferences to be made about the largely covert mechanisms which guide the performance of everyday activities.

1. Even during the execution of well-practised tasks, some degree of attentional investment is necessary to ensure the appropriate or desired outcome. These attentional checks are particularly important when planned actions deviate from customary practice; when sense data are attenuated or ambiguous; and when intentions must be encoded into prospective memory, or retrieved from it at the right moment.

2. Attention (whatever it might be) is a limited control resource: 'It implies withdrawal from some things in order to deal more effectively with others.' (James, 1890, p. 403). It is this spare self-monitoring capacity which appears to go absent in absent-mindedness.

3. When cognitive operations are *under-specified* (see Reason, 1986), control of the system tends to default to contextually appropriate, high-frequency schemata. There are many possible ways in which cognitive operations may be under-specified (inaccurate or patchy knowledge, losses from prospective memory, ambiguous sense data, impoverished retrieval cues, etc.), but inattention is probably the most important factor in the production of slips and lapses (as distinct from mistakes, or planning failures).

According to this analysis, the key to successful or error-free performance lies in the moment-to-moment management of this limited attentional resource. The higher levels of the cognitive system must be kept out of the control loop during the running of automatic sequences, but brought in at certain critical points. This is an extremely difficult task, and the evidence suggests that no one performs it perfectly, even under optimal conditions. It is not surprising, therefore, that external stressors make matters worse; nor that people, whose cognitive 'management style' renders them excessively error prone, should be less able to cope with such stressors.

A possible way of accommodating both state and trait variation is in terms of a continuum of cognitive resource-management styles, ranging from a pronounced degree of *involuntary attentional fixedness* at one extreme to *voluntary attentional flexibility* at the other (see Reason, 1984; Reason and Lucas, 1984). At the 'fixedness' end of the continuum, the attentional resource may be 'locked on' to just one of the available informational sources, while at the 'flexible' end, it is deployed flexibly at just the right place and just the right time to ensure correct performance. Two other assumptions are necessary. First, that stressors will act to shift all individuals towards the fixedness end of the continuum. Second, that people differ characteristically in their typical position along this continuum, with few, if any, capable of optimal flexible deployment at all times.

The literature on situational stress and attentional management (i.e. state variations), though extensive, is far from uniform in its conclusions (see Chapter 25, this volume). Nevertheless, there is reasonable agreement that (a) stressors affect attentional deployment, and (b) this effect tends to take the form of greater selectivity, or 'fixedness'. The weight of the evidence is thus consistent with the view that stress facilitates slips and lapses by reducing the attentional specification of those ongoing routine activities which fall outside this narrowed focus of concern.

The relationship between absent-mindedness and stress vulnerability is more complex and still highly speculative. However, the findings reviewed in this chapter suggest that both error proneness and the ability to withstand the adverse effects of stress are determined by the same general cognitive factor. The most likely candidate appears to be the characteristic way in which people manage their limited cognitive resources in the face of competing informational demands.

Given a comparable level of everyday activity and 'multiple-tasking', the deciding factor may well be a person's typical position along the attentional fixedness–flexibility dimension. Individuals could adopt a consistently rigid or sluggish management style for a wide variety of reasons: because they are constitutionally or pathologically given to rumination or 'brooding', because their work or intellectual leanings promote abstractedness or 'brown studies' (e.g. Archimedes, Chesterton and 'absent-minded professors' in general), or simply because they have developed this style as an adaptation to a particular set of life circumstances (e.g. solitariness). But whatever the cause, it is but a small step to argue that a relatively inflexible cognitive style is unlikely to promote the best use of coping strategies. Nor is such an individual likely to have the spare resources necessary to sustain the more attention-demanding strategies. And, as cognitive strategies fail, so the adverse effects of stress—the small cracks in the psychological defences—will become increasingly apparent.

SUMMARY AND CONCLUSIONS

This chapter has examined the relationship between stress and cognitive failure, with particular reference to studies employing a wide variety of self-report measures. The principal conclusions of this review are enumerated below.

1. While high levels of stress can, and often do, increase the likelihood of cognitive failure, they are neither a necesary nor a sufficient condition for their occurrence.
2. Self-reported liability to minor cognitive failures is a relatively stable and enduring feature of the individual. The data suggest that susceptibility to these usually inconsequential slips and lapses is governed by some global factor relating to the characteristic way in which an individual manages his or her cognitive affairs.
3. Observations taken from a wide range of samples, exposed to a number of different stresses, provide support for Broadbent's *stress-vulnerability hypothesis*: namely, that relatively high levels of cognitive failure in normal everyday life are associated with increased vulnerability to externally-imposed stresses.
4. Whatever governs a general proneness to everyday slips and lapses also contributes to stress vulnerability. This factor eludes capture by laboratory measures, but it appears to be bound up with the deployment of limited attentional resources.
5. The evidence so far assembled suggests that it is not so much that stress induces a high rate of cognitive failure; rather that certain styles of attentional resource management can lead to both absent-mindedness and to the inappropriate matching of coping strategies to stressful situations.
6. The final section attempts to reconcile two apparently contradictory themes: (a) that stress promotes cognitive failures; and (b) that pronounced absent-mindedness leads to increased stress vulnerability. One way of accommodating both these state and trait variations is in terms of a continuum, ranging from *extreme attentional fixedness* at one end, to *voluntary attentional flexibility* at the other. A relatively inflexible conitive management style, whether stress-induced or characteristic of the individual, is unlikely to lead to either the efficient deployment of limited attentional resources in relation to multiple demands, or to an optimal use of available coping strategies.

REFERENCES

Baars, B.J. (1980). On eliciting predictable speech errors in the laboratory. In V. Fromkin (ed.) *Errors in linguistic performance: slips of the tongue, ear, pen, and hand.* Chichester: Wiley.

Baars, B.J., Motley, M.T., & MacKay, D.G. (1975). Output editing for lexical status in artificially elicited slips of the tongue. *Journal of Verbal Learning and Verbal Behaviour, 14,* 382–391.

Baddeley, A.D. (1972). Selective attention and performance in dangerous environments. *British Journal of Psychology, 63,* 537–546.

Beck, A.T., Rush, A.J., Shaw, B.F., & Emery, G. (1979). *Cognitive therapy of depression.* Chichester: Wiley.

Bell, B.J. (1980). *A review of the literature on psychological stress*. Albuquerque, New Mexico: Sandia National Laboratories.

Berkun, M.M. (1964). Performance decrement under psychological stress. *Human Factors, 6*, 21–30.

Berkun, M.M., Bialek, H.M., Kern, R.P., & Yagi, K. (1962). Experimental studies of psychological stresses in man. *Psychological Monographs: General and Applied, 76*.

Broadbent, D.E., Cooper, P.J., Fitzgerald, P.F., & Parkes, K.R. (1982). The Cognitive Failures Questionnaire (CFQ) and its correlates. *British Journal of Clinical Psychology, 21*, 1–16.

Broadbent, D.E., Broadbent, M.H.P., & Jones, J.L. (1986). Correlates of cognitive failure. *British Journal of Clinical Psychology, 25*, 285–299.

Brown, G.W., & Harris, T.H. (1978). *Social origins of depression: A study of psychiatric disorders in women*. London: Tavistock.

Clare, A.W., & Cairns, V.E. (1978). Design, development and use of a standardised interview to assess social adjustment and dysfunction in community studies. *Psychological Medicine, 8*, 589–604.

Eysenck, M.W. (1982). *Attention and arousal: cognition and performance*. Berlin: Springer-Verlag.

Fisher, S., & Hood, B. (1987). Mobility history and psychological disturbance following transition to university. Unpublished report, University of Dundee.

Fisher, S., Murray, K., & Frazer, N. (1985). Homesickness, health and efficiency in first year students. *Journal of Environmental Psychology, 5*, 181–195.

Fisher, S., Frazer, N., Murray, K., & Hood, B. (1987). The stress of the transition to university: A prospective study of vulnerability to homesickness in first year residential students. Unpublished report, University of Dundee.

Folkman, S., & Lazarus, R.S. (1980). An analysis of coping in a middle aged community sample. *Journal of Health and Social Behaviour, 21*, 219–239.

Goldberg, D.P. (1972). *The detection of psychiatric illness by questionnaire*. Oxford: Oxford University Press.

Grinker, R.R., & Spiegel, J.P. (1963). *Men under stress*. New York: McGraw-Hill (reprinted from 1945).

Harris, J.E., & Wilkins, A.J. (1982). Remembering to do things: a theoretical framework and an illustrative experiment. *Human Learning, 1*, 123–136.

Harris, W., Mackie, R.R., & Wilson, C.L. (1956). *Performance under stress: A review and critique of recent studies*. Los Angeles: Human Factors Research.

Hastings, M. (1981). *Bomber Command*. London: Pan Books.

Herrmann, D.J. (1982). Know thy memory: The use of questionnaires to assess and study memory. *Psychological Bulletin, 92*, 434–452.

Herrmann, D.J. (1984). Questionnaires about memory. In J. Harris & P. Morris (eds), *Everyday memory, actions and absent-mindedness*. New York: Academic Press.

Horowitz, M.J. (1979). Psychological response to serious life stress. In V. Hamilton & D. Warburton (eds) *Human stress and cognition*. Chichester: Wiley.

INPO (1985). *A maintenance analysis of safety significant events*. Atlanta, Georgia: Institute of Nuclear Power Operations.

James, W. (1890). *The principles of psychology*. New York: Longman.

Kane, G. (1987). Studies of coping in stressed populations. Ph.D. thesis, University of Manchester.

Klier, S., & Linskey, J.W. (1960). Selected Abstracts from the Literature on Stress. NAVTRADEVCEN 565–1, Port Wash, NY, U.S. Naval Training Device Center.

Lucas, D.A., Reason, J.T., Maguire, G.P., Goldberg, D., Sellwood, R., & Balwako, L. (1985). Absent mindedness and stress in breast cancer patients. Report to North West Regional Health Authority.

Lucas, D. (1986). Predicting psychiatric morbidity in women treated surgically for breast cancer. Paper given to the Annual Conference of the British Psychological Society.

Mandler, G. (1975). *Mind and emotion*. New York: Wiley.

Mandler, G. (1985). *Cognitive psychology: An essay in cognitive science*. Hillsdale, N.J.: Erlbaum.

Marshall, S.L.A. (1978). *Men against fire*. Gloucester, MA: Peter Smith.

Martin, M., & Jones, G.V. (1983). Distribution of attention in cognitive failure. *Human Learning, 2*, 221–226.

Martin, M., & Jones, V. (1984). Cognitive failures in everyday life. In J. Harris & P. Morris (eds), *Everyday memory, actions and absent-mindedness*. New York: Academic Press.

Morris, P.E. (1984). The validity of subjective reports. In J. Harris & P. Morris (eds), *Everyday memory, actions and absent-mindedness*. New York: Academic Press.

Nature (1986). Coping with the human factor: Chernobyl Report. *Nature, 323*, September.

Norman, D.A. (1981). Categorization of action slips. *Psychological Review, 88*, 1–15.

Reason, J.T. (1979). Actions not as planned: the price of automatization. In G. Underwood & R. Stevens (eds) *Aspects of consciousness*, vol. 1: *Psychological issues*. London: Academic Press.

Reason, J.T. (1984). Lapses of attention. In R. Parasuraman & R. Davies (eds), *Varieties of attention*. New York: Academic Press.

Reason, J.T. (1986). Cognitive under-specification: Its varieties and consequences. In B. Baars (ed.), *The psychology of error: A window on the mind*. New York: Plenum.

Reason, J.T. (1987a). The cognitive bases of systematic human error. In *Contemporary ergonomics 1987*. London: Taylor & Francis.

Reason, J.T. (1987b). The Chernobyl errors. Paper given to the Annual Conference of The British Psychological Society, University of Sussex.

Reason, J.T. & Lucas, D. (1982). The Short Inventory of Mental Lapses (SIML). Unpublished report, University of Manchester.

Reason, J.T., & Lucas, D. (1984). Absent-mindedness in shops: Its correlates and consequences. *British Journal of Clinical Psychology, 23*, 121–131.

Reason, J.T., & Mycielska, K. (1982). *Absent-minded? The psychology of mental lapses and everyday errors*. Englewood Cliffs, N.J.: Prentice-Hall.

Robbins, J.E., McKendry, J.M., & Hurst, P.M. (1961). *Task-induced stress: A literature survey, AD667272*. Ohio: Aerospace Medical Laboratory, Wright-Patterson Air Force Base.

Ronan, W.W. (1953). *Training for emergency procedures in multi-engine aircraft, AIR-153-53-FR-44*. Pittsburgh, Pennsylvania: American Institutes for Research.

Swain, A.D., & Guttmann, H.E. (1980). *Handbook of human reliability analysis with emphasis on nuclear power plant applications*. Albuquerque, New Mexico: Sandia Laboratories.

Wing, J.K., Cooper, J.E., & Sartorius, N. (1974). *The measurement and classification of psychiatric symptoms*. Cambridge: Cambridge University Press.

KEY WORDS

Attention, cognitive failures questionnaires, coping strategies, error proneness, extreme stress responses, mood states, psychiatric illness, stress vulnerability.

Handbook of Life Stress, Cognition and Health
Edited by S. Fisher and J. Reason
© 1988 John Wiley & Sons Ltd.

23

Explanation and Adaptation in Adversity

Chris R. Brewin
Institute of Psychiatry, London

INTRODUCTION

In recent years, psychologists have been very interested in how people explain the behaviour of themselves and other people, and in the consequences of such explanations. There has been considerable controversy about whether people spontaneously try to explain events and actions when they are not specifically asked to do so. It has also been pointed out that the kind of explanations people give for intentional actions are usually couched in terms of reasons (e.g. I ran down the street 'in order to catch the bus'). Whereas actions tend to be explained by reference to the goal that a person is trying to achieve, explanations provided for unintentional events which happen to a person are usually couched in terms of causal factors (e.g. I missed the bus 'because it left five minutes early' or 'because I overslept'). There is, however, general agreement that unexpected or unwelcome events trigger a search for the causal factors that are responsible (Weiner, 1985), a process which has been described in clinical studies of accident victims (Bulman and Wortman, 1977) and cancer sufferers (Taylor *et al.*, 1984).

Given that people do try to explain why misfortune has befallen them, this chapter will explore whether these explanations have an impact on how the person then thinks, feels, and behaves. There is some evidence that simply asking someone for an explanation may be important. Before giving an anagram test, Sherman *et al.* (1981) showed subjects a sample anagram and told them to imagine that they had done either very well or very poorly on the test. Half the subjects were then asked for an explanation of this hypothetical performance, and all subjects went on to estimate how well they expected to do on the test and to complete the test itself. Subjects who had made success explanations expected to do better than control subjects, and subjects who had made failure explanations expected to do worse. Furthermore, these expectations were related to actual performance on the test, higher expectations leading to improved performance. These findings provide experimental evidence that the act of explanation alone may influence behaviour, regardless of the specific conclusion a person arrives at.

We shall begin by examining in more detail the different functions that people's explanations serve and whether certain kinds of explanation are more likely to lead to successful personal adjustment in the face of adversity. Explanations are involved in the labelling of feelings and experiences, in the location of the factors which caused those experiences (the causal attribution process), in the moral evaluation of conduct, and in the presentation of self to others (Antaki and Fielding, 1981; Forsyth, 1980). All these functions are evident in the explanations patients produce for their illnesses and misfortunes.

LABELLING

In the search for explanation, we often have first to describe or label an experience which is ambiguous. For instance, before we can say why we are feeling terrible, we have to decide whether we are depressed, have flu, are tired, or have a hangover. In the same way patients who develop a pain, lump, or other unusual symptom consult a doctor in order to reassure themselves that the symptom can be labelled as harmless. Often it is difficult to discriminate between two experiences (such as indigestion and a heart attack), one of which has an extremely threatening label whereas the other is not at all threatening. Labelling involves categorizing experiences according to the knowledge that we have available, either using our existing categories or creating a new category which can be defined in terms of the existing ones. Each category or label will be associated with its own set of information concerning the frequency of the problem, the likely outcome, and so on, information which may be accurate, inaccurate, or simply missing.

In many cases, therefore, understanding *why* appears to be intimately connected with knowing *what* an experience consists of. The label may then supply useful information about the likely cause. There is an interesting parallel here with Schachter's theory of the emotions (Schachter and Singer, 1962), which claimed that emotional experience consists of an undifferentiated state of physiological arousal which is then assigned a specific label, such as anger or fear, according to the way in which environmental stimuli are appraised. There have been a number of experiments which have attempted to use this principle and achieve some therapeutic benefit by getting people to relabel their experiences in a more helpful way. In a well-known example of this 'misattribution' approach, Storms and Nisbett (1970) gave people suffering from insomnia a pill to take at bedtime. Although the pills were inert, Storms and Nisbett told half the subjects that the pills would calm them down and the other half that the pills would produce feelings similar to those of high physiological arousal. Their reasoning was that insomnia sufferers tend to be tense and highly aroused, which would lead them to worry about the cause of the arousal and so find it more difficult to get to sleep. By providing a new and emotionally neutral label for these feelings, i.e. side-effects of the pills, sufferers should worry less about them and so fall asleep more easily. Consistent with this prediction, the group who were told that the pills would produce symptoms of arousal reported falling asleep faster than the group who were told that the pills would have a calming effect.

The findings of the 'misattribution' studies will not be evaluated in detail here as this has been done elsewhere (Brewin and Antaki, 1982; Harvey and Galvin, 1984). Suffice it to say that their results have been difficult to replicate, and that clinically significant effects have not been established. In part this must be because of the inherent implausibility of many of the manipulations, in which subjects were presented with novel environmental stimuli and expected to relabel fairly familiar experiences. It is hardly surprising that subjects were loth to abandon their original (and presumably plausible) categories in favour of new and untested ones. In principle, however, there is no reason why people who have wrongly or unhelpfully categorized their experiences should not benefit from having them reassigned to a less threatening category. An example of an appropriate and powerful use of relabelling comes from recent work on the treatment of panic attacks.

It has often been noted that the effects of overbreathing or hyperventilation are similar to the experience of a panic attack. In both conditions the person has an intense feeling of apprehension or impending doom accompanied by distressing physical sensations such as vertigo, blurred vision, palpitations, numbness, tingling in the hands and feet, and breathlessness. According to a recent model of panic attacks (Clark *et al.*, 1985; Salkovskis and Clark, 1986), some individuals increase their respiratory ventilation and overbreathe when under stress, which produces a range of these unpleasant sensations. These are then labelled by the patient as symptoms of a heart attack or other medical emergency, or as indications that the patient is going mad.

The frightening consequences of these labels lead to further apprehension, to further increases in ventilation, and so on in a vicious cycle. Their treatment consists of helping patients to relabel their sensations as symptoms of hyperventilation rather than of some more catastrophic condition. Patients first practise voluntary overbreathing, then introspect on their sensations and compare them to those experienced during panic attacks. The therapist then gives an explanation of how overbreathing can induce panic attacks and trains the patient in a pattern of slow breathing which is incompatible with hyperventilation. Although this treatment contains a number of disparate elements, so that improvement need not be the result of relabelling, Salkovskis and Clark argue that the extremely rapid initial reduction in panic attack frequency and self-reported anxiety points to the importance of the cognitive element.

Rodin (1978) has described labelling errors which arise because of inattention to chronic physical states, such as the physiological changes associated with ageing, and metabolic changes which arise from overeating. There seems no reason not to recognize relabelling as a powerful clinical tool, providing the new label is less threatening and is supplied in a convincing way. The process is probably widely applicable and should not be thought of as synonymous with the more restricted 'misattribution' studies, which struggled under the self-imposed requirement to mislead people rather than to enlighten them.

Before leaving the topic of labelling, it should be noted that sociologists have written extensively about the effect on patients of the labels that society uses for their behaviour (e.g. Field, 1976). Part of the knowledge one has about the world includes expectations about the effects of such diseases as epilepsy, diabetes, and schizophrenia, and it has been argued that patients tend to respond to social pressures and act in conformity with the public stereotypes associated with a particular label (the concept of secondary deviance). So people with epilepsy may come to regard themselves as unreliable and even dangerous if consistently treated in this way by others. Just as patients may have difficulty in labelling internal sensations, observers may not know whether to label behaviour as an intentional act, as a symptom of a disease, as a drug side-effect, and so on. To take one example, an elderly person who walks out of a shop with an article that has not been paid for may be shoplifting, may be confused, or may have had a specific memory lapse. Explanation typically cannot proceed until the nature of the event has first been understood.

CAUSAL ATTRIBUTION

The sort of explanation with which psychologists have been most concerned is how people decide what causes have led to a particular event they have experienced, or, in other words, what causal attribution to make. In this research the nature of the event is usually clearly defined, and the focus of interest is on how causes are most commonly described, how people arrive at their causal attributions, and what effect those attributions have on their subsequent behaviour. Theories which are concerned with the consequences of these causal perceptions are sometimes called 'attributional' theories to distinguish them from the 'attribution' theories which concentrate on the antecedents of causal judgements. In this section we shall have most to say about the 'attributional' theories, but first a few words are in order about how people make attributions.

Following Fritz Heider's *The psychology of interpersonal relations*, published in 1958, a distinction has been drawn between causes which reside within the person (internal) and those causes to do with other people, luck, or circumstances (external). Most events, whether becoming ill, getting promotion, or being run over by a car, can be attributed to internal or to external causes, or to a mixture of the two. Becoming ill might be attributed to the external cause of exposure to another person's germs, for instance, or to the internal cause of not taking enough care of oneself and becoming run down. What cause we actually subscribe to depends on a number of factors. When we have experience of several similar situations, it has been suggested by Kelley (1967) that we carry out a 'covariance analysis', that is, we work out which causes are present when a particular outcome occurs and only when it occurs, and we eliminate those causes which are sometimes present without the outcome occurring. So if our spouse is angry one day about something we have failed to do, we search for similar examples of their bad temper and see whether there are consistent factors present, such as a frustrating day at work.

Kelley proposed that three different kinds of information are particularly relevant to determining whether the cause is perceived as being internal or external to the person: consistency information, i.e. how often does the person experience this outcome when in the same situation; consensus information, i.e. how many other people experience this outcome when in the same situation; and distinctiveness information, i.e. how typically does the person experience this outcome in similar situations. Attributions to the person tend to be made when an outcome is highly consistent, low in consensus, and low in distinctiveness. To take our previous example, the sort of information that would help us to make an internal or an external attribution for our spouse's bad temper would be our knowledge of how often he or she is annoyed with us for failing to do something, how often other people get annoyed with us over this, and how often our spouse gets annoyed with us in other situations.

Unfortunately, causal attribution cannot be reduced to a number of simple rules. The idea that for every event there is one cause which can be arrived at logically is idealistic. In reality, people may entertain several possible causes and shift from one to the other. Covariation analysis may be impossible because the necessary information is missing or unreliable. In any case, people will be influenced by pre-existing causal schemata: their internally represented knowledge of causal relationships which has been built up over the years. In addition to the impact of prior expectations, people are likely to be influenced by the salience of certain types of information, and by the social situation in which they find themselves. The making of causal attributions is undoubtedly a complex process, and for further discussion of these issues the reader is referred to Jaspars *et al.* (1983), and Kelley and Michela (1980). We now turn to the question of whether attributions, by whatever means they are arrived at, influence the person's subsequent feelings and behaviour when faced with illness or misfortune.

The Attributional Reformulation of Learned Helplessness Theory

In 1978, the current version of learned helplessness theory underwent a radical change of emphasis. Seligman (1975) had proposed that when people or animals experience an event which they cannot control, they develop an expectation of lack of control (specifically, lack of contingency between their actions and outcomes) in similar situations. In those situations, they then demonstrate a number of 'learned helplessness' effects, such as failure to initiate escape responses from an aversive environment and failure to learn from successful escape experiences. Research in which human subjects were first given an insoluble helplessness induction task and then required to carry out a second test task indicated a number of problems with this simple account. It was found that people often (1) performed better rather than worse after helplessness induction, (2) showed helplessness effects in some situations but not in others, and (3) were affected by instructions about how other subjects had done on the task. Abramson *et al.* (1978) therefore proposed that following an experience of uncontrollability, a person's response depends on their understanding of why it occurred. If the cause is perceived as being permanent rather than temporary ('stable' rather than 'unstable' in the terms of Abramson *et al.*), then helplessness effects in that particular situation are likely to be long lasting. If the cause is perceived as influencing many situations rather than just that one situation ('global' rather than 'specific'), then helplessness effects are likely to generalize to other situations. Finally, if the cause is perceived as being internal ('personal helplessness') rather than external ('universal helplessness'), then that person is likely to suffer a loss of self-esteem.

Let us illustrate these ideas with an example. A woman is criticized for a piece of work by her boss. If she attributes this to an unstable cause such as her boss being in a bad mood, she is less likely to experience helplessness than if she attributes it to a stable cause such as her inability to handle this type of work. If she attributes it to a specific cause such as difficulty with this particular superior, any helplessness she experiences will generalize less to other situations than if she had attributed it to a global cause such as difficulty in relationships with all superiors. Finally, if she attributes it to an internal cause ('My boss is only critical of me'), she will experience lower self-esteem than if she makes an external attribution ('My boss is critical of all the women who work for him'). For a similar attributional account of learned helplessness, see Miller and Norman (1979).

As with previous versions of the theory, it has been proposed that the reformulation provides a model for certain instances of depression. Although Abramson and her colleagues recognized that depression may have a number of causes (e.g. biochemical ones), they suggested that there is a substantial subset of 'helplessness' depressions in which the expectation of uncontrollability plays an important role. They viewed depression as a complex disorder made up of at least four classes of deficits: motivational (reduced initiation of voluntary responding), cognitive (impaired learning of the association between a person's actions and contingent events), self-esteem, and affective (sadness). Depressed affect comes about when a person loses something highly desirable, or experiences something very unpleasant. The importance of this event will influence the intensity of their emotion, as will the strength or certainty of their belief that the event is uncontrollable. The more stable their attribution for the event, the longer lasting the depressive deficits will be; and the more global the attribution, the more generalized the deficits will be. According to the model, people may become depressed whether their attributions are internal or external, but internal attributions (personal helplessness) will lead to the specific depressive deficit of low self-esteem.

This model emphasizes the potential role of attributions in the *onset* of a depressive episode. A number of other attribution–depression relationships are possible, however (Brewin, 1985), and these are shown in Figure 23.1. Peterson and Seligman (1984) have suggested that certain individuals have a 'vulnerable attributional style', in other words, a general tendency to attribute their positive experiences to external, unstable, and specific factors, such as good luck, while attributing their negative experiences to internal, stable, and global factors, such as incompetence or lack of intelligence. Peterson and Seligman suggest that when a person with such a vulnerable style has a failure or setback, they will be more likely to make an internal, stable and global attribution and to suffer a more severe depressive reaction. In addition to this *vulnerability* model, it is possible to outline three additional models. The *recovery* model does not require that attributions be involved in the onset of depression, but holds that people who make internal, stable, and global attributions will take longer to recover from the depressed state. The *coping* model makes even fewer assumptions, predicting

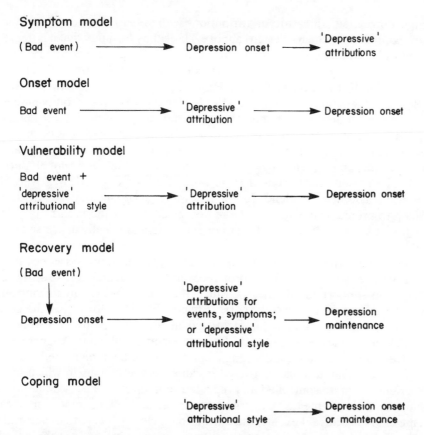

FIG. 23.1   Alternative relations between causal attributions and depression (from Brewin, 1985). © The American Psychological Association.

simply that the depressive attributional pattern will be associated with lower resistance to depression, whether or not the person is depressed to start with. Note that neither the recovery nor the coping model requires the person to have necessarily experienced any negative event. Finally, the *symptom* model, the only one to be completely incompatible with learned helplessness theory, holds that depressive attributions are a symptom of the clinical state of depression and play no causal role either in its onset or maintenance.

Critique of Attributional Theories of Depression

In spite of a large research effort put into testing the reformulated learned helplessness model of depression, empirical support for the theory is equivocal. One recent review of the evidence concluded that the model was supported (Peterson and Seligman, 1984), while another found little support for it (Coyne and Gotlib, 1983). The reason for this discrepancy is not hard to find. Neither of these reviews considered separately the various attribution–depression relationships outlined above. They also included a large number of studies which simply correlated a measure of attributions with a measure of depression at the same point in time. Such a design cannot exclude the possibility that it is depressed mood which influences a person's attributions (the symptom model) rather than the other way round, and so does not provide an adequate test of the theory. When evidence for the five models shown in Figure 23.1 is examined separately (Brewin, 1985), it appears that there is no support for the onset or vulnerability models. In part, this is undoubtedly because these two models make the largest number of assumptions and so are most difficult to test. In contrast, there was evidence that people's mood affected their causal judgements (the symptom model), attributions for negative events being more internal, stable, and global during a depressive episode and becoming more 'normal' after the episode was over. There was also encouraging evidence for the recovery and coping models. Attributions helped to predict who would be more depressed weeks and months later, even when it was taken into account that not everyone was equally depressed to start with.

It does seem, then, that the depressive pattern of attributions is associated with weakened resistance to, and poorer recovery from, depression. But there has been little support for models in which the occurrence of an uncontrollable aversive event was a necessary part. It is possible, therefore, that the account provided by the reformulated model to explain depressive onset is erroneous or only seldom applicable. This may be because cognitions about the triggering event are irrelevant or because the wrong cognitions have been measured.

The reformulated model is rooted in laboratory situations in which aversive experiences can be controlled and repeated (e.g. electric shocks, loud noise, or failure on an insoluble task). Attributions are assumed to be important because, in the case of recurrent events, the attribution is closely linked to expectations of successful performance next time the situation is encountered. Are these the kind of experiences that normally precede clinical depression? The work of Brown and Harris (1978) particularly identifies such experiences as being characterized by moderate or severe long-term threat, i.e. bad consequences lasting longer than one week. These events, such as bereavement, redundancy, or an unpleasant revelation about a loved one, usually involve loss or disappointment and tend in the short term to be non-recurring. With this sort of event, causal attributions are unlikely to be so closely related to future adjustment. For example, attributions about the cause of a close friend's death may be less relevant to adjustment than one's expectations of being able to cope without him or her. Hammen (e.g. Hammen and deMayo, 1982) has provided evidence that the causes of events may not always be as important as their consequences.

We have been arguing that some events may have such a major impact on their own account that causal cognitions are relatively unimportant. There are two possible counter-arguments here. First, epidemiological studies such as that of Brown and Harris may only have identified major events preceding depression. It may be that numerous cases of depression are precipitated by a series of more minor events, such as family rows, but that such events have not shown up in the large-scale studies because they are only significant to some individuals and not to others. Alternatively, loss events such as divorce and death may be important because they *do* represent a recurrence of an early experience in a person's life (Brown and Harris reported that women who had lost their mothers before the age of 12 were more vulnerable when they experienced a severe event). In both these cases the learned helplessness model, with its emphasis on recurrent events, would appear to be appropriate. At present, however, there is doubt about whether Abramson *et al.* (1978) are correct in their assumption that an analysis of recurrent events in the laboratory can be used to explain the effects of real-life events which recur seldom if at all.

We have also raised the possibility that, as far as events are concerned, the wrong cognitions are being measured. These might, for instance, be self-evaluative rather than causal perceptions. In other words, people might be more concerned with the adequacy of their own conduct and with possible transgression of their own standards than with the fact that their actions played some part in a causal chain leading to the uncontrollable event. Learned helplessness research tends to confound these two kinds of judgement, not considering that one may make an internal causal attribution without the feeling that one has necessarily acted foolishly, recklessly, or incompetently (Brewin, 1986). In support of this point, two studies (Janoff-Bulman, 1979; Peterson *et al.*, 1981) have reported that depressed mood is not related to greater self-blame for one's actions but only to greater self-blame for one's character. Characterological self-blame involves feelings of guilt and deservingness and thus appears to be an evaluative as well as a causal judgement. This analysis of self-blame into causal and evaluative elements may help to explain why some recent studies have linked depressed mood in college students to perceiving negative events as more controllable (Hammen and Mayol, 1982; Harvey, 1981), another finding which is contrary to learned helplessness theory. Seeing events as more controllable is related to guilt, i.e. to feeling that one has transgressed one's standards of conduct (Weiner *et al.*, 1982). Thus events may be important in precipitating depression for reasons other than their perceived causal properties.

Causal Attribution and Health-Related Behaviour

We have devoted a great deal of space to examining attributional theories of depression because it is these which have received most attention to date. These theories can be applied just as successfully, probably more successfully, to patients whose disorders are predominantly physical. Whereas, with depression, attributions for events in general were thought to influence the disorder, in the case of physical medicine researchers have been interested in the impact of attributions for the disorder itself on its future course and on the patient's adjustment to it. Just as in the case of depression, however, patients often experience a single event, the onset of illness, which they do not expect to recur. Even if the illness is one with an expectation of recurrence, as in cancer or heart disease, the causes of the first episode may not be perceived to be the same as those of subsequent episodes. For instance, the probability of future heart disease may be substantially determined by the degree of damage to the heart and arteries sustained in previous episodes.

Health contexts provide a rich variety of combinations of circumstances, each of which must be individually analysed. Victims of minor accidental trauma, for instance, usually have to cope with the situation in which their accident originally occurred, whether this be at home, at work, or on the roads. Major trauma such as spinal injury, on the other hand, frequently means that the person's whole environment or way of life changes, so that they never encounter that situation again. One would therefore expect causal judgements about minor accidents to be more relevant than judgements about major accidents in predicting future adjustment. Patients with chronic diseases such as diabetes mellitus can make causal attributions both about the onset of their disorder and about recurrent events such as hypoglycaemic episodes and blackouts which reflect the day-to-day course of the disorder. Once again, one would neither expect that these attributions be similar in content nor expect that their consequences would be the same. Attributions about day-to-day events should theoretically stand the best chance of predicting adjustment and health behaviour, and this may explain why some studies of attributions for disease onset have not found the predicted relationship to adjustment (e.g. Taylor *et al.*, 1984).

One much-quoted study which appears to go against this principle is that of Bulman and Wortman (1977). These researchers interviewed accident victims with severe spinal injuries that had left them with varying degrees of paralysis. Patients rated by their therapists as coping most successfully with their condition (1) tended to blame themselves for their accident, (2) were less likely to blame other people, and (3) believed they were less able to prevent their accident. There are, however, a number of difficulties in interpreting these results. All interviews were carried out at a similar point in time, so we cannot say whether attributions affected adjustment or vice versa. There is also an evident contradiction between holding beliefs (1) and (3) at the same time: if one blames oneself more, one should believe oneself *more* able to prevent the accident, not less able. A subsequent study (Brewin, 1984) measured the attributions of patients for accidents at work. These were accidents involving minor fractures needing an average of 4 to 5 weeks at home before patients returned to work. Upon their return, victims who felt that they had caused the accident reported themselves to be less tense and anxious, and more alert and active. Some evidence about the direction of causation was obtained from the small minority of accidents where there was some clearly identifiable environmental fault or failure which acted as a precipitating agent. Patients who had been involved in this type of accident rated themselves as less causally responsible immediately after the accident, took longer to get back to work, and appeared more poorly adjusted when they did so.

Causal perceptions may be associated with a variety of other behaviours such as choice of treatment. Bradley *et al.* (1987) investigated the psychological factors which were associated with choice of a new treatment for diabetes, continuous subcutaneous insulin infusion (CSII), versus a more traditional regimen of daily or twice-daily self-injections. CSII treatment involves having an insulin pump strapped to the body which automatically releases insulin throughout the day. Using a set of scales specifically developed to measure patients' attributions of controllability for day-to-day events connected with their diabetes (Bradley *et al.*,

1984), it was found that choice of CSII was predicted by the perception that medical staff had a greater degree of control over the patient's diabetes, whereas patients choosing injection regimens perceived higher levels of personal control. The scales also predicted how successful patients would be at controlling their diabetes during the following year. In another study (King, 1982), patients were more likely to attend a screening for high blood pressure if they perceived the causes of the condition to be external but controllable.

Causal Attribution and the Maintenance of Behavioural Change

So far we have examined the effects of attributions for illness and misfortune. Some of the most promising evidence for the importance of attributional processes comes from studies of how successful people are at modifying behaviours such as smoking or overeating. Sonne and Janoff (1982) gave overweight clients two alternative weight-loss programmes, one emphasizing self-control and one external control by the therapist. Both programmes were equally effective during the treatment period, but the self-control group had maintained their progress significantly better at follow-up. Furthermore, weight loss during the 11-week follow-up period was predicted by clients' self-attributions for improvement measured immediately after the treatment programme: the more they credited themselves with the improvement, the more they were able to maintain it.

Chambliss and Murray (1979) gave subjects who wished to give up smoking a placebo capsule to complement their efforts at self-control. The placebo was variously described as increasing, decreasing, or having no effect on symptoms of withdrawal. In the second phase of the study, half the subjects were told that the drug was inactive and that they had reduced their smoking through their own efforts, while the rest of the subjects were not debriefed at all. The debriefed group, and in particular those with an internal locus of control, went on to reduce their smoking by a significantly greater amount than the others. In a similar study using more orthodox methods to reduce smoking, Colletti and Kopel (1979) also reported that the more subjects attributed their improvement to their own efforts, the less they were smoking one year later.

MORAL EVALUATION

Understanding and explaining events is not simply a matter of locating a cause, however. When faced with misfortune, a person is likely to want to know not only whether his or her actions produced the outcome, but also how reasonable or appropriate those actions were. As we have already seen in our discussion of depressive attributions, it is quite possible to blame oneself in the causal sense but not in the moral sense, as for instance when you make some perfectly understandable error of judgement. It is quite another matter when you try to cut corners, ignore the normal procedures, or take unnecessary risks. Under these circumstances, when disaster subsequently occurs, you know that you ought to have acted differently, and the self-recriminations are likely to be painful and prolonged. The essence of this aspect of explanation is the question of what you *ought* to have done, rather than the consequences of what you did do.

To date, few clinically relevant studies have examined causal and moral attribution separately. One exception is the previously mentioned study of accident victims (Brewin, 1984). In the sample as a whole, greater causal self-blame was associated with victims feeling less tense and anxious, whereas greater moral self-blame was associated with a more rapid return to work. These two effects were quite separate from each other even though, as one might expect, the two kinds of self-blame tended to occur together. In another recent study, Furnham *et al.* (1985) investigated the causal and moral judgements typically made by people with a hard-driving, impatient, coronary-prone (Type A) personality compared with people with a more relaxed, unambitious, and non-coronary-prone (Type B) personality. Both groups were given a questionnaire describing a number of negative experiences, such as not being able to get work done or being accused of gossiping about a friend, which came about through either controllable or uncontrollable circumstances. The major differences between the groups were confined to the uncontrollable negative outcomes: Type A subjects were more likely to feel angry with themselves and to judge that their actions had fallen short of their standards. Even in situations beyond their control, Type A subjects seemed to feel that they ought to have done better, although they did not reveal any more causal self-blame than the Type Bs. Another way of expressing this finding is that the Type A personality sets high standards and makes less allowance for circumstances when evaluating how he or she has done relative to these standards.

Self-evaluation or moral judgement appears to be important in many other clinical contexts, although the research has often been described using the language of attributions. For instance, Storms and McCaul (1976) proposed a common mechanism to account for the exacerbation of a variety of anxiety-related behaviours such as stammering, insomnia, male impotence, shyness, and blushing. This mechanism involves: (a) seeing the cause of unwanted behaviour as one's own negative dispositions or characteristics, (b) an increase in an unpleasant emotional state such as anxiety or depression following from this negative self-evaluation, and (c) a consequent exacerbation of the same unwanted behaviour which gave rise to the initial attribution. They reported evidence that negative self-evaluation is common among stutterers, who often have low self-esteem and experience intense anxiety about speaking.

Storms and McCaul's exacerbation model appears to be describing moral rather than causal judgements because they are describing people who feel that they *ought* not to be displaying the unwanted behaviour, of which they will in many cases be ashamed. Shame is a common reaction to many problems which people bring to psychologists and doctors. Storms and Nisbett (1970) reported anecdotal evidence that people with insomnia were prone to worry about the disorder and view it as a serious personal problem, possibly indicative of pathology. In a test of this model, Lowery *et al.* (1979) compared two types of attributional treatment with a no-treatment control condition. In the 'misattribution' treatment, subjects were induced to relabel their symptoms of arousal as a drug side-effect, while in the 'non-pejorative self-attribution' treatment they were persuaded that their arousal was due to autonomic activity which was somewhat above average but that they were otherwise completely normal. Lowery *et al.* found that subjects in both treatment groups said they fell asleep more easily than did the controls, but only the group whose self-evaluation had been manipulated reported that they also fell asleep more quickly.

SELF-PRESENTATION

A number of writers have drawn attention to the fact that making explanations is often a public activity and has the function of enhancing how one appears in the eyes of other people. Whether or not they are aware of it, people may also try to enhance their own view of themselves by making self-protective or esteem-enhancing attributions. Snyder *et al.* (1978) refer to this tendency as 'egotism', and suggest that, faced with the possibility of failure on a task, individuals may employ the tactic of not trying or giving up prematurely. This has the advantage that they are able to attribute failure to lack of effort, a less distressing cause than lack of ability. Other behaviours, such as lack of assertiveness, overdependency, and excessive use of drugs, may also represent attempts to control attributions about the self through the use of 'self-handicapping' strategies (Jones and Berglas, 1978). Sportsmen and politicians are noted for their ability to find a face-saving explanation for an unexpected defeat or change of policy, and their pronouncements are often treated with a good deal of scepticism. Should we therefore treat patients' explanations for their problems with a similar degree of scepticism or, alternatively, should we be inclined to believe everything they tell us?

Clearly, the attributions made by patients are unlikely to serve a wholly self-presentational function, or else their ability to predict such things as choice of treatment and speed of return to work would be hard to account for. Also, if patients were solely concerned with giving the most socially acceptable explanation, there would be very little difference between them. It may be argued that the predictive validity of attributions simply comes down to the predictive validity of different self-presentational strategies rather than of sincerely held causal beliefs, but this is a weak argument because self-presentation theories make no predictions about subsequent behaviour whereas attributional theories do. It appears intuitively likely that when attributions serve a largely self-presentational function, they will be of little use for prediction, but there is as yet no evidence with which to test this hypothesis.

At first sight, patients' attributions appear to be completely non-defensive. The self-blame reported by accident victims and depressed patients is diametrically opposite to the typical self-serving pattern of taking credit for success and blaming external causes for failure. As Bradley (1978) points out, however, this self-serving pattern is typically encountered when a person is being evaluated on a single occasion; if he or she anticipates future evaluations, the person may adopt the 'counterdefensive' strategy of appearing cautious and modest so as not to have too positive a self-evaluation publicly invalidated. Tetlock (1980) has shown that this 'counterdefensive' strategy can produce more favourable reactions in other people, thus underlining its potential value in achieving optimal self-presentation.

Depressive attributional style might then be regarded as a self-presentational device to emphasize incompetence and thereby minimize other people's expectations. This would be a logical tactic for someone who was concerned about being found wanting, since it carries the message that the observer should not be disappointed with a low level of performance, and indeed should expect failure. Under some circumstances it might have the additional advantage of earning marks for modesty. Consistent with this view, House (1983) found that self-effacing attributions were only correlated with depression when they were made in the presence of an observer and not when they were made privately.

Other groups of patients demonstrate more obvious self-serving attributions. King (1983) reported that patients with heart disease commonly cited stress, worry, and rheumatic fever in childhood as causes, while tending to ignore other medically accepted factors such as smoking, overeating, and lack of exercise. As she notes, the emphasis on external causation absolves patients from personal responsibility for their illness. The same tendency to attribute negative outcomes to more external and uncontrollable causes than positive outcomes has been demonstrated in diabetic patients by Bradley et al. (1984).

A final example is taken from a study of naturally occurring attributions extracted from family therapy sessions (Stratton et al., 1986). Unsolicited attributions demonstrate very clearly that the definition of the event to be explained is an important factor to be taken into consideration. Father: 'I know I've got to tell him (son) to wash his hands because if I don't he won't.' Here, the event to be explained is expressed in the language of compulsion, i.e. 'I had to do it'. Not only has the speaker already assumed that he had no choice in acting as he did (an attribution that has already taken place), but he assumes that hand-washing is a necessary activity. The causal part of the statement is a claim about the contingent relationship between his actions and his son's actions, one that of course cannot be disproved by the observer. A little later the mother says: 'He (son) was two years younger then so obviously you're going to have to tell him and tell him'. This use of supposedly shared rules or facts as a warrant for an explanation is another common device (Antaki, 1985). It appears likely that individuals in general use the rhetoric of causal explanation in such a way as to present themselves and their actions in the best possible light, and that patients also do this, at least some of the time.

SUMMARY AND CONCLUSIONS

In this chapter we have examined some of the major functions of explanation. The act of explaining is common when people are faced with the unexpected, and this seems particularly true when the unexpected involves illness, accidents, or misfortune. Explanations involve the labelling of experience and the attempt to make sense of it in terms of what we already know about ourselves and the world around us. When we have determined what sort of event we are dealing with, we can try to attribute it to a cause or to a combination of causes. We will be concerned with whether this cause is internal or external to us, whether it is temporary or permanent, and whether it is controllable or uncontrollable. These judgements are likely to affect our self-esteem and our perceptions of future control in similar circumstances. In addition, our attributions for progress in changing our behaviour will contribute to maintaining that change. We will also be concerned with evaluating our behaviour against our own standards of conduct, and in determining what we ought to have done. Finally, we will in some cases want to portray ourselves in a positive light to the outside world, so that the explanations we offer to others may not be the same as we make to ourselves.

Although the evidence is quite strong that explanations mediate a variety of responses to illness and accidents, their role in determining the specific response of depression following stressful life events is far from clear. There is little reason at present to believe that an attribution about the cause of a specific event will influence whether or not a person suffers a depressive onset following that event. Attributional style does appear to be a predictor of subsequent depression, but this effect is not a mediational one, occurring in the absence of stressful events as much as in their presence. Attributions may mediate some component of depression, such as its chronicity, the amount of active coping attempted, or the utilization of social support, but this possibility awaits further research.

In summary, the act of explanation is not a matter of idle armchair reflection. In times of trouble it is an attempt to re-establish our control over the world and to determine what changes need to be made. Sometimes the changes will need to be to ourselves and sometimes to our environment, and sometimes no changes will be possible. Sometimes we may fall back on explanations which relieve us from the burden of taking any action at all. In any event, explanation is almost certain to be an integral part of our reaction to adversity.

REFERENCES

Abramson, L.Y., Seligman, M.E.P., & Teasdale, J.D. (1978). Learned helplessness in humans: critique and reformulation. *Journal of Abnormal Psychology, 87,* 49–74.

Antaki, C. (1985). Ordinary explanation in conversation: Causal structures and their defence. *European Journal of Social Psychology, 15,* 213–230.

Antaki, C., & Fielding, G. (1981). Research into ordinary explanation. In C. Antaki (ed.), *The psychology of ordinary explanations of social behaviour.* London: Academic Press.

Bradley, C., Brewin, C.R., Gamsu, D.S., & Moses, J.L. (1984). Development of scales to measure perceived control of diabetes mellitus and diabetes-related health beliefs. *Diabetic Medicine, 1,* 213–218.

Bradley, C., Gamsu, D., Moses, J.L., Knight, G., Boulton, A.J.M., Drury, J., & Ward, J.D. (1987). The use of diabetes-specific perceived control and health belief measures to predict treatment choice and efficacy in a feasibility study of continuous subcutaneous insulin infusion pumps. *Psychology and Health, 1,* 133–146.

Bradley, G.W. (1978). Self-serving biases in the attribution process: A re-examination of the fact or fiction question. *Journal of Personality and Social Psychology, 36,* 56–71.

Brewin, C.R. (1984). Attributions for industrial accidents: Their relationship to rehabilitation outcome. *Journal of Social and Clinical Psychology, 2,* 156–164.

Brewin, C.R. (1985). Depression and causal attributions: What is their relation? *Psychological Bulletin, 98,* 297–309.

Brewin, C.R. (1986). Internal attribution and self-esteem in depression: A theoretical note. *Cognitive Therapy and Research, 10,* 469–475.

Brewin, C.R., & Antaki, C. (1982). The role of attributions in psychological treatment. In C. Antaki & C.R. Brewin (eds), *Attributions and psychological change*. London: Academic Press.

Brown, G.W., & Harris, T. (1978). *The social origins of depression*. London: Tavistock.

Bulman, R.J., & Wortman, C.B. (1977). Attributions of blame and coping in the 'real world': Severe accident victims react to their lot. *Journal of Personality and Social Psychology, 35*, 351–365.

Chambliss, C., & Murray, E.J. (1979). Cognitive procedures for smoking reduction: Symptom versus efficacy attribution. *Cognitive Therapy and Research, 3*, 91–95.

Clark, D.M., Salkovskis, P.M., & Chalkley, A.J. (1985). Respiratory control as a treatment for panic attacks. *Journal of Behavior Therapy and Experimental Psychiatry, 16*, 23–30.

Colletti, G., & Kopel, S.A. (1979). Maintaining behavior change. *Journal of Consulting and Clinical Psychology, 47*, 614–617.

Coyne, J.C., & Gotlib, I.H. (1983). The role of cognition in depression: A critical appraisal. *Psychological Bulletin, 94*, 472–505.

Field, D. (1976). The social definition of illness. In D. Tuckett (ed.), *An introduction to medical sociology*. London: Tavistock.

Forsyth, D.R. (1980). The functions of attributions. *Social Psychology Quarterly, 43*, 184–189.

Furnham, A., Hillard, A., & Brewin, C.R. (1985). Type A behavior pattern and attributions of responsibility. *Motivation and Emotion, 9*, 39–51.

Hammen, C.L., & deMayo, R. (1982). Cognitive correlates of teacher stress and depressive symptoms: Implications for attributional models of depression. *Journal of Abnormal Psychology, 91*, 96–101.

Hammen, C.L., & Mayol, A. (1982). Depressive and cognitive characteristics of life event types. *Journal of Abnormal Psychology, 91*, 165–174.

Harvey, D.M. (1981). Depression and attributional style: Interpretations of important personal events. *Journal of Abnormal Psychology, 90*, 134–142.

Harvey, J.H., & Galvin, K.S. (1984). Clinical implications of attribution theory and research. *Clinical Psychology Review, 4*, 15–33.

Heider, F. (1958). *The psychology of interpersonal relations*. New York: John Wiley & Sons.

House, W.C. (1983). Variables affecting the outcome between depression and attribution of outcomes. *Journal of Genetic Psychology, 142*, 293–300.

Janoff-Bulman, R. (1979). Characterological versus behavioral self-blame: Inquiries into depression and rape. *Journal of Personality and Social Psychology, 37*, 1798–1809.

Jaspars, J., Hewstone, M., & Fincham, F.D. (1983). Attribution theory and research: The state of the art. In J. Jaspars, F.D. Fincham & M. Hewstone (eds), *Attribution theory and research: Conceptual, developmental, and social dimensions*. London: Academic Press.

Jones, E.E., & Berglas, S. (1978). Control of attributions about the self through self-handicapping strategies: The appeal of alcohol and the role of underachievement. *Personality and Social Psychology Bulletin, 4*, 200–206.

Kelley, H.H. (1967). Attribution theory in social psychology. In D. Levine (ed.), *Nebraska Symposium on Motivation, Vol. 15*. Lincoln: University of Nebraska Press.

Kelley, H.H., & Michela, J.L. (1980). Attribution theory and research. *Annual Review of Psychology, 31*, 457–501.

King, J.B. (1982). The impact of patients' perceptions of high blood pressure on attendance at screening: An attributional extension of the Health Belief Model. *Social Science and Medicine, 16*, 1079–1092.

King, J.B. (1983). Attribution theory and the Health Belief Model. In M. Hewstone (ed.), *Attribution theory: Social and functional extensions*. Oxford: Blackwell.

Lowery, C.R., Denney, D.R., & Storms, M.D. (1979). Insomnia: A comparison of the effects of pill attributions and nonpejorative self-attributions. *Cognitive Therapy and Research, 3*, 161–164.

Miller, I.W., & Norman, W.H. (1979). Learned helplessness in humans: A review and attribution theory model. *Psychological Bulletin, 86,* 93–119.

Peterson, C., & Seligman, M.E.P. (1984). Causal explanations as a risk factor for depression: Theory and evidence. *Psychological Review, 91,* 347–374.

Peterson, C., Schwartz, S.M., & Seligman, M.E.P. (1981). Self-blame and depressive symptoms. *Journal of Personality and Social Psychology, 41,* 253–259.

Rodin, J. (1978). Somatopsychics and attribution. *Personality and Social Psychology Bulletin, 4,* 531–540.

Salkovskis, P.M., & Clark, D.M. (1986). Cognitive and physiological approaches in the maintenance and treatment of panic attacks. In I. Hand & H.-U. Wittchen (eds), *Panic and phobias.* Berlin: Springer-Verlag.

Schachter, S., & Singer, J.E. (1962). Cognitive, social, and physiological determinants of emotional state. *Psychological Review, 69,* 379–399.

Seligman, M.E.P. (1975). *Helplessness: On depression, development, and death.* San Francisco: Freeman.

Sherman, S.J., Skov, R.B., Hervitz, E.P., & Stock, C.B. (1981). The effects of explaining hypothetical future events: From possibility to probability to actuality and beyond. *Journal of Experimental Social Psychology, 17,* 142–158.

Snyder, M.L., Stephan, W.G., & Rosenfield, D. (1978). Attributional egotism. In J.H. Harvey, W.J. Ickes, & R.F. Kidd (eds), *New directions in attribution research,* Vol. 2. Hillsdale, N.J.: Erlbaum.

Sonne, J.L., & Janoff, D.S. (1982). Attributions and the maintenance of behavior change. In C. Antaki & C.R. Brewin (eds), *Attributions and psychological change.* London: Academic Press.

Storms, M.D., & McCaul, K.D. (1976). Attribution processes and the emotional exacerbation of dysfunctional behavior. In J.H. Harvey, W.J. Ickes & R.F. Kidd (eds), *New directions in attribution research,* Vol. 1. Hillsdale, N.J.: Erlbaum.

Storms, M.D., & Nisbett, R.E. (1970). Insomnia and the attribution process. *Journal of Personality and Social Psychology, 16,* 319–328.

Stratton, P., Heard, D., Hanks, H.G.I., Munton, A.G., Brewin, C.R., & Davidson, C. (1986). Coding causal beliefs in natural discourse. *British Journal of Social Psychology, 25,* 299–314.

Taylor, S.E., Lichtman, R.R., & Wood, J.V. (1984). Attributions, beliefs about control, and adjustment to breast cancer. *Journal of Personality and Social Psychology, 46,* 489–502.

Tetlock, P.E. (1980). Examining teacher explanations of pupil performance: An examination of the self-presentation position. *Social Psychology Quarterly, 43,* 283–290.

Weiner, B. (1985). 'Spontaneous' causal thinking. *Psychological Bulletin, 97,* 74–84.

Weiner, B., Graham, S., & Chandler, C. (1982). Pity, anger, and guilt: An attributional analysis. *Personality and Social Psychology Bulletin, 8,* 226–232.

KEY WORDS

Explanation, adaptation, adversity, misfortune, illness, accidents, labelling, causal attribution, learned helplessness, depression, moral evaluation, self-blame, self-presentation.

Handbook of Life Stress, Cognition and Health
Edited by S. Fisher and J. Reason
© 1988 John Wiley & Sons Ltd.

24

Early Loss of Parent and Depression in Adult Life

GEORGE W. BROWN
Royal Holloway and Bedford New College, University of London

INTRODUCTION

Almost all research on the question of early experience and risk of clinical depression has concentrated on the question of whether or not parental loss in childhood plays any aetiological role. Three recent reviews have been sceptical about the possibility (Granville-Grossman, 1968; Crook and Eliot, 1980; Tennant *et al.*, 1980), although one group has since put its negative conclusions in less absolute terms (Tennant *et al.*, 1982). Most reviews have concentrated on death of a parent. A comprehensive review of the impact of separation and divorce on children states 'if effects exist they must be relatively weak or the studies would have been able to demonstrate them much more consistently' (Richards and Dyson, 1982, pp. 35–36). Only one recent review is at all positive, and this admits the evidence is not overwhelming (Lloyd, 1980, p. 534). This bleakness on the part of commentators is both discouraging and puzzling. For, as will be seen, there is in fact now reasonable evidence that an effect does exist; a conclusion that is persuasively reflected in John Bowlby's third volume on *Attachment and loss* which appeared in 1980, albeit relying a good deal on case-history material. It is argued in this chapter that these negative reviews and the inconsistent results that fill the literature are probably the result of shortcomings in method, theory and understanding. First, despite initial appearances, the study of the long-term effects of loss is a highly complex matter, and its proper execution requires considerable subtlety in measurement and design. Second, it now appears clear that it is not loss as such that is critical, but experiences preceding it and, particularly, what follows it in terms of inadequate care. In this sense loss as such is only part of a complex causal chain, and in a particular study there may be various reasons why loss of a parent has not been associated with inadequate care and therefore has not raised the risk of depression. We have, in other words, yet another manifestation of the classic indicator-concept problem. Thus, in a

441

traditional family-based culture, loss of a mother may be typically linked with a range of good alternative avenues of support; alternatively, a particular study may select women who have had inadequate care following loss because such women tend to gravitate, say, to inner city areas, although in the society at large early loss correlates much less highly with inadequate substitute care. The paradox is that failure for such reasons to document a link between early loss and depression would in fact be evidence in favour of the aetiological importance of some experiences of early loss. In more general terms, perhaps the greatest shortcoming of research has been its general failure to consider the highly complex chain of experience that is likely to link loss of a parent with later depression. There has been a failure to consider either the key final link between current adversity and depression, or the history of the person linking early and late experiences. The likely consequences of ignoring the final link between current adversity and development of depression will be considered first.

Recent research, concentrating on psychosocial influences, has suggested a basic model of depression as follows:

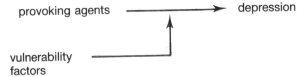

Certain current provoking agents determine when an episode of depression takes place. Most significant are severely threatening events that usually involve an important loss or disappointment, if this is understood to encompass not only loss of a person but loss of a role or even an idea (Brown and Harris, 1978a; 1978b; 1986a). (Loss in the sense of bereavement forms only a small minority of events associated with onset of depression, at least among women in urban settings.) A second and somewhat less important agent concerns ongoing major difficulties such as might be brought about by poor housing or by a husband who drinks heavily. Evidence for the aetiological role of such agents is now impressive. Many research centres have demonstrated the critical role of such severe life events and have shown that onset usually occurs within a month or so of the event (e.g. Finlay-Jones, 1981; Paykel, 1973; Brown and Harris, 1986a).

Such provoking agents probably bring about at least 60% of all episodes of depression among psychiatric patients, and between 80% and 90% among women developing depression in the general population (Brown and Harris, 1986a). However, the chance of such experiences bringing about depression is greatly influenced by the presence of vulnerability factors, such as lack of social support. The bottom arrow in the diagram represents the fact that these factors increase risk only in the presence of the provoking agent, but have no impact without it. There is now good evidence that lack of an intimate tie with a husband acts as a vulnerability factor for women—that is, the risk of depression is increased in its presence once a provoking agent occurs (Brown and Harris, 1986b). Under certain circumstances, having three or more children under the age of 15 living at home can act in this way (e.g. Brown and Harris, 1978a; Campbell et al., 1983;

Martin, 1982; Murphy, 1982; Paykel *et al.*, 1980; Surtees and Ingham, 1980). There is some suggestion that lack of employment may also play such a role, although evidence suggests this process is more complicated. But which factors act in this way is in any case bound to be influenced by the cultural setting (Brown and Prudo, 1981; Prudo *et al.*, 1981).

The importance of taking account of such aetiological factors occurring around the time of the onset of disorders is that the impact on risk of depression of early loss may be masked if 'counterbalancing' influences from current favourable circumstances are not considered. This can be illustrated by results from the first inquiry carried out among women living in Camberwell, an inner-city area of London, with the well-recognized social problems of such areas. In a random sample of women aged between 18 and 65, a definite association emerged between early loss of a parent and psychiatric 'caseness' in the year before our inquiry, i.e. symptoms were of a severity comparable with that seen in out-patient practice. This was established by a clinical-type interview (to be discussed later). When type of early loss was considered, only that of loss of mother before age 11, by either death or separation lasting at least 1 year (and not due to war, which was not considered), had a clear association with depression in the year of our inquiry; the proportion with a loss of a father between birth and 10 years, or between 11 and 16 years, was not statistically different between depressed and other women. Of those with depression, 22% had lost a mother before age 11, compared with 6% of other women (see Brown *et al.*, 1977, for details).

However, the most important result to emerge from this early study concerned evidence that one way in which early loss of a mother relates to onset of depression is through its role as a vulnerability factor. To test for such a vulnerability effect it is essential to deal only with women not already depressed at the start of the year investigated, and to consider whether increased risk of depression is only associated with early loss of a mother when a provoking agent has also occurred. Table 24.1 shows that this is just what happened among women in the general population. There was a much increased risk of depression in the year of inquiry among those who lost their mothers before the age of 11 in the presence of a provoking agent, but no raised risk without such an agent. In fact, none of the 15 women with an early loss of mother but without a provoking agent developed depression, compared with 7 of the 15 with such an agent.

However, if the presence of a provoking agent is ignored, as in the row giving totals, the difference in risk of depression by loss of mother is much attentuated and falls far short of statistical significance.

The second point concerned the effect of ignoring the intervening life history between early loss and current depression. This is likely to be less dramatic in a statistical sense, but its probable impact on theoretical understanding could be even more devastating. For a start, such an approach tends to assume by default that the consequences of early loss are in some way internalized and then carried forward until a provoking agent occurs in adult life. Although such a dormant effect is certainly possible, it seems most unlikely as a general explanation. Fortunately there has been increasing interest in such intervening experiences.

The work of Bowlby (1969; 1973) suggests that while the disruption of parental

Table 24.1 Percentage of women in Camberwell who suffered onset of depression in the year (chronic cases excluded)

| | Loss of mother before age 11 years | |
	Yes	No
	Percentage onset	Percentage onset
Severe event or major difficulty	47 (7/15)[a]	17 (26/149)
None	0 (1/15)[a]	2 (4/240)
Total	23 (7/30)	16 (30/189)

[a] p <0.05, other comparisons n.s.

bonds in childhood is likely to lead to psychopathology in adulthood, certain characteristics of the disruption are of particular aetiological importance. Bowlby emphasizes the role of mourning, but also discusses a number of other factors, particularly the quality of replacement care. The work of Rutter and his colleagues also points to the importance of substitute care (Rutter, 1981; 1982; Quinton et al., 1984; Quinton and Rutter, 1984a; 1984b), particularly discord in the home in childhood: and suggests that these, rather than the experience of loss itself, may be the crucial pathogenic factors (Rutter and Madge, 1976, pp. 205–208).

THE WALTHAMSTOW STUDY

Particular attention will be paid to the results of a study in Walthamstow, North London, specially designed to tackle such a long-term perspective (Harris et al., 1986). Although the study was based on a general population sample, there was deliberate over-selection of women with parental loss in childhood. Demographic features known to relate to affective disorder were monitored during sample selection to ensure that any differences between the loss and no-loss groups could not be explained away as due to contamination. Both current and previous psychiatric symptomatology were recorded. Possible interference from effects due to sex were accounted for by deciding from the outset to study only women. The interview lasted on average 4 hours and was usually carried out in the woman's own home. Semi-structured tape-recorded interviews allowed the kind of flexibility required for the combination of exploratory and confirmatory research that was planned (Brown, 1974). Previous experience with this style of data collection had shown that high levels of validity and reliability could be achieved (Brown, 1974; Brown and Harris, 1978a; 1986b; Tennant et al., 1979; Parry et al., 1981), that respondent bias could be controlled by using a contextual form of measurement, and that investigator bias could be minimized by the use of consensus ratings (Brown and Harris, 1979; 1986b). This style of interviewing had been developed to bridge the gap between the systematic, but often somewhat mechanical, measurement procedures of epidemiology, and the clinical insights of the case-history method.

Current depression was assessed using a semi-structured clinical-type interview, the Present State Examination (PSE; Wing *et al.*, 1974). The PSE has as its core a glossary of terms and definitions about specific symptoms, and it has been established that medical and non-medical interviewers can reach satisfactory reliability in rating specific items (Cooper *et al.*, 1977; Wing *et al.*, 1977). A number of further stages were added to these initial ratings. One of these was to rate women considered to have experienced a definite psychiatric syndrome in the year before interview as cases, and those with lower levels of disturbance as borderline cases. The threshold which underlay the distinction between a case and a borderline case was based on the level of severity of symptoms commonly met with in out-patient psychiatric clinics.

In order for a woman to be considered a case there had to be both depressed mood and four or more of the following ten symptoms: hopelessness, suicidal ideas or actions, weight loss, early waking, delayed sleep, poor concentration, neglect due to brooding, loss of interest, self-depreciation, and anergia. Usually many other PSE symptoms were also present. These items have been shown statistically to underlie our clinical criteria of depression (Finlay-Jones *et al.*, 1980). Recent research suggests that this threshold for caseness is comparable to, if perhaps a little higher than, other thresholds in use such as ID level-5 when using the CATEGO programme with the PSE and RDC criteria for major depression (Dean *et al.*, 1983; Brown *et al.*, 1985). (For further reference to CATEGO and ID level see Wing and Sturt, 1978.) The great majority of the conditions were entirely depressive or involved an important depressive component. For the purpose of this chapter I will henceforth simply refer to depression, although in some surveys this included a few disorders in which anxiety was primary.

After obtaining information about current symptoms, the interviewer asked whether the respondent had ever experienced certain key symptoms at any point in her life. These key symptoms included depressed mood, hopelessness, suicidal feelings, panic attacks and other bouts of anxiety, agitation and nervous debility or exhaustion (op. cit. for details). We were aware that information about symptoms as far back as this would be bound to be subject to error; instead of the three-point grouping 'case', 'borderline case', and 'normal', previous episodes were grouped on a four-point scale: 'probable case', 'possible case', 'probable borderline case' and 'probably no episode'.

Table 24.2 provides a simplified summary of the basic findings in terms of type of parental loss and caseness of depression in the 12 months before interview (see Harris *et al.*, 1986, Table 1, for full version). As in the original Camberwell finding, the overriding importance of loss of mother is confirmed; but in this larger series there was a clear suggestion that the influence could extend beyond the age of 11, although it is probable that the impact between the ages of 11 and 17 is somewhat less strong. Rates were high both for loss of mother by death and for loss by separation. However, the separations included a number which we named 'aberrant' because they involved definite elements of rejection or stigma (for example, where the children were sent away because they were illegitimate), and these had a particularly high rate of current depression. There was therefore already at this early stage of the analysis an implication that it may not be

Table 24.2   Type of parental loss in childhood and caseness of depression in the 12 months before interview — Walthamstow series

Age at loss (years)	Percentage with depression		
	0–10	11–17	All ages
Loss of mother (including any who also had loss of father)	26 (24/94)	16 (6/45)	22 (30/139)[a]
Loss of mother only	30 (6/20)	17 (5/29)	22 (11/49)[b]
Loss of father only	10 (4/41)	Not studied	
Comparison series	4 (2/45)[a,b]		

[a] $p < 0.02$.
[b] $p < 0.05$.

separation as such which is the critical factor, but circumstances surrounding the loss. Loss of father, as in the Camberwell Study, was by contrast unimportant, although there was a hint that loss of a father by separation might be related to a somewhat raised risk.

When the lifetime experience of depression was considered, the same patterning of results emerged. But separation from father without loss of mother emerged in a clearer light: 10% had been in-patients compared with none of those without loss ($p < 0.05$). Such in-patient experience was also raised in the separation from mother group, but was only 3% in the death of mother group (see Harris et al., 1986, Table 2).

One possible objection to these results stems from the size of the comparison series, which was deliberately kept small. Fortunately, it was possible to make a further test, which provides a more convincing confirmation. In the course of work on a different project, another section of the research team interviewed 70 married women also living in Walthamstow, selected at random and aged between 18 and 45; and it is possible to use them to provide a second comparison series (O'Connor and Brown, 1984). When women who had lost their mother by death before the age of 17 were matched with this second series in terms of social class, age, marital status, and stage of family development, the rate of depression of those with a loss was almost four times greater—7/19 versus 6/59 ($p < 0.02$).

EARLY LOSS OF MOTHER AND EXPERIENCE OF LACK OF CARE

As an explanation of these results concerning loss of mother, we have placed particular weight on the quality of care given to children after the loss of their mother. Table 24.3 suggests that experience of high parental indifference, peak experience of suggested stigma, and overall long-term emotional change are the most critical experiences. The degree of overlap between these three scales was high—not unexpectedly, given that experience of parental indifference was often exactly the change in atmosphere which had led to the high score on overall long-term emotional change, and that the stigma was often suggested by none other than the surrogate parent whose verbal abuse of the child had caused the

Table 24.3   The relationship between certain global measures of care in childhood and current depression, Walthamstow series (loss of mother group only)

High values in:	Percentage with depression	
	Factor present	Factor absent
Overall practical change in childhood	28 (13/47)	18 (17/93) n.s.
Overall emotional change in childhood	31 (16/52)	16 (14/87) p <0.05
Peak experience of suggested stigma	36 (10/28)	18 (20/11) p <0.05
Peak experience of rejection	33 (8/24)	19 (22/115) n.s.
Peak experience of discord	20 (11/54)	22 (19/85) n.s.
Peak experience of anxiety in the home	21 (8/38)	22 (22/101) n.s.
Any experience of high parental indifference	36 (15/42)	15 (15/97) p <0.01
Any experience of low parental control	29 (9/31)	19 (21/108) n.s.
Any experience of low parental control *excluding* those with high parental indifference	35 (7/20)	10 (8/77) p <0.01
Any experience of parental indifference	35 (22/62)	10 (8/77) p <0.001

high score on indifference. This overlap with high scores on parental (or parental surrogate) indifference occurred for most of the other variables in Table 24.3 except for experience of 'low' parental control. We therefore formed an index combining high indifference and low control, as the measure most predictive of current depression. Aggregating these two particular variables also made theoretical sense since they both implied a lack of positive experiences, unlike the other factors in Table 24.3 which involved definite negative experiences. Both represent inadequacy in the way the surviving or substitute parent related to the child after the loss, and indicate neglect of the child, materially as well as emotionally. 'Low control' arose when the supervision of the child was so negligent that she was apparently allowed to do more or less what she liked. The unusual phrase 'we ran wild' recurred spontaneously in several accounts rated low on control. This rating was most often made where the father alone was responsible for the child and appeared to be too busy or preoccupied to be able to look after her properly.

Thirty-five per cent (22/62) of women with either or both these experiences were currently depressed compared with only 10% (8/77) among the remaining women with loss of mother. The association was identical for the death and separation groups. It has already been noted that there was a particularly high rate of depression among girls whose separation from mother was 'aberrant'. In this group of eighteen, the child was sent away from both parents at a time when there was no obvious socially acceptable reason for the separation. In six of the eighteen, the girls had been removed from their families where they were being neglected, battered or interfered with sexually; in four instances they had been illegitimate and were left with the maternal grandmother; in four there was no clear reason why the mother had sent the child away, and in another four a miscellany of reasons of a rejecting nature applied, for example, the paternal

Table 24.4 Depression and index of lack of care by type of loss — Walthamstow series

Lack of care index	Percentage with depression					
	Death of mother	Separation from mother	Separation from father (without loss of mother)	Death of father (without loss of mother)	No loss of parent	No loss of mother
Lack of care	34 (13/38)	36 (12/33)	50 (2/4)	0 (0/1)	13 (1/8)	21 (3/13)
Adequate care	10 (4/40)	4 (1/28)	12 (2/17)	0 (0/19)	3 (1/37)	4 (3/73)
	$p < 0.01$	$p < 0.01$	$p < 0.10$	n.s.	n.s.	$p < 0.01$

grandmother and three single aunts wanted to have a child and 'borrowed' her for years. In an attempt to characterize the rather unusual, stigmatizing character of these eighteen separations, we have called them *aberrant separations*, and the rate of depression of 44% (8/18) among them was greater than the 12% (5/43) among the remaining separations. The joint index of parental indifference and low parental control showed only a moderate relationship to such separations (gamma 0.30). That it is not closer probably stems from the fact that the measure of indifference and control in the Walthamstow women applied to the period *after* the initial loss, which for some who had experienced an aberrant separation was an improvement on the original family situation. The two measures had also been used only to characterize the behaviour of parents and parent surrogates, and not the different situations obtaining in institutional care. Since some of the women with aberrant separations went into institutions and stayed there throughout childhood, they had not been considered at all in terms of the parental measures and were scoring zero when there was evidence that they had received inadequate care. To take account of this, aberrant separation was included with the two other measures in a trial threefold index of *lack of care*.

Lack of care defined by the index is highly related to current depression (see Table 24.4), and works in a parallel way in both the death of mother and the separation from mother groups. The very low rate of lack of care in the death of father group explains the very low rate of depression in that group. When those with lack of care are excluded, the rate of depression in the mother-loss group is the same as the overall rate for those with no loss of parent; in other words, it is lack of care rather than loss of mother itself that is important.

These results have recently been replicated in their essentials in a quite different survey in Islington, London, based on a random survey of working-class women (or single mothers) with a child living at home (Bifulco *et al.*, 1987). Parental indifference and control were measured over the whole of childhood and in this sense any aberrant separation automatically became an index of parental indifference and was thus an unnecessary measure. Unlike the study in Walthamstow, the Islington survey collected material on provoking agents and the onset of depression in the follow-up year, and a direct test of the role of lack of care as a vulnerability factor was therefore also possible. There were 45 women in the sample with lack of care who were not depressed at first interview and could thus be included in the vulnerability analysis. Among women with a provoking agent in the follow-up year, 33% (10/30) with lack of care became depressed compared with 17% (20/120) of remaining women (p = 0.07; Table 24.5). The presence of lack of care in childhood also doubled the likelihood of experiencing a provoking agent and therefore appears to have increased the risk of depression in two ways.

These results are so clearcut that they must raise a question about the validity of the lack of care measure. With this in mind in the Walthamstow enquiry, 20 pairs of sisters were separately interviewed about arrangements after the death of their mother. When compared for periods in which they experienced the same household arrangement, agreement concerning the quality of care was high (Bifulco, 1985). Additional evidence for validity is provided by the associations between lack of care and some of the simpler, 'harder' measures involving family structure

Table 24.5   Loss of mother and lack of care as vulnerability factors for onset of depression
            — Islington series

	Percentage with onset of depression	
	Provoking agent present	Provoking agent absent
(1) High parental indifference and low control	43 (3/7) ⎫	0 (0/13) ⎫
(2) High parental indifference only	33 (7/21) ⎬ 30 (10/30)	0 (0/1) ⎬ 0 (0/17)
(3) Low control only	0 (0/2) ⎭	0 (0/3) ⎭
(4) Neither	17 (20/120)	1 (2/136) n.s.

Rows (1)+(2)+(3) vs (4): $p = 0.07$, 1 d.f.
Rows (1)+(2) vs (3)+(4): $p < 0.05$, 1 d.f.

such as whether women had lived with surrogate siblings for a year or more at any time. Where there had been a definite refusal by another relative to take in the child after the loss of the mother, lack of care had been rated twice as often. Some simple indicators of family structure also emerged as underpinning the softer measure of lack of care, for example whether the young girl had to run the household herself, how efficiently it was run, how surrogate parents treated surrogate siblings in comparison to their treatment of the subject and so on. (For further discussion see Bifulco, 1985.)

It may not be accidental that the studies which have produced a similar patterning of results used identical categories to those employed in Walthamstow and concentrated only on women (Roy, 1978; 1981). Roy used the same one-year duration threshold for separations as in the original Camberwell survey, and took the same age range for the span of childhood. He found maternal loss of both types to be associated with depression. Separation from father, but not death of father, was also associated with depression.

There has been no suggestion that death of a mother leads to a greater risk of subsequent disorder among women than separation from her. But since the relative frequency of the various kinds of separation, especially of the aberrant kind, will probably differ between populations, it would be hazardous to place much weight on the *lack* of a difference in prevalence of depression between deaths and separations. The important conclusion is that *type* of separation appears to be related to depression, and that this is a reflection of the importance of lack of care. Separation from mother due to illness or parental divorce may be associated with depression in some populations if the substitute arrangements exhibit lack of care. (For the impact of parental divorce on children see Wallerstein and Kelly (1975) and Hetherington *et al.* (1978) who describe as crucial certain aspects of parental behaviour closely akin to indifference and low control.)

The highlighting of lack of care as the feature contributing most powerfully to the impact upon rates of current depression helps to explain the differences between losing a father and a mother. It has been, at least until quite recently, easier for a mother to take on the breadwinning role after the death of her husband, and to combine this with a continuity in her caregiving role as a mother, than it is for a father to combine adequate 'mothering' with the role of chief provider. The low rate of lack of care in the death of father group (as compared with the no-loss-of-parent group) bears witness to this. It does not follow, of course, that the patterning of results concerning type of loss and depression will obtain in all societies. Moreover, if the implications of the finding on lack of care are followed through, then, as family 'role reversals' continue to become more prevalent through the 1980s, the differences in the experiences of depression may become more evenly distributed between the mother-loss and father-loss groups.

These data on lack of care, loss of mother and depression accord with two other studies concerned with quality of upbringing after parental loss. Birtchnell reported interesting results concerning the quality both of the replacement experience after losses of mother in childhood and of the pre-separation maternal relationship, suggesting that poor relationships influence the degree and character of depression and dependency (Birtchnell, 1980; Kennard and Birtchnell, 1982). Adam found not only a significantly higher rate of loss of parent before age 25 among those attempting suicide than among his comparison group, but also that this effect was potentiated by a 'chaotic' family environment after the loss (Adam et al., 1982). His case descriptions suggest that what distinguishes his 'chaotic' from his 'unstable' category is similar to our lack of care: it is the *emotional* stability that seems crucial, not just the absence of *practical* changes in the family environment. In the Walthamstow study, discord in the home was not importantly related to adult depression, contrary to the predictions of Rutter and Madge (1976). Lack of care may prove to be specific to depression, and discord in the home may well turn out to play a much more important role in bringing about other forms of psychiatric disorder, particularly conduct disorder in children and its sequelae in adulthood. It is also necessary to take into account that we have been dealing with female samples and that boys have been shown to be more susceptible to the effects of discord in the home than girls (Rutter, 1982; Hetherington, 1979).

The importance for depression in adulthood of the dimensions of parental indifference and low control has also emerged with the use of two other research instruments. Crook and colleagues, using Schaeffer's Children's Reports of Parental Behaviours Inventory (Schaeffer, 1963), found hostile detachment more closely related to depression than rejection by mother; depression was also associated with both lax discipline and extreme autonomy, although the authors found this 'somewhat surprising' since patients also scored higher than normals on subscales such as hostile control and control through guilt, which reflected tight parental control (Crook et al., 1981). The dimensions of care and control in Parker's 25-item checklist Parental Bonding Instrument (PBI) are very similar, although the lack of care index might be considered a harder measure as it is based on the more detailed information of an interview with specific probes designed to obtain a narrative account of experience. Low care, as measured by the PBI, related to depression and anxiety in adults (Parker, 1979; 1981; 1983). The similarity of these dimensions to the lack of care index is also encouraging in another respect, namely, evidence as to their validity, since in retrospective studies there is always the possibility that reporting bias might have contributed to the association of such measures with depression through the selection of negative memories consequent upon the disordered mood state. Parker found that reports given by mothers as to how they had formerly treated their now adult children were correlated with reports of the mothers' caregiving given by the children themselves (Parker, 1981). The result of our own validity study with twenty pairs of sisters is equally encouraging. Furthermore, some form of construct validity is suggested since the index of lack of care is theoretically appropriate within our cognitive model of depression (Brown and Harris, 1978a, pp. 264–269). This proposed that the level of self-esteem was crucial in determining the cognitions of women experiencing stressors which typically provoke depression. Those with low self-esteem would be more likely to generalize any feelings of hopelessness arising in reaction to the provoking agent and would thus be more likely to experience the cognitive triad which Beck has identified as the core feature of clinical depression (Beck, 1967). This model has now been tested in a prospective study where low self-esteem measured at time 1 was confirmed as an important predictor of depressive onset between time 1 and time 2 (Brown and Bifulco, 1985; Brown et al., 1986c). It was proposed that intimate confiding in a marriage worked as a protection against depression through its prior impact upon self-esteem as much as through its prediction of practical support in a crisis. In the same way, since the regard of others is often a source of one's own self-regard, those exposed to deficient care in childhood are likely to place a lower estimate on their own worth, even perhaps when childhood is past, and will thus prove more vulnerable to depression in the face of provoking agents.

A LIFE HISTORY APPROACH

However, the account so far has not faced the critical question of how experiences surrounding lack of care manage to increase risk of depression so many years later. Some picture of what might be occurring begins to emerge, but first it is necessary to place what we have discussed so far in a more theoretical context. No account can ignore the seminal contribution of John Bowlby.

Bowlby's recent review of childhood antecedents of disordered mourning and of clinical depression and anxiety notes how the nature of attachment and how disruption of the initial bond with mother may influence subsequent personality development (Bowlby, 1980; see also Bowlby, 1969; 1973). In the third volume of his trilogy on *Attachment and loss*, he argues that even young children are capable of successful mourning, but that at any age mourning can take a pathological course in terms of either chronic mourning or the absence of conscious grieving. Children are particularly likely to experience pathological mourning because of their dependence on adults for comfort and for information to help them understand the reasons for the loss. Often this support is not forthcoming, perhaps as a result of the surviving parent's own grief, and the child finds it more difficult to accept the fact of the loss.

Bowlby considers a current sense of helplessness or hopelessness as the key characteristic of depression. He relates the likelihood of experiencing such feelings in adult life to three kinds of experience in childhood: never attaining a stable and secure relationship with parents; being told repeatedly that one is unlovable, inadequate, or incompetent; and experiencing loss of a parent with other disagreeable consequences that are not easily changed. His emphasis on the importance of pathological mourning fits in here, although these three types of experiences might occur before, or indeed without, the loss of parent. All are important in so far as they impart 'cognitive biases' of a kind that lead to seeing later loss in terms of personal failure or to seeing oneself as doomed to frustration in restoring or replacing what has been lost. In his final volume, he appears to change somewhat the emphasis of his earlier formulations by giving greater weight to external circumstances in determining whether or not mourning following loss is pathological. In childhood such 'unfavourable' circumstances are stated to include poor family relationships before the loss, separation from the surviving parent after the loss, having to fend for oneself, and having to look after a parent.

Loss in childhood associated with such unfavourable circumstances increases the chance of disordered mourning; and a failure to complete the work of mourning means that the child does not withdraw attachment from the lost parent and therefore cannot reinvest in any substitute parent. The importance of unsuccessful mourning therefore lies not so much in a failure to express grief, but in a predisposition to distortion in subsequent relationships and to various cognitive biases that continue into adult life. It is through these cognitive biases that distortions in later attachment behaviour tend to occur. Bowlby (1980) outlines three types of cognitive bias that result from disordered mourning in childhood; compulsive care-giving relationships, ambivalence and anxiety in relationships, and a show of independence from close ties ('compulsive self-reliance'). However, the perspective is far from being couched in deterministic terms. The impact of such bias can be avoided, or the bias corrected, if the person happens to make a secure attachment at some point. Bowlby suggests that favourable experience can push a person away from pathological development; unfortunately, the circumstances that are conducive to such a reorientation are as yet poorly formulated and little documented.

Others emphasize far more the importance of the favourable circumstances dealt with by Bowlby. Rutter's review of research has been particularly influential. In the second edition of *Maternal deprivation reassessed*, published in 1981, he discusses research relating to personal loss, particularly in relation to institutional care and its link with childhood disorders such as affectionless psychopathy and delinquency. Rutter is critical of Bowlby's emphasis on the disruption of the bond with a mother as such, and underlines the importance of social circumstances surrounding the loss that bring disruption and disturbance rather than the loss itself. The actual distress experienced by children when separated from their mothers can be moderated if adequate substitute care is provided. Rutter distinguishes failure to make the original bond with mother in the first place from the disruption of the relationship. He argues that the former is likely to be more damaging, pointing to evidence that very young children put into care show more signs of disturbance. He also emphasizes the critical importance of the nature of family relationships in the home before the loss. Where loss of a parent has come from separation, this is often linked to ongoing family tension and discord, and in such instances delinquency among children is more likely to occur than in families where a parent has been lost by death and perhaps ongoing tension and discord have been relatively low. He also makes the important general point that it is necessary to characterize losses by their surrounding circumstances: that, for instance, separations due to holidays or physical illness have fewer disturbing effects than those of family break-up.

Indeed, both Rutter and Bowlby show a tendency to move away from the role of early loss to emphasize early experience in general. This may well be correct, and the implications of the results concerning lack of care do just this—that is, emphasize the importance of studying early loss as a way of introducing us to the general impact of childhood experience in adult depression (see Table 24.4, which shows a high rate of depression among those with lack of care but no loss of mother). Rutter cites a study in London in which children from broken homes were less disturbed than those in intact but disturbed homes (Rutter, 1971). However, methodological pitfalls are everywhere in this research and, as Richards and Dyson (1982) point out, the tension in the disturbed homes is contemporaneous, while the separation may have taken place some time ago and the disturbance that followed it may, to some extent, have abated. To draw any conclusion about relative impact, it would be essential either to deal with children coping with a recent separation or to take account of the time element in some other way. Comparative studies of the quality reported by Rutter are extremely rare, and it would therefore meanwhile be wise to retain the possibility that loss of a parent can be a peculiarly potent stress factor for a child.

This very brief overview is sufficient to make the point that differences between the views exemplified by Bowlby and Rutter are probably best seen as related to emphasis. We see at present no reason why their formulations should not eventually prove compatible. Nonetheless, it is important to recognize that there are differences in emphasis that research will need to explore.

While we have been much influenced by Bowlby's formulation, we are much in favour of Rutter's central concern with the role of social circumstances leading to, surrounding, and following the loss. We are sympathetic not only because we believe it to be correct, but because we see no effective way for research to proceed in this extraordinarily complex field without the detailed documentation of the circumstances surrounding the loss and the subsequent biography of the person as child and adult up to the time of any depressive disorder. The cognitive biases emphasized by Bowlby will be difficult to study because their measurement is likely to be influenced by the very thing we wish to understand—depression in adult life. Emphasis on environmental circumstances is therefore critical, if only because their documentation is less likely to be subject to bias due to the presence of current psychiatric disorder; and insofar as they can be shown to link to cognitive biases, they are likely to provide the most convincing evidence, albeit indirect, of the presence of the intrapsychic processes emphasized by Bowlby.

While Bowlby's and Rutter's views are consistent with the results so far presented, it may be useful to distinguish two possible chains of explanation inherent in their formulations. First, that it is the cognitive biases resulting from the experiences surrounding early loss that are the critical intervening factors; and that it is these which leave a woman vulnerable to later depression following a major disappointment. Such biases will probably be reflected in the relationships she has formed, but it is the underlying cognitive sets that are critical. A second view would downplay cognitive bias as such and place overriding weight upon the external circumstances in later life—while not denying that cognitive biases may have played a significant role in creating these. Thus, to continue our example, let us take a key variable which is related to depression in adult life, namely premarital pregnancy. Certain cognitive biases, perhaps expressed as a wish to be looked after, may relate to early experience and may also increase chances of a premarital pregnancy. However, whether or not this leads to depression in adult life will entirely depend on how things turn out. How 'suitable' is the man involved in the pregnancy? Does she get married? How does the marriage turn out? Does the fact of the premarital pregnancy lead to a long history of adverse experiences, say, a series of pregnancies in a short space of time, unsuitable and overcrowded housing, continual tension with mother-in-law, and so on. Consistent with this emphasis would be the assertion that the experience of premarital pregnancy, whether or not there were associated enduring cognitive biases, would be associated with depression as long as the depression resulted in adverse later experiences. Pushing this more sociological, less psychological strand of explanation further back in time, it could be argued that the premarital pregnancy itself need not in any way be the result of a cognitive bias, but could be entirely determined by untoward experiences in adolescence. Thus some women might be at greater risk of premarital pregnancy simply because, through circumstances resulting from the loss, they find themselves at the time of finishing their schooling with no settled base, perhaps because they do not get on well with their stepmothers or because they have nowhere to go when they emerge from institutional life.

Figure 24.1 depicts these two strands of explanation, extending the original Camberwell aetiological model of depressive onset to take account of the role of the inner world of the individual along the bottom line and the outer world along the top. The mutual interdependence of these worlds, in fact, persists throughout the person's life span, but for simplicity's sake the vertical arrows representing these influences have only been included at the time just before onset. This is the point where the level of ongoing self-esteem may prove critical in determining whether or not onset of depression occurs, and it is the consequence of both strands. It is when the roles available to a woman in her particular social setting determine her ongoing level of self-esteem, and at this point also her self-esteem influences the use she chooses to make of the resources available to her in her social environment. My own view is that both processes are at work and that there is a great deal of interplay between enduring cognitive biases and later experience, and it is to some of this evidence I now turn.

The Walthamstow enquiry has produced reasonably convincing evidence about some possible linking strands between loss of mother, lack of care and subsequent depression that places a good deal of weight on early relationships with the opposite sex and current class position (Harris *et al.*, 1987). These factors might be

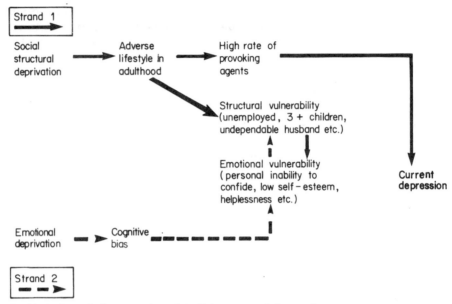

FIG. 24.1   Speculative causal model of the onset of depression.

expected to occur in the top strand 1 of the schematic outline. Figure 24.2 deals
with structural deprivation and adverse lifestyles and fills in some of the bare
outline. For understanding the commentary on this figure it is important to bear in
mind that premarital pregnancy was associated with early loss of mother and lack
of care, and also highly related to current depression, but *only* among working-
class women.

A simple index was devised to reflect coping with such a premarital pregnancy.
It was based upon the idea that premarital pregnancies may operate as a trap in
which a woman may become ensnared by marrying a man she would not otherwise
have chosen. It grouped together, on the one hand, reactions such as seeking a
termination, only marrying the father if he had already been intended as the
future spouse, or choosing as a husband a man who was not the father of the child,
and on the other, marrying the father only because of the illegitimate conception,
becoming a long-term single parent, or bearing the child only to have it adopted
later. The former group of reactions we called 'effective' and the latter 'less
effective'.

With the link of premarital pregnancy and depression occurring only among
working-class women in mind, the figure shows that in Walthamstow low class
father is barely associated with lack of care, and the two are not shown as directly
linked. Therefore, although lack of care is highly associated with premarital
pregnancy, the actual size of the association between father's class and premarital
pregnancy is negligible, and again no link is shown with father's class. It is only the
style of coping with premarital pregnancy which gives importance to father's class
position in the model—when the father was working class and coping less
effective, almost all were currently working class, and this in turn was highly
related to depression.

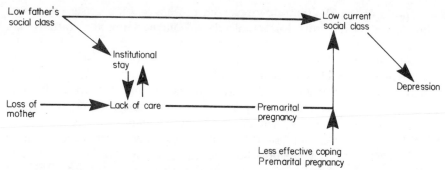

FIG. 24.2 Diagram to represent links from loss of mother to current depression via premarital pregnancy and low social class.

Why should less effective coping play this role? As we defined it in this particular study, a woman's class status is almost entirely determined by her husband's occupation. Therefore such interaction between father's working-class status and less effective coping with premarital pregnancy may simply be indicating a woman's failure, for varying reasons, to have become involved with a man who would achieve middle-class status. One explanation for the link between premarital pregnancy and current working-class status would thus involve the range and kind of social contacts of the girls at the time of the pregnancy. However, there is also the added possibility that the circumstances surrounding the birth and its consequences may have hindered some of the men with whom the women went on to live from achieving middle-class status.

It is, however, the links with depression that are critical, and here the findings are complex, particularly insofar as current social class is involved. Although some research.workers have questioned the link between working-class position and depression, there has been a growing body of evidence to confirm the association, and it was not surprising to find it replicated in the Walthamstow survey (Brown and Harris, 1982). It has already been noted that premarital pregnancy plays a crucial part in the class results, and this association is critically determined by a woman's relationship in adulthood with members of the opposite sex, both in early adulthood (premarital pregnancy) and currently (undependability of partner), since these factors are associated both with depression and with working-class status. It is notable that, once current class is taken into account, effectiveness of the coping with premarital pregnancy is unrelated to depression. For working-class women, it is therefore the mere fact of premarital pregnancy, whether or not there was effective coping, that is most important for depression. This implies that it is the longer-term consequences of a premarital pregnancy, rather than the experience of the pregnancy itself and the immediate coping reactions to it, which contribute most to depression. In other words, the high rate of depression among those who showed less effective coping with premarital pregnancy stems from the fact that they are much more likely to be currently working class with low intimacy and undependable husbands, and also with more provoking agents. Coping with premarital pregnancy does not add anything to the association between working-class status and depression over and above premarital pregnancy itself.

The reports of the Walthamstow research present a complex set of results, including certain predictors for middle-class women. However, rather than pursue these, further evidence concerning such long-term links will now be considered. Of particular relevance is a prospective study following 81 women who were in care in childhood into adulthood (Quinton et al., 1984). This identified a very similar aetiological pathway to the one just described, although focusing upon the women's current parenting rather than upon depression. A short courtship and a teenage pregnancy were more common among the women who had been in care in childhood than in a quasi-random general population comparison group, and contributed to poorer psychosocial functioning and breakdown in parenting behaviour as indicated by admission into care of the next generation (see also Rutter et al., 1983). Premarital pregnancy as such was not examined, but may well have underlain these findings. In a parallel study of 44 families with a child currently in care and a randomly selected comparison group of 49 families in the same borough, Quinton and colleagues were able to characterize the spouses, or cohabitees, of their subjects at a time before marriage or cohabitation, and it emerged that even before their partnerships began, the spouses of the women who had been in care had more 'deviant histories' than those in the comparison group (Quinton and Rutter, 1984a; 1984b). Not only had they experienced more disruption in childhood (being sent to institutions, or subject to parental discord and police contact), but they had already exhibited signs of disturbance themselves, such as persistent truanting or leaving home for a negative reason before the age of 19. These studies suggest that the emphasis of our earlier interpretation of the links between premarital pregnancy and undependability of partner may need to be shifted further towards the earlier characteristics of the men with whom women may become 'trapped', and away from too narrow a concentration upon the impact of settling down too soon. Clearly, however, there is no compulsion to favour one of these aetiological pathways over the other; in the end, it is probably the combination of many of the factors identified which pushes a woman into depression.

One of the limitations of the Walthamstow enquiry was that 'soft' variables concerning cognitive sets were collected retrospectively and provoking agents in the current situation were not collected at all. For a picture of how early experience might relate to the inception of new cases of depression it is necessary to return to the subsequent Islington enquiry. It should, however, be kept in mind that the women were selected as a high-risk group for depression and included 20% with a single-mother status, a figure a good deal higher than the general UK population.

In line with the conception of strand 1 (external) and strand 2 (internal), the Islington enquiry provides a series of measures of the women's circumstances, attitudes and behaviour which could be seen as covering strand 1 and 2 factors at the time of our first contact with the women. The instrument, the Self Evaluation and Social Support Schedule (SESS), deals not only with external manifestations, but also with how activities are internally represented (O'Connor and Brown, 1984; Brown et al., 1986b). Following the Camberwell model, we first considered vulnerability in terms of self-esteem, taking as an index *negative evaluation of self* (based just on negative comments the woman made about herself during the course of the first interview). It was possible to show that it did act as a vulnerability factor—that is, there was an increase in risk of depression associated with it *only* in the presence of a stressor (see Brown *et al.*, 1986, for details). This cumbersome label has been used, rather than low self-esteem, to emphasize that it is based only on negative comments. Depression was over twice as likely to occur following a stressor among those with such negative evaluation.

The quality of relationships at the time of first interview was measured in many ways. One of the simplest was an index of interpersonal difficulty and tension in the home, based on the presence of negative interaction with child or husband in the home or a difficulty involving them lasting at least 6 months.

Figure 24.3 illustrates that, for those without current difficulties or tension, the proportion with negative evaluation of self is the same, regardless of whether or not there was lack of care or premarital pregnancy. (This is shown by the lines that meet in the extreme left of the diagram.) But *with* difficulties and tension, negative evaluation of self increases disproportionately among those with pre-marital pregnancy or lack of care. The important message would seem to be that the past *can* have an influence on negative evaluation, but *only* in so far as it is linked via troubles in the present.

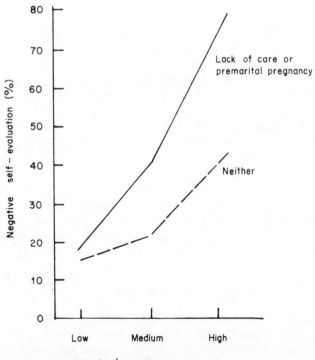

FIG. 24.3 Percentage with negative self-evaluation at first interview, by difficulty/negative interaction index and early adversity.

More complex analyses have produced essentially comparable results (e.g. Brown, 1987). The effect of adverse early experience on later risk of depression appears to be very largely moderated by current adversity. However, it would be foolish not to recognize that the issues are extraordinarily complex, and at present such results must be seen as exploratory. There is, for example, some hint that early adversity may link with a certain style of attachment which may indirectly raise risk of depression. In a recent study, a small group of women was identified who had early inadequate care *and* who had shown 'non-optimal' confiding at the time of our first contact—that is, who had developed relationships with people in whom they confided (in a fashion), but in which confiding did not elicit support and which often let them down in a crisis (Andrews and Brown, 1987). Early 'lack of care' was highly related to such non-optimal confiding. Those with such early lack of care and non-optimal confiding at first contact had a particularly high risk of depression during the following year. We strongly suspect, but as yet have no systematic evidence, that the pattern of non-optimal confiding goes back some way in time. Therefore there is some possibility that the high risk of depression among this group of women once a provoking agent has occurred is related to a persistent style of attachment which in turn is related to experiences of rejection in childhood.

Although attachment theory had its roots in the study of clinical issues, there is no systematic evidence as yet linking it to the development of specific psychiatric disorders such as depression (Cummings, 1987). There are, of course, many fairly obvious possible links with the framework just outlined. There is, for example, a parallel between the cognitive biases and insecure internal working models of attachment and the kind of cognitive schema that appears to play a direct role in the onset of adult depression (Bretherton and Waters, no date). A major challenge is to try to sort out how far contributions from the past are via long-term cognitive sets, perhaps largely outside awareness, and how far they are via environmental conditions, to which, of course, such sets may well have contributed. In the end, the answer is likely to be both are at work, but formulating questions at this stage in such oppositional terms may be helpful. In short, the kind of research that has been outlined potentially fits well into the new approach of developmental psychopathology. This studies the long-term pathways to disorder in the context of the study of individual adaptation and maladaptation rather than in terms of group trends (Rutter *et al.*, 1986; Cummings, 1987), and progress on the antecedent factors to adult depression can be confidently expected over the next decade.

SUMMARY AND CONCLUSIONS

The evidence reviewed indicates that early loss of a mother can be powerfully linked to depression in adult life. However, there is every reason to believe that the size of this link will be related to the kind of population studied. Thus, Birtchnell's finding of a lack of any association in middle-class Sussex is understandable in terms of the class distribution of provoking agents and vulnerability factors. The same general point holds for the distribution of aberrant separation xperiences. It is highly unlikely that the kind of extreme experiences involved are andomly distributed among those undergoing a separation from a mother; such eparations are almost certainly more frequent among women in just those areas vhere there are more provoking agents anyway. (The study of psychiatric patients ntroduces additional complications—Brown *et al.*, 1986.)

Two main lines of influence have been suggested which may well interact to ıave a joint impact on current feelings of self-esteem and risk of depression. The nost convincing evidence concerns strand 1, which has been described in terms of he notion of a conveyor belt of adversity. The specific form taken by these nfluences is, of course, likely to differ according to time and place. The signifi- :ance of premarital pregnancy as defined by us may well be changing. However, in _ondon in the recent past at least, there are links between unsuccessful coping vith a premarital pregnancy and current working-class status. Such a class status is :nown to increase the rate of provoking agents and vulnerability factors. How- :ver, in the Walthamstow enquiry based on women with an early loss of mother, ıo social-class difference in depression was found once women with a premarital ıregnancy were excluded. The most parsimonious explanation lies in the critical ,econdary effect of premarital pregnancy on choice of marriage partner and on the :ourse of the marriage. A person's level of education is usually crucial for social nobility, but, in fact, we found little relationship with subsequent social class and ıone with depression. This negative finding suggests that, for women, factors :oncerning husbands and marriages may have a greater impact on their psychi- ıtric state than their own educational and work achievements (see Harris *et al.*, 1986; 1987).

At present, the case for personality characteristics comprising the enduring :ognitive sets and coping styles of strand 2 are perforce less convincing, and ıecause of this little weight has been placed on them in this review. However, they ıre potentially of considerable importance, and there is some evidence to suggest hat important links may exist (see Harris *et al.*, in preparation); and, it would ndeed be implausible if the strand 1 factors were not paralleled to a certain extent ıy internal strand 2 factors. The crucial task is to establish how far strand 2 factors nake some kind of independent affect—either in past or present. Whether the atter can have a 'life on their own'. The need to relate such research to attachment :heory has already been noted.

The most crucial measure in our model is lack of care in childhood, which is ikely to span both strands of explanation. It proved more discriminating than any ɔf the measures surrounding the actual loss (Harris *et al.*, 1986). This may mean ıo more than that our various measures have so far failed to identify pathogenic :h'ldhood mourning experiences. However, even if such experiences can later be ıdentified, inevitably they will be highly correlated with lack of care, since this is so highly linked with depression. It may be taken as a sign that in terms of the two theoretical perspectives we contrasted earlier of Bowlby and Rutter, there is more ≥vidence for the role of family environment than for the impact of loss and mourning in producing disorder in adulthood. But it must be recalled that research is in an early stage, and, although the broad outlines of an aetiological model begin to emerge with some clarity, it is too soon to have any confidence about such specific issues, particularly when it is borne in mind that some processes may be multidetermined.

Acknowledgements

1. The research in this chapter was supported by the MRC and ESRC.
2. Tirril Harris and Toni Bifulco were responsible for the Walthamstow Project and, in large part, results reported are the results of their sustained efforts in the field.

REFERENCES

Adam, K.S., Bouckoms, A., & Streiner, D. (1982). Parental loss and family stability in attempted suicide. *Archives of General Psychiatry, 39*, 1081–1085.

Andrews, B., & Brown, G.W. (1987). Social support, onset of depression & personality: an exploratory analysis. *Social Psychiatry*, (in press).

Beck, A.T. (1967). *Depression: clinical, experimental, and theoretical aspects*. London: Staples Press.

Bifulco, A. (1985). Death of mother in childhood and depression. Doctoral thesis, University of London.

Bifulco, A., Brown, G.W., & Harris, T.O. (1987). Childhood loss of parent, lack of adequate parental care and adult depression: a replication. *Journal of Affective Disorders, 12*, 115–128.

Birtchnell, J. (1980). Women whose mothers died in childhood: An outcome study. *Psychological Medicine, 10*, 699–713.

Bowlby, J. (1969). *Attachment and loss*. Vol. 1: *Attachment*. New York: Basic Books.

Bowlby, J. (1973). *Attachment and loss*. Vol. 2: *Separation: Anxiety and anger*. New York: Basic Books.

Bowlby, J. (1980). *Attachment and loss*. Vol. 3: *Loss: Sadness and depression*. New York: Basic Books.

Bretherton, I., & Waters, E. (no date). Growing points of attachment theory and research. In *Monographs of the Society for Research in Child Development*. 50: Nos. 1–2.

Brown, G.W. (1974). Meaning, measurement and stress of life events. In B.S. Dohrenwend & B.P. Dohrenwend (eds), *Stressful life events: Their nature and effects*. New York: Wiley.

Brown, G.W. (1987). Causal paths, chains and strands. In M. Rutter (ed.), *The power of longitudinal data: studies of risk and protective factors for psychosocial disorders*. Cambridge University Press (in press.)

Brown, G.W., & Bifulco, A. (1985). Social support, life events and depression. In I. Sarason (ed.), *Social support: Theory, research and applications*. Dordrecht: Martinus Nijhoff.

Brown, G.W., Craig, T.K.J., & Harris, T.O. (1985). Depression: disease or distress? Some epidemiological considerations. *British Journal of Psychiatry, 147*, 612–622.

Brown, G.W., & Harris, T.O. (1978a). *Social origins of depression: A study of psychiatric disorder in women*. London: Tavistock Publications; New York: Free Press.

Brown, G.W., & Harris, T.O. (1978b). Social origins of depression: A reply. *Psychological Medicine, 8*, 577–588.

Brown, G.W., & Harris, T.O. (1979). The sin of subjectivism: a reply to Shapiro. *Behavioural Research and Therapy, 17*, 605–613.

Brown, G.W., & Harris, T.O. (1986a). Establishing causal links: the Bedford College studies of depression. In H. Katschnig (ed.), *Life events and psychiatric disorders: controversial issues*. Cambridge: Cambridge University Press.

Brown, G.W., & Harris, T.O. (1986b). Stressor, vulnerability and depression: a question of replication. *Psychological Medicine, 16*, 739–744.

Brown, G.W., Harris, T.O., & Bifulco, A. (1986). Long-term effect of early loss of parent. In M. Rutter, C. Izard & P. Read (eds), *Depression in childhood: Developmental perspectives*. New York: Guilford Press.

Brown, G.W., Harris, T.O., & Copeland, J.R.M. (1977). Depression and loss. *British Journal of Psychiatry, 130,* 1–18.

Brown, G.W., & Prudo, R. (1981). Psychiatric disorder in a rural and an urban population: 1. Aetiology of depression. *Psychological Medicine, 11,* 581–599.

Campbell, E.A., Cope, S.J., & Teasdale, J.D. (1983). *British Journal of Psychiatry, 143,* 548–553.

Cooper, J.E., Copeland, J.R.M., Brown, G.W., Harris, T.O., & Gourley, A.J. (1977). Further studies on interviewer training and inter-rater reliability of the Present State Examination (PS.E.). *Psychological Medicine, 7,* 517–523.

Crook, T., & Eliot, J. (1980). Parental death during childhood and adult depression. *Psychological Bulletin, 87,* 252–259.

Crook, T., Raskin, A., & Eliot, J. (1981). Parent–child relationships and adult depression. *Child Development, 52,* 950–957.

Cummings, E.M. (1987). *Towards a developmental psychopathology of attachment and depression.* Presented at Attachment Conference. Bayswater, London. (West Virginia University), June 1987.

Dean, C., Surtees, P.G., & Sashidharan, S.P. (1983). Comparison of research diagnostic systems in an Edinburgh community sample. *British Journal of Psychiatry, 142,* 247–256.

Finlay-Jones, R.A. (1981). Showing that life events are a cause of depression—A review. *Australian and New Zealand Journal of Psychiatry, 15,* 229–238.

Finlay-Jones, R.A., Duncan-Jones, P., Brown, G.W., Harris, T.O., Murphy, E., & Prudo, R. (1980). Depression and anxiety in the community: Replicating the diagnosis of a case. *Psychological Medicine, 10,* 445–454.

Granville-Grossman, K.L. (1968). The early environment of affective disorder. In A. Coppen & A. Walk (eds), *Recent developments in affective disorders.* London: Headley Brothers.

Harris, T.O., Brown, G.W., & Bifulco, A. (1986). Loss of parent in childhood and adult psychiatric disorder: The Walthamstow Study 1. The role of lack of adequate parental care. *Psychological Medicine, 16,* 641–659.

Harris, T.O., Brown, G.W., & Bifulco, A. (1987). Loss of parent in childhood and adult psychiatric disorder: the role of social class position and premarital pregnancy. *Psychological Medicine, 17,* 163–183.

Harris, T.O., Brown, G.W., & Bifulco, A. (in preparation). *Loss of parent in childhood and adult psychiatric disorder: The role of situational helplessness.*

Hetherington, E.M. (1979). Divorce. A child's perspective. *American Psychologist, 34,* 851–858.

Hetherington, E.M., Cox, M., & Cox, R. (1978). The aftermath of divorce. In J.H. Stevens Jr & M. Matthews (eds), *Mother–child, father–child relations.* Washington, DC: National Association for the Education of Young Children.

Kennard, J., & Birtchnell, J. (1982). The mental health of early mother separated women. *Acta Psychiatrica Scandinavica, 65,* 388–402.

Lloyd, C. (1980). Life events and depressive disorder reviewed. 1. Events as predisposing factors. *Archives of General Psychiatry, 37,* 529–535.

Martin, C.J. (1982). Psychosocial stress and puerperal psychiatric disorder. Presented to the Marce Society.

Murphy, E. (1982). Social origins of depression in old age. *British Journal of Psychiatry, 141,* 135–142.

O'Connor, P., & Brown, G.W. (1984). Supportive relationships: fact or fancy? *Journal of Social and Personal Relationships, 1,* 159–175.

Parker, G. (1979). Parental characteristics in relation to depressive disorders. *British Journal of Psychiatry, 134,* 138–147.

Parker, G. (1981). Parental representations of patients with anxiety neurosis. *Acta Psychiatrica Scandinavica, 65,* 33–36.

Parker, G. (1983). Parental 'affectionless' control as an antecedent to adult depression. *Archives of General Psychiatry, 40,* 956–960.

Parry, G., Shapiro, D., & Davies, L. (1981). Reliability of life-event ratings: an independent replication. *British Journal of Clinical Psychology, 20,* 133–34.

Paykel, E.S. (1973). Life events and acute depression. In J.P. Scott & E.C. Senay (eds), *Separation and depression.* Washington, DC: American Association for the Advancement of Science.

Paykel, E.S., Emms, E.M., Fletcher, J., & Rassaby, E.S. (1980). Life events and social support in puerperal depression. *British Journal of Psychiatry, 136,* 339–346.

Prudo, R., Brown, G.W., Harris, T.O., & Dowland, J. (1981). Psychiatric disorder in a rural and an urban population. 2. Sensitivity to loss. *Psychological Medicine, 11,* 601–616.

Quinton, D., & Rutter, M. (1984a). Parents with children in care: 1. Current circumstances and parenting skills. *Journal of Child Psychology and Psychiatry, 25,* 231–250.

Quinton, D., & Rutter, M. (1984b). Parents with children in care: 2. Intergenerational continuities. *Journal of Child Psychology and Psychiatry, 25,* 231–250.

Quinton, D., Rutter, M., & Liddle, C. (1984). Institutional rearing, parenting difficulties and marital support. *Psychological Medicine, 14,* 107–124.

Richards, M.P.M., & Dyson, M. (1982). *Separation, divorce and the development of children: A review.* London: Department of Health and Social Security.

Roy, A. (1978). Vulnerability factors and depression in women. *British Journal of Psychiatry, 133,* 106–110.

Roy, A. (1981). Role of past loss in depression. *Archives of General Psychiatry, 38,* 301–302.

Rutter, M. (1971). Parent–child separation. Psychological effects on the children. *Journal of Child Psychology and Psychiatry, 12,* 233–260.

Rutter, M. (1981). *Maternal deprivation reassessed,* 2nd edn. Harmondsworth, Middlesex: Penguin.

Rutter, M. (1982). Epidemiological-longitudinal approaches to the study of development. In W.A. Collins (ed.), *Minnesota symposium on child psychology,* Vol 15. Hillsdale, N.J.: Lawrence Erlbaum Associates.

Rutter, M., Izard, C., & Read, P. (eds) (1987). *Depression in childhood: Development perspectives.* New York: Guilford Press.

Rutter, M., & Madge, N. (1976). *Cycles of disadvantage.* London: Heinemann.

Rutter, M., Quinton, D., & Liddle, C. (1983). Parenting in two generations: looking backwards and looking forwards. In N. Madge (ed.), *Families at risk.* London: Heinemann Educational.

Schaeffer, E.S. (1963). Children's reports of parental behaviour: an inventory. *Child Development, 36,* 413–424.

Surtees, P.G., & Ingham, J.G. (1980). Life stress and depressive outcome: application of a dissipation model to life events. *Social Psychiatry, 15,* 21–31.

Tennant, C., Bebbington, P., & Hurry, J. (1980). Parental death in childhood and risk of adult depressive disorders; a review. *Psychological Medicine, 10,* 289–299.

Tennant, C., Hurry, J., & Bebbington, P. (1982). The relation of childhood separation experiences to adult depressive and anxiety states. *British Journal of Psychiatry, 141,* 475–482.

Tennant, C., Smith, A., Bebbington, P., & Hurry, J. (1979). The contextual threat of life events: the concept and its reliability. *Psychological Medicine, 9,* 525–528.

Wallerstein, J.S., & Kelly, J.B. (1975). The effects of parental divorce: experiences of the preschool child. *Journal of the American Academy of Child Psychiatry, 14,* 600–616.

Wing, J.K., Cooper, J.E., & Sartorius, N. (1974). *The measurement and classification of psychiatric symptoms.* Cambridge: Cambridge University Press.

Wing, J.K., Nixon, J.M., Mann, S.A., & Leff, J.P. (1977). Reliability of the PSE (ninth edition) used in a population study. *Psychological Medicine, 7,* 505–516.

Wing, J.K., & Sturt, E. (1978). *The PSE–ID–CATEGO system—A supplementary manual* (mimeo). London: Institute of Psychiatry.

KEY WORDS

oss of parent in childhood, depression, lack adequate parental care, psychiatric disorder, ss of parent by death or separation, loss of mother in childhood, premarital pregnancy, ck of care, parental neglect, vulnerability to depression, stress and depression, self-steem.

Handbook of Life Stress, Cognition and Health
Edited by S. Fisher and J. Reason
© 1988 John Wiley & Sons Ltd.

25

Trait Anxiety and Stress

Michael W. Eysenck
Royal Holloway and Bedford New College, University of London

INTRODUCTION

It is generally accepted that the amount of psychological stress (i.e. a negative subjective, behavioural and physiological state) experienced by an individual at any given moment is determined interactively by the current environmental demands and by characteristics of the individual concerned. For example, one person may feel that he or she possesses the resources needed to cope with a given situation, and thus experience relatively little stress, whereas another person confronted with precisely the same situation may feel unable to cope, and so experience considerable stress.

Despite the general agreement that there may well be important individual differences in susceptibility to psychological stress, most stress research has ignored such individual differences. The reasons for this neglect are difficult to ascertain, and will not be discussed here (this issue is discussed in M. Eysenck, 1986). If one wants to consider such individual differences, then an obvious personality dimension to investigate is that of trait anxiety or neuroticism. While these two dimensions have been regarded as separate, the fact that they correlate highly with each other (approximately + 0.70) indicates that they are actually closely related (c.f. Watson and Clark, 1984). Trait anxiety has been defined in various ways. However, a representative definition was offered by Spielberger et al. (1970), who defined it as 'relatively stable individual differences in anxiety proneness'. The general assumption is that those who are high in trait anxiety (or neuroticism) are more susceptible to stress than those who are low in trait anxiety.

There has been some degree of controversy concerning the factors responsible for individual differences in trait anxiety. Spielberger (1972) has emphasized the role of early childhood experiences, whereas H. Eysenck (1967) has claimed that heredity is of major importance. Various studies indicate quite strongly that heredity does play a part in determining an individual's level of trait anxiety or neuroticism. For example, Shields (1962) discovered that dizygotic twins brought up together had an intraclass correlation coefficient of +0.11 for neuroticism, monozygotic twins brought up together had a correlation of +0.38, and mono-zygotic twins brought up apart had one of +0.53. Thus, monozygotic twins were much more similar than dizygotic twins in their level of neuroticism, and mono-zygotic twins brought up apart resembled each other in neuroticism considerably more than dizygotic twins brought up together, despite the fact that there was much greater environmental similarity in the latter group. In general, it seems that genetic factors account for approximately half of the variance.

How does heredity affect an individual's level of trait anxiety or neuroticism? According to H. Eysenck (1967), individual differences in neuroticism depend upon the functioning of the so-called visceral brain, which consists of the hippocampus, amygdala, cingulum, septum, and hypothalamus. Those who are high in neuroticism generally have more active visceral brains than those who are low in neuroticism. Gray (1981) has also favoured a physiological explanation. He argued that an individual's level of trait anxiety is determined by the behavioural inhibition system, which includes the septohippocampal system, its neocortical projection in the frontal lobe, and its monoaminergic afferents from the brain-stem.

Despite the theoretical differences between them, H. Eysenck (1967) and Gray (1981) are in general agreement that individual differences in susceptibility to stress are due in great measure to individual differences in the responsiveness of certain physiological systems. How adequate is this conceptualization? One of its major limitations is that it clearly implies that those individuals who have especially responsive physiological systems should tend to be rather anxious and stressed in most, or even all, stressful situations, whereas those with unresponsive physiological systems should characteristically experience relatively little anxiety in any situation. In fact, the evidence indicates that this unidimensional view of trait anxiety should be replaced by a multidimensional conceptualization. Endler (1983) has argued that five different dimensions of trait anxiety can be identified, but the two dimensions of social evaluation and physical danger are the only ones for which there is convincing empirical support.

According to the multidimensional view of trait anxiety, the increase in state anxiety produced by a threatening or stressful environment will be greater among those high in trait anxiety than among those low in trait anxiety only when there is *congruence* between the nature of the threat and the dimension or facet of trait anxiety which is being considered. This prediction has been confirmed a number of times, especially when social evaluation and physical danger have been investigated (e.g. Donat, 1983; Kendall, 1978).

The notion that trait anxiety is determined in large measure by heredity is in danger of ignoring the dynamic changes in trait anxiety which occur. Conley (1984) has evaluated the longitudinal evidence in detail, and concluded that trait anxiety and neuroticism show reasonable consistency over time, but rather less than is the case for intelligence. The nature of the problem which such findings pose for the traditional view of trait anxiety or neuroticism was spelled out clearly by Gray (1982): 'Studies . . . of the personality trait of neuroticism and ex-traversion . . . estimate the contribution of heredity to these conditions at about 50 per cent of the variance. But that means, of course, that another 50 per cent of the variance remains to be accounted for; and it is likely that learning (of as yet unknown kinds) plays a determining role in this respect' (p. 438).

The emphasis which H. Eysenck (1967) and Gray (1981) place on the physiological system in their theoretical accounts means that they tend to de-emphasize the roles played by other systems in anxiety. A more fruitful approach to conceptualizing trait anxiety may evolve from the theoretical position adopted by Lang (e.g. 1971). He argued that there are three separate response systems involved in anxiety, which he termed the behavioural, the physiological and the verbal. It is of particular importance to distinguish among these (or similar) response systems because they frequently fail to respond concordantly. Failures of concordance were shown rather clearly by Craske and Craig (1984) in a study of competent pianists. Measures belonging to the same response system tended to correlate significantly with each other, but measures from different response systems mostly failed to correlate. If concordance is the exception rather than the rule, then it means that we must simultaneously consider all of the various systems involved in anxiety in order to achieve a full understanding of its complex nature.

THE COGNITIVE APPROACH

Basic Assumptions

Despite the obvious value in considering anxiety, and individual differences in trait anxiety, from the multisystem viewpoint favoured by Lang (1971) and by others, there is also merit in an in-depth investigation of each system separately. This is perhaps especially true of the cognitive system, which has received remarkably little systematic empirical and theoretical attention. Why might the cognitive system play an important role in determining individual differences in anxiety? In essence, the cognitive system is involved in the selective allocation of processing resources to stimuli present in the environment, and in assigning meaning to those stimuli which are processed. These functions of the cognitive system presumably affect subsequent activity within the physiological system. Thus, in a sense, the cognitive system acts as a gateway to the physiological system. Of course, this is only part of what is involved. There are undoubtedly complex effects of the cognitive system on the physiological system, and vice versa, but the crucial point is that both systems need to be considered. It is probably true to say that the theories of trait anxiety or neuroticism proposed by H. Eysenck (1967), Gray (1981), and Spielberger (1972) de-emphasize the role of the cognitive system, and are thus inadequate.

Some theorists (e.g. Markus et al., 1982) have incorporated the cognitive system into personality theory by emphasizing the self-schema. It is assumed that the self-schema depends on the personal significance or salience of any given trait dimension to the individual concerned. The contrast between the self-schema approach and the traditional trait approach was described in the following terms by Markus (1977): 'Systematic effects in social behaviour depend less on people having some amount of a particular substantive attribute, such as independence or dependence, and more on the readiness or ability to categorize behaviour along certain dimensions.' (p. 77).

Self-schema theories have often successfully predicted behaviour (e.g. Markus, 1977; Markus et al., 1982), but they seem to suffer from important limitations. A particular problem concerns the issue of the discriminability of self-schema from overall trait level. Measures of self-schema and of overall trait level are usually not independent of each other, and sometimes the correlations are so high that measures of self-schema appear to be simply alternative measures of trait level (Burke et al., 1984).

Despite these problems with self-schema theory, it can still plausibly be argued that this theoretical approach has potential value in terms of explaining some individual differences in personality. Instead of regarding the self-schema as separate from trait level, it probably makes more sense to argue that the self-schema constitutes part of the cognitive mechanism mediating the effects of trait level on behaviour.

One of the basic assumptions made in this chapter is that there are important individual differences between those high and low in trait anxiety in the content of the information which they have stored in long-term memory. To that extent, we are in agreement with the self-schema approach. This theoretical assumption is supported indirectly by two important phenomena: mood-state-dependent retrieval (Bower, 1981) and mood-congruent learning (e.g. Bower et al., 1981). Mood-state-dependent retrieval is demonstrated when information which is learned in one mood state has a higher probability of subsequent recall when the mood state at recall is similar rather than dissimilar to that at the time of learning. Mood-state-dependent retrieval has sometimes proved to be a somewhat elusive phenomenon (e.g. Bower and Mayer, 1985), but it can usually be obtained provided that the learner perceives there to be a causal link between the information which is to be learned and his or her current mood state (Bower, 1985). The relevance of mood-state-dependent retrieval in the current context is that it indicates that information about current mood state is often stored in long-term memory. There is overwhelming evidence that individuals high and low in trait anxiety usually differ in their mood states (Watson and Clark, 1984), and thus the content of long-term memory should vary systematically as a function of the level of trait anxiety.

A very similar argument can be applied to the phenomenon of mood-congruent learning. In this phenomenon, emotionally charged material is learned best when its affective value is congruent with the learner's current mood. Thus, the fact that individuals high and low in trait anxiety differ in their characteristic moods means that what is learned will be affected in predictable ways by the level of trait anxiety.

The assumption that the nature of the information stored in long-term memory varies in a systematic fashion as a function of the level of trait anxiety may obviate some of the problems which have beset the traditional theories of trait anxiety. Firstly, it provides a plausible reason for many of the changes in trait anxiety obtained in longitudinal studies. The contents of long-term memory change over time, and these changes may either increase or decrease the level of trait anxiety depending on whether the memories concerned are mainly happy or anxiety-related ones. Secondly, a theoretical approach to trait anxiety which emphasizes the role of long-term memory is well able to account for the fact that many individuals are anxious in some stressful situations but not in others. An individual's previous experiences in stressful situations of any given type will determine the information stored in long-term memory, and this in turn will affect that individual's susceptibility to anxiety in that type of situation.

We have seen so far that one important way in which the cognitive system may be involved in trait anxiety is in terms of the information stored in long-term memory. However, it is also probable that individuals high and low in trait anxiety also differ in the functioning of their cognitive processes. Thus, a full account of trait anxiety from the cognitive perspective requires consideration of both the *structure* of the cognitive system (e.g. the organization of long-term memory) and the *processes* involved in cognition (e.g. attentional processes).

In sum, it is argued that a complete theory of trait anxiety would indicate how the physiological, cognitive, and behavioural systems combine to determine how each individual deals with threatening and stressful situations. Theories such as those of H. Eysenck (1967) and Gray (1981) have been too physiologically oriented. As a result, they have emphasized the role of heredity, the unidimensional nature of trait anxiety, and the longitudinal stability of trait anxiety. In contrast, the cognitive approach to trait anxiety emphasizes the role of environmental determinants of anxiety, the multidimensional nature of trait anxiety, and systematic changes in trait anxiety over time. A synthesis of the two theoretical approaches offers hope of providing an adequate conceptualization of trait anxiety.

Previous Theory and Research

A theoretical position which is of especial relevance to the theme of this chapter was proposed by Byrne (1964). In essence, he devised a questionnaire (the Repression–Sensitization Scale) to measure individual differences in personality having an obvious cognitive component. Those scoring high on this scale (the sensitizers) allegedly tend to approach threatening stimuli, whereas those scoring low on the scale (the repressors) tend to avoid threatening stimuli. In other words, the extent to which threatening stimuli are processed plays a part in defining a major personality dimension.

The reason why Byrne's (1964) theoretical approach is relevant here is that his Repression–Sensitization Scale is essentially a measure of trait anxiety. Standard tests of trait anxiety (e.g. Spielberger's State–Trait Anxiety Inventory; Taylor's Manifest Anxiety Scale) correlate approximately +0.80 to +0.85 with the Repression–Sensitization Scale (Watson and Clark, 1984). It may thus be assumed that those identified on the Repression–Sensitization Scale as sensitizers are also high in trait anxiety, whereas those identified as repressors are also low in trait anxiety.

If the empirical evidence supported Byrne's hypothesis, it could then be concluded that the initial processing of threatening stimuli is associated with individual differences in trait anxiety. What does the evidence actually indicate? This evidence is reviewed in detail by Eysenck (in press), and so a review will not be provided here. The evidence was also evaluated by Watson and Clark (1984). They argued that scales of repression–sensitization and trait anxiety can both be regarded as measures of negative affectivity, and they considered the association between negative affectivity and approach–avoidance tendencies to sexually provocative stimuli, to taboo words, and to painful or gruesome stimuli. Their review led them to the following unequivocal conclusion: 'The results have been overwhelmingly negative. Taken together, they indicate that NA [i.e. negative affectivity] is unrelated to the approach/avoidance of these types of threatening stimuli' (p. 481).

Watson and Clark (1984) based their conclusion mainly on the results of studies which have investigated perceptual defence, which is said to occur when taboo or emotionally threatening stimuli have higher recognition thresholds than affectively neutral stimuli. It has often been assumed that perceptual defence occurs because there is partial avoidance of the threatening stimuli. If that assumption is correct, then it seems natural to predict, on Byrne's (1964) hypothesis, that repressors (those low in trait anxiety) should show greater evidence of perceptual defence than sensitizers (those high in trait anxiety).

No significant differences between repressors and sensitizers were found in most of the relevant studies of perceptual defence. Furthermore, no support for Byrne's hypothesis was obtained in the two studies (Van Egeren, 1968; Wagstaff, 1974) in which systematic attempts were made to obtain measures of perceptual sensitivity which were uncontaminated by any response bias effects. It is possible that approach and avoidance tendencies in the presence of threat manifest themselves only at the later stages of perceptual processing. Since the perceptual defence paradigm requires only relatively 'early' and low-level perceptual processes, no evidence of differences between repressors and sensitizers should be expected. However, this interpretation is untenable in view of the results from other studies in which the duration of visual attention to threat-related pictures of mutilated bodies and corpses and to neutral pictures was compared. Despite the fact that these pictures were looked at for an average duration of approximately 10 seconds, and thus were presumably thoroughly processed, there was no difference between repressors and sensitizers in duration of attention to either the threat-related or neutral stimuli (Carroll, 1972; Lewinsohn et al., 1972).

An alternative interpretation is to argue that the perceptual defence paradigm is an unrepresentative one because only one stimulus is presented at a time. Repressors would only have higher recognition thresholds than sensitizers if there were the equivalent of a volume control associated with information processing. In other words, repressors turn down the volume control whenever a threatening stimulus is presented, whereas sensitizers turn it up. Since the predicted results have not been obtained, this cannot be an accurate conceptualization of what is involved. A more plausible notion is that there are individual differences in some selective mechanism rather than in a volume control. That is to say, the allocation of processing resources to two or more concurrent stimuli may well differ in a relatively systematic fashion from one individual to another. More specifically, if a threatening and a neutral stimulus were presented concurrently, then repressors or those low in trait anxiety might selectively allocate processing resources to the neutral stimulus rather than to the threatening stimulus, whereas sensitizers or those high in trait anxiety might selectively allocate processing resources in exactly the opposite fashion. These selective biases would, of course, produce the approach and avoidance tendencies postulated by Byrne (1964).

In sum, while the theory put forward by Byrne (1964) seems to be a reasonable one, the experimental evidence has largely failed to support it, various possible reasons for which have been discussed. The next section of the chapter deals with recent research which has been carried out in an attempt to elucidate matters, and to decide whether a modified version of Byrne's hypothesis is tenable.

Current Theory and Research

The hypothesis that those high and low in trait anxiety or repression–sensitization differ in terms of a selective bias was first put to systematic experimental test by Christos Halkiopoulos (reported in M. Eysenck et al., 1987). He used a modified dichotic listening task in which pairs of words were presented concurrently, one to each ear. All of the words which were presented to one ear (the attended channel had to be shadowed (i.e. repeated back aloud), whereas all of the words presented to the other ear (the unattended channel) were to be ignored. A mixture of threat-related (e.g. grave, fail) and neutral words was presented to the attended channel; on the unattended channel all of the words were neutral in affective tone. A tone to which the subjects were asked to respond as rapidly as possible was presented on occasion very shortly after a pair of words had been presented. This tone was presented half of the time on the attended channel and the other half of the time on the unattended channel. The crucial theoretical assumption was that the speed of responding to the tone would provide an approximate index of the allocation of processing resources: the faster the response was, the greater was the implied allocation of processing resources to the channel on which the tone was presented. All of the subjects were administered the Facilitation–Inhibition Scale (Ullmann, 1962), which is a personality test which correlates very highly with Byrne's Repression–Sensitization Scale and with standard tests of trait anxiety.

The results were almost precisely as expected on the basis of the selective bias version of Byrne's (1964) hypothesis. Facilitators (i.e. those individuals high in trait anxiety) preferentially allocated processing resources to the channel on which a threat-related word had just been presented. This was revealed by rapid responding to the tone when it followed a threat-related word in the same ear, together with slow responding to the tone when it followed a threat-related word in the other ear. Inhibitors (i.e. those individuals low in trait anxiety) exhibited the opposite pattern of response times to the tone, and thus appeared to be avoiding allocating processing resources to the channel on which a threat-related word had just been presented.

A visual version of the auditory task discussed above has been used in a number of subsequent studies. MacLeod et al. (1986) investigated the allocation of processing resources between concurrent threat-related and neutral stimuli in generalized anxiety disorder patients and in normal controls. In essence, the anxious patients responded faster to the visual signal or probe when it replaced a threat-related word than when it replaced a neutral word, whereas the control subjects showed the opposite pattern. These results are very similar to those reported by M. Eysenck *et al.* (1987). The visual version of the task has also been used with normals high and low in trait anxiety, and the results have been in line with those discussed above (Broadbent, personal communication; M. Eysenck, in preparation).

These studies indicate convincingly that there is an element of truth in Byrne's hypothesis that high-anxiety individuals will approach threatening stimuli or situations, whereas low-anxiety individuals will avoid them. However, the predominantly negative findings reported in the literature mean that Byrne's hypothesis must be modified in order to account for the data. It may be argued provisionally that those high and low in trait anxiety differ in terms of selective biases in favour of or against threatening stimuli, and that these selective biases are used only when at least one threatening and one neutral stimulus are presented concurrently. When only a single stimulus is presented at a time, the selective biases cannot be used, and so systematic individual differences in approach and avoidance strategies with threatening stimuli are not found.

An issue of obvious relevance concerns the kinds of threatening stimuli which produce these systematic biases. In particular, it might be anticipated that biases would be greater where the nature of the threat-related word was closely connected to the particular worries and concerns of the individual subject. This was considered by Macleod *et al.* (1986). The threat-related words which they presented to their subjects were divided into those which referred to physical health concerns (e.g. injury, agony) and those which referred to social threats (e.g. criticized, ashamed). The patients with a diagnosis of generalized anxiety disorder were divided into two groups on the basis of whether they indicated that physical health or social concerns formed the main source of their worries. In fact, the amount of selective bias in speed of responding to the visual signal was unaffected by whether or not the nature of the threatening stimulus matched the primary area of concern of the patient. The reason for this may be that the specific nature of the threat is important only at later, post-attentional stages of processing than those investigated in their study. It is probably relevant in this connection to mention a finding obtained by Mathews and MacLeod (1986). They found with a dichotic listening task that selective bias could be obtained even when the subjects appeared to have no conscious awareness of the threat-related words which were presented on the unattended channel. This suggests that selective biases can operate at a rather early, pre-attentive level.

Are these selective biases of general significance in everyday life? They probably are, because the minor threatening stimuli of everyday life are usually accompanied by other, non-threatening stimuli, and thus the conditions for the operations of the selective biases occur frequently. In contrast, the conditions in which individual differences in approach to and avoidance of threat are not found (i.e. only one stimulus present at any moment) are probably rather rare in everyday life. The operation of these selective biases would make the environment appear subjectively much more threatening to high-anxiety individuals than to low-anxiety individuals, and this could help to account for the fact that individuals high in trait anxiety are generally higher in state anxiety than individuals low in trait anxiety, even under relatively neutral conditions.

It is improbable that the only important difference in cognitive functioning between those high and low in trait anxiety is in pre-attentive selective biases. It seems intuitively reasonable to assume that there would also be systematic individual differences in the interpretation of ambiguous stimuli or situations which can be interpreted in either a threatening or a neutral fashion (e.g. 'The chest was opened'). There are a few studies in the literature which have explored differences in interpretation of ambiguity as a function of repression–sensitization. The basic prediction is that sensitizers tend to approach threat and repressors to avoid threat, and so sensitizers should be more likely to interpret ambiguous stimuli in a threatening fashion. Modest support for this prediction has been obtained (e.g. Blaylock, 1963; Haney, 1973).

Interpretation of ambiguity as a function of trait anxiety was investigated by M. Eysenck *et al.* (1987). They presented homophones having both a threat-related meaning and spelling and a neutral meaning and spelling (e.g. die, dye; guilt, gilt). The homophones were presented auditorily, and the subjects' task was simply to write down the spelling of each word. Those high in trait anxiety interpreted more of the homophones in the threatening fashion than did those low in trait anxiety; the correlation between trait anxiety and the number of threatening interpretations selected was +0.60. The threatening interpretation referred to social threat for half of the homophones, and to physical health concerns for the others. However, the nature of the threatening interpretation associated with the homophones did not interact with the primary concerns of the subjects, i.e. threatening interpretations were not selected more frequently when the nature of the threat and the nature of the primary concerns matched than when they did not.

In sum, despite the generally negative findings which were obtained when Byrne's (1964) hypothesis was tested experimentally during the 1960s, it appears that sensitizers or high-anxiety individuals do differ from repressors or low-anxiety individuals in their cognitive functioning in a number of significant ways. In particular, sensitizers (or high-anxiety individuals) have a pre-attentive selective bias favouring the allocation of processing resources to threatening stimuli, and they also tend to provide threatening interpretations for ambiguous stimuli. Repressors (or low-anxiety individuals), on the other hand, have a pre-attentive selective bias producing avoidance of processing threatening stimuli, and they tend to provide neutral interpretations for ambiguous stimuli. It should be noted, however, that the reported interpretations of ambiguous stimuli may be affected by response biases as well as by interpretative mechanisms *per se*. While the precise processes involved in producing these individual differences in cognitive functioning remain unclear, it is of great importance to have established that those high and low in trait anxiety differ both in terms of *what* stimuli are processed and *how* stimuli are processed.

Vulnerability to Clinical Anxiety

The characteristics of cognitive functioning discussed above are of particular consequence because they may help to account for the development of anxiety neurosis. The issues involved are dealt with at some length by M. Eysenck and Mathews (1987) and by Mathews and M. Eysenck (1987), but the main thrust of the argument will be summarized here. In essence, it is assumed that individuals high in trait anxiety are more vulnerable to clinical anxiety than are individuals low in trait anxiety. In addition, it is assumed that at least part of this vulnerability depends upon aspects of cognitive functioning which are characteristic of those high in trait anxiety, but not of those low in trait anxiety. For example, it seems plausible that those who selectively allocate processing resources to threatening stimuli and who typically interpret ambiguous stimuli in a threatening fashion regard the environment as being very threatening and so experience generally high levels of state anxiety. As a consequence, they may be especially vulnerable to clinical anxiety.

Our strategy is to compare the cognitive task performance of currently anxious patients with a diagnosis of generalized anxiety disorder, individuals who have recovered from clinical anxiety at least 6 months prior to taking part in any of the experiments, and normal controls. The basic rationale is that those cognitive measures reflecting stable characteristics associated with vulnerability to anxiety should distinguish the matched controls from the other two groups. While individuals who have recovered from clinical anxiety resemble normal controls in much of their cognitive functioning (including the interpretation of ambiguous stimuli), they appear to find it more difficult than normal controls to avoid processing a threatening word when they have been instructed to attend only to a concurrent neutral word, and the same is true of currently anxious patients. This suggests that the pre-attentive selective bias favouring the allocation of processing resources to threatening stimuli is present in normal individuals high in trait anxiety, in currently anxious patients, and in those who have recovered from clinical anxiety. On the basis of these findings, it may provisionally be concluded that this bias constitutes one of the vulnerability factors predisposing to anxiety neurosis.

It is less clear that the tendency to produce threatening interpretations of ambiguous stimuli is associated with vulnerability to anxiety. Since currently anxious patients tend to produce such threatening interpretations, but those who have recovered from clinical anxiety and normal controls undifferentiated for trait anxiety do not, the most reasonable conclusion is that the bias in favour of threatening interpretations shown by currently anxious subjects is a function of their current mood state rather than reflecting a vulnerability factor.

At a somewhat speculative level, the evidence which is accumulating from the research programme suggests that earlier, possibly automatic, processes are resistant to change during and after therapy, whereas later processes (e.g. interpretation of ambiguity) are much less resistant to change.

There are important advantages associated with considering cognitive task performance in a variety of different groups of subjects. A comparison of cognitive task performance between normals high and low in trait anxiety allows one to identify differences in cognitive functioning as a function of trait anxiety. However, it is improbable that all of these differences in cognitive functioning have the same theoretical and practical significance. In order to decide which of these differences are enduring characteristics of cognitive functioning and which are transient and mood dependent, and also to decide which are associated with vulnerability to clinical anxiety and which are not, it is essential to collect additional data. As we have seen (Mathews and M. Eysenck, 1987), there is provisional evidence indicating that the pre-attentive selective bias may be associated with vulnerability to clinical anxiety, whereas biased interpretation of ambiguity may not.

In sum, an important reason for investigating cognitive functioning in normals high and low in trait anxiety is that such research may shed light on some of the aspects of cognitive functioning which predispose to clinical anxiety. For reasons which are by no means clear, research on cognition as a function of trait anxiety has proceeded along almost entirely separate lines from research on cognitive functioning in clinically anxious patients. It is to be hoped that in future most strenuous efforts will be made to bring together findings from these two research traditions, to their mutual benefit. Some of the potential fruits of such a research strategy have been indicated in this chapter.

LOW TRAIT ANXIETY

Theoretical Assumptions

The emphasis in this chapter has been on those individuals who are high in trait anxiety. However, there are reasons for believing that it may be of considerable interest to examine low-anxiety individuals in more detail. At a theoretical level, there have been major disagreements concerning the issue of how well such individuals are. Most theorists (e.g. H. Eysenck, 1967) have argued that susceptibility to maladjustment is lowest among those who are low in trait anxiety. However, Byrne (1964) argued for a very different theoretical position. According to him, it is those who are intermediate on the Repression–Sensitization Scale who are on average the best adjusted. Extreme scorers at the two ends of this scale (i.e. the repressors and the sensitizers) resemble each other in that both groups are very affected by threatening stimulation, although, of course, they do differ in their preferred strategy for coping with such stimulation.

The two theoretical approaches are in broad agreement that a high level of trait anxiety or a high score on the Repression–Sensitization Scale is on average associated with relatively poor adjustment, but they clearly differ substantially in terms of the implications of low trait anxiety or a low score on the Repression–Sensitization Scale for adjustment. Byrne (1964) argued that such individuals tend towards maladjustment, whereas H. Eysenck (1967) argued that they are less maladjusted than any other group. The scattered evidence relating to this theoretical controversy is dealt with in the next section.

Experimental Evidence

Systematic investigation of individuals low in trait anxiety has indicated that they constitute a rather heterogeneous group. Some of them appear to be relatively untroubled by anxiety. They are thus high on adjustment, as predicted by H. Eysenck (1967). On the other hand, there are other individuals low in trait anxiety who are actually very affected by threat and stress, but who respond in a defensive fashion. These individuals obviously correspond closely to Byrne's (1964) conceptualization of repressors, who allegedly need to defend themselves against threat by avoiding it whenever possible.

These two groups of individuals have usually been distinguished by the Marlowe–Crowne Social Desirability Scale. This test is possibly inappropriately named, since it seems to be measuring defensiveness, protection of self-esteem, and affect inhibition. Those who are genuinely relatively low-anxious individuals have low scores on trait-anxiety scales or on the Repression–Sensitization Scale together with low scores on the Marlowe–Crowne Social Desirability Scale. In contrast, defensive repressors have low scores on trait anxiety or repression–sensitization, but high social desirability scores. Weinberger *et al.*, (1979) compared low-anxious subjects and defensive repressors during the performance of a somewhat stressful task. Their key finding was that the defensive repressors appeared to be more stressed than the low-anxious subjects on six different measures (three of which were physiological and three of which were based on task performance). Indeed, on most of these measures the defensive repressors appeared to be rather more stressed than a further group of subjects who were high in trait anxiety.

Further evidence indicating that defensive repressors are highly susceptible to stress was reported by Schwartz (1983). He measured alpha-EEG activity under resting conditions, and discovered that defensive repressors (with low Taylor Manifest Anxiety Scale and high Marlowe–Crowne scores) were more aroused than those high in trait anxiety, whereas genuinely low-anxious subjects (with low Manifest Anxiety Scale and low Marlowe-Crowne scores) were much less aroused than either of the other two groups.

If we can accept the conclusion that there are two very different kinds of individuals who obtain low trait-anxiety scores, then this probably has implications for the research on pre-attentive biases discussed earlier in this chapter. We have discovered that normal individuals low in trait anxiety tend to have a pre-attentive selective bias against threat-related stimuli, but it may be that this bias is much more pronounced in defensive repressors than in genuinely low-anxious individuals. However, the relevant evidence is not available.

THEORETICAL SPECULATIONS

It is almost tautological to claim that individuals high in trait anxiety are more susceptible to stress and to state anxiety than individuals low in trait anxiety. What *is* of theoretical and practical importance is to understand why it is that there are these individual differences in susceptibility to stress. As was pointed out earlier in this chapter, it is virtually certain that the answer will be a complex one, involving the physiological, cognitive and behavioural systems.

So far as the cognitive system is concerned, individuals high and low in trait anxiety differ from each other in both the contents of long-term memory and in various cognitive processes concerned with the allocation of processing resources and attention. Perceptual processing involves bottom-up or stimulus-driven processes and top-down or conceptually-driven processes, and information stored in long-term memory presumably plays an important role in determining the nature of the top-down or conceptually-driven processes which are used. The effects of top-down processes can be seen when the information obtained from bottom-up processes is insufficient to provide a definite interpretation of an external stimulus, as is the case with ambiguous stimuli.

The contents of long-term memory in high-anxiety and low-anxiety individuals probably differ in terms of both broad memory structures such as general schemata and more specific items of information such as worries or concerns. While there is little evidence about schemata in normal populations, it does appear that anxious patients may possess 'danger schemata' (Butler and Mathews, 1983). Anxious patients were found to regard themselves as being significantly more at risk from a great variety of potential environmental dangers than other people, in contrast to normal controls, who did not feel that the environment was more dangerous for them than for others.

At the more specific level of worries, individuals high in trait anxiety tend to worry more than those low in trait anxiety. Indeed, Borkovec *et al.* (1983) reported a correlation coefficient of $+0.67$ between trait anxiety and the percentage of a typical day spent worrying. There are at least two reasons why those high in trait anxiety might worry more than those low in trait anxiety.

a) High-anxiety individuals may have sets of worries stored in long-term memory which are more numerous and more highly organized than those of low-anxiety individuals.

b) The worries of high-anxiety individuals may be more accessible than those of low-anxiety individuals because their characteristically more negative mood states facilitate the retrieval of worries via mood-state-dependent retrieval.

M. Eysenck (1984) made a preliminary attempt to distinguish between these two possibilities. His main finding was that high-anxiety individuals tended to worry more than low-anxiety individuals even when the initial level of state anxiety in the two groups was comparable. This finding is more consistent with the notion that the two groups differ in the structure of long-term memory than that their different rates of worry reflect only current mood state.

If individuals high and low in trait anxiety differ in the anxiety-related schemata and specific worries stored in long-term memory, then it is easy to see why they differ in their cognitive appraisal of ambiguous stimuli and situations. It would also follow that an individual might be very susceptible to stress and to anxiety in some stressful situations but not in others, depending on the particular schemata and worries which were activated in any given situation. Thus, the multi-dimensional nature of trait anxiety is readily explicable from this theoretical position.

There is one characteristic of the experimental evidence which is slightly puzzling from the current theoretical perspective. It is only occasionally in our research that the specific nature of the threat-related stimuli being presented is of importance. There are three plausible explanations for this relative failure of specific effects to occur. Firstly, the emphasis in a number of the experimental tasks used has been on the early stages of processing. It may only be at later stages of processing that fine-grain information about the specific nature of a threatening stimulus is available. Secondly, we have basically focused on only two kinds of threat-related stimuli: those relating to social threats, and those relating to physical health concerns. These two areas of concern tend to be fairly highly correlated in a normal sample, which reduces the likelihood of specific effects occurring. Thirdly, it is possible that specific effects would be observed if a greater variety of areas or domains of threat or concern were sampled.

One of the best established differences in cognitive functioning between those high and low in trait anxiety is in pre-attentive selective biases. However, there is no clear evidence concerning the way in which these biases are established in the first place. Perhaps the simplest explanation is based on the assumption that threatening stimuli above some threshold value of degree of threat are almost certain to be processed or 'approached', since there is obvious biological utility in attending to any stimuli which pose a substantial threat. Let us also assume that threatening stimuli below the threshold are avoided, and that threat-related stimuli are generally perceived as subjectively more threatening by high-anxiety individuals than by low-anxiety individuals. These various assumptions together lead to the prediction that modestly threatening stimuli (as used in our research) would be more likely to exceed the threshold and thus attract resources to themselves in high-anxiety than in low-anxiety individuals.

In sum, the role of the cognitive system in accounting for some of the differences in susceptibility to stress between those high and low in trait anxiety is still unclear. However, it has been established that there are several significant differences in cognitive functioning between high-anxiety and low-anxiety individuals. A task for the future is to endeavour to make theoretical sense of the accumulating data.

SUMMARY AND CONCLUSIONS

Individual differences in trait anxiety have usually been considered from a physiological perspective. However, there is increasing evidence that those high and low in trait anxiety also differ importantly in various aspects of cognitive functioning. More specifically, they differ in terms of what stimuli are processed and how stimuli are processed. Thus, any complete theory of trait anxiety will necessarily consider the cognitive system as well as the physiological and behavioural systems. Those high in trait anxiety are more vulnerable than individuals low in trait anxiety to clinical anxiety, and it is possible that some of the characteristics of their cognitive functioning may help to account for the development of anxiety neurosis.

REFERENCES

Blaylock, B.A.H. (1963). *Repression–sensitization, word association, responses, and incidental recall*. Unpublished Master's thesis, University of Texas, Austin.

Borkovec, T.D., Robinson, E., Pruzinsky, T., & DePree, J.A. (1983). Preliminary exploration of worry: Some characteristics and processes. *Behaviour Research and Therapy, 21*, 9–16.

Bower, G.H. (1981). Mood and memory. *American Psychologist, 36*, 129–148.

Bower, G.H. (1985). Discussant at Mood and Cognition symposium, Cognitive Psychology Section, British Psychological Society, Oxford.

Bower, G.H., Gilligan, S.G., & Monteiro, K.P. (1981). Selectivity of learning caused by affective states. *Journal of Experimental Psychology: General, 110*, 451–473.

Bower, G.H., & Mayer, J.D. (1985). Failure to replicate mood-dependent retrieval. *Bulletin of the Psychonomic Society, 23*, 39–42.

Burke, P.A., Kraut, R.E., & Dworkin, R.H. (1984). Traits, consistency, and self-schemata: What do our methods measure? *Journal of Personality and Social Psychology, 47*, 568–579.

Butler, G., & Mathews, A. (1983). Cognitive processes in anxiety. *Advances in Behavior Research & Therapy, 5*, 51–62.

Byrne, D. (1964). Repression–sensitization as a dimension of personality. In B.A. Maher (ed.), *Progress in experimental personality research*. New York: Academic Press.

Carroll, D. (1972). Repression–sensitization as a dimension of personality. *Perceptual and Motor Skills, 34*, 949–950.

Conley, J.J. (1984). The hierarchy of consistency: A review and model of longitudinal findings on adult individual differences in intelligence, personality and self-opinion. *Personality and Individual Differences, 5*, 11–25.

Craske, M.G., & Craig, K.D. (1984). Musical performance anxiety: The three-systems model and self-efficacy theory. *Behaviour Research and Therapy, 22*, 267–280.

Donat, D.C. (1983). Predicting state anxiety: A comparison of multidimensional and unidimensional trait approaches. *Journal of Research in Personality, 17*, 256–262.

Endler, N.S. (1983). Interactionism: A personality model, but not yet a theory. In M.M. Page (ed.), *Nebraska Symposium on Motivation: Personality—current theory and research*. London: University of Nebraska Press.

Eysenck, H.J. (1967). *The biological basis of personality*. Springfield, Illinois: Charles C Thomas.

Eysenck, M.W. (1984). Anxiety and the worry process. *Bulletin of the Psychonomic Society, 22*, 545–548.

Eysenck, M.W. (1986). Individual differences in anxiety, cognition and coping. In G.R.J. Hockey, A.W.K. Gaillard & M.G.H. Coles (eds), *Energetics and human information processing*. Dordrecht: Martinus Nijhoff.

Eysenck, M.W. (in press). Personality, stress arousal, and cognitive processes in stress transactions. In R.W.J. Neufeld (ed.), *Advances in the investigation of psychological stress*. New York: Wiley.

Eysenck, M.W., MacLeod, C., & Mathews, A. (1987). Cognitive functioning and anxiety. *Psychological Research, 49*, 189–195.

Eysenck, M.W., & Mathews, A. (1987). Trait anxiety and cognition. In H.J. Eysenck & I. Martin (eds), *Theoretical foundations of behaviour therapy*. New York: Plenum.

Gray, J.A. (1981). A critique of Eysenck's theory of personality. In H.J. Eysenck (ed.), *A model for personality*. Berlin: Springer.

Gray, J.A. (1982). *The neuropsychology of anxiety*. Oxford: Clarendon.

Haney, J.N. (1973). Approach–avoidance reactions by repressors and sensitizers to ambiguity in a structured free-association. *Psychological Reports, 33*, 97–98.

Kendall, P.C. (1978). Anxiety: States, traits–situations? *Journal of Consulting and Clinical Psychology, 46*, 280–287.

Lang, P. (1971). The application of psychophysiological methods to the study of psychotherapy and behaviour modification. In A. Bergin & S. Garfield (eds), *Handbook of psychotherapy and behaviour change*. Chichester: Wiley.

Lewinsohn, P.M., Berquist, W.H., & Brelje, T. (1972). The repression–sensitization dimension and emotional response to stimuli. *Psychological Reports, 31*, 707–716.

MacLeod, C., Mathews, A., & Tata, P. (1986). Attentional bias in emotional disorders. *Journal of Abnormal Psychology, 95*, 15–20.

Markus, H. (1977). Self-schemata and processing of information about the self. *Journal of Personality and Social Psychology, 35*, 63–78.

Markus, H., Crane, M., Bernstein, S., & Siladi, M. (1982). Self-schemas and gender. *Journal of Personality and Social Psychology, 42*, 38–50.

Mathews, A., & Eysenck, M.W. (1987). Clinical anxiety and cognition. In H.J. Eysenck & I Martin (eds), *Theoretical foundations of behaviour therapy*. New York: Plenum.

Mathews, A., & MacLeod, C. (1986). Discrimination of threat cues without awareness in anxiety state. *Journal of Abnormal Psychology, 95*, 131–138.

Schwartz, G.E. (1983). Disregulation theory and disease: Applications to the repression/cerebral disconnection/cardiovascular disorder hypothesis. *International Review of Applied Psychology, 32*, 95–118.

Shields, J. (1962). *Monozygotic twins*. Oxford: Oxford University Press.

Spielberger, C.D. (1972). Anxiety as an emotional state. In C.D. Spielberger (ed.), *Anxiety: Current trends in theory and research*, Vol. 1. London: Academic Press.

Spielberger, C.D., Gorsuch, R., & Lushene, R. (1970). *The State–Trait Anxiety Inventory (STAI) Test Manual Form X*. Palo Alto, Calif.: Consulting Psychologists Press.

Ullmann, L.P. (1962). An empirically derived MMPI scale which measures facilitation–inhibition of recognition of threatening stimuli. *Journal of Clinical Psychology, 18*, 127–132.

Van Egeren, L. (1968). Repression and sensitization: Sensitivity and recognition criteria. *Journal of Experimental Research in Personality, 3*, 1–8.

Wagstaff, G.F. (1974). The effects of repression–sensitization on a brightness scaling measure of perceptual defence. *British Journal of Psychology, 65*, 395–401.

Watson, D., & Clark, L.A. (1984). Negative affectivity: The disposition to experience aversive emotional states. *Psychological Bulletin, 96*, 465–490.

Weinberger, D.A., Schwartz, G.E., & Davidson, R.J. (1979). Low-anxious, high-anxious, and repressive coping styles. Psychometric patterns and behavioural and physiological responses to stress. *Journal of Abnormal Psychology, 88*, 369–380.

KEY WORDS

Trait anxiety, cognition, clinical anxiety, selective processing, vulnerability to stress, social desirability, prepression–sensitization, physiology, mood effects, long-term memory, schemata.

Handbook of Life Stress, Cognition and Health
Edited by S. Fisher and J. Reason
© 1988 John Wiley & Sons Ltd

26

Learned Resourcefulness, Stress and Self-Regulation

Michael Rosenbaum
Tel Aviv University

INTRODUCTION

Learned resourcefulness is a personality repertoire which has been defined as a set of behaviors and skills by which individuals self-regulate internal responses that interfere with the smooth execution of an ongoing behavior (Rosenbaum, 1983). This term was first used by Meichenbaum (1977) in conjunction with his 'stress inoculation' program. In stress inoculation training, individuals are instructed in cognitive and behavioral skills which enable them to cope effectively with stressful events. The major components of the stress inoculation program are: (1) self-monitoring of maladaptive thoughts, images, feelings, and behaviors; (2) problem-solving skills; (3) emotion regulation and other self-control skills (Meichenbaum, 1985). Meichenbaum (1977) found that persons who have acquired these skills develop a sense of 'learned resourcefulness', i.e. the belief that they can effectively deal with 'manageable levels of stress'. The personality repertoire that I have labeled learned resourcefulness consists not just of a set of beliefs but also of skills and self-control behaviors which are taught in a typical stress inoculation training program. Research on learned resourcefulness is guided by the underlying assumption that these behaviors are acquired in different degrees by most people without any formal training.

The main instrument used for the assessment of learned resourcefulness is the Self-Control Schedule (SCS; Rosenbaum, 1980a). The SCS is a self-report instrument directed at assessing individual tendencies to apply self-control methods to the solution of behavioral problems. It covers the following content areas: (a) use of cognitions and self-instructions to cope with emotional and physiological responses; (b) application of problem-solving strategies (e.g. planning, problem definition, evaluating alternatives, and anticipation of consequences); (c) ability to delay immediate gratification; and (d) a general belief in one's ability to self-regulate internal events. The schedule consists of 36 items rated on a six-point scale that indicates the extent to which the subjects evaluate the item as characteristic of themselves. Evidence on the psychometric adequacy of the schedule is presented in the appendix at the end of this chapter, in addition to evidence on its construct validity which is presented in the studies cited throughout the chapter. Those who score above the median score of the SCS are referred to as high resourceful persons and those who score below the median score are referred to as low resourceful individuals. In all the studies which have used the SCS, a wide range of scores was obtained, which indicates that there are large individual differences in learned resourcefulness even in rather homogeneous populations.

To explicate fully the role of learned resourcefulness in the self-management of stressful events, the present discussion will begin with a definition of personality repertoires in general and with a description of the role of self-regulation in coping with stress. This will be followed by a discussion of the influence of specific personality repertoires on each of the three phases of the self-regulatory process (representation, evaluation, and action). The hypothesis that learned resourcefulness influences mainly what a person does during a stressful encounter and not how he or she evaluates it will be discussed. Research evidence will be presented to substantiate the claim that high resourceful individuals use more self-control methods during a stressful encounter than low resourceful individuals. In addition, studies on the role of learned resourcefulness in correctional and anticipatory self-regulation will be presented.

DEFINITION OF PERSONALITY REPERTOIRES

The concept of personality repertoires was introduced by Staats (1975), who used it interchangeably with the term 'basic behavioral repertoires'. These he defined as 'constellations of complex skills which are evoked by many situations but also have the quality of providing the basis for additional learning' (Staats, 1975, p. 63). A personality repertoire, is not a personality trait, but rather a set of behaviors, cognitions and affects that are in constant interaction with the social and physical environment of the person. For example, the types of statements a person makes about him or herself may influence the way other people respond to him or her, and at the same time these statements may be modified by the responses of others to them (Staats, 1963). Furthermore, these self-statements are also expected to function as stimuli that control the person's own behavior. Thus the personality repertoire may be treated both as an independent variable (a cause) and as a dependent variable (an effect). Learned resourcefulness is a personality repertoire which in most studies has been treated as an independent variable.

STRESS AND THE THREE PHASES OF SELF-REGULATION

Any effort at coping with stressful events involves attempts at self-regulation (see Nerenz and Leventhal, 1983). In fact, the coping process could not be understood without reference to the self-regulatory process. Self-regulatory processes are activated in situations 'in which reflex or automatic action sequences are unavailable, or have been interrupted, or when several response sequences of nearly equal probability are in conflict' (Kanfer, 1986). The conditions that activate the self-regulatory process are similar to those that have been recognized by stress researchers as conditions of stress. More specifically, Mandler (1982) developed an 'interruption theory' of stress which assumes that most psychologically stressful situations are the result of interruptions of a sequence of habitual acts or thoughts. The immediate consequence of any interruption is autonomic arousal, which attracts the person's attention to it. This is followed by the person's cognitive evaluation of the autonomic signals as being either pleasant or noxious (i.e. stressful). Whether an autonomic signal is evaluated in positive or negative terms is determined by person and situational variables. Thus, according to Mandler (1982), the problem of stress is twofold: 'both the internal autonomic signals and the conditions that generate these signals require some conscious capacity and thereby interfere with the performance of targeted tasks' (p. 92). As will be noted in later sections, the person's level of learned resourcefulness is postulated to determine the extent to which such interferences will occur.

On the basis of theories of stress (e.g. Lazarus and Folkman, 1984; Mandler, 1982; McGrath, 1976) and of Kanfer's three-stage model of self-regulation (Kanfer, 1977; 1986), I propose that the self-regulatory process can be conceptualized as consisting of three phases: representation, evaluation, and action. During the representational phase the individual experiences an emotional and/or a cognitive reaction to real or imagined changes within him or herself, or within the environment. These reactions occur more or less automatically, without any conscious effort. Thus, disruptions of ongoing behaviors, plans and well-established expectations may trigger 'automatic' thoughts about such things as one's self-worth and one's basic beliefs. These automatic thoughts are assumed to originate from deeply rooted cognitive self-schemata, and should not be confused with conscious and deliberate attempts to appraise the situation at hand. For example, a husband who is used to finding his well, accepting wife at home each day when he returns from work may automatically think that his wife is rejecting him when one day he does not find her at home at the regular time. Similarly, disruptions may trigger emotional responses such as anxiety and anger. In fact, it is postulated that the self-regulatory process (i.e. a self-change process) cannot be activated unless there are either emotional or cognitive reactions to the disruption.

The initial automatic reaction to a disruption is followed by a *conscious* evaluation of its meaning for the individual. In the evaluation phase of the self-regulatory process, individuals engage in what Lazarus and Folkman (1984) have labeled primary and secondary cognitive appraisals. In primary appraisal the person evaluates whether the disruption is desirable or threatening. If the person concludes that there is nothing at stake for her in the disruption, she will ignore her reactions to it and the self-regulatory process terminates here. However, if the person feels threatened by the disruption, she evaluates whether anything can be done to minimize its adverse effects and to maximize potential benefits. The latter is referred to by Lazarus and Folkman (1984) as secondary appraisal. Once the individual concludes that she can do something to minimize the negative effects of the disruption she engages in what has been referred to as 'coping' (Lazarus and Folkman, 1984). In the context of the present discussion, coping will be referred to as the action phase of the self-regulatory process.

Thus any effective coping with a stressor involves the three phases of the self-regulatory process. The first is an emotional or a cognitive reaction which we have called the representational phase of the process. This is followed by a conscious evaluation of the stressor, i.e. the evaluation phase of self-regulation. The final phase consists of an active response to minimize negative effects of the disruption, which is the action phase of the self-regulatory process.

THE ROLE OF PERSONALITY REPERTOIRES IN SELF-REGULATION

Although each phase of the self-regulatory process is influenced by both situational and personality factors, the focus of the present chapter is on personality factors, with a particular emphasis on learned resourcefulness.

Individual differences in learned resourcefulness are likely to have little impact on the representational phase of the self-regulatory process. For example, it has been demonstrated that high resourceful subjects do not differ from low resourceful subjects in their initial reactions to an epileptic seizure (Rosenbaum and Palmon, 1984), in their level of seasickness (Rosenbaum and Rolnick, 1983), or in their sensitivity to pain (Rosenbaum, 1980b). However, the differences between these two groups of subjects is mainly in how they cope with their emotional and cognitive reactions to these and other stressors (i.e. the action phase of the self-regulatory process).

There is, however, evidence that other personality repertoires may influence the likelihood and manner in which individuals react to disruptions. For example, individuals who have a strong disposition to attend to the inner, unshared aspects of themselves (i.e. are high on private self-consciousness; Buss, 1980), are more likely to react to changes in their bodily sensations and in their moods. Yet individuals who are high on public self-consciousness (Buss, 1980) are more likely to react to changes in the response of others to them. Hypnotic ability is another personality repertoire that may account for people's reactions to changes within themselves. People who are high on hypnotic ability have been found to be more responsive to psychological and physiological changes (Wickramasekera, 1986).

Once individuals react to a disruption, they consciously appraise its importance to their well-being. This part of the evaluative phase of the self-regulatory process has been referred to, in the context of stress, as primary appraisal (Lazarus and Folkman, 1984). Here again, high resourceful persons are not expected to differ from low resourceful persons in their evaluation of the negative impact of a stressor on their well-being.

Other personality repertoires have been hypothesized to affect the primary appraisal of a stressor. These include the 'sense of coherence' (Antonovski, 1979) and 'hardiness' (Kobasa, 1979). Thus, by definition, individuals with a high sense of coherence are those who usually evaluate stressors in a positive way because they are generally confident that their 'internal and external environments are predictable and that there is a high probability that things will work out as well as can be expected' (Antonovski, 1979, p. 123). Similarly, it is expected that 'hardy' individuals will emphasize the positive aspects of a stressor in particular because they view changes and disruptions in their life as challenging and desirable (Kobasa, 1979). Most studies on the sense of coherence and on hardiness have focused only on the general stress-buffering effects of these personality repertoires. Therefore, it is not clear from these studies whether these personality factors affect the subject's evaluation of the stressor or his or her coping with the interfering effects of the stressor (i.e. the action phase of self-regulation). Nevertheless, from the theoretical expositions of hardiness and the sense of coherence, it can be hypothesized that their main impact is likely to be on the primary appraisal of the stressor.

In sum, although learned resourcefulness, hardiness and the sense of coherence are all personality repertoires which may have stress-buffering effects, they mitigate the effects of stressful events at different phases of the self-regulation process. Whereas hardiness and the sense of coherence are postulated to influence the person's evaluation of the stressful disruption, learned resourcefulness is postulated to influence the person's actions toward reducing the interfering effects of his or her reactions to a stressor and not his or her primary appraisal of the stressor.

The extent to which secondary appraisals and people's self-efficacy beliefs in their ability to cope with a specific stressor (Bandura, 1977) are guided by personality dispositions is not clear. Bandura (1977) has enumerated various conditions which influence an individual's self-efficacy expectations; none of these includes personality factors. Folkman et al., (1986) found only a low correlation between a person's secondary appraisals and Pearlin and Schooler's (1978) Mastery Scale, which assesses people's belief in their ability to control their own behavior. Learned resourcefulness was found to be positively correlated with self-efficacy expectancies mostly in cases where the subjects had a past experience with the stressful task (e.g. Rosenbaum and Ben-Ari Smira, 1986), but not where they had no experience with the stressful task (e.g. Weisenberg et al., 1986). Thus one's level of learned resourcefulness is postulated to influence one's self-control expectancies only under specific situational conditions.

Learned resourcefulness is postulated to have its major impact on the third phase of the self-regulatory process, namely, the action phase. During this phase the person engages in what Folkman et al. (1986) define as 'coping'. These authors define coping as 'the person's cognitive and behavioral efforts to manage (reduce, minimize, master, or tolerate) the internal and external demands of the person–environment transaction that is appraised as taxing or exceeding the person's resources' (p. 542). The cognitive and the behavioral skills required for effective coping are part of the person's learned resourcefulness repertoire. Therefore, how a person evaluates a stressful encounter will determine whether or not he or she will attempt to cope with the stressor. However, without the appropriate repertoire of self-control skills (i.e. learned resourcefulness), coping will be ineffective (Rosenbaum, 1983).

To summarize, learned resourcefulness is postulated to have no influence on the individual's initial emotional and cognitive reactions to a stressor (the representational phase) nor on his or her primary appraisal of the stressor (part I of the evaluation phase). Under certain circumstances, the person's level of learned resourcefulness may influence secondary appraisal (part II of the evaluation phase, i.e. control expectancies). Learned resourcefulness as a personality repertoire is postulated to have its greatest impact on the person's attempts during the action phase to self-regulate internal responses that interfere with the smooth execution of a desired behavior.

LEARNED RESOURCEFULNESS AND THE USE OF SELF-CONTROL METHODS

Our learned resourcefulness model suggests that high resourceful subjects use more self-control methods during a stressful encounter than low resourceful subjects. Because self-control behaviors are private events, the only way to find out whether or not subjects are using them is by questioning the subjects directly. In a number of studies, my colleagues and I have asked subjects immediately following a stressful event what they did to cope with that event. In one such study (Rosenbaum, 1980b), subjects were exposed to a cold pressor. As expected, high resourceful subjects tolerated the cold pressor for longer durations than did low resourceful subjects, but did not differ in rating the intensity of the experienced pain. Moreover, high resourceful subjects reported using self-control methods more frequently and more effectively than did low resourceful subjects.

In another study (Rosenbaum and Rolnick, 1983), we investigated individual differences in learned resourcefulness and coping with seasickness among crewmen serving on missile boats in the Israeli Navy. Although seasick subjects generally performed worse than non-seasick subjects, high resourceful seasick subjects showed significantly less performance deficits in a stormy sea than did low resourceful seasick subjects. Seasickness symptoms, as assessed by peer and self-reports, were unrelated to different levels of learned resourcefulness. Furthermore, in retrospective reports, high resourceful seasick subjects reported more extensive and specific uses of self-control methods to cope with seasickness than low resourceful seasick subjects. Similarly, Gal-Or and Tennebaum (1985) reported that, among novice parachutists, high levels of learned resourcefulness are associated with better performance during the jumps as well as increases in the use of coping self-statements indicating emotional self-control and task orientation. High resourceful parachutists, in comparison to low resourceful parachutists, reported that they more frequently used self-statements that indicate emotional self-control and task orientation.

Two additional studies on coping with stress-related medical problems provide evidence that high resourceful subjects more frequently use self-control methods during stress than low resourceful subjects. The first study examined the effects of learned resourcefulness on coping with epilepsy. In this study (Rosenbaum and Palmon, 1984), high resourceful epileptics who experienced low and medium ranges of epileptic seizures were found to cope more effectively with their seizures than low resourceful epileptics under the same conditions. High resourceful epileptics reported that they have used more self-control methods during their coping with the psychological consequences of an epileptic seizure than did low resourceful epileptics. In the second study, Groves (1986) compared the reactions of high resourceful women with those of low resourceful women during 'natural childbirth' (i.e. without drugs). As expected, high resourceful women reported that they had more control over the delivery process, engaged more often in breathing–relaxation exercises, and used more self-encouraging statements during delivery.

One major problem with the studies cited so far is that they all used retrospective reports. These reports might be confounded with the successful outcomes of the subjects' coping efforts. To circumvent this problem, we conducted a study in which subjects were questioned about their thoughts *during* a laboratory-produced stressful event. Such a procedure is usually impossible during exposure to real-life stressors. The purpose of this study (Rosenbaum and Ben-Ari, 1985) was to investigate the differential reactions of high resourceful and low resourceful subjects to an uncontrollable failure condition which was hypothesized to produce learned helplessness (Abramson *et al.*, 1978). Similar to a typical learned helplessness paradigm, this study consisted of a training phase in which subjects were exposed to uncontrollable failure, and a test phase which consisted of a solvable task. During the training phase of the experiment, we asked subjects to check, from a list of self-referent statements, those statements that best fitted their current thoughts and feelings. As predicted, high resourceful subjects more frequently checked statements indicating positive self-evaluations and task-oriented thoughts than did low resourceful subjects. Further, as expected, only the low resourceful subjects, and not the high resourceful subjects, showed the debilitating effects from the learned helplessness induction on the test task.

In conclusion, there is strong evidence that high resourceful persons, in comparison to low resourceful persons, utilize more self-control methods when faced with a stressful event.

LEARNED RESOURCEFULNESS AND ANTICIPATORY SELF-REGULATION

Kanfer (1986) has recently identified two types of self-regulation: corrective and anticipatory self-regulation. Corrective self-regulation occurs when ongoing behaviors are disrupted and the person's efforts are directed at resuming normal functioning. The discussion so far has dealt mainly with people's attempts at corrective self-regulation. Anticipatory self-regulation, on the other hand, is initiated when the person recalls certain information that disrupts the progress of a planned or a habitual behavior. In this case the disruption is self-generated. For example, after a myocardial infarction an obese person recalls her physician's instruction to reduce weight. Consequently, she initiates self-produced changes and disruptions in various aspects of her life that are related to food consumption. Nerenz and Leventhal (1983), who discussed self-regulation in the context of illness, have labeled this type of self-regulation as 'danger control'. They note that it 'consists of representations of the health threat as objectively perceived and of

plans and reactions for modifying the impact of the threat on the individual'
(p. 15).

Whenever a person engages in anticipatory self-regulation, he delays immediate gratifications for the sake of future consequences, and copes with the
frustrations and stresses produced by the delay. The adoption of health-related
behaviors almost always requires some kind of delay or gratification for the
purpose of maintaining good health in the long run. Individuals who have a rich
repertoire of self-control skills (i.e. have a high level of learned resourcefulness)
are hypothesized to have the ability to cope with the personal difficulties encountered in acquiring and maintaining good health behaviors. This hypothesis is
supported by two studies in which compliance to difficult medical requirements
was investigated. In the first study (Rosenbaum and Ben-Ari Smira, 1986) it was
found that high resourceful dialysis patients adhered more closely to fluid-intake
restrictions than did low resourceful patients. It should be noted that high
resourceful patients did not differ from low resourceful patients in their understanding of the adverse consequences of failure to adhere to fluid-intake restrictions, nor did they differ in their motivation to adhere. In the second study (Amir,
1985), it was found that high resourceful diabetics were more successful in
controlling sugar intake than low resourceful diabetics. In line with these studies,
Katz and Singh (1986) found that high resourceful smokers were more successful
in quitting cigarette smoking on their own than low resourceful smokers. Furthermore, in general, high resourceful persons in comparison to low resourceful
persons were found to comply more closely with psychological treatment requiring self-change (e.g. Achmon, 1988; Biran, in preparation, Rusnak, 1983; Simons
et al., 1985).

Thus, there is research evidence indicating that high levels of resourcefulness
are associated with the effectiveness of both corrective and anticipatory self-
regulation.

IMPLICATIONS

Stress researchers have increasingly focused on the role of personality repertoires
and social support systems in buffering the effects of stressful life events (e.g.
Hobfoll and Leiberman, 1987). Yet most studies have failed to distinguish
between the initial automatic reactions to the disruptive event (i.e. the representational phase), the cognitive evaluation of the event, and the person's activities to
reduce the interfering effects of these reactions on ongoing functioning. Our work
on learned resourcefulness has focused on the last-mentioned. In a number of
studies we have demonstrated that high resourceful individuals do not differ from
low resourceful individuals in their initial reactions to stressful life events, nor in
their evaluation of the stressor, but they do differ in their ability to reduce the
interfering effects of stress reactions on ongoing behaviors.

The present chapter has exclusively focused on the role of personality resources
in coping with stress. Yet, obviously, social resources may be as important in this
process as personality resources. The question is, however, at what stage of the
coping process do social resources play a significant role? It can be argued that

perceived social support is likely to influence mainly the person's evaluation of the stressor but not her attempts at reducing the aversive consequences of the stressor (i.e. the action phase of the self-regulatory process). Partial support for this argument is obtained by the positive correlation that was found by Ganellen and Blaney (1984) between measures of social support and hardiness (Kobasa, 1979). Recall that, according to the scheme presented here, hardiness as a personality repertoire is postulated to have its main effect on the evaluation phase of the self-regulatory process. Furthermore, there is cogent evidence that the stress mitigation effects of social support is in the belief that support is available, irrespective of its use (Lieberman, 1982). Monroe and Steiner (1986) have recently noted that 'whereas high perceived support predicts fewer psychological symptoms, high support utilization predicts greater levels of symptoms' (p. 37). Thus individuals who believe that social support is available when needed may appraise disruptive events as less stressful. On the other hand, individuals who turn to others for help because they lack the necessary self-control skills needed for reducing the interfering effects of stressful events, may not benefit from social support. In fact, I postulate that those who are able to help themselves (i.e. high resourceful persons) will be most helped by others. Yet those who are unable to help themselves (i.e. low resourceful persons) are likely to deplete their social resources by their highly socially dependent behavior (cf. Monroe and Steiner, 1986).

The three-stage model of self-regulation presented in this chapter enables the delineation of the effects of social resources from personality resources on the process of coping with stressful events.

Perhaps the most important question in the study of learned resourcefulness is: how is it acquired? Cognitive–behavioral programs such as those suggested by Meichenbaum (1985) may be one way by which individuals learn to be resourceful. However, my basic premise is that resourcefulness is acquired during childhood through informal training. In fact, learned resourcefulness could be conceived as a stable personality trait, like intelligence. Block and Block (1980) developed the concept of ego resiliency in their work with children which is highly similar to the concept of learned resourcefulness. Ego resiliency is described as a stable personality dimension which is defined by 'resourceful adaptation to changing circumstances and environmental contingencies . . . and flexible invocation of the available repertoire of problem-solving strategies . . .' (Block and Block, 1980, p. 48). Children's ego resiliency was found to predict their social and personal adjustment during adolescence (Funder et al., 1983). Similarly, Mischel (1984) found that children who were able to delay immediate gratification (one major component of learned resourcefulness) during their preschool years developed into adolescents who were 'attentive and able to concentrate . . . responsive to reason, competent, skillful, able to plan and think ahead, and able to cope and deal with stress maturely' (p. 355). Thus there is some evidence to indicate that learned resourcefulness is a stable personality repertoire which is acquired in early childhood.

During the past decades, psychologists directed their efforts at assessing intellectual skills for the purpose of predicting future academic achievements. The time is now ripe for developing effective methods for assessing the person's self-regulatory skills (i.e. learned resourcefulness) and his or her ability to cope effectively with stressful events. The focus of our research should shift from studying the pathological parts of the human beings toward studying the 'healthy' aspects of human behavior to further our understanding on how most individuals remain well adjusted despite their exposure to the stresses and strains of modern life.

SUMMARY AND CONCLUSIONS

Learned resourcefulness refers to an acquired repertoire of self-control skills and is operationally defined as a repertoire of behaviors and skills (mostly cognitive) by which a person self-regulates internal responses, such as emotions, pain, and cognitions, that interfere with the smooth execution of an ongoing behavior. Currently, it is mostly assessed by the Self-Control Schedule (Rosenbaum, 1980a).

The concept of learned resourcefulness originated from Kanfer's theory of self-regulation (Kanfer, 1977; 1986) and from Meichenbaum's stress-inoculation training program (Meichenbaum, 1985). In the present chapter the concept is applied to coping with stress. My basic premise is that any effort at coping with stressful events involves attempts at self-regulation. Disruption of ongoing habitual activities has been postulated by Kanfer (1977) to activate the self-regulatory process, and by a number of stress researchers (e.g. Mandler, 1982) as a precursor of stress. Hence the process of coping with stress has been described in terms of a self-regulatory process which follows an interruption of ongoing behaviors.

The self-regulatory process consists of three phases: representation, evaluation, and action. During the representational phase the individual reacts emotionally and/or cognitively to the disruptions in her ongoing activities, thoughts, or plans. These reactions occur more or less automatically, without any conscious effort. During the second phase, the evaluation phase, the individual consciously and purposely evaluates the meaning of the disruption for her well-being and whether she can effectively cope with it. Whether a specific disruption is considered to be stressful or not is determined by the person's cognitive evaluations of the disruption (Lazarus and Folkman, 1984). The final phase, the action phase, consists of an active response that minimizes or reduces the interfering effects that emotional and cognitive responses have on the performance of a target behavior.

The three-stage model of self-regulation presented in this chapter provides the theoretical framework by which the differential role of various personality and social resources in coping with stress can be elucidated. Specifically, learned resourcefulness is postulated to play a major role in the action phase of the self-regulatory process. Studies are presented which indicate that high resourceful individuals do not differ from low resourceful individuals in their initial reactions to stressful life events, or in their evaluation of the stressor, but that they do differ in their ability to reduce the interfering effects of stress reactions on ongoing behaviors.

APPENDIX: PSYCHOMETRIC CHARACTERISTICS OF THE SELF-CONTROL SCHEDULE (SCS)

Normative Data

The SCS means for three samples of Israeli students ranged from 23 to 27, with standard deviations ranging from 21 to 25 (Rosenbaum, 1980a). Similar means and standard deviations were found with American college students (Redden *et al.*, 1983). Lewinsohn and Alexander (in preparation) gave the SCS to 450 male and 356 female residents of Eugene, Oregon, with a mean age of 63.7 years (S.D.=7.9). The mean SCS score for this sample was 24.6 (S.D.=15.2). In most studies there were no sex differences on the SCS scores.

Reliability

Two kinds of reliability measures were reported: test–retest and coefficient alphas. Rosenbaum (1980a) reported a test–retest correlation after 4 weeks of 0.86, and Leon and Rosenthal (1984), in the US, reported a correlation of 0.77 after an interval of 11 months. Thus the SCS scores are quite stable over time. However, an increase in SCS scores is expected following cognitive–behavior therapy (Simons *et al.*, 1985; Achmon, 1988). The internal consistency of the SCS items was computed on the data obtained from five samples in the Rosenbaum (1980a) study by the use of the Kuder–Richardson formula 20. The alpha coefficient ranged from 0.78 to 0.91. Redden *et al.* (1983) reported a Cronbach coefficient alpha of 0.82.

Factor Analysis and Correlations with Other Scales

In a recent factor analysis performed on the SCS, three factors have emerged: problem-focused coping, mood and pain control, and externality (Gruber and Wildman, 1987).

The convergent and the discriminant validity of the SCS was examined by correlating the SCS scores to scores of various other scales. Rosenbaum (1980a) reported that the SCS had low but statistically significant correlations with the following scales: Rotter's I–E Locus of Control Scale (Rotter, 1966; see also Richards, 1985), the Irrational Beliefs Test (Jones, 1968), and the G Factor ('Self-Control') of Cattell's 16 PF (Cattell *et al.*, 1970). In addition, the SCS was found to correlate with Fitz's Self-Esteem Scale (Michelson, 1985), and with various antidepressant cognitions and behaviors (Lewinsohn and Alexander, in preparation). High correlations were obtained between SCS scores and assessment of specific self-efficacy expectations in situations that require self-control behavior (Leon and Rosenthal, 1984; Rosenbaum and Ben-Ari Smira, 1986). In the Lewinsohn and Alexander (in preparation) study, the SCS was not found to correlate with the Crowne–Marlow Social Desirability Scale, yet Rosebaum (1980a) reported a low (r=0.21) correlation with this scale.

REFERENCES

Abramson, L.Y., Seligman, M.E.P., & Teasdale, J. (1978). Learned helplessness in humans: Critique and reformulation. *Journal of Abnormal Psychology, 87*, 49–74.

Achmon, J. (1988). Hypertensives' response to cognitive and biofeedback treatments as a function of their resourcefulness and heart rate variability. An unpublished doctoral dissertation, Tel Aviv University, Tel Aviv, Israel.

Amir, S. (1985). Prediction of compliance and control in juvenile diabetes through self-control, perceptions and assertive behavior determinants. An unpublished master thesis submitted to the School of Social Work at Tel Aviv University, Tel Aviv, Israel.

Antonovski, A. (1979). *Health, stress, and coping.* San Francisco: Jossey-Bass.

Bandura, A. (1977). Self-efficacy: Toward a unifying theory of behavior change. *Psychological Review, 84*, 191–215.

Biran, M.W. (in preparation). Successful treatment of agoraphobics and resourcefulness. In M. Rosenbaum (ed.), *Learned resourcefulness: On coping skills, self-regulation and adaptive behavior.* New York: Springer.

Block, J.H., & Block, J. (1980). The role of ego control and ego-resiliency in the organization of behavior. In W.A. Collins (ed.). *Development of cognition, affect and social relations: The Minnesota symposium on child psychology,* Vol. 13 (pp. 39–101). Hillsdale, NJ: Erlbaum.

Buss, A.H. (1980). *Self-consciousness and social anxiety.* San Francisco: Freeman.

Cattell, R.B., Eber, H.W., & Tatsuoka, M.M. (1970). *Handbook for the 16 PF questionnaire.* Champaign, Illinois: Institute for Personality and Ability Testing.

Folkman, S., Lazarus, R.S., Gruen, R.J., & DeLongis, A. (1986). Appraisal, coping, health status, and psychological symptoms. *Journal of Personality and Social Psychology, 50*, 571–572.

Funder, D.C., Block, J.H., & Block, J. (1983). Delay of gratification: Some longitudinal personality correlates. *Journal of Personality and Social Psychology, 44*, 1198–1213.

Gal-Or, J., & Tennebaum, G. (1985). The effects of self-control, anxiety, and body image on the performance and the self-talk of novice parachutists. Unpublished manuscript (in Hebrew). The Wingate Institute, Israel.

Ganellen, R.J., & Blaney, P.H. (1984). Hardiness and social support as moderators of the effects of life stress. *Journal of Personality and Social Psychology, 47*, 156–163.

Groves, S. (1986). Learned resourcefulness and coping with childbirth. Unpublished MA thesis, Tel Aviv University, Tel Aviv.

Gruber, V.A., & Wildman, B.G. (1987). The impact of dysmenorrhea on daily activities. *Behavior Research and Therapy, 25*, 123–128.

Hobfoll, S.A., & Leiberman, J.R. (1987). Personality and social resources in immediate and continued stress resistance among women. *Journal of Personality and Social Psychology, 52*, 18–26.

Jones, R.G. (1968). *A factor measure of Ellis' irrational belief systems.* Whichita, Kansas: Test Systems.

Kanfer, F.H. (1977). The many faces of self-control, or behavior modification changes its focus. In R.B. Stuart (ed.), *Behavioral self-management: Strategies, techniques and outcomes.* New York: Brunner/Mazel.

Kanfer, F.H. (1986). Self-regulation and behavior. Paper presented at the Ringberg Symposium on Volition and Action, Schloss Ringberg, West Germany.

Katz, R.C., & Singh, N. (1986). A comparison of current smokers and self-cured quitters on Rosenbaum's Self-Control Schedule. *Addictive Behaviors, 11*, 63–65.

Kobasa, S.C. (1979). Stressful life events, personality, health: Inquiry into hardiness. *Journal of Personality and Social Psychology, 37*, 1–11.

Lazarus, R.S., & Folkman, S. (1984). *Stress, appraisal, and coping.* New York: Springer.

Leon, G.R., & Rosenthal, B.S. (1984). Prognostic indicators of success or relapse in weight reduction. *International Journal of Eating Disorders, 3*, 15–24.

Lewinsohn, P.M., & Alexander, C. (in preparation). In M. Rosenbaum (ed.), *Learned resourcefulness: On coping skills, self-regulation, and adaptive behavior*. New York: Springer.

Lieberman, M.A. (1982). The effects of social support on responses to stress. In L. Goldberger & S. Breznitz (eds), *Handbook of stress: Theoretical and clinical aspects* (pp. 764–783). New York: Free Press.

Mandler, G. (1982). Stress and thought processes. In L. Goldberger & S. Breznitz (eds), *Handbook of stress* (pp. 88–120). New York: Free Press.

McGrath, J.E. (1976). Stress and behavior in organization. In Dunnette, M.D. (ed.) *Handbook of industrial and organizational psychology* (pp. 1351–1395). Skokie, Illinois: Rand McNally.

Meichenbaum, D. (1977). *Cognitive–behavior modification: An integrative approach*. New York: Plenum.

Meichenbaum, D. (1985). *Stress inoculation training*. New York: Pergamon Press.

Michelson, S. (1985). Private self-consciousness interactive effect on the causation of anxiety and depression: Three possible mediating variables. Unpublished MA dissertation, Tel-Aviv University.

Mischel, W. (1984). Convergences and challenges in the search for consistency. *American Psychologist, 39*, 351–364.

Monroe, S.M., & Steiner, S.C. (1986). Social support and psychopathology: Interrelations with preexisting disorder, stress, and personality. *Journal of Abnormal Psychology, 95*, 29–39.

Nerenz, D.R., & Leventhal, H. (1983). Self-regulation theory in chronic illness. In T.G. Burish & L.A. Bradley (eds), *Coping with chronic disease: Research and applications* (pp. 1–37). New York: Academic Press.

Pearlin, L.I., & Schooler, C. (1978). The structure of coping. *Journal of Health and Social Behavior, 19*, 2–21.

Redden, E.M., Tucker, R.K., & Young, L. (1983). Psychometric properties of the Rosenbaum Schedule for Assessing Self-Control. *The Psychological Record, 33*, 77–86.

Richards, P.S. (1985). Construct validation of the Self-Control Schedule. *Journal of Research in Personality, 19*, 208–218.

Rosenbaum, M. (1980a). A schedule for assessing self-control behaviors: Preliminary findings. *Behavior Therapy, 11*, 109–121.

Rosenbaum, M. (1980b). Individual differences in self-control behaviors and tolerance of painful stimulation. *Journal of Abnormal Psychology, 89*, 581–590.

Rosenbaum, M. (1983). Learned resourcefulness as a behavioral repertoire for the self-regulation of internal events: Issues and speculations. In M. Rosenbaum, C.M. Franks & Y. Jaffe (eds), *Perspectives on behavior therapy in the eighties* (pp. 54–73). New York: Springer.

Rosenbaum, M., & Ben-Ari, K. (1985). Learned helplessness and learned resourcefulness: Effects of noncontingent success and failure on individuals differing in self-control skills. *Journal of Personality and Social Psychology, 48*, 198–215.

Rosenbaum, M., & Ben-Ari Smira (1986). Cognitive and personality factors in the delay of immediate gratification of hemodialysis patients. *Journal of Personality and Social Psychology, 51*, 357–364.

Rosenbaum, M., & Palmon, N. (1984). Helplessness and resourcefulness in coping with epilepsy. *Journal of Consulting and Clinical Psychology, 52*, 244–253.

Rosenbaum, M., & Rolnick, A. (1983). Self-control behaviors and coping with seasickness. *Cognitive Therapy and Research, 7*, 93–98.

Rotter, J.B. (1966). Generalized expectancies for internal versus external control of reinforcement. *Psychological Monographs, 80*, No. 1.

Rusnak, J.G. (1983). The effects of learned resourcefulness and autogenic phrases on skin temperature control. Unpublished doctoral dissertation, Arizona State University, Phoenix.

Simons, A.D., Lustman, P.J., Wetzel, R.D., & Murphy, G.E. (1985). Predicting response to cognitive therapy of depression: The role of learned resourcefulness. *Cognitive*

Therapy and Research, 9, 79–90.
Staats, A.W. (1963). *Complex human behavior*. New York: Holt, Rinehart, & Winston.
Staats, A.W. (1975). *Social behaviorism*. Homewood, Illinois: Dorsey.
Weisenberg, M., Wolf, Y., Mittwoch, T., & Mikulincer, M. (1986). Learned resourceful-
ness and perceived control of pain. Unpublished manuscript, Bar-Ilan University,
Ramat Gan, Israel.
Wickramasekera, I. (1986). A model of people at high risk to develop chronic stress-
related somatic symptoms: Some predictions. *Professional Psychology: Research and
Practice, 17*, 437–447.

KEY WORDS

Anticipatory self-regulation, coping process, corrective self-regulation, disruptions, hardiness, individual differences, learned resourcefulness, personality repertoire, primary
appraisal, secondary appraisal, self-control, Self-Control Schedule, self-control skills,
self-efficacy, Self-regulation, self-regulatory process, self-statements, sense of coherence,
social support, stress, stress inoculation.

Handbook of Life Stress, Cognition and Health
Edited by S. Fisher and J. Reason
© 1988 John Wiley & Sons Ltd.

27

Putting the Life Back into 'Life Events': Toward a Cognitive Social Learning Analysis of the Coping Process

SUZANNE M. MILLER and ADINA BIRNBAUM
Temple University, Philadelphia

INTRODUCTION

What makes life events stressful? In the past two decades, a wealth of research has demonstrated that the occurrence of major life events and, perhaps more importantly, of minor daily hassles increases psychological and physical indices of morbidity (Burks and Martin, 1985; DeLongis *et al.*, 1982; Dohrenwend and Dohrenwend, 1974; Monroe, 1983; Sarason *et al.*, 1982). Yet it is clear that only a subset of individuals fall ill or become distressed in response to such events. Recently, therefore, investigators have attempted to delineate when and under what circumstances negative outcomes are precipitated and when they are not. Lazarus and his colleagues (1985) have argued persuasively for a person-by-situation approach to stress that emphasizes the interaction between the environmental situation and the individual's appraisal of that situation. For example, several studies have shown that it is not simply the experience of life events per se that generates stress, but rather the perception of such events as undesirable (Matheny and Cupp, 1983; Sarason *et al.*, 1978; Suls and Mullen, 1981; Vinokur and Selzer, 1975), uncontrollable (Matheny and Cupp, 1983; Suls and Mullen, 1981) and unanticipated (Matheny and Cupp, 1983).

The study of life events may be rendered even more fruitful by delineating the individual difference factors that moderate their impact and that may account for the variability in how such events are perceived. In this chapter, we focus on two promising dispositional dimensions along which individuals' information-processing behavior can vary. The first is the extent to which they seek out and 'monitor' for information about threat, and the second is the extent to which they can cognitively distract from and psychologically 'blunt' threat-relevant information (Miller, 1980a; 1981; in press; Miller and Grant, 1979; Miller and Green, 1985). This research is conducted within a cognitive social learning framework which endorses the value of taking simultaneous account of the interaction between relevant personal dispositions and the specific properties of the situation (Mischel, 1979; 1984; 1986). We first summarize some current approaches to the study of individual differences in information processing, especially relevant to threat and stress stimuli. We next apply the monitoring–blunting perspective to the area of life events, providing dimensions for analyzing individual differences in response to objectively identical sources of stress. We also present data supporting this approach and integrate them with existing literature, exploring the implications for the study of life events.

SOME PROMISING APPROACHES TO INDIVIDUAL DIFFERENCES IN INFORMATION PROCESSING

Several lines of evidence support the role of individual differences in attentional dispositions as a moderator between life events and subsequent physical and psychological dysfunction. Emphasis has tended to shift away from how individuals attend to and process information about the aversive event (e.g. its desirability, controllability, etc.) to a focus on how individuals attend to and process information about themselves (e.g. Carver and Scheier, 1982). Borrowing on recent developments in social, personality, and cognitive psychology, there has been a growing interest in applying control systems theory to an understanding of how people regulate their psychological and physical well-being (Carver and Scheier, 1982; Schwartz, 1983). This approach suggests that whether or not individuals generally take action to cope with their internal states is a function, in part, of the perceived discrepancy between their current state and the 'normal' state. With respect to the experience of negative life events, the degree to which individuals typically tend to focus on themselves is postulated to affect the adaptiveness of their subsequent self-regulatory behaviors. Specifically, it is hypothesized that those who are prone to attend to aspects of the self will be more likely to perceive their own internal reactions to negative life events. This, in turn, should prompt them to take instrumental actions that reduce stress and allow them successfully to negotiate their response to the event. In contrast, those who are not prone to focus attention on the self will fail to perceive their own internal reactions and hence fail to take appropriate instrumental actions. This should make them particularly vulnerable to the impact of negative stressors.

Suls and Fletcher (1985) have obtained data that support this view. Using the private self-consciousness subscale of Fenigstein et al. (1975), they found that the incidence of stressful life events predicted subsequent reports of physical symptoms among persons low in self-focus but not in persons high in self-focus (see also Mullen and Suls, 1982). Although the conceptual and methodological approach developed in their work is heuristic and promising generally, the specific interpretation of these results is problematic. First, the investigators used a self-report measure of physical symptoms rather than direct, objective assessments of actual physical status or health-care-seeking behaviors. Second, in the absence of other measures of arousal, such as psychological distress, it becomes difficult to interpret the pattern of results obtained. Finally, the study provides no direct evidence that self-focused individuals do, in fact, take instrumental actions to deal with their reactions to life stressors. The scale itself assesses the tendency to focus on one's moods, emotions, and feelings but does not address the specific behavioral strategies that individuals tend to employ to cope with aversive events. Since the execution of control actions can include a diverse array of possibly unrelated self-regulatory behaviors, ranging from actual information seeking under threat to problem solving, reinterpretation, planning, and outcome-oriented instrumental behaviors (Folkman and Lazarus, 1980), it may be inappropriate to combine informational preferences and control preferences together. Elsewhere, we have argued that the twin constructs of information and control are each complex and should be kept conceptually and methodologically distinct (Miller, 1979a; 1979b; 1980a; 1980b; 1981; 1987).

A further difficulty with interpreting these data is that a different pattern of results has been obtained by other investigators. Mechanic and his colleagues (Mechanic, 1978; 1980; Mechanic and Volkart, 1961; Tessler and Mechanic, 1978; Tessler et al., 1976) have extensively studied the factors underlying the reporting of psychological distress and physical symptoms as well as the factors that prompt symptomatic individuals to seek medical care. Their work suggests that an important risk factor for increased symptomatology and health-care utilization appears to be the individual's learned pattern to monitor and be sensitive to internal bodily states. Using a measure of introspectiveness, derived in part from the private self-consciousness scale of Fenigstein et al. (1975), Hansell and Mechanic (1985) found that adolescents high in self-focus showed greater psychological distress and more physical symptoms in response to stress than adolescents low in self-focus. Similar results have been obtained in other studies (Greenley and Mechanic, 1976; Mechanic, 1979; 1980; Mechanic and Cleary, 1980). Mechanic (1980) has also found that a variety of maladaptive behaviors (such as smoking, not exercising, etc.) are associated with the reporting of common physical symptoms. Overall, while this work contains some of the problems of the studies cited previously (e.g. a reliance on self-report measures of physical symptoms), the results described here suggest a clear pattern: namely, attention to the self may be a vulnerability, rather than an invulnerability factor, predisposing to increased stress and decreased self-regulatory behaviors.

STYLES OF INFORMATION PROCESSING UNDER THREAT: MONITORING AND BLUNTING

In our previous work we have explored individual differences in the disposition to 'monitor' and to psychologically 'blunt' threat-relevant cues when faced with the prospect of uncontrollable aversive events (Miller, 1980a; 1981; in press; Miller and Grant, 1979; Miller and Green, 1985). Generally, this work has combined the monitoring and blunting dimensions together, categorizing individuals as either high monitors/low blunters or low blunters/high monitors. These studies have indicated that high monitors/low blunters are not overall more state or trait anxious and depressed than are low monitors/high blunters (Miller, 1987; in press; Miller and Mangan, 1983; Phipps and Zinn, 1986; Steptoe, 1986). However, in response to negative but uncontrollable situations, the former group tends to show greater and more sustained physiological, subjective, and behavioral arousal than the latter group (Efran *et al.*, 1981; Gard *et al.*, in press; Lamping *et al.*, 1985; Miller, 1979a: Miller and Mangan, 1983; Phipps and Zinn, 1986). Moreover, dispositional differences in coping style interact with and determine the impact of information in stressful situations, with high monitors/low blunters benefiting from voluminous threat-relevant information and low monitors/high blunters benefiting from more minimal information (Efran *et al.*, 1981; Lamping and Robertson, 1985; Miller and Mangan, 1983; Watkins *et al.*, 1986). Thus the stressfulness of an aversive event depends not only upon its specific qualities (e.g. its intensity and duration) but also upon the context in which it occurs. For some, stress is augmented when the level of information made available is low; while for others, stress is reduced when information is withheld.

More recent research treats the monitoring and blunting dimensions as unique and separable and suggests that there are distinctive features associated with each (Miller, 1987). For example, in a set of studies, the monitoring subscale proved to be a stronger predictor of whether subjects chose to monitor for information about the quality and speed of their performance on an ego-threatening cognitive task than the blunting subscale. In contrast, scores on the blunting subscale proved to be a stronger predictor of the choice to listen for information about the prospect of electric shock or to distract with music (Miller, 1987). In ongoing work, we are continuing to specify more precisely the nature of the two scales, their potential interchangeability, and the conditions under which they provide distinctive information (e.g. Miller *et al.*, in press).

In one line of research, we are further exploring the relations among information-processing styles, health status, and health-seeking behavior. In addition to having to deal with a variety of external environmental stressors, the emergence of internal physical symptoms may represent an important minor life event or chronic hassle to which individuals must continually adapt (Lazarus *et al.*, 1985). The evidence on self-focus presented above suggests that dispositional differences in coping style may affect the individual's attention, interpretation and response to such symptoms. The monitor and blunter dimensions may well be relevant here. Because high monitors and low blunters are more likely to scan for external threat-relevant cues and less likely to distract than low monitors and high blunters, they may also have a lower threshold for attending to 'internal' bodily cues. This would make them more inclined to detect or overinterpret new or changing physical symptoms, which they would find difficult to ignore. This, in turn, should prompt them to report and seek treatment for their symptomatology. Further, consistent with research on patients facing aversive medical procedures, high monitors and low blunters may show less symptom improvement in acute primary care problems and less improvement in their stress-related problems than do low monitors and high blunters (Miller, in press).

A RESEARCH ILLUSTRATION: AIMS AND METHODS

To examine these issues, we studied 118 patients visiting the primary care facility of General Internal Medicine at Temple Hospital for acute onset of medical symptoms in the week preceding their visit (Miller *et al.*, 1988). In order to circumvent some of the limitations of previous work, we obtained physician assessments of the patients' actual physical and psychological status, in addition to the patients' own somatic and psychological self-reports. Measures of patients' psychological distress included both general concerns and their concerns about their specific physical symptoms. We were particularly interested in examining the role of depression, which has been found to be both prevalent in primary care populations and related to increased health-seeking behaviors and poorer health status (Magill and Zung, 1982; Mechanic, 1978; 1980; Nielson and Williams, 1980; Rodin and Voshart, 1986; Scaramella, 1977; Stoeckle *et al.*, 1964). Since information-processing variables such as monitoring and blunting also may be related to initial indices of perceived stress in primary care settings, such as depression, we explored the effects of coping style while controlling for depressed state.

As a secondary aim, we sought to determine patients' actual pre-visit preferences for interventions and information. There is a good deal of evidence that patients vary in their desires for information about the nature and effects of their medical problem and in their desires for medical and psychosocial interventions (Faden *et al.*, 1981; Good *et al.*, 1983; Korsch *et al.*, 1968; Lazare *et al.*, 1975; Reader *et al.*, 1957). Yet, there has been little attempt to specify the underlying coping style dispositions that may account for this variation. High monitors and low blunters may well desire more voluminous information and greater attention to psychosocial factors, whereas low monitors and high blunters may well desire more minimal information and reassurance (Bandura, 1977; 1981; 1985; Miller, 1980a; 1981; in press; Miller and Grant, 1979).

A final issue had to do with delineating more precisely the relation between informational preferences and control preferences. One way of assessing control preferences in primary care settings is to measure how active a role a given patient desires to play in the treatment of his or her medical problem (Strull *et al.*, 1984). To the extent that self-focusers are characterized by a tendency not only to seek information about their internal states but also to use this information to execute instrumental actions, then they should show greater preferences to play an active role in their medical care than do individuals who do not tend to focus on the self. In contrast, if self-focusers tend to scan for internal bodily cues in order to reduce uncertainty or to put themselves in the presence of safety signals (Weiss, 1970), then they should not necessarily show increased desires for control in this setting. Indeed, if anything, playing a more active role might be seen to interfere with the patient's ability to obtain symptom-relevant (reassuring) information from the physician.

To identify information seekers ('high monitors')/information avoiders ('low monitors') and distractors ('high blunters')/non-distractors ('low blunters'), patients were administered the Miller Behavioral Style Scale. Specifically, this scale asks the individual to imagine four stress-evoking scenes that are similar in context to the hospital situation (e.g. 'Imagine that you are afraid of flying and have to go somewhere by plane.'). Each scene is followed by eight statements that represent different ways of dealing with the situation. Four of the statements are of a monitoring or information-seeking variety (e.g. 'I would read and reread the safety instruction booklet.'), and four are of a blunting or information-avoiding variety (e.g. 'I would watch the in-flight film even if I had seen it before.'). This scale has been shown to have good reliability and good predictive validity. It also has good discriminative validity and is unrelated to constructs such as repression–sensitization, internal locus of control and anxiety (Efran *et al.*, 1981; Gard *et al.*, in press; Miller, 1987; Miller *et al.*, 1987a; Miller and Mangan, 1983; Phipps and Zinn, 1986; Steptoe, 1986; Watkins *et al.*, 1986). Preliminary analyses showed the monitoring and blunting subscales to be uncorrelated ($r=-0.07$, n.s.). Further, results obtained with the blunting scale were generally weaker, but in the same direction, as results obtained with the monitoring scale. Since the monitoring dimension has greater conceptual similarity to the self-attention construct than the blunting subscale, results with this latter dimension have been omitted in the interests of space.

MAJOR RESULTS: HEALTH IMPLICATIONS OF MONITORING

Because depression and monitoring were moderately correlated ($r=0.25$, $p<0.01$), analyses of covariance were computed on the dependent variables, with depression as the covariate. Post-visit evaluations by the physicians showed that high monitors actually had less serious medical problems than did low monitors ($p<0.003$). Only 9.4% of low monitors had problems rated 'not at all' serious, whereas twice as many high monitors (20.8%) fell into this category. The two groups had an equal number of problems rated as 'slightly' serious (57.8% of low monitors, 67.9% of high monitors), but almost one-third (32.8%) of the low monitors had moderately serious or quite serious problems, compared with only 11.3% of the high monitors. Indeed, about three times as many low monitors fell into these upper categories as did high monitors. Interestingly, doctor and patient ratings of seriousness were found to be unrelated for high monitors but positively correlated for low monitors ($p<0.03$). Physicians also indicated that high monitors had experienced less dysfunction prior to the visit than low monitors ($p<0.03$) and less discomfort ($p<0.05$).

In spite of the fact that their medical problems were less severe (as rated by the physician), high monitors' self-rated levels of problem seriousness, discomfort, dysfunction, disability, concerns and stress were equivalent to those of low monitors, both before and after the visit. Further, at a 1-week follow-up, high monitors reported significantly less improvement in their stress-related problems ($p<0.01$) than did low monitors. This sustained arousal is consistent with prior work (e.g. Mechanic, 1979; 1980; Hansell and Mechanic, 1985) and parallels our results found with patients facing more short-term medical and laboratory settings (Efran *et al.*, 1981; Gard *et al.*, in press; Lamping *et al.*, 1985; Lamping and Robertson, 1985; Miller, 1979a; 1987; Miller and Mangan, 1983; Phipps and Zinn, 1986).

Thus, the first conclusion is that monitors appear to be as likely to attend to internal 'bodily' symptoms as to external threat-relevant cues. Since high monitors cannot or do not choose to avoid threatening information, they seek out medical care as the most likely means of reducing their distress. These results are similar to those of Suls and Fletcher (1985) and Mechanic and his colleagues

(Greenley and Mechanic, 1976; Hansell and Mechanic, 1985; Mechanic, 1979; 1980; Mechanic and Cleary, 1980), showing that self-focusers tend to be more inclined to perceive the emergence of physical symptoms. However, unlike the Suls and Fletcher data, but consistent with Mechanic's findings, this internal focus is associated with an over-reporting rather than an under-reporting of physical symptomatology. That is, although high monitors appear to present with less severe medical problems, they complain about them equally and are slower to report improvement or to recover.

Perhaps high monitors may be over-sensitive to internal bodily cues because they experience more distress in their lives compared to low monitors (Mechanic, 1980). But note that we obtained these differences in sensitivity even when controlling for initial levels of depression. Moreover, monitoring and depression were only modestly correlated in the present sample (see also Miller, 1987; in press; Miller and Mangan, 1983; Phipps and Zinn, 1986). The present results suggest that, independently of depression, high monitoring may predict greater health-care utilization. This may be because high monitors are more inclined to scan their bodies and are therefore quicker to perceive the emergence of physical symptoms, compared to low monitors. On the other hand, high and low monitors may have similar somatic perceptions, but high monitors may exaggerate the significance of their symptoms—perhaps because they attend more than do low monitors to the potential negative consequences of such symptoms. That is, monitoring may be correlated with risk aversiveness in decision making more generally (Kahneman and Tversky, 1984). Consistent with this possibility, patient evaluations of problem seriousness were correlated with physician evaluations in the low- but not in the high-monitoring group.

The third conclusion concerns interventions and information desired. Higher monitoring scores were seen in patients who were concerned about being treated with kindness and respect ($p<0.01$); wanted tests done ($p<0.002$); wanted a new prescription ($p<0.02$); and who wanted reassurance about the effects of stress on their health ($p<0.03$). In addition to their treatment preferences, higher monitoring scores were found among those who desired information pertaining to: the cause of their medical problems ($p<0.005$); how healthy they were in general ($p<0.01$); how they could prevent future health problems ($p<0.001$); and possible medication side-effects ($p<0.01$). These findings underscore the importance generally of measuring both situational features and individual difference variables (Bandura, 1977; 1981; Miller, 1981; in press).

In the primary care context, results of previous studies suggest that the use of general psychological interventions can reduce medical problems and use of medical facilities (Rosen and Wiens, 1979). The present data further suggest that the management of acute medical problems might include a specific, routine assessment of the patient's preferred coping mode. Information interventions could then be varied accordingly, with low monitors receiving minimal information and high monitors receiving maximal information.

The final conclusion is that high monitors desired a less active role in their medical care than did low monitors ($p<0.01$). More specifically, almost no patients desired to have the final say in their medical care. However, almost ¾

(71.4%) of the low monitors preferred that treatment decisions be made jointly by them and their physicians, whereas under half (48.1%) of the high monitors desired such an active role. Indeed, twice as many high monitors (36.5%) as low monitors (15.9%) desired to play a completely passive role in their own care. Thus, while demanding more tests, information, counseling, etc., from their doctor, high monitors do not appear to seek this information for its instrumental value (Miller, 1979b; 1980b). The results are consistent with evidence showing that while physicians tend to underestimate patient desires for information, they tend to overestimate patient desires to play an active role (Strull *et al.*, 1984).

These data suggest that monitoring does not simply reflect a generalized preference for information and control, but points toward the discriminative nature of this cognitive coping style. In other studies, we have found that high monitors and low blunters scan for information even in the face of uncontrollable threats (Miller, 1979a; 1987; in press). Further, high monitoring and low blunting appear to be unrelated to control-oriented personality dimensions such as the Type A behavior pattern (Miller *et al.*, 1982). The present findings provide further evidence that high monitors may be motivated by a desire to reduce uncertainty and concomitant arousal rather than to exercise controlling actions.

Future research should delineate the circumstances under which high monitors are inclined to engage in adaptive self-regulatory behaviors and when they are not. Of particular interest in the present context is to determine the extent to which they undertake preventive actions and their overall level of health. On the one hand, Steptoe and O'Sullivan (1986) have shown that high monitors/low blunters are more likely than low monitors/high blunters to adhere to recommended regimens such as undergoing annual pap smears and regular breast self-examinations. On the other hand, Miller *et al.* (1987b) have found that high monitors are less inclined to engage in healthy lifestyle practices, such as getting proper sleep, exercising regularly, and keeping their stress levels low. It may be that high monitors are more likely to activate self-regulatory behaviors than entail the reduction of uncertainty (e.g. finding out if one has cervical cancer) but less likely to activate self-regulatory behaviors that involve the effective modulation of stress (e.g. falling asleep without ruminating and worrying).

SOME IMPLICATIONS FOR THE STUDY OF LIFE EVENTS

The cognitive social learning approach illustrated in the present research may have implications for specifying the impact of major and minor life events generally. In order to strengthen the diagnostic and predictive value of life events and hassles, it may be important to tap more than their perceived occurrence, desirability and controllability. Rather, it may be critical to determine the type of cognitive social competencies required to cope with the situation as well as the type of cognitive social competencies available in the individual's repertoire. Individuals facing stressful situations that demand cognitive social competencies incompatible with their predisposing coping style skills may show more physical and psychological distress and poorer overall outcomes. Furthermore, the more individuals feel that they lack the competencies required, the more likely they should be to find the situation undesirable and/or uncontrollable. It is in this sense that the perception of major and minor life experiences may function most potently as a moderator variable. In other words, the greater the mismatch between situational requirements and dispositional abilities, the greater the toll on self-efficacy perceptions and expectations (Bandura, 1977; 1981; 1985). This, in turn, may result in the occurrence of inflexible and seemingly maladaptive behaviors (see, for example, Forsythe and Compas, 1987; Wright and Mischel, 1987).

As applied to individual differences in information-processing styles, the stressfulness of objectively similar situations should differ for high and low monitors, depending on the competencies required. For example, in situations that are largely uncontrollable and/or chronic, high monitors may show the greatest morbidity since they tend to lack the relevant competencies—i.e. the ability to psychologically blunt and distract themselves from threat-relevant cues. In a study of college freshmen, Miller et al. (1987b) found that high monitors judged their problems at work and school to be more stressful than did low monitors. Moreover, they also indicated that these situations required cognitive social competencies that they generally lacked. Specifically, compared to low monitors, they felt that their problems needed the ability to tune out unpleasant situations, delay gratification, tolerate frustration and accept chronic, low levels of satisfaction. Since many of the ongoing stressors to which people fall prey often demand this cluster of cognitive social skills, high monitors may tend to experience more strain on their coping resources than low monitors.

SUMMARY AND CONCLUSIONS

In conclusion, our specific results show that high monitors—who typically seek out threatening information—show greater physical and psychological morbidity in response to uncontrollable stressors than do low monitors—who typically ignore threat-relevant cues. More generally, the present research illustrates how the analysis of the impact of life events can take account of the situational features and cognitive social competencies required by the event as well as of the individual's own dispositional coping skills. In life, the impact of stressful events surely depends both on the event and on the person. It seems time for life events researchers to allow this truism to animate our own investigations.

Acknowledgements

We are deeply indebted to W. Mischel for his invaluable insights on an earlier draft of this paper. We also thank B. Boyer, C. Combs, F. Quintos, M. Rodoletz, and E. Stoddard for their assistance, and E. Gracely for his help with data analysis. This research was partially supported by the Robert Wood Johnson Foundation and by Temple University Grant-In-Aid of Research and Temple University Research Incentive Fund.

REFERENCES

Bandura, A. (1977). Self-efficacy: Toward a unifying theory of behavior change. *Psychological Review, 84*, 191–215.

Bandura, A. (1981). Self-referent thought: A developmental analysis of self-efficacy. In J.H. Flavell & L.D. Ross (eds), *Social cognitive development: Frontiers and possible futures* (pp. 200–239). London: Cambridge University Press.

Bandura, A. (1985). *Social foundations of thought and action. A social cognitive theory.* Englewood Cliffs, NJ: Prentice Hall.

Burks, N. & Martin, B. (1985). Everyday problems and life change events: Ongoing versus acute sources of stress. *Journal of Human Stress, 11*, 27–35.

Carver, C.S., & Scheier, M.F. (1982). Control theory: A useful conceptual framework for personality–social, clinical, and health psychology. *Psychological Bulletin, 92*, 111–135.

DeLongis, A., Coyne, J.C., Dakof, G., Folkman, S., & Lazarus, R.S. (1982). Relationship of daily hassles, uplifts, and major life events to health stress. *Health Psychology, 1*, 119–136.

Dohrenwend, B.S., & Dohrenwend, B.P. (1974). Overview and prospects for research on stressful life events. In B.S. Dohrenwend & B.P. Dohrenwend (eds), *Stressful life events: Their nature and effects* (pp. 313–331). New York: Wiley.

Efran, J., Chorney, R.L., Ascher, L.M., & Lukens, M.D. (1981). The performance of monitors and blunters during painful stimulation. Paper presented at the meeting of the Eastern Psychological Association, New York, April.

Faden, R.R., Becker, C., Lewis, C., Freeman, J., & Faden, A.I. (1981). Disclosure of information to patients in medical care. *Medical Care, 19*, 718–733.

Fenigstein, A., Scheier, M.F. & Buss, A.H. (1975). Public and private self-consciousness: Assessment and theory. *Journal of Consulting and Cinical Psychology, 43*, 522–527.

Folkman, S., & Lazarus, R.S. (1980). An analysis of coping in a middle-aged community sample. *Journal of Health and Social Behavior, 21*, 219–239.

Forsythe, C.J., & Compas, B.E. (1987). Interaction of cognitive appraisal of stressful events and coping: Testing the goodness of fit hypothesis. *Cognitive Therapy and Research, 11*, 473–485.

Gard, D., Edwards, P.W., Harris, J., & McCormick, G. (in press) The sensitizing effects of pretreatment measures on cancer chemotherapy nausea and vomiting. *Journal of Consulting and Clinical Psychology.*

Good, M.D., Good, B.J., & Nassi, A.J. (1983). Patient requests in primary health care settings: Development and validation of a research instrument. *Journal of Behavioral Medicine, 6*, 151–168.

Greenley, J.R., & Mechanic, D. (1976). Social selection in seeking help for psychological problems. *Journal of Health and Social Behavior, 17*, 249–262.

Hansell, S., & Mechanic, D. (1985). Introspectiveness and adolescent symptom reporting. *Journal of Human Stress, 11*, 165–176.

Kahneman, D., & Tversky, A. (1984). Choices, values, and frames. *American Psychologist, 39*, 341–350.

Korsch, B.M., Gozzi, E.K., & Francis, V. (1968). Gaps in doctor–patient communication: 1. Doctor–patient interaction and patient satisfaction. *Pediatrics, 42*, 855–870.

Lamping, D.L., Molinaro, V., & Stevenson, G.W. (1985). The effects of perceived control and coping style on cognitive appraisals during stressful medical procedures: A randomized, controlled trial. Paper presented at the meeting of the Eastern Psychological Association, Boston, March.

Lamping, D., & Robertson, A.L. (1985). An experimental investigation of the effects of social support on coping with stress. Paper presented at the meeting of the Association for the Advancement of Behavior Therapy, Houston, November.

Lazare, A., Eisenthal, S., & Wasserman, L. (1975). The customer approach to patienthood. Attending to patient requests in a walk-in clinic. *Archives of General Psychiatry, 32*, 553–558.

Lazarus, R.S., DeLongis, A., Folkman, S., & Gruen, R. (1985). Stress and adaptational outcomes. The problem of confounded measures. *American Psychologist, 40*, 770–779.

Magill, M.K., & Zung, W.W.K. (1982). Clinical decisions about diagnosis and treatment for depression identified by screening. *The Journal of Family Practice, 14*, 1144–1149.

Matheny, K.B., & Cupp, P. (1983). Control, desirability, and anticipation as moderating variables between life change and illness. *Journal of Human Stress, 9*, 19–23.

Mechanic, D. (1978). Effects of psychological distress on perceptions of physical health and use of medical and psychiatric facilities. *Journal of Human Stress, 4*, 26–32.

Mechanic, D. (1979). Development of psychological distress among young adults. *Archives of General Psychiatry, 36*, 1233–1239.

Mechanic, D. (1980). The experience and reporting of common physical complaints. *Journal of Health and Social Behavior, 21*, 146–155.

Mechanic, D., & Cleary, P. (1980). Factors associated with the maintenance of positive health behavior. *Preventive Medicine, 9*, 805–814.

Mechanic, D., & Volkart, E.H. (1961). Illness behavior and medical diagnoses. *Journal of Health and Human Behavior, 1*, 86–96.

Miller, S.M. (1979a). Controllability and human stress: Method, evidence and theory. *Behavior Research and Therapy, 17*, 287–304.

Miller, S.M. (1979b). Coping with impending stress: Psychophysiological and cognitive correlates of choice. *Psychophysiology, 16*, 572–581.

Miller, S.M. (1980a). When is a little information a dangerous thing? Coping with stressful life-events by monitoring vs. blunting. In S. Levine & H. Ursin, (eds), *Coping and health* (pp. 145–169). New York: Plenum Press.

Miller, S.M. (1980b). Why having control reduces stress: If I can stop the roller coaster I don't want to get off. In J. Garber & M.E.P. Seligman (eds), *Human helplessness: Theory and applications* (pp. 71–95). New York: Academic Press.

Miller, S.M. (1981). Predictability and human stress: Towards a clarification of evidence and theory. In L. Berkowitz (ed.), *Advances in experimental social psychology, Vol. 14* (pp. 203–256). New York: Academic Press.

Miller, S.M. (1987). Monitoring and blunting: Validation of a questionnaire to assess styles of information-seeking under threat. *Journal of Personality and Social Psychology, 52*, 345–353.

Miller, S.M. (in press). To see or not to see: Cognitive informational styles in the coping process. In M. Rosenbaum (ed.), *Learned resourcefulness: On coping skills, self-regulation, and adaptive behavior.* New York: Springer-Verlag.

Miller, S.M., Boyer, B., & Birnbaum, A. (1987a). Psychometric properties of the Miller Behavioral Style Scale. Unpublished manuscript, Temple University.

Miller, S.M., Boyer, B., Rodoletz, M., & Birnbaum, A. (1987b). Health status and health care utilization in adolescents. Unpublished manuscript, Temple University.

Miller, S.M., Brody, D.S. & Summerton, J. (1988). Styles of coping with threat: Implications for health. *Journal of Personality and Social Psychology, 54*, 142–148.

Miller, S.M., & Grant, R. (1979). The blunting hypothesis: A view of predictability and human stress. In P.O. Sjoden, S. Bates & W.S. Dockens (eds), *Trends in behavior therapy* (pp. 135–151). New York: Academic Press.

Miller, S.M., & Green, M. (1985). Coping with threat and frustration: Origins, nature and development. In M. Lewis & C. Saarni (eds), *The socialization of behavior* (pp. 263–314). New York: Plenum Press.

Miller, S.M., Lack, E., & Asroff, S. (1982). Preference for control and the Type A coronary-prone behavior pattern. Paper presented at the meeting of the Association for the Advancement of Behavior Theory, Toronto, Ontario, November.

Miller, S.M., Leinbach, A., & Brody, D.S. (in press). Coping style in hypertensives: Nature and consequences. *Journal of Consulting and Clinical Psychology.*

Miller, S.M., & Mangan, C.E. (1983). Interacting effects of information and coping style in adapting to gynecologic stress: Should the doctor tell all? *Journal of Personality and Social Psychology, 45*, 223–236.

Mischel, W. (1979). On the interface of cognition and personality. *American Psychologist, 34*, 740–754.

Mischel, W. (1984). Convergences and challenges in the search for consistency. *American Psychologist, 39*, 351–364.

Mischel, W. (1986). *Introduction to personality*, 4th edn. New York: Holt, Rinehart and Winston.

Monroe, S.M. (1983). Major and minor life events as predictors of psychological distress: Further issues and findings. *Journal of Behavioral Medicine, 6*, 189–205.

Mullen, B., & Suls, J. (1982). Stressful life events and the ameliorative effects of private self-consciousness. *Journal of Experimental Social Psychology, 18*, 43–55.

Nielson, A.C., & Williams, T.A. (1980). Depression in ambulatory medical patients. *Archives of General Psychiatry, 37*, 999–1004.

Phipps, S., & Zinn, A.B. (1986). Psychological response to amniocentesis: II. Effects of coping style. *American Journal of Medical Genetics, 25*, 143–148.

Reader, J.J., Pratt, L., & Mudd, M.C. (1957). What patients expect from their doctors. *Modern Hospital, 89*, 88–91.

Rodin, G., & Voshart, K. (1986). Depression in the medically ill: An overview. *American Journal of Psychiatry, 143*, 696–704.

Rosen, J.C., & Wiens, A.N. (1979). Changes in medical problems and use of medical services following psychological intervention. *American Psychologist, 34*, 420–431.

Sarason, I.G., Johnson, J.H., & Siegel, J.M. (1978). Assessing the impact of life changes: Development of the life experiences survey. *Journal of Consulting and Clinical Psychology, 46*, 932–946.

Sarason, I.G., Levine, H.M., & Sarason, B.R. (1982). Assessing the impact of life changes. In T. Millon, C. Green & R. Meagher (eds), *Handbook of clinical health psychology* (pp. 377–399). New York: Plenum Press.

Scaramella, T.J. (1977). Management of depression and anxiety in primary care practice. *Primary Care, 4*, 67–77.

Schwartz, G.E. (1983). Disregulation theory and disease: Applications to the repression/cerebral disconnection/cardiovascular disorder hypothesis. Special issue on behavioral medicine. *International Review of Applied Psychology, 32*, 95–118.

Steptoe, A. (1986). Avoidant coping strategies: The relationship between repressive coping and preference for distraction. Unpublished manuscript, St George's Hospital Medical School, London.

Steptoe, A., & O'Sullivan, J. (1986). Monitoring and blunting coping styles in women prior to surgery. *British Journal of Clinical Psychology, 25*, 143–144.

Stoeckle, J.D., Zola, I.K., & Davidson, G.E. (1964). The quantity and significance of psychological distress in medical patients. *Journal of Chronic Diseases, 17*, 959–970.

Strull, W.M., Lo, B., & Charles, H. (1984). Do patients want to participate in medical decision making? *Journal of the American Medical Association, 252*, 2990–2994.

Suls, J., & Fletcher, B. (1985). Self-attention, life stress, and illness: A prospective study. *Psychosomatic Medicine, 47*, 469–481.

Suls, J., & Mullen, B. (1981). Life change and psychological distress: The role of perceived control and desirability. *Journal of Applied Social Psychology, 11*, 379–389.

Tessler, R., & Mechanic, D. (1978). Factors affecting children's use of physician services in a prepaid group practice. *Medical Care, 16*, 33–46.

Tessler, R., Mechanic, D., & Dimond, M. (1976). The effect of psychological distress on physician utilization: A prospective study. *Journal of Health and Social Behavior, 17*, 353–364.

Vinokur, A., & Selzer, L.M. (1975). Desirable versus undesirable life events: Their relationship to stress and mental distress. *Journal of Personality and Social Psychology, 32*, 329–337.

Watkins, L.O., Weaver, L., & Odegaard, V. (1986). Preparation for cardiac catheterization: Tailoring the content of instruction to coping style. *Heart and Lung, 15*, 382–389.

Weiss, J.M. (1970). Somatic effects of predictable and unpredictable shock. *Psychosomatic Medicine, 32,* 397–409.

Wright, J.C., & Mischel, W. (1987). A conditional approach to dispositional constructs: The local predictability of social behavior. *Journal of Personality and Social Psychology, 53,* 1159–1177.

KEY WORDS

Monitoring, blunting, stress, life events, hassles, coping, medical symptoms, self-attention, information processing, information seeking, controllability/uncontrollability, individual differences, self-focus, depression, preventive actions, arousal, person by situation interactions, cognitive social learning theory, instrumental actions, introspectiveness, self-regulation, private self-consciousness, health care utilization, risk aversiveness, cognitive social competencies/skills, desirability/undesirability, control systems theory, health seeking, threat.

Handbook of Life Stress, Cognition and Health
Edited by S. Fisher and J. Reason
© 1988 John Wiley & Sons Ltd.

28

Social Support and Stress: Perspectives and Processes

JACQUES A.M. WINNUBST
State University of Utrecht, The Netherlands
BRAM P. BUUNK
University of Nijmegen, The Netherlands
and
FRANS H.G. MARCELISSEN
TNO Institute of Preventive Health Care, Leiden, The Netherlands

INTRODUCTION

Although the importance of the relationship between social ties and well-being and health has long been recognized by social and behavioral scientists, it has been particularly during the past decade that numerous studies have examined the relationship between the characteristics of people's social relationships and a variety of physical and psychological symptoms. Special attention has been paid to the moderating role that social support can play in the adjustment to such diverse stressful events as divorce, chronic illness, pregnancy, bereavement, job loss and work overload. A main theme in this literature has been that social support can protect or buffer individuals against the negative consequences of stressful circumstances upon mental and physical health, including depression, psycho-somatic symptoms and physical disease.

The first part of this chapter will consist of a discussion of central theoretical and methodological perspectives, focusing upon the role of social support with respect to stress. Thereafter, we will examine some of the social psychological processes involved in the development and maintenance of support systems. Next, we will provide a global review of the research into social support and occupational stress, and describe in detail some of our own studies. These studies include a smaller cross-sectional study and a larger longitudinal extension of the same study. In the longitudinal study we were able to examine causal relationships between variables. Some of the interesting implications of this study for research and theory on social support will be discussed, particularly the fact that social support should be viewed as an interpersonal exhange process that takes place within social and personal relationships.

THE CONCEPTUALIZATION OF SOCIAL SUPPORT:
FOUR PERSPECTIVES

Despite the important advances that have been made in the study of social support, the field is still plagued by some persistent conceptual problems. As Shumaker and Brownell (1984) have pointed out, conceptual ambiguity characterizes research on social support, and predictive validity has been emphasized at the expense of construct validity. For many of the early researchers in the field, the meaning of the term social support seemed so obvious that often *no* attempt was made to give a precise definition of the construct. Furthermore, endeavors to define social support have in some instances led to definitions that are so vague or broad that the concept seems to lose its distinctive meaning (Barrera, 1986). This may be illustrated by the following definition of social support offered by Caplan *et al.* (1975): 'Any input, directly provided by an individual (or group) which moves the receiver of that input towards goals which the receiver desires' (p. 211). Taken literally, this very broad definition includes not only all kinds of informal support, but also diverse types of formal aid, including social benefits, commercial services (such as those delivered by a plumber), and treatment provided by a physician or psychotherapist. As Wortman (1984) has noted, other operational definitions of social support have included such divergent elements as financial resources, self-esteem, and job satisfaction, or—even more problematic— variables such as 'adaptability' or 'crying', which may overlap considerably with the outcomes that are assessed. While such views of social support are not generally accepted, many different conceptualizations still exist, including circular definitions that in fact describe social support as 'support that is social' (Barrera, 1986; Fleming *et al.*, 1984; Thoits, 1985b; House, 1981).

Notwithstanding the foregoing, it is possible to separate a number of valuable theoretical and empirical perspectives on social support that may all be important for understanding the impact of interpersonal relationships upon well-being and health: (1) the view that conceptualizes social support as the individual's degree of social integration; (2) the perspective defining social support as the subjectively experienced quality of the individual's relationships; (3) the concept of social support as the perceived supportiveness and helpfulness of others, and (4) the notion that the term social support refers primarily to the actual enactment of supportive behaviors (see Barrera, 1986; Bruhn and Philips, 1984; Sarason and Sarason, 1985b; Syme, 1984). Although the divergence of the field, as is apparent from these different conceptualizations, is deplored by many authors, the four notions are, in our opinion, not so much contradictory as complementary. We would even like to suggest that the various perspectives denote different *levels* of analysis, and each level can be seen as a precondition for the next level. Thus, the existence of social ties is a necessary, albeit not sufficient, precondition for satisfying relationships; these are in turn presupposed if an individual is to perceive others as potentially supportive. Again, this perceived helpfulness is assumed to be a necessary condition for the actual asking and getting of social support. Furthermore, to a certain extent, the four perspectives may represent different supposed *mechanisms* through which social support affects health (Rook, 1984). For example, social integration, as well as satisfying relationships, seems to have a *direct* effect upon well-being, while perceived as well as actually enacted support may, each in a different way, buffer the individual against the negative consequences of stressful events (cf. Cohen and Wills, 1985). We will now discuss the different perspectives in more detail.

Social Support as Social Integration

In line with the early work of Durkheim, many authors, particularly sociologists, have conceptualized and measured social support in terms of social integration or social embeddedness, i.e. the number and strength of the connections of individuals to significant others in their social environment (Rook, 1984; Barrera, 1986). Such conceptualizations have been referred to as structural or quantitative. In this tradition, two prevalent approaches of measuring social embeddedness can be distinguished. The first method takes into account as indicators for social support the presence of certain social ties such as marriage, friendships or involvement in community organizations. The significance of such variables for health was demonstrated in the well-known longitudinal study of Berkman and Syme (1979), that showed that indicators of social integration can predict mortality to a considerable degree. The second approach focuses upon structural aspects of the individual's social network, such as size, homogeneity, stability, symmetry and complexity (Antonucci, 1985b; Gottlieb, 1981; Turner, 1983).

An important objection to these approaches is that the presence of certain social relationships does not indicate anything about the quality of these relationships, or about the actual helping interactions that do take place. However, it must be noted that some network measures have been devised to assess the social support exchanges between members of the network (Barrera, 1986). A second, related objection is that it is unclear through which mechanisms the presence of social ties influences health. As has been suggested by Rook (1984), the social integration framework supposes that the main contribution of social relationships in this regard consists of social regulation: providing stable and rewarding roles, promoting healthy behavior, deterring the person from ill-advised behavior, and maintaining stable functioning during periods of rapid social change. Although little is known about the actual importance and operation of these mechanisms, it is obvious that social integration is a necessary, though not sufficient, condition for any positive effects of interpersonal relationships.

Social Support as Relationship Quality

While the foregoing approach emphasizes the quantitative aspects of the social support system, the second approach views social support in terms of the subjectively experienced quality of the social relationships of the person, and has therefore sometimes been labeled as qualitative. Thus, Gentry and Kobasa (1984) define social support as '. . . a psychological resource, one that defines the perceptions of an individual as regards the quality of his or her interpersonal relationships', and they contrast this notion with the quantitative concept of social network. In a similar vein, Hobfoll (1985) has suggested that it is not the number of relationships that is important; rather, that one or two intimate relationships are critical in terms of social support, and only those without intimates are at risk. Also emphasizing the qualitative aspects of relationships, Cobb (1976), in an influential paper, described social support as '. . . information leading a person to believe that he is loved and cared for (emotional support), that he is esteemed and valued (esteem support), and that he is part of a network of communication and mutual obligation (network support)'. From a similar perspective, many studies within the field of occupational stress have viewed social support in terms of organizational climate and the quality of the relationships between work associates (Jackson, 1985).

Since the approach under consideration equates social support with the quality of relationships, the degree of social support from the spouse can, viewed from this perspective, be assessed by measuring the quality of marital communication and the level of marital satisfaction (for a review, see Schaap *et al.*, 1987). Indeed, several scales for assessing social support by the family do in fact tap such variables as compatibility, cohesion and consensus (e.g. Billings and Moos, 1982). Satisfying, intimate personal relationships can, in various ways, contribute to health by, for instance, fulfilling affiliative needs, meeting needs for affection, offering a feeling of identity and belonging, being a source of positive self-evaluation, and by giving a sense of control and mastery (Rook, 1984; Shumaker and Brownell, 1984; Thoits, 1985a).

The importance of positively valued, intimate relationships has been particularly emphasized in the case of serious disease. In such a situation, there is a large group of potential support-givers, including spouse, family, friends, neighbors, colleagues, physicians, nurses, pastoral workers, social workers, psychologists and self-help groups. However, the proximity of one person on whom one can count completely and who is to be trusted completely, seems to be decisive for the relative well-being of the patient and his or her capacity to manage the situation as well as possible (Lowenthal and Haven, 1978). Intimacy has a cognitive, an emotional and a behavioral dimension (Hatfield, 1984). The cognitive dimension refers to the fact that intimates are prepared to show their weak sides; they provide each other with personal and confidential information and are prepared to listen to each other's confidences. The emotional dimension concerns the fact that intimates care deeply about each other; instead of indifference, intense, often conflicting emotions are characteristic of an intimate relationship. Finally, the behavioral dimension implies that intimates feel comfortable in direct proximity and therefore call on each other, and touch and caress each other. The absence of such intimacy among persons suffering from a serious illness, coupled with a lack of positive events, seems to leave individuals in a markedly disphoric state (Lefcourt, 1985). Intimacy is not always easy to attain. Many fears can prevent individuals from getting close to one another, including the fear of showing one's weak side and destructive tendencies, the fear of losing or of being exposed to the anger of the other, and the fear of losing one's control and individuality (Hatfield, 1984). In some cases, too much intimacy can be threatening and thus decrease a person's sense of well-being.

Social Support as Perceived Helpfulness and Supportiveness

While neither of the two conceptualizations of social support thus far described focuses upon help-oriented transactions, the third perspective conceives social support as perceived supportivenes and helpfulness—the appraisal that, in case of stressful circumstances, others can be relied upon for such things as advice, information, instrumental help and empathic understanding (Sarason and Sarason, 1985b). For example, in research on occupational stress, questions have been asked about the availability of supervisor support when the situation at work becomes difficult (House, 1981). According to Cohen and Wills (1985), it is precisely the feeling that others can and are willing to help that can prevent a potentially stressful event from being appraised as stressful, and thus hinder the onset of physiological and psychological strains. Lazarus (1966) particularly has shown that threatening situations change into stressors only in so far as the person appraises the situation as such and appropriate coping responses are lacking. Perceived social support might lead to the perception that problems are not particularly threatening. Indeed, the mere presence of a friend may prevent physiological strains in subjects faced with a stressful task in the laboratory (Kissel, 1965).

It should be pointed out that the notion of social support as perceived helpfulness and supportiveness of others is sometimes implicitly equated or confused with the quality of the relationships with these others. Thus, Schaefer *et al.* (1981) included in the same scale statements about the perceived caring by others (relationship quality), as well as items referring to the reliability of others in time of need (perceived helpfulness). In other studies, similar measures have been employed (Etzion, 1984). Although such confounding is quite common and may even be appropriate sometimes, the two notions of social support under consideration are conceptually and empirically distinct. A satisfactory intimate relationship is not necessarily a relationship that is perceived as helpful. For example, people may believe that intimate others are not able to give them the support they need, or may expect assistance in demeaning and debilitating ways (Antonucci, 1985a). Furthermore, in a study of friendship, it was found that for several types of support, particularly instrumental assistance, individuals perceived their family as being more potentially helpful than their friends, even though the relationships with friends were described as much more intimate than those with the family (Buunk, 1985a).

Social Support as the Enactment of Supportive Behaviors

The last notion of social support emphasizes the actual enactment of supportive behaviors. In this perspective, social support is conceptualized as the helpful acts performed for an individual by significant others (Thoits, 1985b), or 'the actions that others perform when they render assistance to a focal person' (Barrera, 1986, p. 417). Some authors have suggested that the use of the term social support is only justified in this context. Thus, Rook (1984) has argued that social ties may have many health-sustaining functions, but that it would be most useful to reserve the term social support exclusively for a subset of these functions, i.e. the help-oriented transactions that occur in response to learning of another's problem. Although such use of the term would, without doubt, contribute to substantial conceptual clarity, it would probably not be agreed upon by a majority of researchers. Nevertheless, the analysis and observation of supportive interactions may constitute one of the most important areas of future research in the social support area.

Many taxonomies of supportive acts have been developed. One of the better known of these is the one proposed by House (1981). According to House, social support refers to all helping social transactions, particularly emotional support (behavior that transmits trust and love), esteem support (behavior that results in information relevant for self-evaluation), instrumental support (support bringing goods and services), and informational support (behavior resulting in direct information). Although similar elements can be found in most other taxonomies, emotional and esteem support are generally considered to be the most important. For example, some authors (e.g. Cobb, 1976) have excluded instrumental and informational support from their definition, while others (e.g. Thoits, 1985b) have emphasized that emotional support plays by far the most crucial role. Once stressful situations have arisen, help-oriented behaviors can buffer the individual against harmful consequences in numerous ways: for instance, by helping derive a solution to the problem, by increasing the coping mechanisms, or by altering helping to manage negative emotions, by reducing such strains as anxiety, and improving another's mood, by influencing the coping mechanisms, or by altering the cognitive appraisal of the problem (Cohen and Wills, 1985; Rook, 1984; Thoits, 1985b; Wilcox and Vernberg, 1985; Wortman, 1984). These processes moderate stress in one way or another *when it has already come into existence*, and are thus different from the buffering process supposed to be operating in the case of perceived support, which is assumed to *prevent the onset* of strains.

Although many professionals would agree that, for instance, scapegoating the person in need can hardly be considered a seriously helpful act (cf. Hobfoll, 1985), it is sometimes difficult to establish whether or not a particular interaction should be viewed as socially supportive. There are many examples of efforts to help a person in need that, although well intended, can nevertheless have destructive, boomerang effects, leaving the distressed person even more upset than before (Thoits, 1985a). This can be the case when well-meaning others try, for example, to cheer up an individual suffering from a serious illness, denying the feelings of grief and anxiety that the person may want to express and deal with (Wortman, 1984). Others, in their endeavors to be helpful, may disrupt a process of selective denial, a coping strategy that may at some point be the only alternative which makes a situation bearable (Wilcox and Vernberg, 1985). Furthermore, there are, without a doubt, individual differences in the type of supportive behaviors preferred and, additionally, a particular behavior that is helpful in a given situation will not necessarily be considered supportive in another situation. As a consequence, concepts of social support should take into account the individual *perceptions* of the actual supportiveness of a given act, and recognize that the perspectives of support-giver and receiver can be quite divergent. Therefore, we can agree with the definition of Shumaker and Brownell (1984) which describes social support as

'. . . an exchange of resources between at least two individuals perceived by the provider or the recipient to be intended to enhance the well-being of the recipient' (p.13).

In general, effects of social support upon well-being seem to occur particularly, or only, when the support provided matches the needs of the recipient. Cohen and Wills (1985) reviewed a large number of studies on the moderating effects of social support with regard to the impact of stressful life events, and concluded that a buffering effect was only found when there was a close tie between the support offered and the nature of the stressors. However, they pointed to the fact that, although there are several large prospective studies on the effects of social support, few used appropriate methods for showing causal effects. In our own research, which will be discussed later on, we have attempted to overcome such problems.

SOCIAL SUPPORT AS A SOCIAL PSYCHOLOGICAL PROCESS

Behind many studies on psychosocial stress lies a model that assumes stressors are a potential cause of strains, and that social support is an aspect of the social environment that can intervene in the causal relationship between stressors and strains. However, the processes linking stress and social support are far more complex than is often supposed. First, stressful situations can *lead to* a deterioration of social support systems. Many stressful circumstances, particularly stigmatizing events, can affect social relationships in a negative way, such as by alienating others or by leading to care-giver burnout. Such circumstances may thus reduce the willingness or ability of others to provide support (Barrera, 1986; Shinn et al., 1984). In this context it is noteworthy that research on interpersonal attraction testifies to the fact that emotionally disturbed individuals are less attractive to others. A second, even more important issue in this context is that social support may be a personality characteristic rather than a feature of the social environment. Social support is always a transactional process, and the degree of social support a person has available seems to be determined by his or her personality to a substantial extent. Thus, measures of social support appear not only to be rather stable over several years, but also to be correlated with personality factors such as neuroticism, low self-esteem and social anxiety. In addition, studies are now appearing that suggest that persons receiving less social support are judged as less attractive and less socially skilled than individuals receiving much social support (Hansson et al., 1984; Sarason and Sarason, 1985b). As Hansson et al. (1984) have noted, studies of lonely people (i.e. people who lack social support) suggest that the personality of these people is reflected in behavioral manifestations which actually reduce the likelihood of friendship formation. According to these authors, individuals differ widely in a variable designated as relational competence, i.e. those personality and behavioral characteristics that facilitate the acquisition, development and maintenance of mutually satisfying relationships. Partially following Hansson et al., we assume that relational competence may affect social support through at least four different processes, and that each of the processes is especially relevant to one of the four conceptualizations of social support elaborated in the foregoing.

1) The *building* of relationships: characteristics such as sociability, assertiveness, and extraversion (cf. Heller *et al.*, 1986), may contribute to the frequency, ease, and success of initial encounters, not only because persons with such characteristics have the skills to deal with such situations, but perhaps also because their personalities are relatively more attractive to others.

2) The *development* and *maintenance* of relationships: these probably are partially different traits and skills than those adequate for the building of new relationships, such as tolerance of intimacy (Wortman, 1984), emotional stability, cooperation, sensitivity, and empathy (Hansson *et al.*, 1984), and other rather complex skills for handling problems in intimate relationships (Schaap *et al.*, 1987).

3) The *conceptualization* of relationships: persons who lack social support appear to have more negative, cynical and pessimistic attitudes towards other people (Hansson *et al.*, 1984). This might not only result in problems with the establishment of intimate relationships, but also in the failure to believe that social support is available. A particularly relevant variable in this context is self-esteem, since many persons with low self-esteem may have a more negative view of others.

4) The *employment* of relationships for the purpose of social support and the ability to mobilize this support system are what really count in times of crisis. Many skills are required for obtaining the actual provision of socially supportive behaviors from others. Persons low in social anxiety and high in self-esteem may find it relatively easy to obtain such support (Hansson *et al.*, 1984), while neurotic and depressed individuals may turn others away (Sarason and Sarason, 1985b). In addition, Shumaker and Brownell (1984) have pointed to the importance of the ability to provide information about one's needs, while Hobfoll (1985) has emphasized the ability to accept support.

Factors other than relational competence affect the enactment of socially supportive behaviors, however. Aside from social skills, and the earlier noted fact that others may turn away from persons under stress, affective factors such as shame, guilt and self-esteem and related feelings can be mentioned as barriers against supportive acts (Hansson *et al.*, 1984; Hobfoll, 1985; Shinn *et al.*, 1984). Asking for social support often implies disclosing feelings of weakness and vulnerability (Buunk, 1985b), which may evoke shame and guilt and which may threaten one's self-concept as a competent and autonomous person.

SOCIAL SUPPORT AND OCCUPATIONAL STRESS

After this general overview of conceptualizations and social psychological processes concerning social support, we will now turn to an analysis of the role of social support in the alleviation of job stress. This analysis will include a presentation of some of the results of studies carried out by our research team. One of the reasons that this topic merits special attention here is that occupational stress is a very prevalent, often protracted phenomenon that affects health and well-being to a significant degree, while at the same time relatively little is known about the role that social support can play in easing or preventing stress at work. Most research on social support has not been conducted within the context of the work situation, but with regard to the impact of important life events and crises. Thus, in a recent review of the various effects of social support, Cohen and Wills (1985) were only able to include three studies on occupational stress out of a total of more than 50 studies. Nevertheless, social support has long been recognized as an important factor in alleviating stressful situations at work (Stouffer *et al.*, 1965).

A Theoretical Model for Analyzing Occupational Stress

The most important theoretical model utilized in current research on social support and occupational stress is the so-called Michigan model. This model was developed by members of the Institute for Social Research of the University of Michigan (Caplan *et al.*, 1975) and has been further validated and elaborated upon in research that has taken place in the Netherlands (Van Dijkhuizen, 1980, 1985; Winnubst *et al.*, 1982; Marcelissen, 1987). In this model, stress is seen as a relationship between the individual and the environment. Two kinds of stress may threaten the individual: (1) he or she may feel an imbalance between the demands from the environment and his or her resources to meet these demands; and (2) the environment may not provide sufficient opportunities to fulfill his or her needs. In the Michigan model, stressors are those demands in the work environment that are perceived by the individuals as being problematic, i.e. workload, role conflict, and future ambiguity. Thus, this tradition of research focuses upon rather chronic problems, as opposed to life events, where the emphasis is placed upon one single event, e.g. job loss, widowhood or retirement (Cobb and Kasl, 1977). Stressors can lead to so-called strains—all those behavioral, physiological and psychological processes that occur under the influence of excessive demands and that indicate a disturbance of normal, healthy functioning. Several strains, such as high blood pressure and high cholesterol level, are considered as precursors for disease, and it is assumed in the Michigan model that strains can eventually lead to illness. In job-stress research, it is generally only the effects upon minor health aspects, in particular psychosomatic complaints, that are studied. The model further suggests that there are two types of variables that moderate the relationship between stressors and strains: (1) personality, e.g. Type A behavior and rigidity (Winnubst *et al.*, 1984), and (2) the social environment, particularly social support.

Direct and Buffer Effects of Social Support

Earlier, we pointed in passing to the direct and buffering effects that social support may have upon the well-being of the individual. A buffer effect refers to the fact that a high level of social support protects the individual against the negative consequences of stressors at work. This implies that among individuals who have access to a strong social support system, such stressors are unlikely to lead to strains and to the deterioration of mental and physical health, while they are assumed to have a negative effect upon well-being among persons who lack adequate social support (House, 1981). Thus, according to this hypothesis, social support is beneficial only in time of crisis. In contrast, the direct effect hypothesis assumes that social support has a general positive effect upon well-being. Two types of direct effects can be distinguished. First, support may directly reduce certain work stressors. It has even been suggested that the main, and perhaps only, function of social support may be in structuring the work role itself (Ganster et al., 1986). For example, supportive managers may prevent role overload by only allocating tasks to their subordinates that these individuals are capable of handling well, and may prevent role ambiguity by giving clear and unambiguous directions. The second direct effect of social support concerns the positive influence one's relationships with others have upon mental and physical health by meeting important human needs for regard, belonging, and understanding.

The empirical support for both hypotheses in work settings, and particularly for the buffer hypothesis, is mixed. One of the most interesting earlier studies in this area was done by Caplan et al., (1975). They analyzed a sample of 2010 men in 23 occupations and studied the relationships between stressors (work overload, role ambiguity, role conflict, lack of participation, underutilization), and a series of job-related and psychological strains. The results showed perceived support from supervisors, subordinates, and co-workers to be negatively correlated with stressors and strains. Pinneau (1976) refined the analysis of the same sample but also expressed some doubts about the current buffering hypothesis. He tested the three hypothesis concerning social support outlined above: social support (a) reduces psychological strain, (b) reduces job stress, (c) buffers psychological and physiological strains against the effect of job stress. The hypotheses (a) and (b) were confirmed, but hypothesis (c) was not. Thus, support did not buffer the stressor–strain relationship. Sears et al. (1983), and Jayaratne and Chess (1984) found no evidence for buffering effects of social support either. However, research by House and Wells (1978), LaRocco et al. (1980) and Etzion (1984) did show some interesting buffering effects.

Nevertheless, even in the studies where buffering effects were found, such effects generally only occurred for some stressors or for some strains (Jackson, 1985). For example, in a study described by House (1981), only 24 out of a total of 140 tests of buffering effects yielded significant results, while in the study of Ganster et al. (1986), no more than three out of 24 regressions analyses showed evidence of interactions between social support and a stressor. Furthermore, negative buffer effects—indicating a relatively high level of strains among individuals with a high level of social support—are by no means exceptional (Jackson, 1985).

Research upon direct effects has also produced many inconsistent findings, even within the same study. In addition to the study of Caplan et al. (1975) mentioned above, several studies on job stress have indeed found negative relationships between job stressors and social support (House, 1981; Pinneau, 1976; Winnubst et al. 1982). However, aside from the issue of the direction of the causality between both variables, it is equivocal whether social support has an effect upon some stressors and not upon others. The same is true with respect to strains. For example, LaRocco et al. (1980) found that social support had a main effect upon job satisfaction and self-esteem, but not upon self-reported illness.

As the foregoing makes clear, much has yet to be learned about the exact role of social support in the alleviation of job stress. This is all the more true since nearly all studies in this field have been cross-sectional in nature. Such designs do not in fact allow causal interpretations, especially with regard to direct effects of social support. In the following, we will first describe a cross-sectional study, then point to the limitations of such studies, and next present a longitudinal extension of this study geared at attempting to overcome the problems inherent in most occupational stress research.

Example 1. The Cross-Sectional Study

Research by LaRocco et al. (1980) supported the buffering hypothesis for psychological and physical strains (anxiety, depression, irritation, and somatic symptoms), but failed to support this hypothesis with regard to job-related strains (job dissatisfaction, boredom, dissatisfaction with workload).

In line with the model of LaRocco et al. (1980), our team analyzed a preliminary sample consisting of 1246 employees from 13 different industrial organizations in the Netherlands (1167 males and 79 females); both blue and white collar occupations were represented. The employees were aged 34–65 years and the mean age was 45 years (Winnubst et al., 1982). A comprehensive instrument, The Organizational Stress Questionnaire (VOS), measured perceived stress in the work environment (role conflict, role ambiguity, role overload, future uncertainty about job and responsibility for persons), perceived strain (irritation, depression, anxiety, threat), behavioral strain (smoking, drinking), health problems (heart complaints, general somatic complaints, systolic blood pressure, diastolic blood pressure, level of cholesterol, and the Quetelet index, which measures the degree to which one is overweight).

Two measures of social support were included: one five-item scale for the degree of social support by the supervisor, referring to the possibility of communication with the superior on work problems; and the availability for supervisor support when things at work became difficult, the regard and esteem provided by the supervisor, the quality of the relationship with him or her, and the frequency of conflicts. A similar scale was employed for social support by the co-workers. These scales are similar to those used in American studies and based upon the Michigan model.

The direct effects of supervisor support on stressors were nearly all strong and highly significant ($p < 0.01$): social support was negatively correlated with role conflict (-0.42), role ambiguity (-0.36), future job uncertainty (-0.28), and role overload (-0.20). In the case of responsibility we found a weaker effect (-0.08). The direct effects of co-worker support showed the same pattern, but were weaker, although still significant.

There were also interesting direct effects upon psychological strains: correlations between supervisor support and these types of strains were, for threat -0.35, for irritation -0.41, for depression -0.26, and for anxiety -0.21 (all $p < 0.01$). The main effects of co-worker support showed the same pattern, with a few small differences. On the other hand, the direct effects of supervisor and co-worker support upon the physiological strains (blood pressure, cholesterol) and on the behavioral strains (smoking, drinking) were lacking.

Regression analysis of stressors × psychological strains did reveal that supervisor support buffers against feelings of threat and irritation in the case of role overload and responsibility. Co-worker support buffers against threat and irritation in the case of role conflict and against feelings of threat in the case of role overload. When thwarted by future uncertainty, the co-worker support buffers against depression, anxiety and excessive smoking. Another interesting buffering effect we found was that among people who feel threatened, depressed and anxious, supervisor support buffered against high blood pressure (see Winnubst *et al.*, 1982).

Three interactions, however, went in the reverse direction and indicated that in some cases the role of social support may be a negative one, e.g. that too much social support is harmful, and thus, in effect ceases to be supportive. This is the case with the responsibility variable; people with high responsibility experience far more depression and smoke more cigarettes when their colleagues attempt to help them, and even experience depression when their supervisors attempt to do so.

In contrast to LaRocco's findings, we found interesting direct *and* buffering effects for different kinds of stressors and strains. Indicators of job-related stress and strain were affected by direct effects and by buffering effects, and we could drawn the same conclusion for the relationship between stressors, support and health outcomes.

The main problem in these kinds of studies is, of course, the lack of insight into the *causal* relationships between variables. Concurrent correlations between measures of social support on the one hand and job stressors and strains on the other, are amenable to several alternative explanations. They may indicate that social support reduces or prevents job stress; that job stress has a negative impact upon the level of social support; or that a third factor, e.g. a certain personality characteristic, influences social support as well as well-being. Additionally, halo effects may be responsible for the correlations between social support and other aspects of the work situation. Use of a longitudinal design overcame such problems.

Example 2. The Longitudinal Study

In the longitudinal study (Marcelissen *et al.*, 1988) the above-mentioned sample was enlarged, with up to 21 Dutch companies. Assessment took place at three different points in time so as to meet the requirements of a longitudinal design. Of the 2034 employees who participated in the first assessment, 409 were also included in the second, and 965 in the third assessment. In addition, 305 employees participated in the second as well as in the third assessment. Only about 20% of the original group of employees that were requested to participate in the study refused to do so. The sample can be regarded as representative of the population of Dutch employees. In this longitudinal study The Organizational Stress Questionnaire (as described earlier) was used once again.

A longitudinal panel design was used in which the sample was investigated at three points in time. We used the linear structure relationship method (LISREL), as developed by Jöreskog (1979). This procedure is related to path analysis, and makes it possible to estimate mutual influence between variables and to investigate causal effects, i.e. the extent to which changes in one variable are *caused* by changes in the other. The results of this study were as follows. First, the professionals and the manual laborers, perceived less support than individuals from other levels in the organization. Second, manual laborers consistently reported that co-workers provide more support than supervisors. On the other hand, social support by the supervisor is far more important for them than support by colleagues, as observed earlier in the cross-sectional study.

The analyses were performed separately for higher and lower occupational levels, as the sample was dichotomized. These results are described in Tables 28.1 and 28.2. For both occupational levels, social support provided by the supervisor was correlated with all stressors, with the exceptions of 'responsibility for others'. However, only in the lower level group did social support by the supervisor have a causal effect upon most stressors and reduce role ambiguity, role overload, role conflict and job future uncertainty. In the higher level group, a two-sided relationship with role ambiguity was found, indicating that this stressor and social support are influenced by one another.

Similar analyses were performed concerning social support by co-workers. However, the number of significant correlations was lower here and there is little evidence for a causal effect of social support by co-workers on stressors. Only in the lower occupational group did co-worker support seem to have some effect, i.e. by reducing the amount of role overload and role conflict.

Continued analyses indicated that in both occupational groups social support was not at all correlated with objective health indices, including systolic and diastolic blood pressure, and level of cholesterol. On the other hand, supervisor support correlated substantially with affective strains and worry, and negatively with health complaints. There were limited causal effects: in the lower group there was a significant effect upon regular health complaints; in both groups, supervisor support seemed to reduce the amount of worrying concerning the job.

Table 28.1 Relationship between social support by supervisor and stressors for lower occupational levels

	Correlations Time			Path coefficient		Misfit
	1	2	3	b1	b2	Chi
Role ambiguity	−0.33	−0.34	−0.38	−0.04	−0.21[b]	5.6
Responsibility	0.13	−0.01	0.02	−0.06	−0.10	2.6
Role overload	−0.21	−0.30	−0.44	0.01	−0.33[b]	5.3
Role conflict	−0.39	−0.16	−0.25	−0.20	−0.51[b]	0.6
Future uncertainty	−0.30	−0.31	−0.19	−0.11	−0.24[b]	6.5

b1 = Causal effect of stressors upon relationship with supervisor.
b2 = Causal effect of relationship with supervisor upon stressor.
[b] = $P < 0.05$.

Table 28.2   Relationship between social support by supervisor and stressors for higher occupational levels

	Correlations Time			Path coefficient		Misfit
	1	2	3	b1	b2	Chi
Role ambiguity	−0.37	−0.47	−0.47	−0.34[a]	−0.50[a]	4.9
Responsibility	0.02	0.04	0.01	0.07	0.12	10.7[b]
Role overload	−0.16	−0.12	−0.21	−0.01	−0.13	6.9
Role conflict	−0.33	−0.25	−0.39	−0.08	−0.16	3.1
Future uncertainty	−0.26	−0.27	−0.07	−0.27	−0.08	10.2[b]

b1 = Causal effect of stressors upon relationship with supervisor.
b2 = Causal effect of relationship with supervisor upon stressors.
[a] = $P < 0.01$.
[b] = $P < 0.05$.

The results of the LISREL analyses again indicated quite a different pattern in the case of co-worker support: in the lower group, affective complaints and worry appeared to influence social support negatively, while, on the other hand, this was the case for the higher occupational group with regard to affective strains and regular health complaints. These results suggest that relationships with colleagues are influenced negatively by strains that individuals experience. We return to this remarkable finding later on. A further noteworthy finding was the nearly complete absence of buffer effects.

Comparison Between the Two Studies

Some common trends and a series of intriguing differences can be observed in comparing the cross-sectional and the longitudinal studies. In both kinds of studies the following results are noteworthy: (a) the special place of the responsibility variable: in the cross-sectional study we see inverse relationships and in the longitudinal study we see a complete lack of correlations with this variable; (b) with only a few exceptions, the lack of correlations involving physiological variables; (c) the importance of supervisor support as compared to co-worker support; and (d) the existence of main *and* interaction effects.

Despite their common findings, important additional information was obtained in the longitudinal study as compared to the cross-sectional study. First, in comparison with the cross-sectional study, we were able to refine the longitudinal analysis by dividing the sample into higher and lower occupational levels. (This was possibly due to the size of the sample.) As a result, we observed striking differences in the effectiveness of support in the different occupational levels: supervisor support has a causal effect upon most stressors in the group with lower occupational levels, whereas this is not the case in the group with higher occupational levels. Secondly, in the longitudinal study for *both* occupational groups, supervisor support was not at all correlated with objective health indices. However, co-worker support played an interesting role in the lower occupational group. In this group, diastolic blood pressures affected social support negatively in the LISREL analysis; so we may conclude that this physiological strain causes the relationships with colleagues to deteriorate. Thirdly, we found that, for both occupational levels, the two kinds of support—supervisor's and co-worker's—show a circular causality with psychological strains such as threat, irritation, anxiety and depression. Fourthly, to our surprise, and in contrast with results in our cross-sectional study, we did not find any buffer effect in our longitudinal study. These findings illustrate how important it is to validate data established in cross-sectional research by employing a longitudinal design. In general, findings from cross-sectional research should be viewed with extreme caution.

An important conclusion seems to be that for people of lower educational levels, social support provided by the supervisor plays an important part in eliminating and reducing stressful circumstances at work, while this is not the case for people higher in the occupational hierarchy. Marcelissen (1987) stated that the greater importance of social support in the lower occupational groups is probably a consequence of a lower degree of autonomy and greater dependency upon the supervisor.

SUMMARY AND CONCLUSIONS

The goal of this chapter was to focus upon the operation of social support in the alleviation of stress. We have tried to explicate the main perspectives on social support and to analyze some of the social psychological processes involved in the building and utilization of social support systems. In the final sections we have dealt with social support and occupational stress. We presented some data from our own cross-sectional and longitudinal research. One of the most intriguing findings from this last study is probably that, in contrast to what is generally assumed in the literature, strains seem to reduce social support by co-workers, and not vice versa. Thus, merely the fact that someone experiences feelings such as anxiety, anger and depression more frequently, seems to lower the degree of social support available to him or her. Although unexpected, these data are quite compatible with our earlier analysis of social competence. As Hansson *et al.* (1984) have noted, the so-called social support environment is a complex interpersonal environment that is not necessarily supportive, and contains a variety of barriers to effective access. For a supervisor, giving support to his subordinates is part of his role; norms in society and the organization expect him to help and support the workers he supervises. On the other hand, the willingness of co-workers to give support may be more dependent upon the feelings of personal attraction for one's colleagues.

In general, we agree with Jackson (1985) that it seems worthwhile to shift attention to look for the way in which help is sought and offered in work-related settings, and for the emotional transactions that take place in this context. Such transactions always occur within relationships, and many aspects of such relationships, including, for example, interpersonal orientations, self-disclosure, trust, communication and equity, seem relevant with regard to social support. Indeed, research on social support in general could substantially benefit from the theories and findings in the emerging field of social and personal relationships.

Acknowledgements

Thanks are due to Adèle Couzijn and Hedy Buunk-Kleijweg for their help in improving the English of this chapter.

REFERENCES

Antonucci, T.C. (1985a). Personal characteristics, social networks and social behavior. In R.H. Binstock & E. Shanas (eds), *Handbook of aging and the social sciences*. New York: Van Nostrand Reinhold.

Antonucci, T.C. (1985b). Social support: theoretical advances, recent findings and pressing issues. In I.G. Sarason & B.R. Sarason (eds), *Social support: theory, research and applications*. Dordrecht/Boston/Lancaster: Martinus Nijhoff.

Barrera, M. (1986). Distinctions between social support concepts, measures and models. *American Journal of Community Psychology, 14*,4, 413–445.

Berkman, L.F., & Syme, S.L. (1979). Social networks, host resistance, and mortality: a nine year follow-up study of Alameda County residents. *American Journal of Epidemiology, 109*, 186–204.

Billings, A.G., & Moos, R.H. (1982). Work stress and the stress-buffering roles of work and family resources. *Journal of Occupational Behaviour, 3*, 215–232.

Bruhn, J.G., & Philips, B.U. (1984). Measuring social support: a synthesis of current approaches. *Journal of Behavioral Medicine, 7*,2, 151–169.

Buunk, B. (1985a). *Vriendschap. Een studie over de andere persoonlijke relatie.* (Friendship. A study of the other personal relationship). Amsterdam: Bert Bakker.

Buunk, B. (1985b). Hiding socially disapproved experiences from the social network. Paper presented at the meeting of the National Council on Family Relations, Dallas, Texas, November.

Caplan, R.D., Cobb, S., French, J.R.P., Van Harrison, R., & Pineau, S.R. (1975). *Job demands and worker health*. US Department of Health, Education and Welfare, HEW (NIOSH) Publication No. 75–160. Washington, DC: US Government Printing Office.

Cobb, S. (1976). Social support as a moderator of life stress, *Psychosomatic Medicine, 38*, 5, 300–314.

Cobb, S., & Kasl, S. (1977). Social support and health through the life course. In M.W. Riley (ed.), *Aging from birth to death: Interdisciplinary perspectives*. Boulder: Westview Press.

Cohen, S., & Wills, T.A. (1985). Stress, social support, and the buffering hypothesis. *Psychological Bulletin, 98*,2, 310–357.

Etzion, D. (1984). Moderating effect of social support on the stress–burnout relationship. *Journal of Applied Psychology, 69*, 615–622.

Fleming, M., Rohmann, S., & Wong, N.W. (1984). Social interaction and social support. *Journal of Social Issues, 40*,4, 55–76.

Ganster, D.C., Fusilier, M.R., & Mayes, B.T. (1986). Role of social support in the experience of stress at work. *Journal of Applied Psychology, 71*, 102–110.

Gentry, W.D., & Kobasa, S.C.O. (1984). Social and psychological resources mediating stress–illness relationships in humans. In W.D. Gentry (ed.), *Handbook of behavioral medicine*. New York: Guilford Press.

Gottlieb, B.H. (ed.) (1981). *Social networks and social support*. Beverly Hills/London: Sage.

Hansson, R.O., Jones, W.H., & Carpenter, B.N. (1984). Relational competence and social support. *Review of Personality and Social Psychology, 5*, 265–284.

Hatfield, E. (1984). The dangers of intimacy. In E. Derlega (ed.), *Communication, intimacy and close relationship*. New York: Springer.

Heller, K., Swindle, R.W. & Dusenbury, L. (1986). Components of social support processes: Comments and integration. *Journal of Consulting and Clinical Psychology, 54*, 4, 466–470.

Hobfoll, S.E. (1985). Limitations of social support in the stress process. In I.G. Sarason & B.R. Sarason (eds), *Social support: theory, research and applications*. Dordrecht/ Boston/Lancaster: Martinus Nijhoff.

House, J.S. (1981). *Work stress and social support*. Reading, Mass.: Addison-Wesley.

House, J.S., & Wells, J.A. (1978). Occupational stress, social support, and health. In A. McLean, G. Black & M. Colligan (eds), *Reducing occupational stress: Proceedings of a conference*. (DHEW-NIOSH Publication No. 78–140). Washington, DC: US Government Printing Office.

Jackson, P.R. (1985). A critical analysis of the stressbuffering role of social support at work. Paper presented at the West European Conference of the Psychology of Work and Organization, Aachen, West Germany.

Jayaratne, S., & Chess, W.A. (1984). The effect of emotional support on perceived job stress and strain. *Journal of Applied Behavioral Science, 20*, 141–153.

Jöreskog, K.G. (1979). Statistical models and methods for analysis of longitudinal data. In K.G. Jöreskog (ed.), *Advances in factor analysis and structural equation models*. Cambridge, Mass.: Abt Books.

Kissel, S. (1965). Stress-reducing properties of social stimuli. *Journal of Personality and Social Psychology, 2*, 378–384.

LaRocco, J.M., House, J.M., & French, J.R.P. (1980). Social support, occupational stress and health. *Journal of Health and Social Behavior, 21*, 202–218.

Lazarus, R.S. (1966). *Psychological stress and the coping process*. New York: McGraw Hill.

Lefcourt, H.M. (1985). Intimacy, social support, and locus of control as moderators of stress. In I.G. Sarason & B.R. Sarason (eds). *Social support: Theory, research and applications*. Boston: Martinus Nijhoff.

Lowenthal, M.F., & Haven, C. (1978). Interaction and adaptation: Intimacy as a critical variable. *American Sociological Review, 33*, 20–30.

Marcelissen, F.H.G. (1987). *Psychological pacemakers in the process of stress*. Leiden, The Netherlands: NIPG/TNO.

Marcelissen, F.H.G., Buunk, B., Winnubst, J.A.M., & De Wolff, Ch.J. (1988). Social support and occupational stress: A causal analysis. *Social Science and Medicine, 26*, (3), 365–373.

Pinneau, S.R. (1976). Effects of social support on occupational stresses and strains. Paper presented at the meeting of the American Psychological Association, Washington, DC.

Rook, K.S. (1984). Research on social support, loneliness and social isolation. *Review of Personality and Social Psychology, 5*, 234–264.

Sarason, I.G., & Sarason, B.R. (1985a). *Social support: Theory, research and applications*. Boston: Martinus Nijhoff.

Sarason, I.G., & Sarason, B.R. (1985b). Social support: Insights from assessment and experimentation. In I.G. Sarason & B.R. Sarason. *Social support: theory, research and applications*. Dordrecht/Boston/Lancaster: Martinus Nijhoff.

Schaap, C., Buunk, B., & Kerkstra, A. (1987). Marital conflict resolution. In M.A. Fitzpatrick & P. Nollen (eds), *Perspectives on marital interaction*. Clevedon and Philadelphia: Multilingual Matters.

Schaefer, C., Coyne, J.C., & Lazarus, R.S. (1981). The health related functions of social support. *Journal of Behavioral Medicine, 4*, 4, 381–406.

Sears, A., McGee, G.W., Serey, T.T., & Graen, G.B. (1983). The interaction of job stress and social support: A strong interference investigation. *Academy of Management Journal, 26*, 273–284.

Shinn, M., Lehmann, S., & Wong, N.W. (1984). Social interaction and social support. *Journal of Social Issues, 40*, 4, 55–76.

Shumaker, S.A., & Brownell, A. (1984). Toward a theory of social support: closing conceptual gaps. *Journal of Social Issues, 40*,4, 11–36.

Stouffer, S.A., Suchman, E.A., Devinney, L.C., Star, S.A. & Williams, R.M. (1965). *The American soldier.* New York: Wiley. (Original printing 1949.)

Syme, S.L. (1984). Sociocultural factors and disease etiology. In W.D. Gentry (ed.), *Handbook of behavioral medicine.* New York: Guilford Press.

Thoits, P.A. (1985a). Self-labelling processes in mental illness: The role of emotional deviance. *American Journal of Sociology, 92*, 221–249.

Thoits, P.A. (1985b). Social support and psychological wellbeing: theoretical possibilities. In I.G. Sarason & B.R. Sarason (eds), *Social support: Theory, research and applications.* Boston: Martinus Nijhoff.

Turner, R.J. (1983). Direct, indirect, and moderating effects of social support on psychological distress and associated conditions. In H.B. Kaplan (ed.), *Psychosocial stress: Trends in theory and research.* New York: Academic Press.

Van Dijkhuizen, N. (1980). *From stressors to strains. Research into their interrelationships.* Lisse, The Netherlands: Swets & Zeitlinger.

Wilcox, B.L., & Vernberg, E.M. (1985). Conceptual and theoretical dilemmas facing social support research. In I.G. Sarason & B.R. Sarason (eds), *Social support: Theory, research and applications.* Boston: Marinus Nijhoff.

Winnubst, J.A.M., Marcelissen, F.H.G., & Kleber, R.J. (1982). Effects of social support in the stressor–strain relationship: A Dutch sample. *Social Science and Medicine, 16*, 475–482.

Winnubst, J.A.M., Marcelissen, F.H.G., Van Bastelaer, A.M.L., De Wolff, Ch.J., & Leuftink, A.E. (1984). Type A behaviour pattern as a moderator in the stressor–strain relationship. In A.M. Koopman-Iwema & R.A. Roe (eds), *Work and organizational psychology.* Lisse, The Netherlands: Swets & Zeitlinger.

Wortman, C.B. (1984). Social support and the cancer patient. *Cancer, 53*, 2339–2360.

KEY WORDS

Buffer effect, co-worker support, depression, direct effect, future uncertainty, health complaints, heart complaints, intimacy, job dissatisfaction, job satisfaction, lack of participation, LISREL, occupational groups, occupational stress, perceived helpfulness, relational competence, responsibility, role ambiguity, role conflict, role overload, self-disclosure, self-esteem, social integration, social network, social relationships, social support, stigmatizing events, strains, stressors, supervisor support, work stressors.

Section IV: Social Cognitive and Biological Models of Stress and Illness

Handbook of Life Stress, Cognition and Health
Edited by S. Fisher and J. Reason
© 1988 John Wiley & Sons Ltd.

29

Stress, Language and Illness

RICHARD TOTMAN
The University of Sussex

INTRODUCTION

This chapter takes as its theme man's unique standing among other social species due to his capacity for the manipulation of signs and symbols. By far the most important system of signs he uses is, of course, language.

There are many different definitions of stress and many psychological theories of how stress may combine with genetic, physiological and physical (environmental) 'risk factors' to cause or exacerbate illness. These theories are really searches for a common denominator to the many different life circumstances linked through research with a threat to health. We can now confidently say that a statistical relation exists between, for example, bereavement and increased illness and mortality (e.g. Bowling, 1987; Chapter 4, this volume), and lack of social support and illness (e.g. Cohen and Wills, 1985; Chapter 28, this volume). But most bereaved people do not get ill and die; neither do most of those lacking obvious sources of social support. So what distinguishes those who suffer adverse effects in these circumstances from those who do not?

A full answer to this question may yet be some way off, but it is a pressing, not to say an intriguing, question and one that taxes the imagination of those working in this area. We should not be shy of theorizing, even speculating, in a field now almost overburdened with correlations and other data. The main problem in setting up a theory of stress and its relation to illness is that stress represents a psychological state whereas illness is mainly regarded in terms of organic pathology. The majority of theories of stress are either pitched squarely within psychology—the 'cognitive' theories that prevail at the present time—or squarely within physiology—they deal with neuroendocrine mediators of organic pathology. There has been occasional talk of the 'interface' between psychological and physiological processes, but no proper exploration of whether this is a sensible notion and if so what it might mean. The aim of this chapter is to outline some ideas which represent a new approach to the problem of stress and illness.

PSYCHONEUROIMMUNOLOGY

The debate about stress and illness is remarkable in that it seems to be expanding continually to involve more and more different disciplines. While this is obviously a good thing, it carries with it a problem that is endemic to specialism. The difficulty in persuading researchers and theorists to take a broader view of issues and problems than the one dictated by the boundaries of their own speciality was nowhere more obvious than at a conference held in Utrecht in December, 1982, organized by the EEC and entitled 'Psychoneuroimmunology'. Immunologists, neurologists and psychologists from throughout Europe were invited together in the hope that some of the interactions implied in the term 'psychoneuroimmunology' would be brought to light and the exchange of ideas between those working in different disciplines would pave the way for new collaborative research. But this hope turned out to be a vain one. There was considerable resistance among the immunologists present to the idea that neuroendocrine activity could affect immune system reactions. They preferred to hold on to the view of the immune system as autonomous. Moreover, there was virtual rejection by both immunologists and neurologists of psychological models, other, that is, than the kind developed by Ader and his associates, based on studies of the pathological effects of conditioned stress in laboratory animals (Ader, 1981).

Nevertheless, the term psychoneuroimmunology, though not elegant, does at least contain the idea that central activity related to stress and unhappiness results in neuroendocrine imbalances which, if sustained, have a disruptive effect upon the normal, adaptive immune response of the organism. It is necessary to amplify what is meant by 'normal immune response' here, since it is known that the immune system is involved not only with the mobilization of defences against antigens from outside, but also with the control of pathological conditions which can arise internally—the so-called autogenic or autoimmune conditions such as multiple sclerosis and some forms of cancer.

There is strong evidence that abnormally high levels of certain hormones can be immunosuppressive, that is, they can adversely affect the normal healthy production of antibodies in response to an invading antigen (e.g. Riley, 1981). But as well as interfering with the immune response itself, it seems neuroendocrine activity may also influence other vital functions of the immune system. For example, a group of leucocytes, known as natural killer (NK) cells, is believed to have a special policing function. These cells circulate in the blood and can become hostile to target cells, including tumour cells, without any prior sensitization. They could therefore play an important part in the control of metastasis. There is some evidence that interferon may be necessary for their effective function (Lipinski *et al.*, 1980). Interferon production is known to be suppressed by stress and by high levels of stress-related hormones such as glucocorticoids (Amkraut and Solomon, 1975), thereby providing a channel of communication for an inhibiting effect of psychological stress on NK cell activity. So it is not outside the realms of possibility that cancer cells arise naturally in the normal healthy body but that their concentration and spread are kept down by immunosurveillance mechanisms that are in turn responsive to stress-related hormones (cf. Hanna and Fidler, 1980).

When talking about the immune system there are good medical grounds for holding on to a distinction between challenge from outside, for example from a virus or bacterium, and internal resistance. During plagues and epidemics it is clearly appropriate to attribute deaths to an exceptionally high concentration of microorganisms in the environment. Conversely, autoimmune conditions are so named because they are thought to occur purely as a result of internal pathogeny. However, attitudes change as knowledge advances, and for the majority of 'everyday' serious illnesses this distinction may turn out to be of limited value. For example, there is growing evidence that viruses play a part in the causation of many types of cancer. Conversely, an increasing number of known antigens, streptococcus for example, are discovered as natural, harmless residents of the healthy body (in this case the mouth), albeit in low concentrations.

The approach generally favoured among those concerned with stress and illness is to regard the majority of the pathological states which arise as part of living in the late twentieth century as the combined result of external challenge and internal resistance. Given the chain of causes and effects that the term psychoneuroimmunology (for a recent review of the field, see Baker, 1987) implies, the range of illnesses susceptible to the influence of psychological stress becomes enormous.

PSYCHOLOGICAL STRESS

But what do we mean by psychological stress, other than a shorthand for 'the mental state that disposes the organism to illness'? The language of psychology is not reducible to that of physiology, and, as psychologists, this is the most central question we are called on to answer. Common sense, together with a very large research literature, warns against too naive a view of stress—stress as overwork, or worry or physical strain. All these are normal components of daily life and most of us who have to endure them manage to stay reasonably healthy most of the time. Neither is it particularly useful turning to animal studies for an answer. We do not need data from research to tell us that the kinds of experience a mouse finds stressful in the laboratory are not commensurate with the stresses that people suffer as the darker side of life.

Nevertheless, there are plenty of studies of people in ordinary situations that give a clue as to what psychological forces are at play to protect someone from, or dispose them to, life-threatening illness.

The most stressful real human environment of which there is any systematic record must be that of the Nazi death camps of the 1930s and early 1940s. 'Systematic', that is, in the sense that a large number of survivors' accounts have been published and these show good agreement over the psychology of camp internees. Prisoners were transported from their homes throughout Europe in cattletrucks, and arrived at a camp to confront genocide, disease, infestation, foul living conditions, extreme brutality and literally hourly threats of gassing or shooting. They were subjects of a systematic regime of overwork, physical abuse, humiliation and slow starvation. The system even extended to a deliberate policy of insufficient toilet facilities. Stangl, commandant of the camp at Treblinka, openly explained the reason for this (Sereny, 1974). The fact that prisoners were contaminated with their own excrement made it easier for the guards to see them as subhuman and so carry out their brutal duties. On any hypothesis of stress as accumulated physical or emotional strain, one would expect the death rate from causes other than killings under these conditions to be highest among those who had endured the camp conditions longest and so had suffered the most. But this was not the case. In all the camps natural death rate (if one can call it such) was highest during the first few weeks of a person's imprisonment (Cohen, 1954; Bettelheim, 1961; Des Pres, 1976).

Such a picture concurs with the general lack of psychological evidence that chronic conditions, however stressful they may appear to an outside observer, produce equivalent destructive effects in a person as does stress brought on by a sudden traumatic change. On their arrival at Auschwitz, one of the larger camps, confronted with the terrible conditions of life and death, most prisoners went into a state of suspended belief which typically lasted for some weeks. 'Nightmare' and 'unreality' are the two words which, according to Des Pres (1976), appear most frequently in survivors' accounts of these first days and weeks: 'All around us were screams, death, smoking chimneys making the air black and heavy with soot and the smell of burning bodies . . . It was just like a nightmare and it took weeks and weeks before I could really believe this was happening.' (Hart, 1962, pp. 92–93.)

Bettelheim makes exactly the same observation: 'Not only during the transport, but for a long time to come, prisoners had to convince themselves that this was real and not just a nightmare' (Bettelheim, 1961, p. 127).

But, as Frankl (1959) says, failure sooner or later to accept the reality of life in the camp was a failure to adapt and carried with it all the dangers that the stress–illness hypothesis would predict. Those prisoners who survived the initial shock and accepted that they really were in a concentration camp and that conditions were as bad, or worse, than they were rumoured to be, developed what is referred to as a 'fighting spirit'. Accounts from survivors consistently relate survival to the taking on of some moral initiative or goal. The form this took varied. Sometimes it simply involved the cultivation of a certain professionalism in the near-impossible art of survival. Sometimes it was planning to escape. Sometimes it was a determination to help others resist, as in the case of this Polish woman whose job it was to index incoming prisoners at Maidenek: 'I know that a person coming to a camp was afraid of everything and everybody, that she was distracted and terrified. The first word was so important. I decided to be patient, to answer all questions, to calm them and give them courage. My life began to hold meaning.' (Zywulska, 1951, p. 113.)

For many others, a sense of commitment was found in a determination to make some kind of record of the conditions in the camp so that, later, others should come to know about them (Des Pres, 1976).

Failure to take upon oneself a role or commitment of some kind was a prelude to death. In the Nazi camps the name for this vast majority, most of whom were new prisoners, was the *muselmanner*—the 'walking dead'. In Soviet labour camps they were known as *dokhodyaga*—the 'goners': 'Their life is short, but their number is endless; they, the *Muselmanner*, the drowned, form the backbone of the camp, an anonymous mass, continually renewed and always identical, of non-men who march and labour in silence, the divine spark dead within them, already too empty to really suffer. One hesitates to call them living; one hesitates to call their death death.' (Levi, 1965, p. 82.)

So much research has been done in the social sciences in connection with stress and illness that we are able to call on a very large library of studies of naturally stressed individuals and populations; studies by sociologists, anthropologists and epidemiologists as well as those by psychologists. It would be inappropriate, indeed impossible, to review these here, but accounts are to be found in this volume and elsewhere (e.g. Totman, 1985). No one theory of stress will ever be able to account for every single observation and correlation. But is it possible to draw any general conclusions from a comprehensive reading of this research? I believe it is, and that the following generalizations are justified by the data.

1) Psychological circumstances which have life-threatening consequences for the individual—the category of 'stressors' we are trying to define—are predominantly social in origin, and are characterized by traumatic social change. They exist over and above the effects of worry per se, physical strain, diet and exercise. This fact is still contested by opponents of the stress–disease hypothesis but there is plenty of evidence for it. The strongest evidence comes from studies of the negative relation between health and bereavement (Bowling, 1987), and the favourable effect on health of social support during times of crisis (Kessler et al., 1985).

2) Active commitment on the part of the individual to a project or cause in terms of which actions are motivated and justified is generally found to be protective of health. This much we can infer from the reports of survivors of concentration camps. Research into conditions of work (e.g. Alfredsson et al., 1982) and the effects on health of unemployment (Brenner, 1979; Levi, 1987), as well as the extensive literature on 'loss' in its various forms, underpin this point.

3) It is the significance of a life event or life change to that individual which defines whether the event is stressful or not. This can be inferred from the fact that correlations between stressful life experience and life-threatening conditions are generally greater in biographically styled studies that take into account the context of the event than in statistical approaches that rely on crude descriptions and checklist questionnaires. This conclusion forms the foundation for the new transactional models of stress, such as that of Lazarus et al. (1985). It is also central to the methods developed by George Brown in the study of depression (Chapter 24, this volume).

4) The category of stressor we are trying to define is not only associated with increased risk of serious illness and death, but also with increased risk of other life-threatening states including suicide attempts, alcoholism, drug abuse, accident proneness and victimization. For example, excess rates of all these conditions, along with excess rates of coronary disease, strokes, infections and cancer, are statistically associated with loss and bereavement (Stroebe et al., 1982). Indirect support for this conclusion is provided by an analysis of all the death statistics available in the United States from 1900 to 1975, which from 1933 to 1975 include records for the entire population. Holinger and Klemen (1982) showed

that mortality rates from suicide, homicide and motor accidents rose and fell in synchrony. That is, when suicides were common, so were accidents and homicides, etc.

These four points add up to a theme which is often reiterated by students of life stress in humans: stress, where this is conceived as a distinct psychological state associated with raised risk of life-threatening illness and self-destructive tendencies, appears in an individual when that individual lacks some kind of social identity. A variety of circumstances could be responsible for this state of affairs—a bereavement, losing one's job, transferring from a familiar culture (or subculture) to an unfamiliar one, lacking the various facilities that come under the general description 'social support'—to take some commonly quoted examples. But a string of other, more esoteric, circumstances could in principle carry just the same stress value, depending upon the individual in question and their meaning to him or her. Nonetheless, repeatedly, descriptions of these circumstances give a picture of the vulnerable person as somehow disengaged, or distanced, from society or some valued division of it, and consequently without the capacity to see life as meaningful and goals and projects as worthwhile.

Is it possible to refine this concept of stress any further? 'Failure to adapt or cope', 'isolation from society', 'loss of self-esteem', 'loss of meaning'—these themes appear frequently in the literature on stress. They are certainly important pointers to an understanding of the psychology of stress, but they do not on their own add up to a theory.

LANGUAGE AND LANGUAGE GAMES

Man is a social species and much of the expression of his social nature is through symbols. The most vital of all his systems of symbols is language. Language gives the opportunity to lay down rules and to set up social and moral orders which can be remembered, acted on and sustained in the absence of immediate physical prompts. In this respect, humans are quite different from any other social species. I have represented psychological stress as a kind of detachment of the individual from social sources; a detachment which can come about as the result of a variety of circumstances. This is to be seen not primarily as a physical detachment—life in the concentration camps was horribly crowded and cramped—but as a symbolic one. The sense of meaninglessness, hopelessness and goal-lessness observed in ill, dying and suicidal individuals can be attributed, on the hypothesis of stress set out here, to the individual's detachment from, or lack of articulation within, any shared system of rules that constitute a moral order.

The proposition that language plays a vital role in establishing and sustaining a person's social identity has a direct counterpart in Wittgenstein's theory of language, especially in his notion of 'language games'. In *Philosophical investigations*, Wittgenstein argues that there is an intimate relation, almost an isomorphism, between the speaking practices of groups of people and the social fabric of such groups. His theory rests on the principle that the meaning of exchanges (i.e.

utterances) between individuals is established by their practice in a community. Meaning, he claims, arises purely and simply out of shared use: 'If we had to name anything which is the life of the sign, we should have to say that it was its *use*' (1958, p. 4). The term 'language game' is coined to refer to the sort of things that are habitually said between individuals. Language games are not just the property of groups and institutions, they are the expression of those groups and institutions. A premise very similar to this lies behind much of the thinking in modern sociolinguistics (e.g. Gumperz, 1982).

The size of the group within which language games are played can be anything from two individuals upwards. But to have a language it is necessary to have a group of some sort, and it is one of Wittgenstein's points of departure that the idea of a private language—an introspective commentary intelligible only to the speaker—is not a sensible one and must be rejected as logically untenable.

From the implausibility of private languages, Wittgenstein argues that there is an essential connection between an individual's social world and his or her speech and mental life. Perhaps the closest thing to a private language are the highly intimate, esoteric forms of small talk which sometimes grow up between two people who share a very close relationship.

In fact, Wittgenstein uses the term 'language games' in a much broader sense than this to typify not only spoken exchanges between people, but all forms of sign-based activity. Wherever there are rules, and activity based on rules, there lurk the conventions and institutions which make up social life.

Using Wittgenstein's phrase, then, we can paint a sort of impressionist picture of the loss of meaning that stress of social origin involves. We can say that the condition of stress, when this term refers to the psychological precursors of life-threatening states, including illness, is a non-participation in any of the language games which are the expressions of a society or some pocket of it. For in these language games lie rules, moral enjoiners to action, and order. In a sense this is no more than saying that unity with others works to protect health and is therefore anti-stressful, and that, in humans, unity with others goes beyond hand-to-hand cooperation and is expressed in plans, discourse and thought. Yet the concept of language games provides us with a neat way of summarizing these ideas.

Returning again to the death camps of Nazi Germany and the comparison between those prisoners who gave up and died and those who survived, the 'language games' of the latter inhere in their commitments, be these religious, political, humanist or the morally pressing urge to bear witness to the conditions of life and death in the camp. Des Pres (1976) insists it was not hope that kept survivors alive. Too much hope led to despair, and you were better off forgetting there was an outside world, not thinking about release, and developing a moral identity that could be applied and acted on then and there: 'The survivor is the figure who emerges from all those who fought for life in the concentration camps, and the most significant fact about their struggle is that it depended on fixed activities: on forms of social bondings and interchange, on collective resistance, on keeping dignity and moral sense alive' (p. viii).

STRESS: MALADAPTIVE AND ADAPTIVE

One of the conditions of stress is widely represented as a life event, or series of life events, which requires the individual to adapt to changed circumstances. This condition is necessary, though not sufficient. As Kessler *et al.* (1985) point out, stress becomes real and dangerous if the person fails to adapt by failing to find some way of coping with their altered circumstances. Such a situation is 'dangerous' because it is associated with a number of consciously and unconsciously driven self-destruct tendencies. Examples of these conscious and unconscious tendencies are, respectively, suicide and inhibition of the normal healthy workings of the immune system. Moreover, I have identified this failure to adapt with a condition of symbolic aloneness, or separateness from any of the communities which make up the complex structure of the human social world. Without a tie to at least one of these communities, the individual has nothing against which to measure and justify his or her actions. He or she has no source of motivation beyond that dictated by biological necessity.

An association between failure to adapt to a changing or changed environment on the part of the individual and threat to that individual's survival has a certain Darwinian flavour to it that is perhaps worth briefly exploring. Biologists concur that social organization in any species provides a powerful aid to survival. A cooperative organization insures that the potential for survival of the group as a whole is greater than the sum of the isolated survival potentials of each constituent member. However, in a social species the interests of the group are not always commensurate with the interests of the individual. There are plenty of examples in the animal world where weak, non-contributing members of a group are discriminated against and banished or murdered (Breuer, 1982). Among humans too, a cohesive group containing a clear structure of roles is a more efficient unit than an unstructured group in which roles are poorly defined. It follows that an articulated and developed social organization will have little use for role-less individuals—that is, individuals who, for whatever reason, are not participants in the cooperative structure. Such individuals contribute nothing to the energy of the group and represent, potentially, a net drain on the group's resources. A genetically programmed contingent link between role-lessness and the self-destructive tendencies that we have seen are associated with psychological stress supplies a means of ensuring cohesion and increasing the chances of survival of the group and therefore of the species.

It can be argued, as Harré (1979), for example, does, that most of human social life in economies that produce a surplus is organized around expressive rather than practical projects. Once the basic needs for food, shelter and a degree of comfort are satisfied, the need for practical cooperation between individuals in a struggle to survive becomes secondary to the need to exhibit oneself as socially worthy and deserving of respect.

In a society that is materially replete in this way, a gene for role-occupancy, assuming such a thing exists, expresses itself not in the kind of physical activity that has a direct bearing on survival, but in what Harré describes as 'ritual markings of respect and contempt': uniforms, prizes, applause and all the numerous more mundane forms of praise and criticism which fill our daily lives. The fact that this hypothetical gene once had direct consequences for survival but in most modern societies no longer does is quite compatible with a teleological explanation of the stress–illness relation. That gene, though redundant, will not just disappear, and will seek expression in some form. The human capacity to make and use artifacts and symbols means that there are available a virtually infinite number of vehicles for the expression of respect and contempt, from a simple handshake or snub to the grander trappings of public investiture. The role-less person in a society where expressive projects take precedence over practical ones is the person who, as a result of change, finds himself with no access to any of these vehicles. It is therefore only to be expected that 'social support' provides a 'buffering effect' against 'stress' at times, such as the death of someone close, when an important source of expressive projects becomes no longer accessible.

The work that has been done in connection with stress and illness therefore forces us to consider the possibility that illness in humans may be more internally regulated, and more under the control of a genetic programme, than had been imagined when germ theory dominated medical thinking. The two facts, (1) that we are prepared to talk about 'stress' as a distinct psychological condition associated with different kinds of life-endangering states, and (2) that the weight of evidence indicates that stress has to do with an individual's standing in relation to the social world, argue for a radical rethink of the notion of disease as a passive yielding of the organism. Forces that are much more active seem to be at play. Of particular significance is the fact that many other life-threatening dispositions beside physical illness are associated with psychological stress. A picture begins to emerge of illness and those other dispositions as regulatory and patterned.

In the previous section, it was argued that human social organization is, unlike any other, complex and sign bound. If this is the case, then the nature of the circumstance in which the 'social' part of the individual breaks down—i.e. the condition of psychological stress—will also be complex and sign bound. Human social organization is pluralistic. We are not all members of one huge homogeneous group with a few dissenters, but rather subscribers variously to a criss-cross of communities, some large, some small, each with its own, often overlapping, opinions, attitudes, moralities and styles. The image I am attempting to build up of the stressed or 'at risk' person is not that of dissenter or revolutionary—one who makes a career of reacting against the wider, more conservative establishment. Far from it; such individuals, like the survivors who fought against the morality (or lack of it) of the concentration camp, are participants in a very potent language game signifying a very strong moral and political code. Their status is that of the active opposition and their lives are charged with meaning and justification.

As was said in the discussion of language games, a 'group' can consist in as few as two individuals. The central point is that a person can never be a group on his or her own, and it is the beached quality of this solitary predicament which better than anything else seems to define stress and its destructive consequences.

It has to be said that there is some controversy among biologists over whether or not it is appropriate to take the principles of natural selection developed in a theory of the individual genotype and apply these, as sociobiologists do, to the group. It would be out of place to go into these arguments here; they are well summarized by Breuer (1982). But whatever the biological arguments, there is no logical reason to prevent us considering mechanisms of natural selection among groups. This is simply a theoretical matter of taking the group not the individual as the basic unit of survival—as the 'organism' for the purpose of the analysis. What this means for the individual genotype is that the process of selection of close-knit communities will favour genes for mutualism and role occupancy.

To classify illness, a suicidal disposition, accident-proneness and drug addiction as maladaptive states of the individual is relatively uncontroversial. Construal of the stress–illness connection as an *adaptive* mechanism in relation to species survival (selection works in favour of more socially disposed individuals and therefore more cooperative and effective groups), may be more contentious but does not in fact present a paradox. There is no paradox here because the two analyses apply to different logical categories of selection. What is good for the group is not necessarily good for the individual. Nevertheless, any idea of human suffering and disease as adaptive, whatever the context in which this is proposed, comes over as an unpalatable and, in a sense, undesirable one. It seems to carry the portent that whatever advances we make in the medical treatment of today's diseases, there will always be a replacement disease, so to speak, just around the corner, waiting to stand in for those conditions we succeed in eliminating. Even if we manage to abolish physical illness altogether, is there not a case, on the preceding argument, that the other more deliberate pathways to death, such as suicide and alcoholism, and even accident-proneness (Holinger and Klemen, 1982), will come to the forefront and prevail as the main causes of death?

Looking back over the past 100 years in the history of medicine, there is indeed some basis for this pessimistic attitude. The main causes of death in 1900—influenza, tuberculosis and pneumonia—were quite different from those of today. Today heart disease and cancer are top of the list and there is widespread (though debatable) concern that tomorrow it will be AIDS. Even more disturbing is Schulz's observation that the difference in life-expectancy between 1900 and now is attributable almost entirely to a much higher rate then of deaths in infancy and early childhood: 'The difference in predicted longevity for 65-year-old people who were born in either 1900 or 1971 is only three years. We can conclude from this that, while we are not living much longer than people did 100 years ago, a greater number of us are attaining old age.' (Schulz, 1978, p. 42).

But the unpalatability or otherwise of a theory is no reason for not acting on that theory. Only if we confront the problem of stress and illness, and stress and the other various life-threatening conditions, as primarily a *social* problem with a *social* solution, as the weight of evidence shows it to be, can we arm ourselves with the appropriate equipment to begin to tackle the problem.

SUMMARY AND CONCLUSIONS

An old convention in concluding essays of this nature is to finish with an enjoiner to further research and the conclusion that data will help confirm or refute some of the ideas which have been proposed. I do not believe this is any longer the case in respect of research on psychological stress. There exists an enormous literature on the subject and a very large reserve of data. It is difficult to imagine that a single theory will ever be able to incorporate and explain all these findings.

Lazarus *et al.* (1985) are not alone in emphasizing the complexity of the concept of psychological stress. They argue that stress is inevitably an 'unclean' variable in that it depends upon a dynamic and changing interaction between person and environment. Whether it is possible to break down such a complex business into interdependent variables, especially when it comes to studies of people in natural, everyday situations, is questionable. Those authors who want to do so (e.g. Dohrenwend *et al.*, 1984) usually find themselves working with rather specific definitions of stress, tailored to their particular research design. So the two alternatives would seem to be either many different definitions of stress, each tied in to a specific situation (via a specific research design), or a more general, theory-based, perhaps less precise definition such as the one outlined in this chapter. There is of course no reason to see these different approaches to the problem as incompatible. But whichever approach one prefers, it is clear that stress for humans is not analogous with stress for animals. Any theory of stress as a failure to adapt or cope on the part of the individual must address itself to social forces and the symbolic forms, especially language, in which these are purveyed.

REFERENCES

Ader, R. (1981). *Psychoneuroimmunology*. New York: Academic Press.

Alfredsson, L., Karasek, R., & Theorell, T. (1982). Myocardial infarction risk and psychosocial work environment: an analysis of the male Swedish working force. *Social Science and Medicine, 16*, 463–467.

Amkraut, A., & Solomon, G.F. (1975). From the symbolic stimulus to the pathophysiological response: immune mechanisms. *International Journal of Psychiatry in Medicine, 5*, 541–563.

Baker, G.H.B. (1987). Psychological factors and immunity. *Journal of Psychosomatic Research, 31*, 1–10.

Bettelheim, B. (1961). *The informed heart*. London: Thames and Hudson.

Bowling, A. (1987). Mortality after bereavement: a review of the literature on survival periods and factors affecting survival. *Social Science and Medicine, 24*, 117–124.

Brenner, M.H. (1979). Mortality and the national economy: a review, and the experience of England and Wales, 1936–1976. *Lancet, 2*, 568–573.

Breuer, G. (1982). *Sociobiology and the human dimension*. Cambridge: Cambridge University Press.

Cohen, E.A. (1954). *Human behaviour in the concentration camp*. London: Jonathan Cape.

Cohen, S., & Wills, T.A. (1985). Stress, social support, and the buffering hypothesis. *Psychological Bulletin, 98*, 310–357.

Des Pres, T. (1976). *The survivor, an anatomy of life in the death camps.* New York: Oxford University Press.

Dohrenwend, B.S., Dohrenwend, B.P., Dodson, M., & Shrout, P.E. (1984). Symptoms, hassles, social supports and life events: problems of confounding measures. *Journal of Abnormal Psychology, 93,* 222–230.

Frankl, V.E. (1959). *From death-camp to existentialism.* (Translated by Ilse Lasch.) Boston: Beacon.

Gumperz, J.J. (ed.) (1982). *Language and social identity.* Cambridge: Cambridge University Press.

Hanna, N., & Fidler, I.J. (1980). Role of natural killer cells in the destruction of circulating tumor emboli. *Journal of the National Cancer Institute, 65,* 801–809.

Harré, R. (1979). *Social being.* Oxford: Basil Blackwell.

Hart, K. (1962). *I am alive.* London, New York: Abelard Schuman.

Holinger, P.C., & Klemen, E.H. (1982). Violent deaths in the United States 1900–1975. *Social Science and Medicine, 16,* 1929–1938.

Kessler, R.C., Price, R.H., & Wortman, C.B. (1985). Social factors in psychopathology. Stress, social support and coping processes. *Annual Review of Psychology, 36,* 531–572.

Lazarus, R.S., Delongis, A., Folkman, S., & Gruen, R. (1985). Stress and adaptational outcomes. The problem of confounded measures. *American Psychologist, 40,* 770–779.

Levi, L. (ed.) (1987). Unemployment and health. *Social Science and Medicine, Special Issue,* Vol. 25, No. 2.

Levi, P. (1965). *The truce.* London: Bodley Head.

Lipinski, M., Virelizier, J-L., Tursz, T. & Griscelli, C. (1980). Natural killer and killer cell activities in patients with immunodeficiencies or defects in immune interferon production. *European Journal of Immunology, 10,* 246–249.

Riley, L. (1981). Psychoneuroendocrine influences on immunocompetence and neoplasia. *Science, 212,* 1100–1109.

Schulz, R. (1978). *The psychology of death, dying and bereavement.* Reading, Mass.: Addison-Wesley.

Sereny, G. (1974). *Into that darkness.* (Translated by R. Seaver.) London: Weidenfeld and Nicolson.

Stroebe, W., Stroebe, M.S., Gergen, K.J., & Gergen, M. (1982). The effects of bereavement on mortality: a social psychological analysis. In J.R. Eiser (ed.), *Social psychology and behavioral medicine.* Chichester: Wiley.

Totman, R.G. (1985). *Social and biological roles of language.* London: Academic Press.

Wittgenstein, L. (1958). *Philosophical investigations.* (Translated by G.E.M. Anscombe.) Oxford: Basil Blackwell.

Zywulska, K. (1951). *I came back.* (Translated by K. Cenkalska.) London: Dennis Dobson.

KEY WORDS

Stress, language, psychoneuroimmunology, immunosuppression, autoimmune, survival, role, commitment, social identity, detachment, social support, suicide, bereavement, loss, goal-lessness, language games.

Handbook of Life Stress, Cognition and Health
Edited by S. Fisher & J. Reason
© 1988 John Wiley & Sons Ltd.

30

Life Events, Social Cognition and Depression

KEITH OATLEY
University of Glasgow

INTRODUCTION

The recent advances in the study of stressful life events and epidemiological psychiatry, as described in this volume, have given psychologists an important challenge: how can we describe the relation between important events in our personal world and our mental schemata, those organizations of knowledge by which we understand our world?

The most general formulation that can be offered, and one that is common to most approaches, although it is not always stated explicitly, is that stressful life events are to be understood in relation to our life goals and plans. Human plans are invariably imperfect. The phrase 'stressful life event' is used in empirical studies for the kind of adversity in which the unwished-for happens and disrupts a person's course through life. A life event is stressful in so far as it damages a plan. People's life plans may be very different, and some of them may be only vaguely formulated. Despite this, research has been able to proceed because, on average, a bereavement interrupts a plan of continuing an important relationship, because, for most people, becoming unemployed involuntarily is a reverse of their aspirations, or because having a teenage child in trouble with the police contradicts the plan of having our children grow up happily.

In general, the schemata that apprehend such life events are the same as those that underlie our plans, where plans are to be understood in the broadest sense of goal-directed projects with an element of anticipation. The idea that plans underlie our relation to the world is at the heart of the cognitive approach to psychology (see, for example, Miller *et al.*, 1960). Interruption of an important plan will be likely, as Miller *et al.* pointed out, to have dysphoric emotional effects. The idea that emotions, and emotional states like depression, arise from interruptions is central to the cognitive approach to emotions (see, for example, Mandler, 1984; Oatley, in press; Oatley and Johnson-Laird, 1987).

One approach to understanding this is to consider that the schemata underlying

543

our actions are entirely general, that we use the same kinds of schemata for our dealings with both the physical and social worlds. A second possibility is that we may have specific social schemata that differ in important respects from the schemata that mediate our relation to the physical world. According to this second possibility, social schemata underlie the conduct of our relationships with others. Understanding the properties of these schemata would then form the basis for understanding the stress of life events that disrupt relationships, and the way in which these events can provoke depression and other psychiatric states.

In the following section a comparison will be made between some of the postulates and properties of both approaches. In relation to depression, both approaches have similar structures: that an adverse event can provoke depression, but that it only does so if the person experiencing the event is vulnerable in a defined way.

INSTRUMENTAL SCHEMATA AND SOCIAL SCHEMATA

The stress of adverse life events may be that of being unable to control important aspects of the world. I will identify this position with Seligman and his group (Seligman, 1975; Abramson *et al.*, 1978; Peterson and Seligman, 1984), and describe this kind of control as instrumental.

The other alternative will be referred to as social. Its postulate is that adverse life events are primarily social, and consist not in a failure of control, but in a disruption of social relationships. I will identify this position with Bowlby (1980), Brown and Harris (1978), and Oatley and Bolton (1985).

Of course, both failures of instrumental control and disruptions of social relationships may be stressful. It is, however, an empirical question as to what kind of theory best accounts for a particular set of evidence. This chapter will mainly deal with the evidence of life-event stress in relation to depression. In relation to other kinds of outcome the issues may be different.

Failures of Control and Learned Helplessness

It has been common in psychology to analyse behaviour in terms of an organism controlling the contingencies of its environment. In this paradigm, reinforcement contingencies are brought under the control of the animal's instrumental performance. This kind of learning is thought to be basic to the learning of higher animals, including ourselves, in most situations. The nature of the reinforcement may be different in different circumstances. Thus, because humans are social animals, social reinforcements may well be particularly important for us. Moreover, human plans may be more complex than those of experimental animals. Nevertheless, the proposal of this research programme is that such differences are quantitative, and do not introduce qualitative changes to any analysis.

An important development of the research on stress came from experiments in which dogs that had been given electric shocks in one apparatus behaved passively when placed in a second apparatus, where they could have learned to avoid shocks (Seligman, 1975). In a colourful and suggestive phrase, Seligman called this learned helplessness, and proposed that it was a basic component of depression. According to this hypothesis, failing to control aversive events is stressful, and potentially depressogenic.

Because the original helplessness theory failed to account for some of the phenomena of event-precipitated depression in humans, concepts from the social psychological theory of attribution were added as vulnerability factors by Abramson *et al.* (1978). According to this reformulated helplessness theory: to fail at an instrumental task is stressful, and depression is likely to result when the person is vulnerable in tending to attribute the failure to the self (an internal attribution), to see it as an example of general failure (an attribution that the failure was global rather than local), and to see such failures as continuing permanently (an attribution of temporal stability). Bereavement, then, becomes the failure to prevent the death of a loved person; unemployment the failure to control one's employer, and so on. Depression is likely to result from such events when a person is vulnerable in having an attributional style likely to produce internal, global and stable explanations of the event.

In cognitive terms, to control an environment requires that the animal (human or otherwise) has a schema, representation or model of the relevant aspects of that environment (see, for example, Oatley, 1985). We may imagine that, in a typical task in which learned helplessness is induced, a human subject first builds a model of some aspect of the environment as both aversive and uncontrollable. Then this model is applied to new situations, although it is not necessarily appropriate to do so. If, moreover, the failure is assimilated to schemata that have perhaps been carried forward from experiences of failure in childhood, as suggested by Beck (1976), then it will be the terms of such schemata that produce interpretations of the self as worthless, the world useless and the future hopeless, with depression being likely to result.

Coyne and Gotlib (1983) have shown that these terms of Beck's depressive triad of worthlessness of the self, uselessness of the world and hopelessness about the future are empirically indistinguishable from the attributional terms of the reformulated helplessness theory of internal, global and stable attributions, and that therefore Beck's and Seligman's theories should be considered together.

Social Schemata

I do not wish to question the proposal by Seligman and his group that important psychological consequences follow from failures in instrumental tasks, or the findings that some of these consequences include dysphoric mood. Nor do I wish to question the common finding that depression involves styles of thinking which are self-denigratory, global and hopeless. There are, however, questions about whether this style is a vulnerability factor or a symptom (see Brewin, 1985; and Chapter 23 in this volume), and whether the general instrumental formulation is adequate to the social aspects of depression (a question also raised in a different way by Gilbert, Chapter 31 in this volume).

I want to propose, first, that there is an alternative to the instrumental formulation of the action of life events, namely, the social formulation, and, secondly, that the question of whether clinically significant depression occurs with instrumental failures, or only with social disruptions, or both, has not yet been answered. The instrumental formulation of Seligman and his group, and the social formulation to be offered here, are not the only ones in the field. For instance, Gilbert (1984) has ably reviewed a wide range of cognitive, behavioural and psychobiological theories of depression. Several of these other approaches are discussed elsewhere in this volume. What I want to propose is that within cognitive theory, there are two broad classes of approach to understanding the significance of life events, instrumental and social. Because they are relatively less developed, theories of the schemata underlying specifically social interactions, and how these schemata produce symptoms, need further exploration.

To understand the schemata that underlie social relationships we need to consider what I will call mutual plans (Oatley, in press), which have several characteristics that are quite different from the instrumental plans of a single actor.

When social interactions take the form of well-practised mutual plans they acquire structure and predictability. They can then be described as roles. Examples are parent–child, friend–friend, student–teacher, employer–employee, etc. The rather suprising proposal of Goffman (1961) is that by enacting a role we bring a microworld alive to our own experience and that our experience of selfhood is drawn largely from taking part in such roles. Thus we may experience ourselves as loving and caring by fulfilling the cultural rules of parenthood in our interactions with a son or daughter. If we have a job with certain responsibilities, then we can experience ourselves as responsible in so far as we perform that job according to the script for the role that is known in our cultural community. The great power of the social–psychological concept of role is that it both allows different individuals to fill the positions defined by roles, in a somewhat interchangeable way, and that role occupancy then confers the role characteristics on the individual who fulfils that role, at least to some extent.

Social schemata, then, are the schemata that underlie our goals and plans in relation to other human actors in our world, including those necessary for enacting role relationships. The plans at issue are not those of single actors; they are mutual. Thus having a job rests on an understanding between employer and employee, partly explicit but partly understood implicitly. The realization of the self in the role of employee requires that both the self and the employer play culturally defined parts which correspond, within limits, to expectations derived from the knowledge we have of them.

For a purely instrumental plan in the physical world, a schema is needed that includes a goal and a model of the world within which searches can be made through simulated states and actions, until a route between the current state and the goal is found. Social schemata underlying roles need, in addition, two further components, a model of the role-other, and also a model of the self.

The model of the other person with whom we enact a role tends to generalize from one situation to another. Thus the ordinary knowledge about how to conduct oneself in relation to others in a particular culture is embodied in what Mead (1964) called the generalized other. In the psychoanalytic tradition of object relations theories (see, for example, Fairbairn, 1952), the argument is that early parental figures form a core for our models of at least some kinds of other people. These models are carried forward, and may be projected onto others who are not, in fact, our parents. Thus someone who became well practised in submitting to the will of a peremptory parent might carry forward a style of deference ready to be applied to other people in authority.

In addition, role theory assumes that some aspects of the models that underlie the enactment of any particular role are more or less specific to that role, and that the script for playing that role (friendship, employment, etc.) will be well understood in any community. In addition, we will build up specific models of individuals on the basis of our experience of carrying out mutual plans with them.

It is perhaps somewhat less intuitively obvious that a model of self is also fundamental to being able to conduct social interactions or mutual plans. According to this idea, which derives from Mead, the self is not a bastion of individuality, but part of the cognitive means by which we integrate our actions with others (Mead, 1964; Farr, 1984). For instance, in order to conduct a mutual plan there needs first to be a mutual goal, which may be either assumed, as in the case of the interactions between an infant and caregiver, or explicitly negotiated, as in some contracts. Most adult mutual goals have both implicit and explicit elements. Then there needs to be an arrangement for building a joint plan: who does what, and how? Such plans, as Power (1984) has shown, involve interreliance, and each knowing that the other knows about arrangements for the plan. This means both forming a model of the other's intention, and forming a model of our own goals and abilities. For instance, to make a promise (the basis for many mutual plans) involves knowing about one's own goals and abilities to carry out a plan.

The model of self, then, is a model partly of our own abilities and characteristics. Some of these are seen only in the social mirror of others' reactions to us. Partly it consists of goals, the most important of which are those by which we define ourselves. Ryle (1982) calls these self-definition goals. Self-definition goals are at the top of a hierarchy of personal goals. They often consist of wanting to being liked or respected by others in a certain kind of way. They tend to pervade much of a person's life. At lower levels in the hierarchy are goals like earning one's living. At yet lower levels, goals may be local to particular role-relationships, and at yet lower levels still, to specific plans and mutual arrangements, like an arrangement to undertake some particular piece of work together.

The model of self also contains rules, distilled from a person's experience and endorsed by him or her, which take the form of conditionals in which the goal will be experienced as fulfilled by the enactment of a certain kind of plan, e.g. 'I will be loved if I do X'. Ryle argues that many self-definition goals and the conditionals that form the model of self are implicit, i.e. unconscious, and that the task of psychotherapy can often best be described as discovering, or infering from our actions, some of the terms of self-definition models. For instance, Ryle describes the case of David, who had entered therapy because of uncertainties about his career, and also with the loss of a relationship with a woman friend with whom he had been living. It emerged that David's self-definition goals were to feel worthwhile in the world, and to feel loved. These goals were pursued with plans of proving his self-worth by being helpful to others. In part this goal had been fulfilled by his work as a nursing assistant in an old-people's home. A similar plan had supported his relationship with his woman friend, but this was now severely disrupted by her departure, leaving him without the sense of fulfilling his major goals, and indeed falling back on their converse: feeling unlovable and feeling that his life was pointless. (Ryle also shows that such plans are rarely simple, for instance David's plan of being helpful to others also tended to contradict other goals because its performance often involved submerging his own needs, and this in turn produced ill-defined feelings of resentment.)

A role relationship is really a sequence of mutual plans, conducted with another person, a structure of habit with a history of shared experience, precedents and negotiations, and with an expected future of further mutual projects. It will be perceived as satisfying by a participant in so far as it allows her or him to fulfil self-definition goals and to continue with plans for such fulfilment.

Goals and plans involving two or more actors, such as those supporting role relationships, are thus more complex than those of a single actor with an instrumental plan in the physical world. Action sequences of one actor must interdigitate with those of others. The sense of joint action and interreliance that is involved is part of the pleasure of relationships. But the coordination of two or more actors in a plan also means that mutual plans can go wrong in many ways that do not occur in the plans of single actors.

Important long-term role relationships are those by which we often fulfil self-definition goals. So for many people, to have a continuing sexual relationship may allow them to feel loved; to be employed may allow them to experience themselves as productive and valued, and so on. The hypothesis of this kind of social–cognitive theory is that we actually experience ourselves as loved, productive, etc., by taking part in such long-term role relationships.

The hypothesis of Oatley and Bolton (1985) was that life events are severe when they disrupt a role that was fulfilling a self-definition goal. If a sexual relationship was the means by which a person accomplished the sense of being loved, then a partner being unfaithful, as had happened with Ryle's patient David, would remove the possibility of fulfilling that self-definition goal, at least as accomplished by that plan. This in turn would tend to undermine the sense of self that had been derived from the relationship.

This formulation of the action of life events is clearly different from the proposal that life events are a failure of control. The idea of oneself and those to whom we are close being predictably reliable is quite different from that of the world being instrumentally controllable. In this social–cognitive theory there is no postulate that it is important to control the other person. Although we may often try to control others in a relationship, this is rarely successful in intimate relationships. Even when it is, the schemata underlying the relationship still require the models of self and other, so that this feature differentiates these schemata from those involved in purely instrumental plans in the physical world.

In this proposal, the symptoms of depression (loss of a sense of self-worth, dysphoric emotions, and plans for restoring the relationship that was lost) arise naturally from the theory (Oatley and Bolton, 1985). The same cognitive processes, which support the performance of roles and mutual plans, explain what happens when the goals and plans of an important role miscarry. In helplessness theory, hypotheses about the self were grafted on to the original idea about controlling contingencies. The self is not postulated as having a function in instrumental control of the environment. It only becomes the recipient of attributions when things go wrong.

The proposal of the social hypothesis is that we enter into role relationships by experiencing ourselves and the other person in a range of joint plans. If the relationship progresses, our model of ourselves and the other in that relationship includes a sense of reliability. Our own and the other's behaviour become, within limits, predictable. But if that relationship is disrupted, the sense of self that was derived from it is lost or negated.

In the next section I will show how this theory can account for some of the epidemiological evidence on the events that provoke depression and the factors that make people vulnerable to the impact of such events.

EVIDENCE FROM STUDIES OF LIFE EVENTS

The main evidence in the study of life events is from the new field of psychiatric epidemiology. In this field, diagnoses and estimates of the severity of symptoms are made on members of the ordinary community, not on samples of patients. As the history of epidemiology of physical illness has shown, to base research on patient samples only is to introduce bias that hampers efforts to understand aetiology. Psychiatric epidemiology is new because only in the last 20 years or so have reliable and valid diagnostic instruments been available.

A threatening life event is an occasion that is capable of provoking clinical depression in a member of the community. As Brown and Harris (1978) have shown, depression typically occurs when two conditions are fulfilled. One is that a threatening event or chronic difficulty is severe, e.g. that something of the magnitude of a bereavement, a divorce, or an eviction from home has occurred. The other condition is that the person is also vulnerable in some way, such as being without social support.

Brown and Harris pioneered a method for detecting events and difficulties in community samples, for making socially based but objective judgements of their significance and severity, and for relating severe events and difficulties to a diagnosis of clinically significant depression. To make diagnoses, the Present State Examination (PSE) was used as a research diagnostic interview. As an index of the severity of the syndrome, Brown and Harris defined a 'case' level, equivalent to the severity of syndromes seen in psychiatric out-patient clinics, and to about midway between points 5 and 6 on the Index of Definition on the PSE (see Dean et al. (1983) for a discussion of research diagnoses and case levels). Using this method, Brown and Harris found that, in a sample of 458 women randomly chosen from a London voters list, 37 (8%) had suffered an onset of depression at the case level within a year before the interview. Of those who had suffered an onset, 89% had experienced a severe event or major chronic difficulty preceding the onset. By comparison, only 30% of women who were not depressed had suffered a severe event or major difficulty.

Oatley and Bolton (1985) presented a table of ten recent studies using Brown and Harris's (1978) methodology or its equivalent. All of these showed an increased rate of onset of depression at the case level with events or difficulties that were severe. All but one showed that this rate was higher when the subject was vulnerable by being without the social support of an intimate or confiding relationship.

Since these cross-sectional studies, there have been longitudinal studies. One was by Brown and his colleagues, of events, difficulties and social support in working-class women with children (Brown *et al.*, 1986; 1987; Chapter 24 in this volume). The findings of this study broadly support the conclusions of the cross-sectional research, though prompting some refinements.

In another longitudinal study, Bolton and Oatley (1987) followed up 49 men who were interviewed within 2 weeks of becoming unemployed, and compared them with 49 men in a matched comparison sample who remained employed. Three categories of outcome for the originally unemployed men were found at a second interview 6–8 months after the first interview. Fourteen could not be traced or refused a second interview; 15 had got new jobs; 20 remained unemployed, of whom 5 had become seriously depressed. The depression scores of these five on Beck's Depression Inventory (BDI, Beck *et al.*, 1961) were less than 10 at the first interview and more than 18 at the second. None of the men in the employed sample or men who had become re-employed had BDI scores of more than 10 at either interview. The continuingly unemployed were significantly more depressed at second interview than either the employed group or those who had become re-employed ($p < 0.01$; there were no significant differences between groups at the first interview). Moreover, we confirmed the hypothesis that low social support makes one vulnerable to a depressive reaction to life events. Among those who became and remained unemployed, small amounts of social contact outside work in the month before unemployment significantly predicted higher levels of depression at the second interview, although there was no association between social support and depression scores in the employed group. (The interaction between employment status and social support on the BDI scores at Time 2 was significant, $p < 0.05$.)

I want to suggest that such epidemiological data provide a corpus of evidence that favours the hypothesis that depression most often occurs with provoking agents that consist of disruption of an important social role in the presence of vulnerability factors that are also socially defined, e.g. the availability of social support.

This involves an oversimplification, because not all severe life events and difficulties are purely social disruptions. Brown and Harris (1978) estimated that, of the 37 women in their sample who had an onset of depression, 88% of those with a severe event had suffered a loss of some kind. For 18 of these women, the event was a separation, loss, or threat of loss of someone close. Eleven of the women had losses with an arguably non-social element, such as an enforced change of residence or a major material loss. In Bolton and Oatley's study of unemployment, loss of work typically involved both a social and an economic element. Moreover, although I have presented data here that bear on social support, since it is the most widely studied vulnerability factor in this field, and that which is most often found to be involved in vulnerability, other vulnerability factors have been found significant in the literature of psychiatric epidemiology. For instance, Brown and Harris found that being without a job outside the home was a vulnerability factor for women, and again this could be economic as well as social.

There is currently a difficulty in comparing the hypothesis of instrumental failures of control with the hypothesis that depression is provoked mainly by social losses in that the bodies of evidence to which the two types of theory are applied scarcely overlap.

In a recent review of work on helplessness, attribution and depression, Peterson and Seligman (1984) described five types of study. These were: (a) cross-sectional studies of correlations between scores on Attributional Style Question-naires (ASQs) and depression scores following 'bad events' in a variety of samples; (b) longitudinal investigations in which ASQs were administered to predict depression at a later time following bad events; (c) experiments of nature, including a study in which an ASQ was used to predict mood changes in students following disappointing marks in a midterm examination, and one in which it was used to predict BDI scores of people in prison; (d) laboratory experiments in which people's attributional styles were measured, and then mood change was assessed after subjecting the people to events like inescapable aversive noise or failures in problem-solving tasks; and (e) case studies. None of the studies reviewed by Peterson and Seligman meets the methodological criteria achieved in the epidemiological work following Brown and Harris's research, of measuring depression of clinical significance in factorial designs, i.e. in people who did and did not suffer a bad event, and who were and were not vulnerable.

The evidence of psychiatric epidemiology and life events is methodologically superior to the other literatures on the aetiology of depression in that it treats unbiased community samples, includes studies assessing whether depression is of clinical significance, and includes factorial designs of events and vulnerability, in both cross-sectional and longitudinal designs. (See, for example, Cohen and Wills (1985) for a review of both methodology and findings in this field.) Despite this, there has been little work on the reformulated helplessness hypothesis within this literature.

In the absence of evidence that depression of clinical significance is most usually caused by events which are uncontrollable in the instrumental sense, occurring to people who tend to make internal, global and stable attributions, it seems safest to conclude that a social formulation is at present more promising when considering depression that reaches clinical significance. It remains to be seen how the evidence of distress following failures of instrumental control is to be integrated with the epidemiological data. Seligman and his colleagues have shown that distress is likely to be more marked when it is explained attributionally in terms of the person's own fault, in a global and/or stable way, but it may be that this is the reaction of people facing failure in an instrumental plan rather than of people becoming depressed in a way that meets research diagnostic criteria for the psychiatric state of depression.

COGNITIVE EVALUATION OF LIFE EVENTS

According to the theory of Oatley and Bolton (1985), depression is the response to the loss of a role by which a person has fulfilled an important self-definition goal, when that person lacks alternative means for fulfilling that goal. It is a state that confronts the self with a problem—to revise that goal or to create a new plan to fulfil it. I will now illustrate this process in relation to the conclusions of Bolton and Oatley's (1987) study of unemployment.

Unemployment in our society is an example of an essential problem confronting the self. It causes a major discrepancy between actuality and expectation in the economic and personal relationship between oneself and one's employer. But when do such events lead to depression as opposed, say, to anger or other emotions, and what is the function of the self-absorbed reflection that depression typically involves? To try to answer these questions, I have represented reactions to an adverse event as a series of three cognitive evaluations that are made (more or less consciously), and which depend on the relation of the person's model of self to his or her perception of external circumstances (Fig. 30.1).

The First Evaluation

At the first evaluation, an adverse event is experienced as severe or non-severe. If non-severe, it can lead to emotional distress and even to a dejected mood. Despite

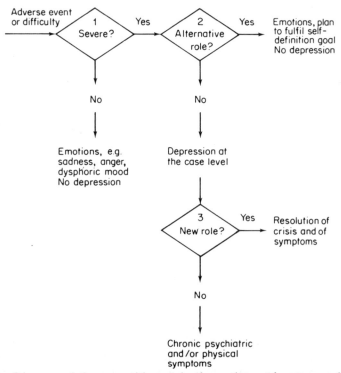

FIG. 30.1   Diagram of three cognitive evaluation points and outcomes following an adverse life event. Each evaluation is depicted by a numbered, diamond-shaped box.

the implication of much research that dysphoric mood engendered by non-severe events is mild depression, the best evidence is that only severe events typically are capable of provoking the qualitatively differentiable state of depression at the case level (see Brown and Harris, 1978; Oatley and Bolton, 1985). Therefore, only if the event is evaluated as severe at this point will it be able to provoke depression.

As Figure 30.1 implies, it is the person suffering the event who makes the cognitive evaluation of severity. But for research purposes another procedure is needed. For Brown and Harris, this involved a process of *Verstehen*— imaginitively understanding the threat of each event that had happened as it would affect the average woman living under those circumstances (see Oatley (in press) for a description of the procedure in these terms). Each event was described to a panel of researchers blind to the psychiatric diagnosis of the subject. Examples of events judged in this way to be severe were bereavement, eviction, divorce, and unemployment. An example of a non-severe event was when a woman's husband had to be away for 3 months to work without returning at weekends. Less severe still would be failing a midterm exam.

Any discrepant event poses a problem, and might lead the person to conscious reflection and the making of new plans, e.g. to keep busy while a spouse is away, or to study harder for the next exam. But in the response to non-severe events there will typically be no revisions of self-definition goals. Only the plans by which they are to be approached will be revised and adapted to the new circumstances.

The Second Evaluation

At the second decision point, an evaluation occurs of whether alternative roles are available, or potentially available, to fulfil the same self-definition goals as the role that has been disrupted by the severe event. If they are, then the person may well experience dysphoric emotions, but his or her life will be channelled into these alternative roles, and/or into the formulation of new plans. According to Oatley and Bolton (1985), people with such alternative roles available or poten- tially available will be protected from becoming clinically depressed. The inverse of being protected is being vulnerable, not having such alternatives available.

In most studies of life events, less than a third of the people afflicted by severe events become depressed; the others have three general types of protection from alternative sources.

First, as well as a role that they have lost, people may have other current roles which allow a sense of self to be maintained. According to this theory, this availability is the basis of the social support that has been found to be protective. For instance, the unemployed men who did not become depressed in the study by Bolton and Oatley had, on average, a wider circle of friends. We inferred that they had other relationships besides employment within which they could experience themselves as worthwhile.

Secondly, some people are more able than others to make effective plans to find a new role to replace one that has been lost. In our unemployment study, some men got new jobs, and none of these were depressed at the second interview. On average, those who got new jobs scored higher on a measure of autonomous self-motivation at the first interview than those who subsequently did not get new jobs.

Thirdly, some people are able to maintain a sense of self without taking part in an important and relatively predictable relationship with others. Such people are relatively well buffered from threatening life events. Although we did not investigate this thoroughly, some of the men in our study seemed to have little alternative social interaction, and yet remained undepressed. We inferred that they had inner resources, not needing so strongly to be sustained by immediate and repeated social interaction. Such people who suffered severe events and had little social support but who remained undepressed were also discovered by Murphy (1982) among the elderly and by Parry (1984) among working-class women.

An example of someone who did become depressed at this second evaluation point was one of the men in Bolton and Oatley's unemployment study. He was unusual in his occupation, though not in respect of the issues that characterized those who became depressed. He had no close friends. He lived with his elderly mother, and saw very few other people. He was a musician, and his group had closed down. Undepressed at first, he was proud of being a good musician (self-definition goal) and thought he would easily get another job. At the second interview, after a number of job applications and some auditions, he had become severely depressed. He had given up making applications and had become withdrawn, and consciously uncertain of his worth.

If, at the second decision point, there are no alternative roles available to fulfil self-definition goals, not only plans but the model of self is threatened, and may need to be re-evaluated, abandoned or changed. The decision at this point implies that the definitions of self implicit in the higher level goals of the model have become a central problem. In other words, severe events can challenge the basis on which a person's model of self is founded. When this happens the person may find thoughts of suicide intruding on consciousness—an indication that no other solution seems possible.

The Third Evaluation

At the third evaluation point, the distress of an acute episode of depression is either resolved or continues chronically. If the person begins to cope, then my hypothesis is that he or she has discovered a new plan that will allow old goals to be fulfilled, or has revised self-definition goals. If the model of oneself in relation to others changes in response to the experience, this also will prompt new plans to meet the new goals. More than 50% of episodes of depression have started to resolve within 4 months (Tennant et al., 1981), but some people remain depressed for long periods. For instance, alongside the 8% of their sample who had experienced an onset within a year of the interview, Brown and Harris (1978) found that a further 7% of their sample had been depressed for more than a year.

If the person remains depressed for some time, this implies that she or he can neither generate new plans to satisfy the old goals nor transform the goal hierarchy. At the same time, depressive plans of relating, e.g. becoming dependent on others, complaining, sulking, withdrawing from certain kinds of interaction etc., can themselves form the basis of roles, while making more productive solutions less likely.

If a depressed person has little sense of worth compiled into the model of self, finds it impossible to transform this model creatively and finds that resources in the outside world are insufficient for forming satisfying new long-term plans, then the episode of depression will be chronic.

Implications

According to this analysis, depression, though profoundly distressing, is also potentially creative. It may challenge people to revise their models of self, their important goals and their plans of how to fulfil these goals. The possibilities for meeting such challenges arise partly from ourselves, but the resources that are protective are not purely psychological. Although some of them may have become psychological as a result of incorporation into models of the self, they also depend critically on available external resources, such as money, mobility, employment and social opportunities. Access to such resources are distributed very unevenly in society. People with more access to them are on average more protected in the three ways defined. In the industrial societies that have been studied, there are higher prevalences of depression among less protected groups. The prevalence of depression is approximately twice as great in women as compared to men, and twice as high in working-class people as compared to middle classes (see, for example, Brown and Harris, 1978; Bebbington et al., 1981). Moreover, the prognosis following a depressive breakdown is also considerably affected by material circumstances (Huxley et al., 1979).

An analysis in terms of planning, including one that involves mutual plans in social relationships and employment, needs a consideration of the cognitive structure of our mental schemata. But these issues cannot be considered in an abstract way, or simulated in the laboratory. They have to be considered in relation to people's ordinary lives and resources of the environments in which we live.

SUMMARY AND CONCLUSIONS

In cognitive theory, threatening life events that can provoke clinical depression are to be considered as reverses in personal plans. On the basis of presently available evidence, miscarriages of these plans that are followed by depression are less well understood as helplessness by single actors attempting to control the world instrumentally, than as disruptions of social roles which are to be understood as mutual plans. Methodologically the best data are from psychiatric epidemiology. A social–cognitive theory of depression has been presented, together with results from a study in which low social support was found to predict depression following unemployment. According to this theory, depression follows loss of a social role that fulfilled self-definition goals when no other plans are available for fulfilling these goals, and there are no resources for starting new ones.

Acknowledgements
I thank Winifred Bolton for her part in the work reported here, and the MRC for supporting it. I am grateful to Jennifer Jenkins for her helpful comments on a draft of the manuscript.

REFERENCES

Abramson, L.Y., Seligman, M.E.P., & Teasdale, J.D. (1978). Learned helplessness in humans: Critique and reformulation. *Journal of Abnormal Psychology, 87*, 49–74.

Bebbington, P.E., Hurry, J., Tennant, C., & Wing, J.K. (1981). Epidemiology of mental disorders in Camberwell. *Psychological Medicine, 11*, 561–579.

Beck, A.T. (1976). *Cognitive therapy and the emotional disorders*. New York: Meridian.

Beck, A.T., Ward, C.H., Mendelson, M., Mock, J., & Erbaugh, J. (1961). An inventory for measuring depression. *Archives of General Psychiatry, 4*, 561–571.

Bolton, W., & Oatley, K. (1987). A longitudinal study of social support and depression in unemployed men. *Psychological Medicine, 17*, 453–460.

Bowlby, J. (1980). *Attachment and loss*. Vol 3: *Loss and depression*. London: Hogarth Press.

Brewin, C.R. (1985). Depression and causal attributions: What is their relationship? *Psychological Bulletin, 98*, 297–309.

Brown, G.W., Bifulco, A., & Harris, T.O. (1987). Vulnerability and onset of depression: some refinements. *British Journal of Psychiatry, 150*, 30–42.

Brown, G.W., & Harris, T.O. (1978). *Social origins of depression*. London: Tavistock.

Brown, G.W., Andrews, B., Harris, T.O., Adler, S., & Bridge, L. (1986). Social support, self esteem and depression. *Psychological Medicine, 16*, 813–831.

Cohen, S., & Wills, T.A. (1985). Stress, social support and the buffering hypothesis. *Psychological Bulletin, 98*, 310–357.

Coyne, J.C., & Gotlib, I.H. (1983). The role of cognition in depression: A critical appraisal. *Psychological Bulletin, 94*, 472–505.

Dean, C., Surtees, P.G., & Sashidharan, S.P. (1983). Comparison of research diagnostic systems in an Edinburgh community sample. *British Journal of Psychiatry, 142*, 247–256.

Fairbairn, W.R.D. (1952). *Psychoanalytic studies of the personality*. London: Routledge & Kegan-Paul.

Farr, R. (1984). Social origins of the human mind. In J.P. Forgas (ed.), *Social cognition: perspectives on everyday understanding*. London: Academic Press.

Gilbert, P. (1984). *Depression: From psychology to brain state*. Hillsdale, NJ: Erlbaum.

Goffman, E. (1961). *Encounters: two studies in the sociology of interaction*. Indianapolis: Bobbs-Merrill.

Huxley, P.J., Goldberg, D.P., Maguire, G.P., & Kingby, V.A. (1979). The prediction of the course of minor psychiatric disorders. *British Journal of Psychiatry, 135*, 535–543.

Mandler, G. (1984). *Mind and body: psychology of emotion and stress*. New York: Norton.

Mead, G.H. (1964). The genesis of the self and social control. In A.J. Reck (ed.), *Selected writings of George Herbert Mead*. Indianapolis: Bobbs-Merrill.

Miller, G.A. Galanter, E., & Pribram, K. (1960). *Plans and the structure of behavior*. New York: Holt.

Murphy, E. (1982). Social origins of depression in old age. *British Journal of Psychiatry, 141*, 135–142.

Oatley, K. (1985). Representations of the physical and social world. In D.A. Oakley (ed.), *Brain and mind*. London: Methuen.

Oatley, K. (in press). *Best laid schemes: a cognitive psychology of emotions*. Cambridge, Mass.: Harvard University Press.

Oatley, K., & Bolton, W. (1985). A social–cognitive theory of depression in reaction to life events. *Psychological Review, 92*, 372–388.

Oatley, K., & Johnson-Laird, P.N. (1987). Towards a cognitive theory of emotions. *Cognition and emotion, 1*, 29–50.

Parry, G. (1984). Psychosocial risk in depression: the role of individual factors. *Bulletin of the British Psychological Society, 37,* A70–71.
Peterson, C., & Seligman, M.E.P. (1984). Causal explanations as a risk factor for depression: Theory and evidence. *Psychological Review, 91,* 347–374.
Power, R. (1984). Mutual intention. *Journal for the Theory of Social Behaviour, 14,* 85–102.
Ryle, A. (1982). *Psychotherapy: a cognitive integration of theory and practice.* London: Academic Press.
Seligman, M.E.P. (1975). *Helplessness: On depression, development and death.* San Francisco: Freeman.
Tennant, C., Bebbington, P., & Hurry, J. (1981). The short term outcome of neurotic disorders in the community: the relation of remission to clinical factors and to 'neutralising' life events. *British Journal of Psychiatry, 139,* 213–230.

KEY WORDS

Life events, bereavement, unemployment, depression, social cognition, learned helplessness, model of self, role relationships, cognitive evaluation, goals and plans, social schemata.

Handbook of Life Stress, Cognition and Health
Edited by S. Fisher and J. Reason
© 1988 John Wiley & Sons Ltd.

31

Psychobiological Interaction in Depression

PAUL GILBERT
Pastures Hospital, Derby

INTRODUCTION

The phenomenon of depression has been recognized for many thousands of years. Well over 2000 years ago, Hippocrates noted a cluster of symptoms which included sadness of mood, pessimistic thoughts and poor appetitive functions. This cluster was labelled melancholia. In fact, throughout the course of human history, depression is ubiquitous. However, depression-like states are not uniquely human concerns. Even in phylogenetically ancient species like the lizard, MacLean (1985) noted that high status lizards who were defeated, lost their brightly coloured appearance and died shortly thereafter. Rats, dogs, mice and primates number among the various species which have been used as experimental subjects in the pursuit of the underlying mechanisms of depressive disorder. Hence, the propensity to respond to environmental events, be these defeats, separations or lack of control over important goals, with patterns which bear some similarity to human depressive states seems ubiquitous in many animal species.

Psychobiology is an integrative discipline which attempts to identify the complex and multiple patterns of activity which correlate with 'various states of mind'. This approach to psychopathology is not new in its philosophy and can, in fact, be traced back to Hippocrates. Freud, in his unpublished 'Project for scientific psychology', sought to develop a psychology of mind derived from evolutionary theory and physiological insight. In America during the early part of this century, Adolf Meyer did much to facilitate the philosophy of psychobiology in psychiatric practice. But it has only been comparatively recently that neurobiological and neuroendocrine mechanisms have been sufficiently well understood to turn this general philosophical desire into a systematic framework.

For the depressive disorders, Akiskal and McKinney (1975) presented one of the first systematic attempts to integrate research and insight from a variety of different approaches and theories of affective disorder. Their general view was that depression constitutes a final, common pathway which could be activated by many and varying psychological, social and/or biological factors. More recently, Whybrow *et al.* (1984), in an outstanding text, have updated and refined this psychobiological approach, Willner (1985) has presented an encyclopaedic review of much of the neurochemical and behavioural biologic work relevant to mood disorders. Gilbert (1984) attempted to describe how various social and psychological factors activate particular, evolved (potential) patterns of psychobiological activity. It was suggested that images, thoughts and appraisals are capable of recruiting certain psychobiological responses which are part of an evolved repertoire for dealing with certain classes of perceived stresses (Gilbert, 1984; in press, a).

In this chapter, some of the psychobiological interactions between social, psychological and biological phenomena are explored. Before proceeding, however, it should be noted that depression itself poses many problems as an area of study.

BIOMEDICAL APPROACHES

By and large, the medical approach to the classification of disease entities has dominated the classification of depression (Kendell, 1975; 1976). The methodology has been varied, and includes: (a) statistical approaches, both cross-sectional and longitudinal; (b) treatment outcome approaches; (c) theoretical approaches; and (d) biological approaches.

The questions addressed by these different approaches are the following. Is depression an illness? According to how this question is answered, a number of subsequent questions follow. First, if depression is an illness, is it a qualitative or quantitative variation from normal, i.e. what is the nature of the distinction between distress, unhappiness and depressive disorder? Second, is there more than one type of depressive order and, if so, are these in turn qualitatively or quantatively distinct from each other? And finally, what is the degree of overlap between the phenomenology of depressive disorders and other disorders such as anxiety states and schizophrenia.

Not all these questions are answered. Kendell (1975) suggests that a quantitative distinction requires a zone of rarity to be demonstrated in the phenomenology between one condition and another. As yet, there is doubt as to whether any zones of rarity have been adequately demonstrated between psychiatric disorders. Nevertheless, the phenomenology of depression has been classified in many different ways. As Kendell (1975) suggests, the reason for classification depends upon the purpose to which it can be put. Table 31.1 outlines some of the various ways in which depressive states can be distinguished. However, it is far from being an exhaustive list; there are many other subclassifications which are possible, especially those which take into account personality characteristics. One of the more recent new distinctions has been rapid versus slow onset depressive disorders (Copeland, 1985).

The general impression is that depression can be classified and subclassified in many different ways: by severity, cyclic form, relation to other disorders, symptom pattern, and so on. Because of this it is possible to use mixed nosologies, e.g. a patient may be described as suffering from an endogenous, retarded, unipolar depressive disorder. It is also the case that 'atypical' forms can occur, as in the

Table 31.1 Ways of classifying depression

Distinction	Schema
Neurotic–psychotic	This distinction is an old one but, in general, is a classification based on the severity of the symptomatology
Exogenous (reactive) Endogenous	Exogenous has sometimes been used to describe precipitated disorder (e.g. by life events), endogenous being unprecipitated; at other times the concept of reactivity has been used to denote disorders in which the patient 'reacts' to events even though depressed. Recent evidence has shown that an endogenous syndrome can be 'precipitated' and may be mild or severe
Unipolar–bipolar	This distinction is applied to the cyclic variation of mood; bipolar illness involves both swings into depression and (hypo)mania
Primary–secondary	Secondary depressions are usually those that exist in relation to other physical or psychiatric conditions. A 'primary' disorder is a disorder of a pure depressive form
Agitated–retarded	This distinction is based on differentiation of a number of psychobiological and psychomotor differences
Type A–Type B	This distinction is made on the basis of presumed neruotransmitter differences and drug responsiveness, i.e. Type A depressions respond to noradrenergic drugs (imipramine); Type Bs to serotonin drugs (e.g. amitriptyline)

recently investigated case of depression which appears to be triggered by seasonal variation (Rosenthal *et al.*, 1984). The very heterogeneity of depression has led to many debates between the dimensionalists and the categorialists.

Nevertheless, there appears to be growing consensus to the view that endogenous–melancholic types of depression can be separated, albeit somewhat loosely, from a multifarious clustering of symptoms which involve depressive shifts in relation to neurotic and personality or general life stress difficulties.

In order to obtain a flavour of the symptom variation of depression, Table 31.2 outlines possible distinctions in phenomenology between endogenous and non-endogenous depressions. This grouping is suggested by Davidson *et al.* (1984), who compared symptoms across five scales for measuring endogenous or melancholic depression. It should be emphasized that this is still a controversial distinction. The core symptoms listed in Table 31.2 may be embedded in a more multifarious disorder—non-specific clustering. Again, these symptoms are not exhaustive, and different combinations can be suggested (e.g. Nelson and Charney, 1980; Whybrow *et al.*, 1984, p. 136). In addition to distinctions based on symptomatology, factors such as duration, frequency and cyclicity of illness play an important part in full nosological descriptions.

A central assumption of many of these distinctions is that there are certain core symptoms that are prominent in melancholic or endogenous disorders but that

Table 31.2   Core symptoms of endogenous depression

Core symptoms
1. Pervasive loss of pleasure (anhedonia)
2. Non-reactivity
3. Distinct quality of mood (beyond feeling, tears etc.)
4. Guilt (can be of psychotic intensity)
5. Major psychomotor change (agitation or retardation)
6. Reduced vegetative activity

Non-specific clustering
1. Diurnal variation
2. Early morning awakening
3. Difficulty falling asleep
4. Suicidal thoughts
5. Loss (or gain) of weight
6. Anxiety (of various forms)
7. Difficulty concentrating
8. Hypochondriasis
9. Self-pity
10. Irritability

these may be embedded in a host of other symptoms that relate to general demoralization or stress responses (e.g. Klein, 1974). Although this introduces a certain neatness, caution should be exercised because recent evidence suggests that types of diagnosis are not stable over time. Individuals may present with one form of depressive phenomenology at one period but have a rather altered presentation if they become depressed some years later (Kendell, 1974; Akiskal *et al.*, 1978). This change in presentation over time causes some difficulties for those who support categorical distinctions.

Epidemiology

The epidemiology of depression rests centrally on the definition and classification of depression. Different classifications based on different phenomenologies give rise to different epidemiological statistics. However, in a major review of studies which have used systematic interview and agreed classificatory procedures, Boyd and Weissman (1981) provide the following epidemiological statistics.

> (1) The point prevalence of depressive symptoms ranges between 9% and 20%.
> (2) The lifetime risk of bipolar disorder is less than 1%. The annual incidence of bipolar disorder is 0.009% to 0.015% for men and 0.007% to 0.03% for women.
> (3) Using the new diagnostic techniques in industrialised nations, the point prevalence of nonbipolar depression is 3% for men and 4% to 9% for women. The life time risk of nonbipolar depression is 8% to 12% for men and 20% to 26% for women, and the annual incidence of nonbipolar depression is 8% for women (however, we have less confidence in the last figure since it is based on only one study). (p. 1044)

Overall then, the gender difference is often between 2 : 1 and 3 : 1, with women suffering the highest rates. Some have suggested that if alcoholism is included, this discrepancy disappears. However, be this as it may, around one-fifth of women and one-tenth of men are likely to suffer depression at some point in their lives. We may conclude, therefore, that depression is multifarious in its presentation and very common. Having sketched out some of these basic issues, attention is now turned to biological considerations, beginning with a brief look at neurobiology and endocrinology.

Neurobiology

The neurobiology of depression is highly complex, as one might expect. However, progress has been made on identifying neurotransmitters that appear to be significantly involved in depressive states, although not necessarily of primary causal significance. Early observations during the 1950s of drugs, such as reserpine, which deplete the CNS of the monoamines—noradrenaline (NA), dopamine (DA) and 5-hydroxytryptamine (5-HT)—showed them to produce depressed-like states in a percentage of individuals. Some suggest that the most vulnerable are those who have personal or family psychiatric histories (Mendels and Frazer, 1974). Iproniazid, used in the treatment of tuberculosis, was found to have mood-elevating properties and research showed that this drug increased the central availability of the monoamines. From these early observations was born the monoamine hypothesis of depression. Stated simply, this suggested that depression was related to a reduction in the central availability of monoamines, while mania was related to heightened activity at monoamine synapses. Research then set about measuring various indices of monoamine function in blood, CSF, urine, the brain of suicide victims and various animals who appeared in depressed states, in an effort to illuminate the pathophysiology of depression. Much has happened since this time (see Whybrow et al. (1984) and Willner (1985) for comprehensive reviews).

It is now believed that monoamine function is indeed intimately tied up with affective disorder, although exactly how remains unclear. Checkley (1978) examined affective change in endogenous depressives subjected to methylamphetamine challenge (methylamphetamine increases the central availability of monoamines). He drew a distinction between euphoric responses and antidepressive responses and suggested that his evidence cast doubt on the simple 'availability theory' of monoamines for depression. Silberman et al. (1981) showed that responses to dexamphetamine infusion in depressives were highly variable in both affective and attitudinal change. Some viewed an antidepressive effect positively, others more negatively.

Although the monoamines have undoubtedly received the bulk of research effort, other workers have suggested that neurotransmitters such as acetylcholine play a central role in a variety of depressive phenomena. Changes in acetylcholine activity and synaptic sensitivity are believed to be involved in sleep disturbance, changes in REM sleep architecture, concentration and psychobiological retardation (Sitaram et al., 1982; Gilbert, 1984; Willner, 1985).

Many researchers now believe that it is a change in the *patterns* of neurotransmitter activity which best accounts for depressive phenomenology. Some researchers suggest that depressive disorders may be distinguished into those with the primary dysfunction residing in the catecholamine systems (NA and DA), in contrast to those depressions with primary dysfunction of 5-HT or acetylcholine systems (Whybrow *et al.*, 1984). In general terms, it is believed that the catecholamines facilitate activated and go-like behaviour, whereas increases in 5-HT and acetylcholine facilitate inhibitory and/or withdrawn behaviour. Hence, some patients may suffer psychobiological deregulation in states of activation, and others may suffer deregulation in states of inhibition. The go–stop model of affective disorders is now gaining greater support (Gilbert, 1984; in press, a; Whybrow *et al.*, 1984). Interestingly, if the nervous system can be classified in terms of two competing systems, activating and inhibiting, then four combinations of deregulation are possible. Pathological states may represent either too little or too much activity in go systems or too much or too little activity in stop systems. Furthermore, various combinations can occur, e.g. having high activity in both go and stop systems simultaneously (like having a car on high revs but going nowhere because the brakes are on). This may be a model for anxious–depressive states, whereas low go and high stop may relate to retarded depressive states (Gilbert, 1984).

Work with antidepressant compounds has further complicated the neurobiological picture. It is now known that acute and chronic treatments with tricyclic compounds have different effects on pre- and post-synaptic monoamine receptors (McNeal and Cimbolic, 1986). Generally speaking, the remission of depression noted for these drugs may result from chronic rather than acute use. Such work has stimulated various theories about altered receptor sensitivity in depression, and recent research has focused on the role of receptors in mediating depressive phenomena.

Neuroendocrinology

The relationship of brain and endocrine responses has also stimulated considerable interest and controversy over the last twenty years. It is known that various hormonal processes have both positive and negative feedback effects on CNS control mechanisms. The brain thyroid axis has received increased attention in recent years and is believed to be disrupted in some depressive states (Whybrow *et al.*, 1984). The most investigated neuroendocrine system, however, has been the hypothalamic–pituitary–adrenal–cortical axis (HPAC) (Kalin and Dawson, 1986). Inputs from various brain areas stimulate the production of corticotropin-releasing hormone from the hypothalamus. This in turn stimulates the pituitary to release adrenocorticotropic hormone (ACTH) plus β-endorphine into the bloodstream. The ACTH circulates in the blood and stimulates the adrenal cortex to produce cortisol. Cortisol can then be measured in blood plasma and is secreted in circadian controlled pulses. It has been known for some time that depressives show heightened secretion of cortisol, sometimes as high as those with Cushing's disease. However, controversy has often revolved around whether this is a non-specific stress response or related to depression per se. Recently, Christie *et al.* (1986) suggested that major alterations in cortisol production are related to various severe symptoms of depression, including psychotic symptoms. Hence, cortisol abnormalities may be more an indicator of severity of psychiatric disturbances than depressive specific (see also Arana *et al.*, 1985). Dolan and colleagues (1985) have demonstrated a positive correlation between the HPAC system, as measured by cortisol, and life events.

In 1981, Caroll and his colleagues presented a procedure to test the specificity of cortisol dysfunction in endogenous depression with the introduction of the dexamethasone suppression test. Briefly stated, 1 mg of dexamethasone suppresses HPAC activity, such that in normals cortisol is suppressed for up to 24 hours. In certain forms of depression, however, individuals demonstrate what is called early escape. That is, these depressed patients demonstrate a capacity to override dexamethasone inhibition and show heightened blood cortisol levels during the subsequent 24 hours. Hyperactivity of the HPAC system is believed responsible for this early escape. The specificity and sensitivity of this test now look rather less impressive than was at first thought, however (Arana *et al.*, 1985). Nevertheless, the dexamethasone suppression test remains an extremely useful research tool for psychiatric research.

There is also growing awareness that many psychobiological patterns show clear cyclic alteration (Weiner, 1982; Whybrow *et al.*, 1984; Eastwood *et al.*, 1985). The manner in which these cyclic alterations in underlying psychobiological patterns of activity interact with psychiatric disorder are still under investigation.

As mentioned earlier, there is growing interest in what is called seasonal affective disorder; that is, certain individuals appear more likely to swing into depression or mania at certain points in the year (Rosenthal *et al.*, 1984). Such individuals may have a hypersensitivity to alterations in light–dark cycles, mediated through the pineal hormone, melatonin. Physiological cycles, as in the menstrual cycle, are also believed to interact with underlying depressive vulnerability (Rubinow *et al.*, 1986). This evidence suggests that there are powerful internal mechanisms controlling various oscillating processes in psychobiological patterns (Weiner, 1982). These mechanisms have profound effects on many psychological variables (Hofer, 1984).

Related to these considerations are the complex interactions that occur between hormone and neurotransmitter systems (Kalin and Dawson, 1986). Leshner (1979), for example, has suggested that in addition to developmental effects of hormones on behaviour, there are two further ways hormones might affect behaviour. The first, and more well known, are feedback effects which relate to changes in behaviour during or after exposure to excitatory stimuli. The second relates to baseline hormonal state which exerts its impact before such exposure. Baseline hormonal state acts to prepare or give preference to certain responses in the presence of a stressor. In other words, in so far as individuals differ in their baseline hormonal state before a stressor is encountered, variations in responsiveness and probably initial appraisals may occur. To make a speculative point, it may be that various social factors (e.g. the availability of a confiding relationship) exert some effect on baseline biological states. Baseline states may act to facilitate certain cognitive appraisal systems over others, and facilitate various affects, both preceding and subsequent to life stressors. It has been suggested, for example, that low status animals are more sensitive and respond more significantly to separation (Rasmussen and Reite, 1982). This may relate to baseline hormonal state associated with the occupation of low social rank. Hence, not only may internal oscillating systems act to shift baseline biological states, but current social interactions may also influence baseline states. This points to complex interactions which combine (e.g. internal shifting of baseline states and social mediation of baseline states) and prepare the individual for certain classes of response to stressful stimuli. The idea that animals respond to stimuli from some neutral, homoeostatic state is therefore doubtful. Moreover, after a stress an animal may come to rest (biologically) in a different, though possibly stable, state. For example, a defeated animal will not settle back into the same biological state as existed while he occupied top rank. Such data may help us more clearly understand the timing of disorder onset and why an individual can cope with a stressor at one time in life but not at another.

More speculatively, some individuals may suffer hypersensitivity to their own biological reactions to stress. This suggestion requires more research than it has at present received. It is possible that the physiological changes that occur in stress in some individuals act to amplify and maintain certain psychological processes which feed back in a state-dependent way to amplify the depressive state. The fact that Cushing's patients show depressive-like and psychotic symptoms secondary to cortisol dysfunction suggests that, perhaps, some depressive symptoms are also the consequence of increased cortisol secretion. Some patients may have autohormonal sensitivities or dysfunctions to their own stress hormones. This speculation awaits further research, although it is not a new idea (Whybrow, 1984).

The notion that particular kinds of stress may activate certain biological patterns which then feed back to amplify or recruit certain psychological-evaluation processes is important. In brain state theory (Gilbert, 1984; in press, a, b), it is suggested that rather than thinking of cognitive structures as kinds of entities within the CNS, we might be better served in viewing learning, encoding, retrieval and storage in state-dependent ways (Reus et al., 1979). In this view, latent schemata represent state-dependent patterns of psychobiological activity (see Iran-Nejad and Ortony (1984) for a biofunctional view of cognitive processes). Once a particular psychobiological pattern is switched on, the next sequence of events will be determined by genetic and learning history. Activation of the physiological responses to threat of interpersonal loss, for example, may, in state-dependent ways, bring back memories and styles of encoding events from an earlier age which further accentuate the perception and experience of loss. This in turn accentuates psychobiological processes (e.g. cortisol response).

Having illuminated some of the neurobiological and endocrine changes in depression, let us now switch attention to the psychological level.

ENVIRONMENT–ANIMAL INTERACTIONS AND PSYCHOBIOLOGICAL PROCESSES

Learned Helplessness

The theory of learned helplessness arose from a typical research procedure in psychobiological research. This involves doing something to the animal, keeping other factors constant as far as possible, and then measuring the effects in a multitude of domains (cognitive, behavioural, physiological). The method of inducing helplessness is now well known and is only stated briefly here. Helplessness can be induced in animals by subjecting them to trauma that they cannot control. Exposure to uncontrollable trauma has been shown to invoke serious disruptions in active avoidance learning, changes in the propensity for aggressiveness, behavioural withdrawal and passivity, vegetative changes and major changes in monoamine functioning (Seligman, 1975). One of the problems with the learned helplessness model of depression is that it is rather unclear which kind of depression it most closely mimics. Depue and Monroe (1978), for example, suggest that the syndrome that results from chronic helplessness is more akin to endogenous depressive phenomenology. This need not be too much of a problem, since Akiskal et al. (1978) have shown that endogenous depression can be precipitated.

The biological changes that are involved in helplessness are complex, but what is clear is that how an animal experiences trauma (i.e. whether it perceives it has control or not) has major consequences for many biological changes. Anisman (1978) has provided an excellent summary of these neurochemical changes associated with control or non-control over stress. Briefly, it is suggested that moderate levels of stress, where control is possible, do not affect the levels of NA and 5-HT, although there is an increase in the turnover (synthesis and release) of these neurotransmitters. If stress continues with no coping option being available, then deficits in the transmission of NA occur. This may be due to the fact that synthesis can no longer keep up with utilization and release. Also, various stress hormones such as cortisol increase. There are also alterations in monoamine oxidase activity and, if the stress is prolonged, acetylcholine activity increases.

Taken together, these biological alterations seem to switch the animal first into a go, or activated, state designed to search for and facilitate escape and coping responses, and next, if this search proves fruitless, into a more inhibitory or stop state. In 1984, I suggested that activated states are associated with hyperactivity in catecholamine systems whereas stop states, or psychobiologically retarded states, are associated with hyperactivity in acetylcholine systems and hypoactivity in catecholamine systems. Go and stop systems can be operated relatively independently and both can be turned on at the same time. This suggests that mixtures of inhibitory and activated psychobiological patterns may occur in the same individual (see also Whybrow et al., 1984).

As a model of depression, learned helplessness has received considerable attention. However, it suffers from a number of weaknesses. First, it is unclear exactly what phenomenology it is supposed to mimic. Second, it treats all traumata as relatively equivalent. Hence, it cannot predict the social behaviour of an animal under stress. This is because threat to social incentives is more likely to activate different behavioural patterns than threat to non-social incentives. Hence, to anticipate our argument for a moment, if stress involves social events and contexts, then efforts at coping will generally be social. For example, loss of control over a loved object will ignite a pattern of searching directed at the lost object. However, it is open to debate under what conditions other forms of uncontrollable event would invoke such other-seeking behaviour. Young children may seek out loved others to help cope with many or all forms of stress. But adults may not. Loss of control of status-related incentives may invoke status searching and activate behaviours designed to overcome the threats to status. These may be aggressive, competitive and classical Type A behaviours (Price, 1982). It remains a question for research whether loss of control over status-related incentives activates the same other-seeking and nurturant-eliciting responses that loss of control over a loved object would. I suggest elsewhere (Gilbert, in press, a, b) that the learned helplessness model seems to be tapping into general go–stop systems which may be involved in many forms of psychopathology, not just depression. It does not predict what kinds of events for which kinds of people are likely to be most stressful. To anticipate for a moment, loss of a significant relationship may be more biologically disruptive in a social-dependent personality (Beck, 1983). Loss of status or control over prestige opportunities may be more biologically disruptive for an autonomous personality and lead to completely different behavioural, affective and cognitive patterns. Hence, the kinds of incentives and goals that an individual pursues will have a very direct bearing on the kinds of physiological changes and ways of handling stress that loss of control invokes. Before we proceed to articulate these ideas we must review current psychological thinking, as these distinctions will be shown to be important. Although loss of control remains a central dimension of depression, different syndromes may relate to the different types of incentive over which a loss of control is experienced.

Psychological Approaches to Depression

The psychological theories of depressive disorders are many and varied. Some are easily linked with neurobiological aspects, others less so. Operant theorists emphasize the low emission of positive reinforceable behaviour (Ferster, 1973; Lewinsohn et al., 1979). Classical conditioning theorist, Wolpe (1979), on the other hand, distinguishes neurotic from psychotic depression and subclassifies neurotic depression into four types based on conditioned anxiety. Klinger's (1975; 1977) incentive disengagement theory shares many elements with learned helplessness and suggests that depression occurs when an individual loses or is forced to disengage from valued incentives.

Other psychological theorists have focused more specifically on the types of incentive that are lost, and suggest that individuals differ in their vulnerability in relation to the dominant incentives they are pursuing in life. The existential psychotherapist Yalom (1980) draws a distinction btween those whose dominant goals in life centre on the securing of important relationships. This type is labelled the 'pursuit of the ultimate rescuer'. A second type pursue goals and incentives designed to bring a sense of specialness through achievement and distinction from others. This is called the 'pursuit of specialness'. In a very similar vein, the ego analysts Arieti and Bemporad (1980) suggest a distinction of depressive types in terms of those who seek dominant others and those who seek dominant goals. The former are linked to a passive, anger-avoidant, and clingy interpersonal style, while the latter tend to be more arrogant, aggressive, aloof and compulsive. Beck (1983) has proposed similar distinctions in the cognitive organization of depressive-prone people. These he labels sociotropic (socially dependent) and autonomous types. The cognitive organization of the former is attuned to maintaining help and interpersonal supplies, while that of the latter is attuned to autonomy and avoidance of constraint. He also suggests differences in symptom patterns and coping styles when these people become depressed. Bowlby (1980) also notes distinctions in the organization of affectional relationships which predispose to depression. This develops out of disturbances in the early attachment relationship of child and parent and leads to the affectional and attachment styles of 'other reliant' versus 'compulsive self-reliant'. Blatt et al. (1982) approach this issue from analytic theory. They suggest distinctions between anaclitic and self-critical depressions. The former is developmentally an earlier vulnerability related to the oral stage of personality. This distinction has clear overlaps with those above. Gilbert (1984) suggested that the central distinction relates to the mechanisms of what is controlled. Care-eliciting types attempt to control the behaviour of others to ensure supplies, whereas others attempt to control interpersonal transactions by distinguishing self from others and being of value to others, indispensable, and so on.

All of these formulations share considerable degrees of overlap, even though the underlying theoretical paradigms from which they have grown are very different. Furthermore, this consensus is potentially very useful to a psychobiological approach. Following the work of Seligman (1975) on loss of control, much research has shown this dimension to be of major importance in depressive states. From the psychological theories outlined briefly above, we can also posit that what incentives are sought out may also be of major significance in determining depressive type, and the pursued coping responses. For example, 'autonomous' or 'special' types may be most unwilling even fearful of eliciting care from others in case this detracts from their autonomy or threatens loss of status. Let us therefore consider the idea that the dominant incentive structure of an individual (e.g. sociotropic or autonomous) tends to operate through biological modes of functioning which have been encoded with the CNS during evolution. The suggestion here is that the sociotropic type tends to operate in the interpersonal mode related to attachment formation and linking up with others. The autonomous type, on the other hand, operates through the interpersonal mode related to 'distinguishing' self from others, i.e. spacing. This mode probably relates to a dominance–power form of interpersonal behaviour.

We know that loss of control is importantly related to depression, but here we add the dimension of social content. Moreover, although we often write about self-esteem as a unitary concept, people may have low self-esteem only when they lose control over their dominant incentives. In other words, when an individual believes he can no longer control or exert influence in his dominant interpersonal mode he may appraise himself negatively, both in terms of his own desires, standards and aspirations and in relation to how he compares himself with his fellows. Yet this negativity may be incentive specific, as in the case of the man who believes his wife loves him, but downrates himself because he cannot maintain performance standards; or the man who can still function competitively but evaluates himself as unloved. Elsewhere Gilbert (in press, b) has suggested that if the go–stop mechanism becomes disrupted because of loss of control over dominant incentives, then, since other interpersonal modes tend to be energized by this general system, the 'depression' may spread across the whole interpersonal behavioural repertoire.

From the above we can argue that loss of control and self-esteem needs to be broken down into subgoals and incentives. In 1984, I suggested three main areas in which loss of control results in different abandonment perceptives. Individuals may experience abandonment: (a) through perceived physical illness or deteroriation—the wander off to die theme; (b) through loss, separation or death of another—the loss of a significant other theme or major source of social reinforcement; and (c) due to loss of status with the consequent loss of influence over inpersonal events—the loss of status theme (e.g. unemployment). These themes are not mutually exclusive.

What is suggested here, then, is that there are two psychobiological aspects that need to be considered: (1) the dimension of control which relates to a general stress system involving changes in the go–stop systems; and (2) running parallel to this, more specific changes in interpersonal mode of functioning (e.g. attachment versus autonomy/status). Symptoms will therefore relate both to general stress and to the specific dominant incentive structure that is threatened or over-whelmed. To add to this skeleton, let us return to an examination of neurobiology in the domains of loss of attachment object and loss of status. The psychobiology of attachment and defeat may map onto the sociotropic versus autonomous styles mentioned earlier.

Isolation

When young infants are separated from their primary care-givers, characteristic changes in the psychobiological patterns of activity tend to occur. The first response to separation is often labelled 'protest', and involves agitated behaviour, increased distress vocalizations and marked changes in many physiological processes (Reite et al., 1981). If reunion with the loved object or care-giver substitute is not possible, a new state emerges in which distress vocalizations decrease, agitated behaviour is replaced with retarded behaviour, and a different pattern of vegetative activity occurs. Much of the work on the psychobiology of attachment and the behavioural effects of the disruption of attachment have been excellently outlined in a series of papers edited by Reite and Field (1985). What is interesting in the protest–despair sequence is that many of the biological changes parallel or overlap those observed in learned helplessness. However, the behaviours associated with protest are potentially quite different to the behaviours associated with escape from non-social trauma like shock or cold water swims, which may differ again from threats to status.

McKinney (1985) has outlined many of the neurochemical changes that are associated with the protest–despair cycle. Again, it appears that major changes in catecholamine functioning occur. Importantly, unlike status defeat, 5-HT is less reactive to this type of social stress (although it may play an important role in social affiliative behaviour). During protest states there is increased activity in catecholamine systems, but during despair this activity falls considerably. Moreover, there is a significant interaction between the biological changes that take place and the infant's history, social housing conditions and the presence of available or alternative caring others. Hence, the social separation model suggests that disruption in important social bonds appears to activate neurochemical processes. Moreover, these appear to be similar to those associated with depressive phenomenology.

The research on the endocrinology of social separation is also very relevant to our psychobiological exploration. Coe *et al.* (1985) have studied the endocrine responses to separation. They studied the effects of isolation in two conditions. In the first, monkeys lived in groups of four infant–mother dyads. In the second condition, infant–mother dyads were housed alone. The cortisol response to separation is very significant but does not correlate with distress vocalizations (i.e. cortisol is higher in despair although distress vocalization has decreased). If the mother is removed from the cage but significant others remain, the cortisol response is still noted but significantly attenuated. On the other hand, removal of the mother when the infant is left alone significantly accentuates the cortisol response. Moreover unfamiliarity with the environment, e.g. a novel cage, also has a significant effect on the cortisol response. Coe *et al.* suggest that it is the presence of familiar others which tends to inhibit the higher cortisol responses noted in separation for isolates. If separated infants are placed with unfamiliar others, then, in fact, the cortisol response is actually aggravated rather than diminished. What this psychobiological research shows is that separation is biologically very disruptive. However, the social environment plays a significant role in the degree of activation of the HPAC system. Such work would have very clear implications for stress research, especially on homesickness (see Chapter 3 in this volume). This may be taken to suggest that stress occurring in the context of a supportive and caring environment will have a very different biological outcome to stress occurring in a non-supportive or unfamiliar environment. The one caveat to this is that in humans it may be appraisal of support, not actual support, that makes the difference. Nevertheless, work on life events showing the importance of a close confiding relationship (Brown and Harris, 1978) would seem to be supported by psychobiological research.

Social Defeat

In social-living mammals, who share access to various resources, a means must be found of organizing competitive endeavour. Generally speaking, this occurs in relation to the development of a dominance hierarchy. Individuals who obtain and maintain dominance show characteristic behaviours which include upright posture, non-gaze avoidance and a preparedness to challenge and approach various survival-relevant resources (territory, food, mates). High and low status animals can also be distinguished in terms of a number of neurochemical and neuroendocrine differences (Henry and Stephens, 1977). Raleigh *et al.* (1984) have shown that blood levels of 5-HT are highly responsive to the status position of monkeys. In one case, a dominant male had blood levels of 5-HT twice as high as those of other males. Various differences in catecholamine mechanisms are also noted according to status position (Weiss *et al.*, 1982). Cortisol responses are generally regarded as being lower in high status as compared with low status animals. There are also differences in the activity of the sympathetic nervous system (Henry and Stephens, 1977).

Low status animals, on the other hand, are characterized by increases in avoidance behaviour, gaze aversion, low body posture, appeasement grin and reduced initiation behaviours, especially approach behaviours, to survival-relevant resources. Low status animals may be particularly sensitive to separation stress (Rasmussen and Reite, 1982). The biology of low status remains unclear, but it appears that blood levels of 5-HT are lower in low status as compared with high status animals. There are, as mentioned previously, differences in monoamine function, and cortisol levels are considerably higher in low status animals. Of interest in these and other studies is that the loss of status invokes a sequence of psychobiological changes, many of which have also been implicated in depressive phenomenology. In humans, loss of status is mirrored in a specific domain of inferiority related to dominance–submissive appraisal. Gardner (1982; in press) has suggested a model of bipolar illness based on dysfunction in mechanisms co-ordinating dominance behaviour.

Price, in 1972, was amongst the first to suggest that loss of status invoked a depressive-like psychobiological pattern which inhibited the animal from making further attacks. This idea has recently been extensively developed into important theoretical concepts (see Price and Sloman, 1987; Price, in press). Loss of status tends to invoke reduced behavioural reactivity, reductions in challenge behaviour and various approach behaviours and an increase in general submissive and avoidant behaviour. Raleigh *et al.* (1984) have shown that removal of dominant males from their group had the effect of markedly changing blood levels of 5-HT. They suggest that in the monkeys they studied, blood levels of 5-HT were a state-dependent consequence of the active occupation of a dominant position. Hence, they demonstrated a considerable variation in 5-HT associated with changes in status. However, as noted earlier, 5-HT appears far more reactive to status loss than to separation—although this does not mean 5-HT is not also involved in separation responses (McKinney, 1985). One may speculatively consider whether 5-HT mechanisms are similarly responsive to 'appraised' changes in status. It would probably be too neat a speculation to suggest that differences in attachment versus status-linked depression map into the Type A and Type B depressions noted earlier (Maas, 1975), but it warrants further research.

In terms of neuroendocrinology, it is known that various changes in the sympathetic and parasympathetic nervous systems occur, as do changes in the HPAC system, as a result of status defeat. Generally speaking, there is a large increase in HPAC activation and cortisol following status defeat (Henry and Stephens, 1977; Leshner, 1978). Interestingly, it has not yet been reported whether defeated animals engage in distress call. There may be some evidence that defeated animals do indeed attempt to make some kind of adaptive response to the dominant other, e.g. in seeking to groom, touch, cuddle, comfort and so on.

As yet we do not fully understand the relationship between these types of behaviour. However, unlike 5-HT, cortisol appears equally sensitive to both separation and defeat, suggesting that both operate through a general stress mechanism related to the HPAC axis. However, the HPAC system is controlled by many different neurotransmitters. This almost certainly means that it is a final pathway of a stress system. It should also be considered that 5-HT activity has been suggested as a biological marker of suicide and auto-aggression in a way that the catecholamines have not, although evidence remains inconclusive (van Praag, 1986). This may mean that it is the socially competitive (dominance–power) modes of interpersonal functioning which bear most centrally on the kinds of depression which involve suicide and high (auto) aggressive components.

In humans, the disruption that may occur in psychobiological state in relation to competitive defeat is well described by Gary Kasparov, a world chess champion who says:

> Chess is life in miniature. Chess is struggle, chess is battle. If you have a theory to prove, if you think you have a better position, if you think you are strong, please use chess. It is much better than really fighting!
> Usually, I win. If I win a tournament or match, or the world championship there is great celebration. But I do not lose myself in happiness because maybe someone else will go in front of me very soon . . . If I lose, it is very bad. I can't eat, can't sleep and I must understand why this has happened. It is very important to look closely at the game to understand, but I never blame my coaches or anyone else because I know it is my fault. Maybe I say to myself some bad words. (Kasparov, 1986, p.50.)

HUMAN APPRAISAL AND SYMBOLIC CODES

Kasparov's description aptly demonstrates the human capacity to turn many social situations into symbolic codes of status contest. Moreover, once the game of chess (in this example) has the symbolic relationship to status, then we see that defeat does indeed invoke a number of vegetative and physiological symptoms. Gary Kasparov says a lot about the psychological and biological interaction in status defeat mechanisms.

The capacity for humans to create internal models of the world and their relation to it, and then respond to these models as if they were real, is a cornerstone for an approach to psychotherapy called cognitive therapy (Beck *et al.*, 1979). I think that Whybrow *et al.* (1984) put the point very well.

> . . . this ability to conceive, abstract and plan in the psychological sphere adds a complication. We are quite capable of dreaming up dangerous situations that do not really exist within existing patterns of social interaction. We can fall short of unrealistically conceived goals and therefore judge our true ability unreasonably harshly. We can believe ourselves to be unworthy and unloved when there is little objective evidence to support the notion. Our physiological response to these symbolic situations is no different from that which would occur if there had been a real bodily assault, a demanding physical fight for dominance with another member of the herd or the true loss of an essential nurturing parent. (p. 114.)

Such a viewpoint is central to a truly psychobiological perspective. Just as we can create sexual fantasies in our heads and then experience a precise pattern of physiological arousal, there is no reason to assume that images of ourselves as defeated, unloved, abandoned or rejected cannot also invoke powerful physiological effects. Once patterns of physiological activity are turned on, it may be very difficult to turn them off again. Once we have fantasized ourselves into states of sexual excitement, we may be affected by intrusive thoughts or sensations even after we have decided not to take our images any further. A more radical example comes from studies of grief. Even though a person may know a spouse has died, he may still be impelled to search for the lost spouse (Parkes, 1986). This is an example of biological changes which, invoked by loss, activate searching behaviour and images which are very difficult to override with rational thought. Indeed, as discussed elsewhere (Gilbert, in press, a, b), the manner in which various 'searches' are made and the purpose of a search depend jointly on the type of incentive lost or threatened and the degree of psychobiological activity.

TOWARD A PSYCHOBIOLOGICAL MODEL

At the beginning of this chapter we examined some of the current classification issues of depression. We then proceeded to look briefly at the neurobiology and endocrine changes believed to be associated with depression. From there we noted how loss of control (helplessness) appeared to invoke changes in physical state not dissimilar to those investigated in depression. We made the criticism of learned helplessness that it was too general a model in that most experimentation did not involve social events and it did not distinguish between types of event. Yet different types of event (interpersonal loss, defeat) will call forth different coping strategies and different search routines and probably involve subtly different neurochemical changes. From these we looked at some psychological classifications which did appear to separate interpersonal–abandonment themes from defeat and loss of autonomy themes. Building on this, we explored the psychobiology of these dimensions of stress as they have been experimentally investigated.

What can we now do to pull these threads together? First, loss of control over any valued incentive invokes a plethora of stress responses. As the individual gives up, the CNS appears to engage in a de-investment programme which inhibits further effective action (e.g. catecholamine levels fall). There is a switch away from go to stop modes of action. Cognitively, the individual focuses on what not to do, on inhibiting effort which usually manifests as 'there is no point in trying', i.e. now is not the time to invest in incentive pursuit. Yet there is more to the story than this. In addition to the general changes in stress profiles, we see other effects of the different modes and systems which have become de-energized. Now attention swings to the dominant mode or incentive structure which has become disrupted and non-functioning. When the dominant incentive structure centered on interpersonal attachment concerns, the changes invoked by loss of control affect those systems in the brain primarily involved with attachment behaviour. As the individual swings into depression, we will note characteristic changes of a protest–despair cycle. As this proceeds, a kind of bottom-up form of information processing occurs such that cognitive processes are at first tuned in to searching for the lost other with the affective state maintaining the search (pining). In the absence of successful restoration of the lost object or substitutes or a switch to an alternative incentive structure, despair ensues which immobilizes the individual for a period of time. On the other hand, when the dominant incentive structure has been autonomy or dominance, the cycle into depression is different. First, it is the brain systems controlling dominance behaviour that are primarily affected, rather than attachment systems (at least in the first instance). Second, during the downswing into depression the individual may attempt to increase his dominance behaviour, becoming more competitive, aggressive, isolationist and secretive. Cognitive schemata are tuned to the possibility of defeat and social evaluative concerns. Such individuals are unlikely to express needs for care if this is in direct opposition to the incentive of specialness and autonomy. As these efforts fail, the individual suffers a de-energizing of the dominant (dominance) mode and loses his 'will to fight'. Beck (1983) has articulated the patterns of symptoms that may relate to the sociotropic versus autonomous types when depressed.

The suggestion is, therefore, that depression involves psychobiological changes in two key dimensions: first in general stress systems and second in the dominant modes of functioning that the individual has been pursuing. It is changes in the second of these dimensions that will reflect the coping style during the pre-depressive phase. We might also add that this way of discussing psychobiology might allow us to link borderline and dependent personality disorders with disturbances in attachment modes of functioning, whereas narcissistic and compulsive personality disorders reflect more of a disorganization in dominance (status) systems. Hence shame is important in understanding narcissistic disorders, because shame is primarily related to dominance–submissive difficulties (Gilbert, in press, b).

As in all cases of model building, we split things up in order to study them more fully, but we must not forget to put them back together. In discussing these different modes of functioning we should not lose sight of the fact that the brain is a system. It is therefore unrealistic to take too literally the idea of separate modes, and these distinctions should be regarded dimensionally rather than categorically (Price and Sloman, 1984). It is for this reason that I prefer the term brain state because this more naturalistically captures the 'whole system' idea—that of shifting patterns. For example, in a kaleidoscope of (say) three colours, one colour may be more dominant and more central to the pattern than another, but this does not mean the other colours are absent. Rather, they change in relationship to the dominant colour.

Psychobiology is still comparatively new and plagued by (dominance) professional disputes between organic versus psychological models. I believe this dichotomy is no more than an accident of history and the way professional boundaries have been artificially drawn up. Hopefully, in the future we may become more able to work co-operatively, recognizing our theories are stronger when we act and think together rather than alone behind our professional divisions.

SUMMARY AND CONCLUSIONS

This chapter began with a brief review of the heterogeneity and epidemiology of depression. Depression is a common experience for up to 20% of the population over their life span. Some of the interactions between psychological and biological factors were examined, with recourse to three models: (1) learned helplessness, (2) separation, and (3) social defeat. The learned helpless model provides a general model by which loss of control over major incentives can be seen to provoke psychological changes believed to be associated with depression. A more detailed examination of the psychology of depression reveals two main routes into depression. The first relates to loss of control over dominant and supportive others. In these cases the psychobiological routines to loss relate to attentional and cognitive–behavioural searching and seeking for the lost other. These routines represent the coping efforts during entry into depression. The psychobiological model fitting this group is the separation model. The second route into depression relates to social defeat. The loss of control over status (incentives) leads to psychobiological routines for regaining status, with attentional and cognitive–behavioural searching and seeking being focused on these endeavours. When these coping efforts fail, depression ensues. The relationships between these routes into depression are given in more detail elsewhere (Gilbert, in press, b).

In humans, the capacity for symbolic thought and internal models of self–other relationships allow us to respond psychobiologically to these internal representations as if they were real (although depression is often associated with life events—loss of control). Depression represents the activation of psychobiological response patterns that have been wired into the human brain through evolution, the origin of which may be as far back as reptilian life forms. Our greatest challenge is to work together to understand more clearly the way psychological processes (internal models) work on and through innate biological mechanisms and the relevant feedback processes.

REFERENCES

Akiskal, H.S., & McKinney, W.T. (1975). Overview of recent research in depression: Integration of ten conceptual models into a comprehensive frame. *Archives of General Psychiatry*, *32*, 285–305.

Akiskal, H.S., Bitar, A.H., Puzantian, V.R. *et al.* (1978). The nosological status of neurotic depression: A prospective three to four year follow up examination in the light of the primary–secondary and unipolar–bipolar dichotomies. *Archives of General Psychiatry*, *35*, 756–766.

Anisman, H. (1978). Neurochemical changes elicited by stress. In H. Anisman & G. Bignami (eds), *Behavioural correlates in psychopharmacology of aversively motivated behaviour*. New York: Plenum Press.

Arana, G.W., Baldessarini, R.J., & Ornsteen, M. (1985). The dexamethasone suppression test for diagnosis and prognosis in psychiatry. *Archives of General Psychiatry*, *42*, 1193–1204.

Arieti, S., & Bemporad, J. (1980). The psychological organisation of depression. *American Journal of Psychiatry*, *137*, 1360–1365.

Beck, A.T. (1983). Cognitive therapy of depression: New perspectives. In P.J. Clayton & J.E. Barrett (eds), *Treatment of depression: Old controversies and new approaches*. New York: Raven Press.

Beck, A.T., Rush, J.A. Shaw, B.F., & Emery, G. (1979). *Cognitive therapy of depression*. New York: Wiley.

Blatt, S.J., Quinlan, D.M., Chevron E.S., McDonald, C., & Zuroff, D. (1982). Dependency and self criticism: Psychological dimensions of depression. *Journal of Consulting and Clinical Psychology, 50*, 113–124.

Bowlby, J. (1980). *Loss: Sadness and depression*. Vol.3: *Attachment and loss*. London: Hogarth Press.

Boyd, J.H., & Weissman, M.M. (1981). Epidemiology of affective disorder. *Archives of General Psychiatry, 38*, 1039–1046.

Brown, G.W., & Harris, T. (1978). *Social origins of depression*. London: Tavistock.

Carroll, B.J., Feinberg, M., Greden, J.F. *et al.* (1981). A specific laboratory test for the diagnosis of melancholia. *Archives of General Psychiatry, 38*, 15–22.

Checkley, S.A. (1978). A new distinction between the euphoric and anti-depressant effects of methylamphetamine. *British Journal of Psychiatry, 133*, 416–423.

Christie, J.E., Whalley, L.J., Dick, H., Blackwood, D.H.R., Blackburn, I.M., & Fink, G. (1986). Raised plasma cortisol concentrations are a feature of drug-free psychotics and are not specific to depression. *British Journal of Psychiatry, 148*, 58–67.

Coe, C.L., Weiner, S.G., Rosenberg, L.T., & Levine, S., (1985). Endocrine and immune responses to separation and maternal loss in nonhuman primates. In M. Reite & T. Field (eds), *The psychobiology of attachment and separation*. New York: Academic Press.

Copeland, J.R.M. (1985). Depressive illness and morbid distress. *British Journal of Psychiatry, 146*, 297–307.

Davidson, J., Turnbull, C., Strickland, R., & Belyea, M. (1984). Comparative diagnostic criteria for melancholia and endogenous depression. *Archives of General Psychiatry, 41*, 506–511.

Depue, R.A., & Monroe, S.M. (1978). Learned helplessness in the perspective of the depressive disorders: Conceptual and definitial issues. *Journal of Abnormal Psychology, 87*, 3–20.

Dolan, R.J., Calloway, S.P., Fonagy, P., DeSouza, F.V., & Wakling, A. (1985). Life events, depression and hypothalamic–pituitary–adrenal axis function. *British Journal of Psychiatry, 147*, 429–433.

Eastwood, M.R., Whitton, J.L., Kramer, P.A., & Peter, A.M. (1985). Infradian rhythms: A comparison of affective disorders and normal persons. *Archives of General Psychiatry, 42*, 295–299.

Ferster, C.B. (1973). A functional analysis of depression. *American Psychologist, 29*, 857–870.

Gardner, R. (1982). Mechanisms in manic-depressive disorder: An evolutionary model. *Archives of General Psychiatry, 39*, 1436–1441.

Gardner, R. (in press). Psychiatric syndromes of infrastructures for intraspecific communication. In M.R.A. Chance (ed.), *Social fabrics of the mind*. London: Lawrence Erlbaum.

Gilbert, P. (1984). *Depression: From psychology to brain state*. London: Lawrence Erlbaum.

Gilbert, P. (in press, a). Emotional disorders, brain state and psychosocial evolution. In W. Dryden & P. Trower (eds), *Recent developments in cognitive psychotherapy*. London: Lawrence Erlbaum.

Gilbert, P. (in press, b). *Human nature and suffering*. London: Lawrence Erlbaum.

Henry, J.P., & Stephens, P.M. (1977). *Stress, health and the social environment*. New York: Springer-Verlag.

Hofer, M.A. (1984). Relationships as regulators: A psychobiologic perspective on bereavement. *Psychosomatic Medicine, 46*, 183–197.

Iran-Nejad, A., & Ortony, A. (1984). A biofunctional model of distributed mental content, mental structures, awareness and attention. *Journal of Mind and Behavior, 5*, 171–210.

Kalin, N.H., & Dawson, G. (1986). Neuroendocrine dysfunction in depression: Hypothalamic–anterior pituitary systems. *Trends in Neurosciences*, June, 261–266.

Kasparov, G. (1986). A life in the day of Gary Kasparov. *Sunday Times Colour Magazine*, August 10th, 50.

Kendell, R.E. (1974). The stability of psychiatric diagnosis. *British Journal of Psychiatry*, *124*, 352–356.

Kendell, R.E. (1975). *The role of diagnosis in psychiatry*. London: Blackwell Scientific.

Kendell, R.E. (1976). The classification of depression: A review of contemporary confusion. *British Journal of Psychiatry*, *129*, 15–28.

Klein, D.F. (1974). Endogenomorphic depression: A conceptual and terminological revision. *Archives of General Psychiatry*, *31*, 447–454.

Klinger, E. (1975). Consequences and commitment to aid disengagement from incentives. *Psychological Review*, *82*, 1–24.

Klinger, E. (1977). *Meaning and void*. Minneapolis: University of Minnesota Press.

Leshner, A.I. (1978). *An introduction to behavioural endocrinology*. New York: Oxford University Press.

Leshner, A.I. (1979). Kinds of hormonal effects on behaviour: A new view. *Neuroscience and Biobehavioural Reviews*, *3*, 69–73.

Lewinsohn, P.M., Youngren, M.A., & Grosscup, S.J. (1979). Reinforcement and depression. In R.A. Depue (ed.), *The psychobiology of depressive disorders: Implications for the effects of stress*. New York: Academic Press.

Maas, J.W. (1975). Biogenic amines and depression: Biochemical and pharmacological separation of two types of depression. *Archives of General Psychiatry*, *32*, 1357–1361.

MacLean, P. (1985). Brain evolution relating to family, play and the separation call. *Archives of General Psychiatry*, *42*, 405–417.

McKinney, W.T. (1985). Separation and depression: Biological markers. In M. Reite & T. Field (eds), *The psychobiology of attachment and separation*. New York: Academic Press.

McNeal, E.T., & Cimbolic, P. (1986). Antidepressants and biochemical theories of depression. *Psychological Bulletin*, *99*, 361–374.

Mendels, J., & Frazer, A. (1974). Brain biogenic amine depletion and mood. *Archives of General Psychiatry*, *30*, 447–451.

Nelson, J.C. & Charney, D.S. (1980). Primary affective disorder criteria and the endogenous reactive distinction. *Archives of General Psychiatry*, *37*, 787–793.

Parkes, C.M. (1986). *Bereavement: Studies in grief in adult life*, 2nd edn. Harmondsworth: Penguin.

Price, J.S. (1972). Genetic and phylogenetic aspects of mood variation. *International Journal of Mental Health*, *1*, 124–144.

Price, J.S. (in press). Alternative channels for negotiating asymmetry in social relationships. In M.R.A. Chance (ed.) *Social fabrics of the mind*. London: Lawrence Erlbaum.

Price, J.S., & Sloman, L. (1984). The evolutionary model of psychiatric disorder (letter). *Archives of General Psychiatry*, *41*, 211.

Price, J.S. & Sloman, L. (1987). Depression as yielding behavior: An animal model based on Schjelderup-Ebbe's pecking order. *Ethology and Sociobiology*, *8*, 85–98.

Price, V.A. (1982). *Type A behaviour pattern: A model for research and practice*. New York: Academic Press.

Raleigh, M.J., McGuire, M.T., Brammer, G.L., & Yuwiler, A. (1984). Social and environmental influences on blood serotonin concentrations in monkeys. *Archives of General Psychiatry*, *41*, 405–410.

Rasmussen, K.L.R., & Reite, M. (1982). Loss-induced depression in an adult Macaque monkey. *American Journal of Psychiatry*, *139*, 679–681.

Reite, M., & Field, T. (eds) (1985). *The psychobiology of attachment and separation*. New York: Academic Press.

Reite, M., Short, R., Seiler, C., & Pauley, J.D. (1981). Attachment, loss and depression. *Journal of Child Psychology and Psychiatry*, *22*, 141–169.

Reus, V.I., Weingartner, H., & Post, R.M. (1979). Clinical implications of state-dependent learning. *American Journal of Psychiatry*, *136*, 927–931.

Rosenthal, N.E., Sack, D.A., Gillian, C.J. *et al.* (1984). Seasonal affective disorder: A description of the syndrome and preliminary findings with light therapy. *Archives of General Psychiatry, 41,* 72–79.

Rubinow, D.R., Roy-Byrne, P., Hoban, C.M. *et al.* (1986). Premenstrual mood changes: Characteristic patterns in women with and without premenstrual syndrome. *Journal of Affective Disorder, 10,* 85–90.

Seligman, M.E.P. (1975). *Helplessness: On depression development and death.* San Francisco: Freeman.

Silberman, E.K., Reus, V.I., Jimerson, D.C., Lynott, A.M., & Post, R.M. (1981). Heterogeneity of amphetamine response in depressed patients. *American Journal of Psychiatry, 138,* 1302–1307.

Sitaram, N., Nurnberger, J.I., Gershon, E.S., & Gillin, C.J. (1982). Cholinergic regulation of mood and REM sleep: Potential model and marker of vulnerability to affective disorder. *American Journal of Psychiatry, 139,* 571–576.

van Praag, H.M. (1986). Biological suicide research: Outcome and limitations. *Biological Psychiatry, 21,* 1305–1323.

Weiner, H. (1982). The prospects for psychosomatic medicine: Selected topics. *Psychosomatic Medicine, 44,* 491–517.

Weiss, J.M., Bailey, W.H., Goodman, P.A. *et al.* (1982). A model for neurochemical study of depression. In M.Y. Spiegelstein & A. Levy (eds), *Behavioural models and the analysis of drug action.* Amsterdam: Elsevier.

Whybrow, P.C. (1984). Contributions for neuroendocrinology. In K.R. Scherer & P. Erkman (eds), *Approaches to emotion.* Hillsdale, N.J.: Lawrence Erlbaum.

Whybrow, P.C., Akiskal, H.S., & McKinney, W.T. (1984). *Mood disorders: Towards a new psychobiology.* New York: Plenum Press.

Willner, P. (1985). *Depression: A psychobiological synthesis.* Chichester: Wiley.

Wolpe, J. (1979). The experimental model and treatment of neurotic depression. *Behavioural Research and Therapy, 17,* 555–565.

Yalom, I.D. (1980). *Existential psychotherapy.* New York: Basic Books.

KEY WORDS

Abandonment, acetylcholine, autonomous, catecholamines, classification, cognitive therapy, cortisol, defeat, despair, dominance, epidemiology, evolution, existential, grief, learned helplessness, hormone, 5-hydroxytryptamine, hypothalamus, incentives, melancholia, monoamines, neuroendocrine, noradrenaline, protest, psychoanalytic, retardation, sociotropic, specialness, symptoms.

Handbook of Life Stress, Cognition and Health
Edited by S. Fisher and J. Reason
© 1988 John Wiley & Sons Ltd.

32

Life Stress, Control Strategies and the Risk of Disease: A Psychobiological Model

SHIRLEY FISHER
The University of Dundee, Scotland

LIFE STRESSES AND HEALTH

Social contexts such as low social and occupational status have long been associated with increased risk of nearly all disease conditions and with shorter life expectancy. Specific conditions such as personal loss, bereavement, job loss and conditions of marital status and mobility are similarly associated with risk of illness. In historical perspective, these findings formed the foundation of psychosomatic medicine (see Weiner, 1982), in contrast to the more traditional medical or disease model in which greater weight was given to constitutional and genetic factors and the role of disease agents. More recently, the balance has shifted towards recognition of the importance of psychogenic factors in mental and physical disorders and there is increasing interest in the psychobiological states which mediate. It is this interest which is manifest as one of the main themes of this handbook.

In this chapter, the main concern is not to itemize the evidence of all the associations between personal life events and illness, but to seek to provide understanding of the mechanisms whereby the risk of illness is changed. The main approach will be to consider some of the proposed common denominators in the conditions associated with high risk of illness and then to present a particular synthesis of ideas, developed by Fisher (1986) and based on physiological and psychological studies, which assumes that decisions about control create and maintain differential hormone states which form the basis of ill-health.

Social Change and the Opportunity for Infection

The occurrence of epidemics during social change created, for example, by industrialization and mass migration, has long been recognized but tends to have been attributed to the stressful contexts created as a result of such factors as

exposure, poor housing and overcrowding. Sigerist (1932) pointed to the prevalence of specific diseases in historical epochs and emphasized cultural determinants. The Middle Ages were characterized by plague and leprosy. In the
Renaissance, the predominant problem was syphilis. In the Baroque period, the
prevailing diseases were due to deficiencies such as camp fever, scurvy or so-called
luxury diseases such as gout, dropsy and hypochondria. Tuberculosis was identified with the industrialization of Western society.

Cultural climates may increase the risk of disease by changing dietary, exercise
or living habits. Human behaviour patterns may additionally increase the
chances, either directly, as in the case of syphilis (and now AIDS), or less directly,
as when survival pressures force individuals to migrate or live in crowded
industrial communities in order to gain work.

Social Change and Stress

Research evidence also suggests that stress is an important feature of social
change. In particular, mass migrations and industrialization may create periods of
stress and anxiety. Tuberculosis has long been of interest in that statistically, the
evidence supports a strong association with conditions of war, migration, relocation, industrialization, urbanization and poverty. There are numerous citations in
the research literature. For example, increases in tuberculosis morbidity and
mortality were recorded for the Navjo and Sioux Indians who were relocated
within the United States. The relocation of Irish immigrants to the USA and of
Bantu natives in South Africa from the vicinity of Johannesburg into the outskirts
of the city are other examples (McDougall, 1949; Moorman, 1950). When
immigrants returned to their native villages, the infections were established there
too. However, the link with stressful transition is underlined in that although up to
73% of village children were affected, mortality remained low. In the case of the
Irish immigrants there is greater support for a link with stress because although
they encountered a more affluent and potentially positive living environment, the
tuberculosis incidence levels were 100% more than in those left behind in Ireland.

An important contribution is made by the research literature demonstrating that
moves have important psychological effects on individuals (see Chapter 3, this
volume). Unfortunately, but perhaps unavoidably, studies of relocation have
confounded a number of potentially stressful circumstances, making it difficult to
determine whether moving itself is a critical factor or whether circumstances
created by moving are responsible for adverse psychological effects. Thus,
although a positive association between moving and the risk of mental and
physical ill-health has been indicated (Chapter 3, this volume), the reason is not
easily identified. For example, Faris and Dunham (1939) established that residential status in a large city (defined by home ownership as compared with rented
accommodation) was related to mental health, since the incidence of schizophrenia and depression was greater in the rental population. However, rented
accommodation locations corresponded with areas of the city where there were
high levels of social disorganization and poverty. Moreover, the possibility of
self-selection by downward mobility, or 'social drift' through incapacity, could not
be ruled out.

Evidence for the effects of moves on psychological state was, however, provided by Fried (1963) in a study of enforced slum clearance. Adverse psychological effects akin to grief and depression were experienced by those forced to move to new housing. By demonstrating adverse psychological changes in circumstances were change leads to better housing opportunity, the stressful aspects of moves are underlined. Also, moves are the third most frequently reported precipitants recalled by clinically depressed patients (Leff *et al.*, 1970), which emphasizes the close relationship with mental disorder.

The relationship between mobility and physical illnesses (such as the proclivity to heart disease), although established in the research literature, has confounded the same variables identified from studies of mobility and mental health (above). However, one or two studies have probed mobility history as a predictor of physical ill-health following a move. An important longitudinal study by Stokols *et al.* (1983) showed that, in general, individuals with a high mobility history were more likely to report illness symptoms following a relocation for a new job than those reporting a low mobility history.

Evidence of the importance of marital status as a factor influencing health is indicated by a number of epidemiological studies. Figure 32.1 illustrates some of the epidemiological data provided by Berkson (1962) which show a statistical association between marital status and physical ill-health amongst US citizens. The effects, generally apparent for both males and females, confirm the increased vulnerability of the divorced and the single as compared with married individuals. The data also illustrate that accidents and homicide rates are similarly affected, suggesting, perhaps, that the *behaviour* of the individual has an important role. The fact that comparable marital status differences are apparent for suicide, provides a strong indication that the factor of importance is stress (although see critical analysis by Cochrane, Chapter 8, this volume).

Dodge and Martin (1970) investigated marital status in the context of between-state differences in chronic disease incidence in the USA. In 1950, USA statistical records showed that the death rate for the white male population aged 35–44 varied in terms of marital status. The divorced had the highest rates and the widowed had the next highest rates, followed by the single. Dodge and Martin found that, although at all age levels the death rate for widowers was higher than for married individuals, the gap closed with increasing age. They favoured the view that marital status is a mediating factor because it represents the degree of social integration but they also conceded that self-selection could be involved— the most robust and healthy might be more likely to become married. An explanation in terms of mediating states such as loneliness suggests that the married are protected because of the marital support offered. However, this does not account for the differences between the non-married groups.

National Health records in the UK (Connolly, 1975) have also provided evidence on the interaction of marital status and age as vulnerability factors: widowers over the age of 55 have mortality rates above the expected levels for age-matched married men. In the 6 months following bereavement, the risk levels are particularly elevated. It may be that the psychological state of grief is linked with increased risk of ill-health. Bereavement has been linked with the increased risk of a variety of diseases, including coronary disease and heart failure, tuberculosis, diabetes, and cancer (see Clegg, Chapter 4 in this volume).

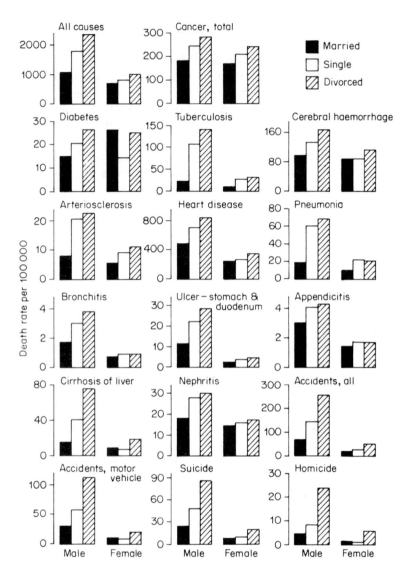

FIG. 32.1 Standardized death rates for different causes of death in the United States. (Data redrawn from Berkson (1962) (deceased) with the permission of the American Medical Association. From Fisher, 1986.)

Life Change Units—Stress and Disease

A series of studies by Holmes and Rahe arising from the clinical observation that life events such as job loss, divorce and bereavement seemed to feature in the protocols of patients being treated for illness, led to the construction of a scale—the Schedule of Recent Experiences. This consisted of a spectrum of personal, social and occupational life events. A stress level weighting factor was introduced: judges were provided with a list of 42 life changes, one of which—

'marriage'—was given the value of 500, and asked to provide relative life change unit values (LCUs) for the rest of the life events—death of a spouse, divorce, marital separation, death of close family member, and detention in jail occupied the top places in terms of perceived stressful qualities.

Early retrospective studies (e.g. Holmes and Rahe, 1967) showed that there was an increase in LCUs in the first 2 years prior to illness. The effect was non-specific and did not predict the type of illness. The studies suggested that below LCU values of 150, there was no reason to expect ill-health; between 150 and 300 LCU, approximately half the individuals reported an illness in the following year. For 300 LCU the level was 70%. A later study involving 2500 US Navy officers (see Rahe, 1972) identified a build-up of LCUs prior to illness. Following the illness, LCU totals remained elevated. The life change unit indexes stress level in terms of the amount of adjustment required by change. The power of this scale to predict the risk of major illness has been given detailed consideration by Rahe (see Chapter 17 in this volume).

Factors Influencing the Risk of Disease as a Response to Life Events

Figure 32.2 illustrates a conceptualization of processes by which the experience of a life event might increase the risk of infectious or chronic disease. First, the life event might create adverse prevailing conditions (poverty, overcrowding, etc.) resulting in more antigen encounters or more encounters with new antigens. The second possibility is that the individual's behaviour changes as a response to stress and that the risk of bodily malfunction or antigen encounter changes as a result. Finally, irrespective of the nature of the life event, the mental and physical state of the individual changes as a function of stress: a person may become more biologically aroused or more worried and preoccupied.

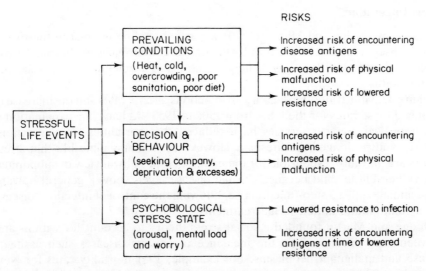

FIG. 32.2 Conceptual model of factors increasing the risk of disease following a stressful life event, e.g. migration, relocation, bereavement, marital separation and divorce.

MODELS OF COMMON DENOMINATORS OF LIFE STRESS EVENTS

Social Disruption and Anxiety

One emphasis taken by those seeking to understand the relationship between stress and ill-health is that of social disruption. There are a number of slightly different focuses, but the general argument is that the individual exists in a social context and life events create changes within this context which lead to and maintain raised anxiety.

Wolff (1952) formulated four main postulates which he argued could provide the basis for understanding the increased risk of illness as a response to change. (i) Changes affect the folklore and taboos of a culture; (ii) the threats created by these taboos often become overexaggerated and create anxiety; (ii) formalized methods for dealing with those threats are part of the culture; and (iv) cultural change reduces the possibility of the use of familiar methods for dealing with threat.

Wolff gives as one example the Hopi Indian taboo of avoiding treading on a snake's track. Infringement of the taboo results in pain to the feet and normally would be treated by the medicine man. Cultural change led to the loss of the medicine man, with the result that there was no treatment for infringement of this taboo.

Wolff argues that situations of rapid cultural change create cultural pressures but remove anxiety-reduction techniques: 'The participant mistrusts habits and intuitions, and social experience no longer leads to a common sense of values' (p. 15). Industrialization and family destabilization are regarded as sources of threat in modern society. They are assumed to be exacerbated by competitive pressures.

Status Integration

Research by Dodge and Martin (1970) was stimulated by interest in the rise in chronic disease levels in the USA, by within-state differences in chronic disease levels, and also by differences in subpopulations as a function of age, race and marital status.

Figure 32.3 illustrates the decrease in infectious disease rates and the increase in chronic disease rates for the USA from 1900 to 1953. At least one explanation is that improved medical services have reduced the mortalities from infectious diseases and prolonged the lifespan. However, it remains plausible that stress factors are partially responsible for the increase, especially in view of subpopulation vulnerabilities and because chronic disease levels show a general upward trend and not a just a step-function rise following the control of infectious disease by inoculation and antibacterial treatments.

Dodge and Martin founded a social stress theory to account for within- and between-state differences in the incidence of chronic diseases such as heart disease and malignant neoplasms. For example, 1951 mortality rates for New York were 938.5 (per 100 000) for heart disease and 238.9 (per 100 000) for malignant disease, whereas in Mississippi rates were 488.4 and 163.3, respective-

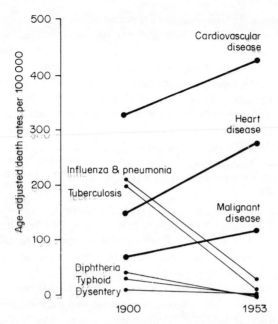

FIG. 32.3   Illustration of the decreased incidence of infectious disease and the increased incidence of chronic disease from 1900 to 1953. (Data provided by the USA Department of Health, Education and Welfare, National Office of Vital Statistics.)

ly. Because both stress levels and medical services were found to differ between states, Dodge and Martin developed an ingenious technique for trying to establish whether the differences in disease levels could be attributed to the stress levels or to the medical services. They used infant mortality levels as a measure of the level of general health due to medical services, and suicide rates as a measure of stress. The two death rate statistics then provide a basis for explanation of chronic disease levels in terms of 'health milieu' or 'social stress'. In the case of both heart disease and malignant disease, the incidence levels across states were correlated with suicide levels rather than with infant mortality levels, thus supporting a stress hypothesis.

On the basis of these correlational patterns, a social disruption hypothesis was proposed. Life experiences, partly created by living conditions (competitive pressures, goals, aims), impose pressures on individuals but social factors dictate the extent of effects. Thus, the poorly integrated marital groups (single and divorced) are more at risk because of the lack of stable and durable relationships. The authors envisage an aetiological complex of three elements: (1) the disease-provoking agent; (2) the nature of the environment in which host and agent are brought together; and (3) the resistance and susceptibility of the host, in turn determined by social integration level.

Social Consistency and Rule Breakdown

The position taken by Totman (1979) has features in common with the Dodge and Martin model because of the emphasis on social breakdown and disharmony following life changes. Totman notes that social factors exert a protective influence on health. The individual becomes at risk for illness when social mobility or status incongruity occurs. Totman proposes a structural theory which assumes that people make sense of each other's actions in terms of social rules and conventions. Thus, each individual is equipped with a set of prescriptive rules. For these rules to exist they must be resistant to change, although some clarification or refinement can occur as the result of social interactions. Social change creates a situation of rule breakdown. Exits, losses, marital breakdown could all be seen in terms of the breakdown of rules. For example, a bereaved person, in addition to grieving for a lost loved-one, may also lose an aspect of his or her identity and has to evolve new status in the community. Oatley (Chapter 30, this volume) develops a similar approach.

The details of how social disharmony creates increased risk of illness need to be explored. One possibility is that anxiety levels increase and that there is long-term damage to health because of persistent states of preoccupation which cause distress and unhappiness. However, there may be different psychobiological dynamics as a function of time following social change. Gilbert (see Chapter 31 in this volume) has considered the importance of loss of social status for a psychobiological theory of depression. He proposes a 'go–stop' model of the reaction to situations of failure and loss, including loss of status. The 'go' phase involves active searching, accompanied by raised anxiety, whereas the 'stop' phase involves giving up and helplessness. An initial phase of struggle which is not successful is later followed by loss of volition and apathy, perhaps with accompanying distress.

The Control Model

Fisher (1986) proposed that life events create changes in the level of demand together with reduction of control over various aspects of the new lifestyle. Reduction of control occurs when a person feels unable to produce a set of actions that will restore perceived discrepancy between reality and aims or ambitions. Change both creates discrepancies and, because of novelty, may decrease the level of control a person experiences in relation to the new environment. Laboratory studies of animals and people suggest that power or mastery over the environment is likely to have an ameliorating effect on threat: animals provided with the instrumental means for avoiding punishment generally show fewer signs of physical lesion and disease than those who do not. Human beings are more likely to choose to have control over noxious stimulation and are more likely to be tolerant of unpleasant stimulation if it is self-delivered. For those who do not choose direct control, more complex strategies may be operating (see Fisher, 1986; Chapter 2).

Karasek (1979) reported that job strain in working environments can be defined with respect to two dimensions—demand (or work load) and discretion (control). Job strain is reported when demand is high and control is low. Perceived challenge is more likely when demand and control are both high. On this analysis, a major life event might be argued to create a 'job strain' environment. The bereaved person has to cope with the strain of living a life without the help and protection of the partner; the relocated have to find out how to cope with life in a new place.

However, it has also been argued by Fisher (1986) that control and perceived demand should be regarded as interactional concepts rather than as passive properties of situations. In other words, it is how individuals perceive demand and control levels which determines whether a life event is interpreted as benign, challenging, or distressing. This would imply that the individual's reaction to a life event should be set in the context of previous life experiences.

THE BIOLOGICAL STATES OF STRESS

If we are to understand how psychological states of the individual might influence the risk of antigens becoming established or chronic diseases developing there needs to be some attempt to link psychological states with biological states. We might begin to imagine that psychological states are rich and varied and link with biological activity in such a way as to raise the risk of particular diseases. Biological states are now known to be highly complex, and it is possible that ways of thinking about the world might create patterns which are associated with particular illnesses.

The effect of stress on biological activity was first described in terms of a unitary state of increased arousal, implying that any number of different kinds of stressful experience (e.g. bereavement, failure, surgical operations, public speaking, illness, job loss) would be associated with non-specific arousal effects (Selye, 1956). Cannon (1932; 1936) was one of the first to make sense of the biological state which accompanied the experience of stress in terms of the need to restore equilibrium. The biological response to the disequilibrium produced by stress was assumed to provide the power to restore the balance. However, this did not change the basic assumption of the non-specificity of the biological state. The question of why one man reacts to stress with ulcers and another with heart disease (Malmo and Shagass, 1949) provided an early challenge to this assumption.

Perhaps the attempt to link even physiological states to disease proclivities must remain fanciful. Weiner (1982) points out that in any population some individuals are at risk for disease but the illness never materializes. One example is the presence of elevated levels of pepsinogen isoenzymes which is a biological marker for peptic duodenal ulcer. Such a marker can occur in persons who remain well. Weiner concludes that the individual is programmed for disease by a multitude of predisposing markers and psychological sensitivities. However, it might be possible to begin to probe the medium in which markers exist. Perhaps the person with a biological marker favouring a peptic ulcer remains well unless creating or encountering stresses which produce changes in gastric activity. A risk model based on *compatibility* and *synchrony* of biological and psychological patterns might be the answer. Also, existing biological markers which should predispose towards illness might be created and sustained by stressful life experiences. It then requires a further life event to create the synchronous existence of sufficient risk factors for a particular kind of illness.

There has been an increasing realization that physiological responses are capable of rich patterning which may reflect the features of the stress (fear provoking, anger provoking), or the idiosyncracies of the individual (self-blaming, external blaming). On the basis of drug and ablation studies, Lacey (1967) suggests that biological arousal is not a uniform state; temporal parallelism exists between cortical, autonomic and behavioural arousal states, and fractionation is possible.

Stress and the Sympathetico Medullary Route

The autonomic nervous system provides the basis of a complex system which controls the release of the catecholamines adrenaline and noradrenaline via the adrenal medulla. Raised sympathetic activity is associated with increased cardiac output, vasoconstriction, changes in gastric motility, reduction of bodily secretions, increased muscle tension, changes in respiratory rate, mobilization of glycogen, and release of fats into circulation.

Chronic, elevated levels of catecholamines can create structural changes in systems. In the cardiovascular system, the depositing of cholesterol and fatty acids decreases the lumen of blood vessels. Therefore, stresses which are prolonged or which involve uncontrollable problems are likely to create conditions which might prepare for structural changes leading to chronic disease. Dietary fat may raise serum cholesterol levels, and hence stress-related behaviour leading to obesity may be another risk factor in cardiovascular disease. Yet Japanese immigrants in the USA who eat high-fat diets but maintain a traditional way of life are less prone to heart disease than those who do not (Marmot and Syme, 1976). Thus, the effect of stress and that of dietary fat may be independent as well as interactive risk factors in cardiovascular disease.

In an analysis of the underlying causes of heart disease in the Western world, Carruthers (1974) examined a high risk group of racing-car drivers. Physiological measures indicated high levels of noradrenaline during and after a race. Carruthers concluded that such an 'arousal-jag' is actively sought by drivers. However, because there is no accompanying physical activity, preparation for massive energy release is not accompanied by sufficient activity, and therefore elevated levels of cholesterol and fats, together with constriction of the cardiovascular system at a time of raised cardiac output, increase the risk of structural damage.

The body's defence system is extremely complicated, and is controlled by systems of messenger substances which enable the necessary defences for up to 30 000 possible antigens to be maintained. The system is remarkably efficient and yet subject to the influence of stress hormones, particularly those associated with the corticoid hormones (see next section). However, increased catecholamine levels may also have a suppressing effect on the body's defence system in the long term, because of suppressed lymphocyte production (Wang *et al.*, 1978). Equally, changes in cyclic nucleotide levels observed to accompany anxiety states (Horovitz *et al.*, 1972) may affect lymphocyte activity levels more directly.

Stress and the Corticoid Hormone Route

The production of corticoid hormones is more likely to be associated with severe acute or chronic stress and is triggered by the production of adrenocorticotrophic hormone (ACTH) released in the brain and acting on the adrenal cortex. Selye (1956) concentrated on the corticoid response pattern in rodents exposed to chronic low temperature stress. An early alarm phase, accompanied by increased cortisol and high discharge of fat granules on first exposure, was followed by a period of resistance in which the adrenal glands were found to be laden with hormones and fat. By the third 'exhaustion' phase, these resources were depleted and the animal was not able to survive further stress.

An important aspect of the cortisol response is that there is evidence that it directly suppresses the immune response. Amkraut and Solomon (1975) showed that ACTH injected into animals increased the risk of antigen infection. The vulnerability of animals distressed by electric shock, constraint or loud noise (120 dB) was well demonstrated by Rassmussen (1957), who investigated susceptibility to a wide range of infectious agents in prestressed animals and reported an increased risk of herpes simplex, poliomyelitis, Coxsackie B and polyoma virus infections. The effect was attributed to increased cortisol level.

The precise mechanisms by which raised cortisol levels might have immunosuppressant consequence are currently being explored. An analysis of the consequences of acute physical stress (Nieburgs *et al.*, 1979) showed that there may be a decrease in the number of small lymphocytes and an increased level of medium-sized lymphocytes in circulation. One possibility is that acute physical stress activates immature lymphocytes and so the number of uncommitted cells is small and not sufficient to cope with the range of possible specific viruses.

However, it has also been shown that chronic stress can have immunofacilitatory properties: when food availability to animals was limited to 2 hours per day for a week, there was enhanced T-cell-dependent immune response (Solomon and Amkraut, 1979). More interestingly, exposure to chronic noise caused facilitation in T and B cell systems, but when the noise was acute the effect was one of immunosuppression. One important implication is that the timing and features of the stress itself may be a determinant of reaction (Sklar and Anisman, 1979, 1981).

The importance of timing of the occurrence of stress and antigen occurrence was further confirmed by the finding that immunological suppression to the antigen flagellin was only apparent if the stress occurred at the time of flagellin inoculation (see Monjan and Collector, 1977). The explanation which makes sense of this is that cortisol precipitates the commitment of the bodily defence system in advance. If this occurs prematurely without the necessary cues for specificity, then the population of lymphocytes may be wasted. On the other hand, if this occurs at the appropriate time, the defences could be efficiently committed to prevent attack. It is not hard to see that there could be survival advantages to a system which allowed stressful conditions to have access to bodily defence mechanisms in this way.

Other influences of cortisol on the immune response have been identified. They include thymus involution as well as reduction of spleen and lymph nodes, and there may be reduction of natural killer cells (NK), which are believed to provide challenge to developing malignancies (Riley 1979; Riley *et al.*, 1979).

Hormone Characteristics and Disease Susceptibility

Decision and the Overriding of Autoregulatory Devices

The main effects of the hormones which are released in stressful conditions are to mobilize and activate a number of bodily resources. The side-effects which occur may directly result from these changes and may be interpreted as illnesses. Thus, dizziness, tension, stomach cramps, palpitations and respiratory problems may be part of the state of hyperarousal created by stress. The individual who is uninformed about the effects of stress on bodily systems may label the symptoms as being part of some more profound disease or disorder and there may be self-confirming aspects.

Adverse long-term effects on biological function could be encouraged by factors which increase the level and duration of stress hormones. Moderate levels of catecholamine are characteristic of daily life. However, chronic circulation of these elevated hormone levels increases risk of structural disorder. Experience of threatening but intractable problems or events characterized by low control should provide ideal conditions in this respect. As many of the chapters in this volume illustrate, life stresses often tend to provide such conditions.

The human capacity to re-experience unpleasant events in reflective thinking or to anticipate and hence experience much of the threat of an impending event in advance, provides a major means of driving and maintaining states of pathological arousal. One consequence is persistent functional abuse of bodily systems. Sterling and Eyer (1981) describe a number of autonomous regulatory controls which act to self-limit the physiological response (see also Chapter 34 in this volume). For example, a rise in the concentration of glucose in the blood stimulates the pancreas to secrete insulin. Insulin encourages the uptake of sugar by muscle fat and liver cells, thus creating a negative feedback loop which results in a drop in the level of glucose in the blood. Such autoregulatory systems should, if correctly functioning, protect against functional abuse of bodily mechanisms. Unfortunately, as Sterling and Eyer point out, neural system can override these self-regulatory systems. The authors argue that the facility for the overriding of autononous systems enables adaptive and anticipatory response to fluctuating circumstances to occur. The argument is an important one; the brain's response to threat or elevated demand is to overrule autoregulatory processes, and thus the risk of long-term penalties in terms of illness is raised.

In addition, wear and tear take some toll on bodily activity. Sterling and Eyer review evidence to suggest that the hormones suppressed during high arousal are those which promote synthetic or anabolic processes requiring energy. Thus there is reduced capacity for cell repair and maintenance of immunological systems. The levels of cholesterol and of fatty acids are not controlled. Equally, catabolic activity rises, resulting in more free fatty acids, raised blood sugar levels, drop in cellular activity, shrinkage of the thymus and swelling of the adrenal glands to maintain hormone production. Thus, if human decision overrides the autoregulatory loops which prevent persistent high levels of catabolic activity, the risk of 'somatization', or functional abuse leading to structural change, increases.

States of preoccupation and worry are associated with life stress experiences (see Fisher, Chapter 3, Pennebaker, Chapter 36, and Wegner, Chapter 37, this volume). They have the potential to increase the risk of illness. First, the period of elevated arousal may be driven and maintained, resulting in a protracted stress experience. Secondly, a preoccupied person is likely to be rendered incompetent and thus may inadvertently create more stresses as well as being unable to cope effectively with the initial threat. Fisher (1984) argued that stresses create a demand for accurate, productive activity, whilst simultaneously creating mental states in which competence levels are often reduced. A number of feedback loops resulting in progressive loss of control were identified, which lead towards a state of complete incompetence or crisis. The failure to act competently may increase the threatening properties of the life event unless it is self-limiting. Moreover, the individual may become aware of his own inabilities to cope and this could result in further self-focused preoccupation.

Decision and Specific Hormonal Consequences

Decisions about control in specific situations may directly determine hormone balance and hence the propensity to different categories of illness. As will be apparent from the previous section, although catecholamines and corticoid hormones do not have mutually exclusive jurisdiction over aspects of bodily function in stress, there is some evidence of 'division of labour'. Raised cortisol has more immediate influence on the immune response system, whereas catecholamine levels have a predominant effect on biological arousal.

From studies involving catecholamines in stressful environments, there is both direct and indirect evidence to suggest that the balance of adrenaline and noradrenaline is a variable influenced by human decision. Ax (1953) distinguished anger- and fear-producing situations in terms of adrenaline–noradrenaline characteristics; the anger profile was linked with increases in both hormones, whereas the fear profile was associated with raised adrenaline.

Funkenstein *et al.* (1957) examined the effects of contrived public failure on competitive college students and reported two distinguishable response patterns which could be predicted with great accuracy by a close associate of each student. The first response style, termed 'anger-in', was a self-blaming style associated with a physiological pattern typical of raised adrenaline. The second response style, termed 'anger-out', was associated with changes symptomatic of raised noradrenaline.

Work involving direct catecholamine measurement by Frankenhaeuser and colleagues has identified different balances of adrenaline and noradrenaline as a function of work context. For example, Frankenhaeuser and Gardell (1976) investigated jobs in a sawmill and showed that conditions of repetition and short-cycle operations are more likely to be associated with lack of subjective well-being and raised adrenaline, whereas conditions of restricted work posture are more likely to be associated with increased irritation and raised levels of noradrenaline.

Frankenhaeuser and Rissler (1970) showed that increasing situational control was accompanied by a preponderance of noradrenaline to adrenaline. Weiss (1968) demonstrated increased noradrenaline levels in rats to avoid shock, but not in yoked controls. Mason *et al.* (1968) confirmed that novelty and uncertainty were more likely to be associated with raised adrenaline, whereas stereotyped situations were more likely to be accompanied by raised noradrenaline.

The implications of different ratios of adrenaline–noradrenaline balance for the risk of illness have yet to be worked out. Collectively, chronic elevated levels of catecholamines increase the risk of cardiovascular and gastrointestinal changes. In the former case, hormone balance may be influential: noradrenaline is more likely to raise blood pressure through vasoconstriction, whereas adrenaline is more likely to act via increased cardiac output.

A recent analysis by Fisher (1986), based on physiological evidence from Frankenhaeuser and Johansson (1982) and psychological evidence from Karasek (1979) suggested that decisions about whether control is possible have implications for the ratio of circulating catecholamines and corticoid hormones. The individual makes strategic decisions concerning level of control when confronted with demanding or threatening events. When there is high control the individual should experience challenge, whereas when there is no control there is risk of helplessness accompanied by distress if there are punishing consequences. In ambiguous situations, decisions about control may involve protracted worry, as the individual seeks to explore the consequences of possible courses of action. Life stresses may create states of 'mental chess', in which the individual rehearses possible moves and countermoves in order to decide on a course of action.

Psychophysiological research (Frankenhaeuser and Johansson, 1982) has provided support for the importance of decision in stressful environments, although unfortunately based on comparisons afforded by different laboratory tasks. A 1-hour vigilance task involving changes in intensity of a weak light was stated to be designed so as to involve low control over outcome. Performance was accompanied by raised subjective effort and perceived distress. The predominant hormone was raised cortisol. By comparison, a choice reaction time task with a high degree of personal control over stimulus rate was associated with raised self-reported effort but no distress. The predominant hormones were catecholamines.

A field study by Johansson and Sanden (1982) involved a group of operators engaged in planning production and control where there was a high degree of control over the work. By contrast, process controllers in the same industry worked under monotonous conditions, remained passive but were required to detect critical signals associated with disturbances in the process. The study showed that the active planning task was associated with primarily positive feelings and raised catecholamine levels, whereas the passive, understimulating process-monitoring task was associated with unease, with some small increase in adrenaline and cortisol levels.

The above studies do not provide proof that perceived control is the direct determinant of hormone pattern, but the reported relationship between effortful situations and raised catecholamines and distressing situations with elevated cortisol and catecholamines is supported. The implications are that differential decision about controllability may turn out to be a major factor influencing prevailing hormone states and hence the proclivity to certain illnesses.

Ursin *et al.* (1978) investigated stress in parachute jumping. One group, who had poor performance, had elevated cortisol and catecholamine levels. A second group performed well, enjoyed the challenge and were characterized by raised catecholamine levels and growth hormone, but not cortisol. This fits well with the idea that performing well and experience of challenge are related to high perceived control, whereas poor performance will create alarm and distress. However, a third group who responded poorly were characterized by a fall in testosterone and an increase in prolactin. This warns against simplistic accounts of the relationship between control and hormone states.

For some disorders there is a research literature suggesting that personal response styles and decision are influential, but there is little information about how this might link with circulating hormone levels. Wolff (1952) conducted investigations of patients with gastric fistulas and concluded that there are two patterns of gastric hypodynamic reactions. The first is a pattern associated with a sense of fear and catastrophe or abject grief and depression. In these cases gastric function ceases. A second pattern is associated with feelings of disgust and defence. In this pattern, although gastric activity is reduced, mucous production increases and skeletal muscles normally involved in vomiting are active.

Patients with ulcerative colitis are further described as outwardly calm and peaceful but with a great deal of underlying feelings of dependency, hostility and guilt. These feelings are associated with increased gastric motility, increased vascularity, turgescence and lesions of the colon. The combined effect of hyper-motility, hypervascularity and fragility of the mucous membrane paves the way for ulcers.

The interesting question is how these reaction patterns are implemented and sustained. Perhaps personal style has implications for gastric response patterns and the risk of different types of gastric disorder. The outward-anger response style and the fear response style already distinguished in terms of adrenaline-like and noradrenaline-like physiological pattern (above) may be responsible for different colonic consequences. However, the failure to express hostility even following conditions of responsibility and frustration which seem to characterize the ulcerogenic person does not seem easily accounted for within this framework.

Animal studies have suggested a relationship between instrumentality or control and ulcerogenic stress. This directly implicates the role of selective decision. Brady (1958) reported that executive monkeys given the means for avoiding repeated shock were more likely to develop ulcers than their yoked, helpless counterparts. The Brady design has been faulted because of the selection procedure for the executive and helpless groups. Also, the result has not been confirmed by studies of helpless and instrumental rodents which generally indicate increased stomach lesions in helpless animals (see Weiss, 1968). A possible explanation of the Brady result as reported is that although the executive monkeys have control, the nature of the avoidance task is such that they do not receive feedback about success. Thus, Fisher (1984) argued that such forms of control may be stressful.

Figure 32.4 illustrates the basis of the control hypothesis developed by Fisher (1986). If the decision is made that control is possible, effort and challenge are

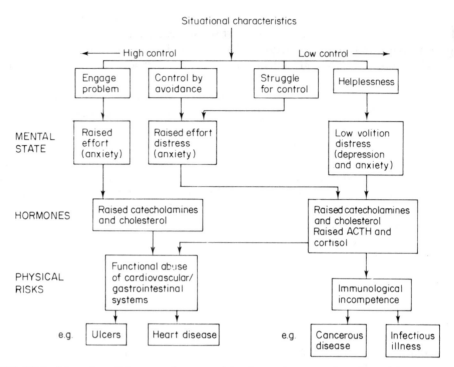

FIG. 32.4   Map of possible routes from cognitive factors in perception of control to mental disorder and physical illness.

features and the hormone balance would favour elevated catecholamines. The implications for illness would be increased risk of chronic disease. By contrast, decision that the situation is uncontrollable results in raised effort and distress if the individual struggles to gain control, or to passivity and distress if the individual fails to become committed and is overwhelmed. In the former case, there should be raised catecholamines and raised cortisol levels; in the latter situation, catecholamine levels would be expected to be low, whereas distress levels and hence cortisol levels could still be elevated. If it is assumed that catecholamines predominantly increase the risk of chronic illness later in life and that corticoid responses predominantly increase the risk of immunological suppression (depending on timing), then we can link decision and control strategy to illness risk.

However, the evidence reviewed on adrenaline–noradrenaline balance in different environments encountered by individuals leads to the conclusion that even in situations where a person has low control, the balance of adrenaline and noradrenaline may reflect psychological factors. Studies by Frankenhaeuser and Gardell (1976), in an industrial setting, showed that uncontrollable work pace was associated with feelings of irritation and preponderance of noradrenaline, whereas uncontrollable work cycle durations were more likely to influence well-being and adrenaline levels. Perhaps a hierarchical model is needed in which the level of control dictates the balance of catecholamines and cortisol in circulation, but features of the uncontrollable 'punishment' are further distinguished by decision which results in adrenaline–noradrenaline balance.

STRESS, DECISION AND THE PROCLIVITY TO ILLNESS

Weiner (1982) formulated a number of questions of interest to the future of psychosomatic medicine. The first is why particular social situations and contexts are associated with a variety of illnesses and diseases. The second is why one person might become ill but another person does not. The third concerns individual differences in health risks.

These are taxing questions and as yet the answers are only speculative. The control model would provide some explanation of why different contexts may be associated with different illness risks because it would assume that different assessments of control are involved. The model could explain individual differences in susceptibility to illness in terms of idiosyncracies in the assessment of control and differences in selected strategy. The specificity of disease remains a problem: there may be behavioural routes which increase chance encounters with antigens and carcinogens; illness categories are distinguished by interpretation of level of control. The existence of biological markers, whether because of genetic factors or lifestyle dictates, might provide a basic risk level tuned to a particular illness; life stresses occur against this background and decisions about control become influential.

Figure 32.5 illustrates the likely influences which have been identified as risk factors in chronic and infectious disease. The figure first illustrates that a stressful life event has the potential to create behaviours which encourage encounters with antigens. It also illustrates the hypothesized influences of specific decisions about control on aspects of disease processes. As already described, decisions concerned with level of control are hypothesized to have selective influence on stress hormone balance, which in turn influences differentially the risk of particular illnesses.

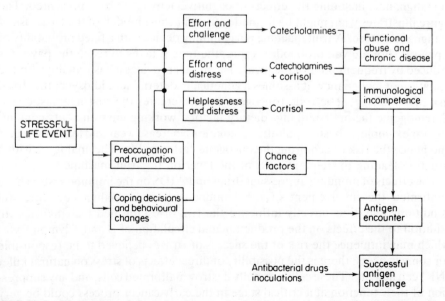

FIG 32.5 Illustration of the role of strategic decisions in the risk of successful antigen challenge and chronic disease.

The figure also illustrates the hypothesized influence of ruminative activity, whether reflective or anticipatory in character. Continuous rehearsal of a stressful problem drives states of pathological arousal and is a perfect way of retaining the hormone states created by decision. If we were to program a computer to increase the risk of disease, it would be necessary to create a harmful agent and then create a state of the computer which gave the agent maximum chance of success. A system in which a state of lowered counter-harm resources was constantly being produced in the computer by its own activity would be ideal for increased disease risk. On first consideration, evolutionary pressures should not favour the survival of such a system, but such a system also has benefits which outweigh the negative features and the costs. Ruminative activity may enhance the consolidation of previously encountered stressful experiences (Fisher, 1984). These advantages may need to be set against the costs of the biological states created as a result.

Two excellent reviews of the role of stress factors in cancerous disease (Cox and Mackay, 1982; Sklar and Anisman, 1981) have indicated the importance of sex and growth hormones as well as stress hormones as factors in the development of malignancy. The stress–cancer relationship is further complicated by the fact that cancers vary in type, responsiveness and development characteristics. Malignancy may occur because of direct genetic malfunctions or because of the effects of carcinogens and viruses. The process of malignancy may occur over a protracted period of time: some estimates have suggested that a single neoplastic division could occur 20 years before the development of any observable tumour, thus affording a changing basis for complex hormone interplays. A developing tumour requires a blood supply, and the communication processes necessary to achieve this may be hormone influenced. Finally, hormones may influence the development of metastases.

Figure 32.6 provides a conceptual format which enables some of the risk factors in malignancy, including the effects of cognitive activity, to be represented. The figure illustrates what might be termed a 'fruit machine model' of the basic risk of malignant disease. A fruit machine is a gambling device with a fixed probability of a pay-off. For a given probability value, the time it takes to reach the pay-off is reduced by frequent pulls of the lever. The model provides a basic analogy for the initiation of malignancy: it assumes a genetically determined, idiosyncratic, fixed risk of a faulty genetic code (oncogene) which creates the first neoplastic cell. Carcinogenic factors (smoking, dietary factors, working environments containing, for example, asbestos, pollution, radiation) increase wear and tear, cell repair and hence the risk of acquiring the oncogene earlier in life. The analogy is with a situation leading to frequent pulls of the lever on the fruit machine.

The effects of immunosuppressant drugs and AIDS on the immune system have confirmed the involvement of the immune system in malignancy. Stressful conditions may thus directly influence the risk of established malignancies. In addition to the effects on the production and circulation of B and T lymphocytes which may influence the risk of the success of viruses believed to be responsible for some cancers, there is the possibility of direct effects of stress on natural killer (NK) cell activity. These cells normally destroy malformed cells, and any suppression of their function at a critical stage in the early cancer process could be very

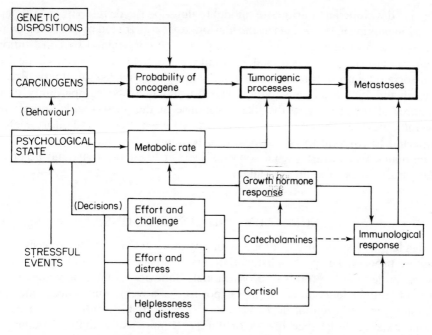

FIG. 32.6   Possible role of stress and decision in the risk of malignant disease.

significant. The NK cells may not only afford defences against tumour cells, they may prevent metastases (Hanna and Fidler, 1980). Injections of hydrocortisone in mice suppress some aspects of NK activity (Hochman and Cudkowicz, 1979).

The control hypothesis would predict that those who react to life stresses with perceived low control should be at risk for cancerous disease. Sklar and Anisman (1979, 1981) reported that exacerbation of tumour growth is evident following acute exposure to uncontrollable as compared with controllable stress. Acute exposure to uncontrollable stress is reported as a major exacerbating factor.

In Chapter 20 (this volume), Cooper points to the vulnerability of the repressed personality, characterized by lack of ability to express emotion. This finding seems to occur repeatedly in studies of life events and cancer. This may reflect a constitutional disposition to respond to life events with passivity. Nieburgs et al. (1979) have shown that women with repressed hostility had the most marked lymphocyte population changes, indicative of immunosuppression. Perhaps hostility which is expressed is terminated, whereas unexpressed hostility continues to be a focus for ruminative activity and drives adverse hormone states.

Thomas et al. (1974, 1979) demonstrated that lack of closeness to parents was more likely to have characterized the life history of those with malignancies. However, the degree of closeness did not distinguish the person likely to incur malignancy from the potential suicide or depressed individual. So there may be a need for a more complex explanation, if different forms of illness are to be predicted.

One possible explanation is that life experiences create styles of behaviour which change the possibility of effective coping with life stresses. Fisher (1986,

Ch. 11) developed a 'marionette' model to describe the development of styles in decision making in stress. Just as the marionette is constricted by the strings which dictate styles of dance, so the individual may be constrained by constitutional factor and life experiences to make certain types of decision. The bias in decision is associated with hormone balance and the differential risk of illness. Psychological and biological sensitivities develop and it is the compatibility of the features of the stress and the likely response of the person which determines overall outcome. Thus the person whose style favours action and effort might be expected to respond to the demise of a terminally ill relative by seeking new treatments. By contrast, the person who is less inclined to activity may accept the standard medical treatment available.

SUMMARY AND CONCLUSIONS

This chapter has been concerned with cognitive activity in the genesis of the disease process. The probabilistic relationship between stress and disease can be better understood in terms of a risk model. Behavioural links may increase the risk of antigen encounter or the exposure to adverse substances, including carcinogens. Differential decisions concerning available control reflect in hormone balance and hence in risk of illness. Ruminative activity is assumed to provide the necessary conditions for persistent adverse biological states and hence to provide a further risk factor in all types of illness.

REFERENCES

Amkraut, A., & Solomon, C.F. (1975). From the symbolic stimulus to the pathophysiologic response immune mechanisms. *International Journal of Psychiatry in Medicine, 5*, 541–563.

Ax, A.F. (1953). The physiological differentiation between fear and anger in humans. *Psychological Medicine, 15*, 433–442.

Berkson, J. (1962). Mortality and marital status. Reflections on the derivation of aetiology from statistics. *American Journal of Public Health, 52*, 1318–1333.

Brady, J.V. (1958). Ulcers in 'executive monkeys'. *Scientific American, 199*, 95–100.

Cannon, W.B. (1932). *The wisdom of the body*. New York: Norton.

Cannon, W.B. (1936). *Bodily changes in pain, hunger, fear and rage*. New York: Appleton-Century-Crofts.

Carruthers, M. (1974). *The western way of death*. London: Davis-Poynter.

Connolly, J. (1975). Circumstances, events and illness. *Medicine, 2*,(10), 454–458.

Cox, T., & MacKay, C. (1982). Psychosocial factors and psychophysiological mechanisms in the aetiology and development of cancers. *Social Science and Medicine, 16*, 381–396.

Dodge, D.L., & Martin, W.T. (1970). *Social stress and chronic illness. Mortality patterns in industrial society*. London: University of Notre Dame Press.

Faris, R.E.L., & Dunham, H.W. (1939). *Mental disorders in urban areas*. Chicago: University of Chicago Press.

Fisher, S. (1984). *Stress and the perception of control*. London, New Jersey: Lawrence Erlbaum.

Fisher, S. (1986). *Stress and strategy*. London: Lawrence Erlbaum.

Frankenhaeuser, M., & Gardell, B. (1976). Underload and overload in working life: Outline of a multidisciplinary approach. *Journal of Human Stress, 2*, 35–46.

Frankenhaeuser, M., & Johansson, J. (1982). Stress at work: Psychobiological and psychosocial aspects. Paper presented at the 20th International Conference of Applied Psychology, Edinburgh, July 25–31.

Frankenhaeuser, M., & Rissler, A. (1970). Effects of punishment on catecholamine release and the efficiency of performance. *Psychopharmacologia, 17*, 378–390.

Fried, M. (1963). Transitional functions of working class communities: implications for forced relocation. In M.B. Kantor (ed), *Mobility and mental health* (Chapter 6). Springfield, Illinois: Charles C Thomas.

Funkenstein, D.H., King, S.H., & Drolette, M.E. (1957). *Mastery of stress*. Cambridge, Mass.: Harvard University Press.

Hanna, N., & Fidler, I.J. (1980). Role of natural killer cells in the destruction of circulating tumor emboli. *Journal of the National Cancer Institute, 65*, 801–809.

Hochman, P.S., & Cudkowicz, G. (1979). Suppression of natural toxicity by spleen cells of hydrocortisone treated mice. *Journal of Immunology, 123*, 968–976.

Holmes, T.H., & Rahe, R. (1967). The social readjustment rating scale. *Journal of Psychosomatic Research, 11*, 213–218.

Horovitz, A.P., Beer, B., & Clody, D.E. (1972). Cyclic AMP and anxiety. *Psychosomatics, 13*, 85–92.

Johansson, G., & Sanden, P. (1982). Mental load and job satisfaction in control room operators. *Rapporter* (University of Stockholm), No. 40.

Karasek, R.A. (1979). Job demands, job decision latitude and mental strain: implicated for job redesign. *Administrative Science Quarterly, 24*, 43–48.

Lacey, J. (1967). Somatic response patterning and stress: Some revisions of the activation theory. In M.H. Appley & R. Turnbull (eds), *Psychological stress: issues in research*. New York: Appleton-Century-Crofts.

Leff, M.J., Roatch, J.F., & Bunney, W.E. (1970). Environmental factors preceding the onset of severe depressions. *British Journal of Psychiatry, 33*, 293–311.

Malmo, R.B., & Shagass, C. (1949). Physiologic study of symptom mechanisms in psychiatric patients under stress. *Psychosomatic Medicine, 11*, 25–29.

Masmot, M.G., & Syme, S.L. (1976). Acculturation and coronary heart disease in Japanese-Americans. *American Journal of Epidemiology 104*(3), 225–247.

Mason, J.W., Tolson, W.W., Brady, J., & Gilmore, L. (1968). Urinary epinephrine and norepinephrine responses to 72 hour avoidance sessions in the monkey. *Psychosomatic Medicine, 30*, 640–665.

McDougall, J.B. (1949). *Tuberculosis—a global study in psychopathology*. Baltimore: Williams & Wilkins.

Monjan, A.A., & Collector, M.I. (1977). Stress-induced modulation of the immune response. *Science, 196*, 307–308.

Moorman, L. (1950). Tuberculosis on the Navaho Indian Reservation. *American Review of Tuberculosis, 61*, 586–596.

Nieburgs, H.E., Weiss, J., Navarrete, M., Strax, P., Teirstein, A., Grillione, G., & Siedlecki, B. (1979). The role of stress in human and experimental oncogenesis. *Cancer Detection and Prevention, 2*, 307–336.

Rahe, R. (1972). Subjects' recent life changes and their near future illness reports. *Annals of Clinical Research, 4*, 250–265.

Rassmussen, A.F. (1957). Emotions and immunity. *Annals of the New York Academy of Sciences, 254*, 458–461.

Riley, V. (1979). Cancer and stress: Overview and critique. *Cancer Prevention and Detection, 2*, 163–195.

Riley, V., Spackman, D., McClanahan, H., & Santisteban, G.A. (1979). The role of stress in malignancy. *Cancer Detection and Prevention, 2*, 235–255.

Selye, H. (1956). *The stress of life*. London, New York, Toronto: Longmans Green.

Sigerist, H. (1932). *Man and medicine* (trans. M. Boise). New York: W.W. Norton.

Sklar, S.L., & Anisman, H. (1979). Stress and coping factors influence tumor growth. *Science, 205*, 513–515.

Sklar, S.L., & Anisman, H. (1981). Stress and cancer. *Psychological Bulletin, 89*,3, 369–406.

Solomon, G.F., & Amkraut, A.A. (1979). Neuroendocrine aspects of the immune response and their implications for stress effects on tumor immunity. *Cancer Detection and Prevention, 2*, 197–223.

Sterling, P., & Eyer, J. (1981). Biological basis of stress related mortality. *Social Science and Medicine, 15E*, 3–42.

Stokols, D., Schumaker, S.A., & Martinez, J. (1983). Residential mobility and personal well being. *Journal of Environmental Psychology, 3*, 5–19.

Thomas, C.B., & Duszynski, K.R. (1974). Closeness to parents and the family constellation in a prospective study of five disease states: Suicide, mental illness, malignant tumour, hypertension and coronary heart disease. *Johns Hopkins Medical Journal, 134*, 251–270.

Thomas, C.B., Duszynski, K.R., & Shaffer, J.W. (1979). Family attitudes reported in youth as potential predictors of cancer. *Psychosomatic Medicine, 41*, 287–302.

Totman, R. (1979). *Social causes of illness*. London: Souvenir Press.

Ursin, H., Baade, E., & Levine, S. (1978). *Psychobiology of stress: A study of coping men*. New York: Academic Press.

Wang, T., Sheppard, J.R., & Foker, J.E. (1978). Rise and fall of cyclic AMP required for the onset of lymphocyte DNA synthesis. *Science, 201*, 155–157.

Weiner, H. (1982). The prospects for psychosomatic medicine: Selected topics. *Psychosomatic Medicine, 44*, 6, 491–517.

Weis, J.M. (1968). Effects of coping responses on stress. *Journal of Comparative Physiological Psychology, 65*, 251–266.

Wolff, H.G. (1952). *Stress and disease*. Springfield, Illinois: Charles C Thomas.

KEY WORDS

Life stress, health, social change, life change, control, demand, effort and distress, job strain, disease, malignant disease, infectious disease, chronic disease, social disruption models, control model, arousal, ruminative states.

33

Psychobiological Factors in Stress and Health

TOM COX
University of Nottingham

INTRODUCTION

It is a common assumption, if not a 'cultural truism' (Leventhal and Tomarken, 1987), that the experience of stress is necessarily associated with the impairment of health. However, while any suggestion that 'the experience of stress can be good for you' should be vigorously debated, it is not correct that it is inevitably detrimental to health. Much of the person's response to the experience of stress, both psychological and physiological, is comfortably within the body's normal homeostatic limits and, while taxing the psychobiological mechanisms involved, need not cause any lasting disturbance or damage. At the same time, it is obvious that *all* negative emotional experiences, stress included, detract from the general quality of life and from the person's sense of well-being. Thus the experience of stress, while necessarily reducing that sense of well-being, does not inevitably contribute to the development of more serious psychological or physical disorder.

However, for some the experience of stress may well affect this process. Such an effect will be but one part of a two-way interaction between the experience of stress and the state of the person's health. Thus, while stress may affect health, there is also evidence that a state of ill-health can (a) act as a significant source of stress in itself, or (b) sensitize the person to other sources of stress by reducing his or her ability to cope. Anecdotal evidence suggests that this relationship can, at any point in time, operate in both directions, establishing a positive-feedback loop, or 'vicious circle'. A simple correlation between self-reported stress and ill-health can therefore only reflect the existence of this interaction and say nothing about causality.

Within these limits, the common assumption of a relationship between the experience of stress and poor health is justified. However, for such an hypothesis to have any social importance or practical usefulness it has to be examined in greater detail. Such an examination must address not only the fact of that relationship, but also the nature of the psychobiological mechanisms that might underpin it. These mechanisms are discussed in this chapter in terms of the nature of stress and health, and the measurement of suboptimum health, the alleged effects of stress on the immune system and cancer(s), and the nature and origin of the post-traumatic stress syndrome.

THE DEFINITION OF HEALTH

The definition of health has been no less a subject for debate than that of stress (see later), although the broad view espoused by the World Health Organisation (1946) is often cited as a starting point for further discussion and development. In its constitution, the WHO offered a dynamic and positive definition of health in terms of psychological and social as well as physical well-being, and emphasized that it is both dynamic and changeable (like the weather). Somewhat later, Rogers (1960) proposed that the health state was a function both of the individual's heredity, and of the accumulated and current effects of the person's environment as 'they act upon the psyche and body'. This offered an alternative approach to the traditional medical emphasis on constitutional and genetic factors. Rogers (1960) also suggested that health might be usefully viewed as a continuum, the opposing poles of which are 'complete well being' and 'death', with a significant watershed existing at the point where the person is recognized as being obviously ill or injured. Accepting this simple model immediately highights the area between complete well-being and obvious illness; an area which Rogers (1960) referred to as suboptimum health, and the advertizing world of the early 1960s discussed in terms of being 'one degree under'.

For most people, the day-to-day variation in their state of health occurs within this 'grey' area of suboptimum health, and therefore it may be changes in suboptimum health which reflect similar variation in the impact of the environment on the person, and any subsequent experience of stress.

THE NATURE OF SUBOPTIMUM HEALTH

There are several different questionnaire instruments which have been used to tap into subjects' suboptimum health, and which, by the nature of their scales and internal structure, offer some description of that area of health (Gurin et al., 1960; Crown and Crisp, 1966; Goldberg, 1972; Derogatis et al., 1974).

Studies at Nottingham have also attempted to map suboptimum health using self-reported symptoms of general malaise. Initially, a compilation of general non-specific symptoms of ill-health was produced from existing health questionnaires (see above) and from diagnostic texts. These symptoms included reportable aspects of cognitive, emotional, behavioural and physiological function, none of which was clinically significant in itself. From this compilation, a prototype checklist was designed with each symptom being associated with a five-point frequency scale ('never' through to 'always') which referred to a 6-month response window. In a series of classical factor analytical studies on British subjects, now variously reported (Cox et al., 1983; 1984), two clusters of symptoms or factors were identified (Table 33.1). These factors were derived as orthogonal.

Table 33.1 Original analysis and factor model (derived from Cox *et al.*, 1983)

Initial factor analysis: factors and associated Eigenvalues

Factor number	Eigenvalue	Variance (%)	Cumulative variance (%)
1	7.151	21	21
2	6.637	19.5	40.5
3	1.334	3.9	44.4
4	1.267	3.7	48.2
5	1.168	3.4	51.6
6	1.009	3.0	54.6
7	0.945	2.8	57.4

Item loading on the 2 factor scale

Item number	Loading	Item content
Factor 1	*Worn out*	
26	0.78	Have your feelings been hurt easily?
18	0.78	Have you got tired easily?
4	0.72	Have you become annoyed and irritated easily?
27	0.69	Has your thinking got mixed up when you have had to do things quickly?
25	0.67	Have you done things on impulse?
24	0.65	Have things tended to get on your nerves and wear you out?
12	0.66	Has it been hard for you to make up your mind?
6	0.59	Have you got bored easily?
1	0.58	Have you been forgetful?
11	0.54	Have you had to clear your throat?
8	0.54	Has your face got flushed?
7	0.53	Have you had difficulty in falling or staying asleep?
15	0.43	Have you had pains or soreness in your eyes?
Factor 2	*Up-tight/ tense*	
33	0.78	Have you worn yourself out worrying about your health?
44	0.66	Have you been tense and jittery?
38	0.65	Have you been troubled by stammering?
32	0.65	Have you had pains in the heart or chest?
40	0.62	Have unfamiliar people or places made you afraid?
31	0.61	Have you been scared when alone?
2	0.60	Have you been bothered by thumping of the heart?
9	0.60	Have people considered you to be a nervous person?
16	0.59	When you have been upset or excited has your skin broken out in a rash
34	0.57	Have you shaken or trembled?
41	0.47	Have you experienced loss of sexual interest or pleasure?
43	0.47	Have you cried easily?
28	0.43	Have you been having a good stiff drink?
20	0.42	Have you had numbness or tingling in your arms or legs?
39	0.32	Have you bitten your nails?

The first factor (GWF1) was defined by symptoms relating to tiredness, emotional lability, and cognitive confusion; it was colloquially termed 'worn out'. The more cognitive items would appear to imply difficulties in decision making (in the specific context of feeling 'worn out'): (a) has your thinking got mixed up when you have had to do things quickly? (b) has it been hard for you to make up your mind? and (c) have you been forgetful? These may have implications for personal problem solving and coping (see later; also Cox, 1987). The second factor (GWF2) was defined by symptoms relating to worry and fear, tension, and physical signs of anxiety; it was colloquially termed 'up-tight and tense'. This model of suboptimum health appeared to have some face validity in that it was acceptable to a conference audience of British general practitioners and medical and psychological researchers (see Cox *et al.*, 1983).

A questionnaire was derived from this factor model, and has now been used in a number of studies conducted by the Stress Research Group at Nottingham, and elsewhere by other researchers.

Scores on both scales have been shown to be determined by the nature of the person, and by the nature of his or her work and work environment. For example, a study of 300 schoolteachers revealed that 'neuroticism' scores on the Eysenck Personality inventory were significantly related to scores on the general well-being questionnaire, concurrently administered. Between 37% and 41% of the variance in well-being was accounted for by 'neuroticism' (emotional instability). However, there was no significant relationship between 'extraversion' and well-being (Cox *et al.*, 1983). Significant sex differences have been reported for workers engaged in semiskilled and unskilled work (Cox *et al.*, 1984). Working women were shown to report poorer well-being than working men, controlling for the age of the worker. Within this sample, well-being scores were shown to be related to the nature of the work on which the person was employed, e.g. repetitive versus non-repetitive (Cox, 1985b). Scores on the general well-being questionnaire have also been shown to influence the person's response to his or her work measured in other ways. Cox, Davis and Cook (unpublished) have shown that the effects of routine computer-based work (data entry) on the report of 'muscular aches and pains' are conditioned by the subjects' scores on GWF1, but not by those on GWF2.

The questionnaire has thus been used in the Nottingham studies in two different ways, to provide not only (a) a dependent measure related to health, but also (b) a moderator or covariable for effects on other health (and performance) measures.

New data have been collected by Cox and Gotts through a series of linked studies in Britain and Australia. These data have recently been re-analysed and the model and its associated scales have been slightly amended to increase their robustness in relation to this international sample (and also to diverse homogeneous samples).

A number of symptoms have now been deleted from the two original scales, although no new symptoms have been added. The two new 'international' scales are now defined by twelve symptoms (Table 33.2), but retain their essential nature: 'worn out' and 'up-tight and tense'. The deleted symptoms were among the weaker ones in terms of scale definition (and item loadings). New norms have been computed for the 'international' scales and are to be published elsewhere (Cox and Gotts, unpublished); the conversion weights for transforming the old scores into new international scale scores are also to be published.

It is thus suggested that suboptimum health, the 'grey area' between complete well-being and obvious illness, is made up of two states, one related to being 'worn out', and the other related to being 'up-tight and tense'. The former has an interesting cognitive component, possibly related to decision making and coping, while the latter is partly defined by physical symptoms of anxiety and tension. It has been shown that people vary in the extent to which they report these feelings, both between individuals and across time, and it has been suggested that this variation may not only reflect the experience of stress, but also affect other responses of stress, such as self-reported mood (see Mackay *et al.*, 1978; Cox and Mackay, 1985).

THE DEFINITION OF STRESS

The various approaches to the definition and study of stress have been reviewed elsewhere (for example, Lazarus, 1966; Appley and Trumbull, 1967; McGrath, 1970; Cox, 1978; Cox and Mackay, 1981; Laux and Vossel, 1980). The present

Table 33.2 Items defining scales: international analysis

GWF1	International scale

Have your feelings been hurt easily?
Have you got tired easily?
Have you become annoyed and irritated easily?
Has your thinking got mixed up when you have had to do things quickly?
Have you done things on impulse?
Have things tended to get on your nerves and wear you out?
Has it been hard for you to make up your mind?
Have you got bored easily?
Have you been forgetful?
Have you had to clear your throat?
Has your face got flushed?
Have you had difficulty in falling or staying asleep?

GWF2	International scale

Have you worn yourself out worrying about your health?
Have you been tense and jittery?
Have you been troubled by stammering?
Have you had pains in the heart or chest?
Have unfamiliar people or places made you afraid?
Have you been scared when alone?
Have you been bothered by thumping of the heart?
Have people considered you a nervous person?
When you have been upset or excited has your skin broken out in a rash?
Have you shaken or trembled?
Have you experienced loss of sexual interest or pleasure?
Have you had numbness or tingling in your arms or legs?

statement concentrates on what appears to be a developing consensus of scientific opinion around an essentially cognitive model of stress.

The term 'stress' refers to the *psychological* state which derives from the person's appraisal (Lazarus, 1966) of the success with which he or she can adjust to the demands of their environment (Cox, 1985a). Thus, stress is not a dimension of the physical or psychosocial environments; it cannot be defined simply in terms of workload or the occurrence of events determined by consensus to be stressful. Equally, it cannot be defined in terms of responses that are sometime consequences of stress, such as physiological mobilization or performance dysfunction. Stress resides in the person's perception of the balance, or 'goodness of fit', between the demands on them and their ability to cope with those demands. The absolute level of demand is therefore not the important factor in determining the experience of stress at work. What is important is the *discrepancy* that exists between the person's perception of those demands and their ability to cope with them.

A central feature of such 'transactional' approaches to stress is the process of cognitive appraisal (Lazarus, 1966), which Holroyd and Lazarus (1982) have defined as 'the evaluative process that imbues a situational encounter with meaning'. The present author has suggested that this process involves a continual *monitoring* of at least four aspects of the person's transactions with their environment, and a continual *evaluation* of the balance between them (Cox, 1987). Cognitive appraisal appears to take account of people's perceptions of:

(a) the demands on them,
(b) their personal characteristics and coping resources—their knowledge, attitudes, behavioural and cognitive skills, and behavioural style,
(c) the constraints under which they have to cope, and
(d) the support they receive from others in coping.

The situation which is typically perceived and experienced as stressful is one in which the person's resources are not well matched to the level of demand placed on them, and where there are constraints on how they can cope, and little social support for coping.

In addition to any consideration of its cognitive and perceptual elements, the state of stress is often defined by the person's experience of negative emotion, unpleasantness and general discomfort.

COPING AND CONTROL

Together, an awareness that a problem exists and an associated negative emotional experience normally initiate a cycle of changes in the person's perceptions and cognitions, and in their behavioural and physiological function. Some of these changes are attempts at mastering the problem, or attenuating the experience of stress, and have been termed 'coping' by Lazarus (1966). Coping usually represents either an adjustment *to* the situation or an adjustment *of* the situation. Elsewhere, the author has described the process of coping with stress within a 'problem-solving' framework, drawing from the literature on rational problem solving and decision making (Cox, 1987).

The concepts of coping and mastery imply the exercise of *control* over events. Fisher (1986; chapter 32, this volume) has suggested that people are more likely to *choose* to have control over aversive events than not, and are more likely to be tolerant of such unpleasant stimulation if it is self-delivered (presumably because of the potential for control that that implies—author). Fisher suggests that more complex strategies may be operating for those who do not choose such direct control.

It may be important to note that this notion of control could be of relevance to contemporary stress theory in at least three ways. First, demands and pressures may arise because the person has little control over important events. Second, the ease and success with which the person manages those demands and problems are partly determined by the constraints that he or she operates under, and thus the control over his or her own coping activities. Third, if the person fails to manage the demands being made on him or her, then this implies some continued lack of control over the total situation, which in turn opens up the possibility of a vicious circle being established (see first point).

It is obvious that the concepts of control and constraint, on the one hand, and demand, on the other, although theoretically discrete, are in a real or practical sense confounded. The person's perception and description of the demands that they face will be coloured by their perceived level of control, and questions about that level of control can only be meaningfully answered in relation to the recognition of demand. Furthermore, as implied in most 'transactional' approaches to stress, and made explicit by Fisher (1986), the perception of control and demand is dependent on the wider person × situation interaction, and neither is a passive property of the situation.

In addition to these psychological responses to stress, there may be significant changes in physiological function, some of which might facilitate coping, at least in the short term, but in the longer term may threaten physical health.

THE LIKELY MECHANISMS RELATING STRESS AND HEALTH

Not only is there a need to demonstrate that changes in the state of health are related to the experience of stress in a statistical sense, but there is also a need to describe the psychobiological mechanisms which might underpin such a relationship.

Part of the answer to this problem lies in the level of detail at which that answer is attempted. As one example, the issue of criterial measures needs to be addressed. Research has to recognize: (a) the different types of negative health outcome which exist, (b) the possible specificity of effect across types, (c) the different stages which occur in the process by which ill-health develops, is recognized, expressed and treated, and (d) the different ways, both direct and indirect, in which these different factors can be measured. It is unlikely that the experience of stress will have an equal effect on each cell in this complex matrix. A similar requirement for detail exists in relation to all the other elements in the study of the relationship between stress and health, and, possibly, through this more focused research, a knowledge base of real practical importance might be developed and newspaper headlines such as 'Psychologist proves stress causes breast cancer' might be avoided. Interesting discussions of these and other related methodological issues have been published by Contrada and Krantz (1987) and Kasl (1987), and by Beehr and O'Hara (1987) and Komaki and Jensen (1986) in relation to stress in the workplace.

What might those underlying psychobiological mechanisms look like? The changes in physiological and psychological function and in behaviour which can accompany the experience of stress may provide the different mechanisms by which it translates into pathology. Cox *et al.* (1983) have suggested that there may be at least four ways in which stress can contribute to poor health.

(1) The behavioural strategies that the person develops to cope with the experience of stress may increase his or her exposure to health-damaging agents and health-risk behaviours, or decrease the frequency of those behaviours which promote or maintain health.

(2) The physiological response to the experience of stress may initiate or promote changes which directly contribute to the disease process by disrupting normal physiological function, for example high plasma noradrenaline levels may disrupt intermediary fat metabolism and promote the deposition of fat in the (coronary) arteries.

(3) The physiological response may also suppress the body's natural defences, hormonal or cell mediated, and allow the spread of infection or contribute to a failure to contain malignant growths.

(4) Coping and the more general psychological response to stress may involve a distortion of normal cognitive, emotional and perceptual processes, contributing to the development of an abnormal pattern of behaviour, isolation and a disruption of normal life.

These different mechanisms obviously have the potential for interaction, and common to those that affect physical health is the involvement of neuroendocrine mechanisms as intermediate but critical pathways.

COMMON PATHWAYS: PHYSIOLOGICAL RESPONSES TO STRESS

The physiological response to stress, like all other types of response, represents a change in some on-going activity and not an elicitation of activity in an otherwise quiescent system. More important, the overall physiological system is comprised of a heterarchy of interacting subsystems variously involving a variety of feedback (control) loops. Much of the response to stress is well within the operating limits of such control. As such, it may not pose any threat to the integrity of the overall system. However, it is possible that the response will exceed these limits and assume some pathological significance for one of at least two reasons: (a) the intensity of the challenge and response, or (b) the overriding of the control mechanisms by higher (cognitive) processes. Often the latter is of immediate value, facilitating behavioural coping, but, somewhat paradoxically, might, at the same time, offer its own longer term threat.

Endocrine Mechanisms

Interest in the physiological response to the experience of stress can be traced back through the early pioneering work of Cannon (1929) and Selye (1950), and has tended to focus on activity in two neuroendocrine systems: the sympathetic–adrenal medullary system and the pituitary–adrenal cortical system. The adrenal glands, and their associated hormones, have thus been central to discussions of stress physiology and psychophysiological theory (Cox *et al.*, 1983; Cox and Cox, 1985). Particular interest has been expressed in the behavioural and physiological functions of the catecholamines, adrenaline and noradrenaline, and in those of the corticosteroids.

Catecholamines

The physiological effects of the catecholamines are ubiquitous, but generally involve cardiocirculatory and metabolic effects similar to those occurring at the beginning of exercise. Indeed, this observation may provide a clue to their behavioural function. The main effects of adrenaline are the mobilization of glucose as a source of energy, and an increase in heart rate and cardiac output. Noradrenaline, by contrast, is a more potent vasoconstrictor, and is particularly important in the maintenance of blood pressure through changes in peripheral resistance. Increased blood pressure may serve, in turn, to decrease heart rate. Both hormones accelerate the rate and increase the depth of respiration, and both affect smooth muscle.

The behavioural function of the sympathetic–adrenal medullary system, and the catecholamines, was first explored by Cannon (1929). The evidence accumulated since his early studies suggests that increased activity in this system prepares the body for 'flight' or 'fight', and thus facilitates rapid powerful and sustained coping. The flight-or-fight reaction appears to be elicited when an animal is threatened or its power to control access to important objects is challenged. However, it may only occur when it is perceived that some sort of response is feasible and the threat or challenge can be met by effective action. Flight and fight have also been described as 'defensive aggression' and 'escape behaviour', respectively.

There is some evidence to suggest that the two catecholamines are differentially sensitive to behavioural and situational factors. Several dimensions have been suggested which may distinguish between the activities of the two hormones: passive–active coping (Elmadjian *et al.*, 1958); fear–anger (Funkenstein, 1956); psychological–physical effort (Dimsdale and Moss, 1980a; 1980b; Cox *et al.*, 1982). S. Cox and her colleagues (1982), for example, examined the effects of short-cycle repetitive work on urinary catecholamine excretion in women workers, using an adaptation of Diamant and Byers' (1975) analysis. She found that the hormones were differentially sensitive to various features of this type of work, such as different pay schedules and pacing requirements. On the basis of the available experimental evidence and other observations, it was suggested that noradrenaline levels were related to two things: first, the activity inherent in the different tasks under study, and second, the constraints (and frustrations) present in repetitive work. By contrast, adrenaline levels appeared related to feelings of emotional effort and stress. These suggestions are consistent with observations made by Frankenhaeuser and Gardell (1976) on Swedish sawmill operators.

By way of summary, Henry (1982) has implied that the behavioural correlates of noradrenergic activity tend to be more active and are characterized by anger and defensive agression. By contrast, the correlates of adrenergic activity tend to be more passive, and are characterized by anxiety and escape behaviour.

It has been variously suggested that increased activity in the sympathetic–adrenal medullary system, if not appropriately utilized, may contribute in some way to the development of a range of different disorders, not least of all coronary heart disease (see, for example, Surwit *et al.*, 1982).

However, despite a significant and continuing commitment to research into the psychosocial and behavioural factors involved in coronary heart disease, interest is now focusing on the second neuroendocrine system, the pituitary–adrenal cortical system, and on the glucocorticoids. There may be many different reasons why this is so, but undoubtedly one is the success attributed to research into coronary heart disease and the range of psychosocial and behavioural interventions that it has opened up. Another is the way current interest in the psychology of *control* (see Fisher, 1986) has married with the developing status of that concept in psychophysiology, particularly in relation to the pituitary–adrenal cortical system and the glucocorticoids.

Glucocorticoids

Increased levels of the glycocorticoids, cortisol or corticosterone, have a major effect on carbohydrate metabolism, but these vary with the target organ. In muscle, adipose and lymphoid tissue it is catabolic, but in liver they stimulate the synthesis and storage of glycogen (see, for example, O'Riordan *et al.*, 1982). Briefly, they bring about an increased production of glucose from tissue protein (gluconeogenesis), an increased deposition of glycogen in the liver, and a depression of fat synthesis from carbohydrates. The glucocorticoids also enhance the release of free fatty acids from adipose tissue and facilitate the absorption of insoluble fats through the stomach lining.

The metabolic effects of the glucocorticoids are largely catabolic, bringing about the release of energy. In this respect they share a common property with, at least, adrenaline. Furthermore, cortisol (and corticosterone) can enhance and maintain vascular reactivity to the catecholamines and thus bring about minor increases in blood pressure. They may also influence the metabolism of the catecholamines.

There is evidence that the glucocorticoids can affect immune system function (see Cox and Mackay, 1982; Cox, 1984); this may be of major importance to the discussion of stress and health and is discussed in some detail below.

STRESS AND THE IMMUNE SYSTEM

The alleged effects of stress on the immune system warrant more than passing attention, and the work of Riley is worth reviewing for two reasons. First, it provides a useful example of the animal studies which have been conducted in this area, and second, it provides some basis for describing the possible dynamics of the stress–cancer(s) relationship which need to be considered in the design of research studies in this general area.

The Research Studies of Riley

Not many experimental programmes have considered the effects of different sources of stress on hormone levels, markers of immune system function, and tumour growth. However, research on mice at the Pacific Northwest Foundation by Riley and his colleagues (Riley, 1979; 1981; Riley and Spackman, 1977; Riley *et al.*, 1979; 1981) has provided important data based on this paradigm.

Riley and his colleagues have demonstrated that exposure to non-traumatic stressors, such as rotation and handling, can significantly increase plasma corticosterone levels in mice. The relationship between speed of rotation and hormonal response was shown to be linear, as was the relationship between duration of handling stress and hormonal response. The latter data also indicated the rapidity of the corticosteroid response. Two points are of importance here: first, the stressors investigated were relatively mild and non-traumatic, in comparison with those used in the early studies on stress (see Selye, 1950), and second, the provision of what is effectively dose–response data for the stress–health relationship was an important methodological advance on many of the other studies in this area.

Two markers of immune competence were investigated in subsequent studies. It was shown that exposure to intermittent rotation significantly depressed leucocyte numbers (leucopenia) compared with unstressed controls. A 50% reduction occurred within 2 hours of exposure. Animals subjected to such stress also showed a marked reduction in thymus weight, which reached a nadir the day after exposure. There is evidence to suggest that thymocytes are destroyed by increases in plasma corticosterone such as have been shown to accompany exposure to stress.

Riley (1981) also considered the direct effects of exposure to rotation on the growth of implanted tumours. It was demonstrated that, in two substrains of C3H mice, exposure to rotation enhanced the growth of a lymphosarcoma which was non-histocompatible with the host (lack of tissue compatibility), but had little effect when the two were histocompatible. Mice, with implanted and non-histocompatible tumours, were exposed to intermittent rotation on days 4 to 6 after implantation. Tumour volume in the stressed mice increased significantly compared to their controls. A strong effect of corticosterone implants on tumour growth was also demonstrated. In subsequent experiments (Riley, 1981), it was shown that stress, in the form of viral challenge, accelerated the growth of a non-pigmented melanoma in the C57B1/6 line of mouse, but had no effect on the development of the pigmented melanoma, which is more histocompatible.

Interestingly, the timing of exposure to corticosterone, and possibly stress, appeared important. When a synthetic corticoid was injected into the mice 7 days before tumour implantation, an enhancement of immunological competence was observed. However, when administration occurred 7 days after implantation, tumour growth was accelerated, suggesting immunosuppression. Riley's (1981) data also suggest that young mice are more capable of resisting tumour growth than older ones.

Irwin and Anisman (1984), while conceding that these data are impressive, have emphasized that alternative interpretations of the experiments are possible based on differences in the growth rates of the various tumours studied and in the reactivity of the mouse strains to aversive stimuli, particularly in relation to their physiochemical states. They also point out that Peters and Kelly (1977) had somewhat earlier demonstrated that manipulations, such as adrenalectomy, do not prevent the effects of exposure to stressors on tumour development. Furthermore, stress-induced enhancement of tumour growth has been seen using syngeneic tumours (that is, where the cell line and host are compatible) and this effect could not be reversed by reconstitution of syngeneic spleen cells (Jamasbi and Nettesheim, 1977). It would therefore seem possible that, in addition to corticosterone-induced immunosuppression, these may be other mechanisms by which exposure to stress might enhance tumour growth.

Other Hormones

The adrenal cortical hormones are not the only ones known to be sensitive to exposure to stress, and similarly those other hormones may also be important in mediating the effects of stress on the immune system (see Cox, 1984; Irwin and Anisman, 1984). Growth hormone (GH), for example, is known to be sensitive to the experience of stress in humans (Charters et al., 1969; Yalow et al., 1969; Noel et al., 1972), and to exposure to stressors in other primates (Brown and Reichlin, 1972). Furthermore, the GH response is often dissociated from that of the glucocorticoids (Yalow et al., 1969), and appears to be more related than those hormones to individual differences in personality and behavioural style. For example, GH responders have been reported to score higher than non-responders on measures of social engagement (Greene, 1970; Kurokawa et al., 1977), field dependence (Brown and Heninger, 1976) and type A behaviour (Friedman and Rosenman, 1971). The GH response also appears to be related to neuroticism (Miyabo et al., 1976). These relationships are of particular interest because there is also evidence that GH may enhance the immune response (Pierpaoli et al., 1969; Fabris et al., 1971; Gisler, 1974; Denckla, 1978). Snell–Bagg mice, a strain with cogenital hypoactivity of the pituitary and consequently low levels of GH, display decreased antibody reactions to sheep red blood cells (SRBC) and deficient rejection of transplanted tissue. Both can be reversed through the administration of GH (and thyroxine) (Pierpaoli et al., 1969; Fabris et al., 1971). Likewise, the suppression of humoral responses to SRBC, following the administration of glucocorticoids, can be restored with GH (Gisler, 1974). Somewhat similarly, there is evidence linking the fluctuations in the levels of thyroid hormones, testosterone and the catecholamines both to exposure to stressors and to the competence of the immune system.

A MODEL OF STRESS AND CANCER

The majority of the studies reviewed above have necessarily used animals as subjects, and it is difficult to conceive of a single study which could convincingly demonstrate all facets of the relationship between the experience of stress and the accelerated development of cancer(s) in humans. The analogy has been used (Cox and Mackay, 1982) that progress in this area is therefore dependent on piecing together a complex jigsaw puzzle of animal studies, clinical studies and observation, and psychophysiological experiments on healthy humans. However, some of the pieces have yet to be identified, let alone fitted into the emerging pattern. Despite this, on the basis of the developing evidence, the following model of the relationship between stress and cancer is proposed—as first described by Wayner *et al* (1979) and then modified by Cox (1984).

There are at least two different ways in which the experience of stress (humans), or exposure to stressors (animals), could effect the production of cancer(s).

First, the behavioural strategy which the person adopts or develops to cope with stressful situations may affect exposure to carcinogenic stimuli, for example through increased smoking (possibly combined with increased alcohol consumption), or through unsafe working procedures in environments where there are known carcinogenic hazards. Exposure to stressful situations may thus effect the *initiation* of the cancer process. Furthermore, both these behaviours and the person's physiological response to stress may act to facilitate the effects of existing carcinogens. This may involve changes in the general nature of the cellular and hormonal environments, resulting in them becoming more favourable for the malignant transformation of cells.

Second, the physiological response to stress may *promote* the malignant transformation and further development of cancer cells through the suppression of immune system function. It appears that these effects are most probably mediated by stress-sensitive hormones, in particular the glucocorticoids, although others may also be involved, for example growth hormone. Stress-associated blockade of immune effector cells may increase the probability of early transformed cells slipping through the host's defences. However, stress effects on antitumour activity could occur later in the development of cancer(s); at an early stage, spontaneous tumours may not be sufficiently different from self to be recognized by immune effector cells.

All such responses may be partly conditioned by covert personality traits or differences in behavioural or cognitive style, for example in the use of denial or repression as a cognitive coping strategy.

One particularly important question remains: how biologically significant, for humans, are these immunological effects of stress, most obviously demonstrated in laboratory experiments on animals? This question remains largely unanswered, although, as a sensible caution, it is worth noting remarks made by Fox (1981): '. . . compared to other . . . biological events, PF [psychosocial factors] may contribute a smaller amount in humans than in animals, assuming there is a contribution'.

STRESS AND OTHER DISEASES

Despite this, it might be worth asking whether this model of the stress–cancer relationship can be usefully generalized to other disease states. Once again, there is evidence to suggest that a variety of infections and other diseases are subject to the effects of stress, and that these effects are mediated by changes in endocrine activity (see Cox, 1984; Irwin and Anisman, 1984). Rasmussen (1969) has, for example, demonstrated that daily exposure to avoidance situations prior to viral inoculation significantly increased susceptibility to several different viruses— herpes simplex virus, poliomyelitis virus, Coxsackie B virus and polyoma virus. The immunosuppressive response appeared to be related to elevated levels of glucocorticoids. Furthermore, several different experiments have shown that handling, housing regimes, and mild aversive stimulation such as footshock, noise, restraint and isolation, can variously modify the rate of tumour growth in mice (Ader and Friedman, 1965; Levine and Cohen, 1959; Marchant, 1967; Ebbesen and Rask-Nielsen, 1967) and susceptibility to a wide range of diseases, including leukaemia, influenza, respiratory infection, malaria, infection with salmonella, and adjuvant arthritis (see Irwin and Anisman, 1984).

Stress and AIDS

In the light of this evidence, it is undoubtedly tempting to stretch the model too far and explore its application to acquired immune deficiency syndrome (AIDS).

AIDS, as the name suggests, is a complex combination of different diseases and symptoms that each contribute to the overall state of ill-health. It is basically a disorder affecting the cellular, or T cell, immune system. AIDS patients not only have fewer helper T cells than normal, but some of those that do exist have intrinsic defects. These changes are brought about by the human T cell lympho-trophic virus type III/lymphadenopathy-associated virus (HTLV III/LAV). The diseases which characterize AIDS are associated with defective T cell immunity, such as viral and fungal infections, and cancer(s). AIDS patients appear, at the moment, to fit into three general categories: some have only Kaposi's sacroma (KS) and no other symptoms, others have only severe opportunistic infections, such as *Pneumocystis carinii* pneumonia (PCP) or candida (thrush); and a third group has both KS and opportunistic infections. In general, patients in the third group suffer the most severe changes in their immune system, and patients with KS alone, the least (see Grierson, 1986).

T cell function is known to be affected by exposure to a variety of different stressors (Folch and Waksman, 1974; Kort and Weijma, 1982; Monjan and Collector, 1977; Laudenslager *et al.*, 1983; Teshima *et al.*, 1982). It is not clear, however, whether this effect is mediated by the glucocorticoids (see Irwin and Anisman, 1984, and, for example, Bartrop *et al.*, 1977). Furthermore, changes in T cell function have been observed in the absence of changes in T cell numbers. Significant changes in *responsiveness* were observed by Bartrop *et al.* (1977) in 26 bereaved spouses 6 weeks after their bereavement. These changes in T cell activity were not associated with any changes in cortisol, or thyroxine, prolactin or growth hormone.

While it is most unlikely that the effects of stress could rival those of HTLV III/LAV in their magnitude or clinical significance, is it possible that individuals whose T cell function is already affected by the experience of stress are the more susceptible to infection by HTLV III/LAV, or to the rapid development of its effects on T cell function after infection? If the effects of stress and HTLV III/LAV on T cell function are simply additive, then it is unlikely that stress will have any significant role to play in AIDS. However, if they are better described by an interactive model, then the position may be very different.

It might also be worth asking whether the development of AIDS after infection with the virus is part of the inevitable progression of the disease, or a triggered event, and if so whether any hormonal (or other stress-sensitive) factors operate on that trigger mechanism. Even if the development of AIDS after infection is inevitable, then, because it occurs at different rates in different individuals, it is still possible that external factors may have an influence. It is of interest to note that, at least in Europe and North America, the 'at-risk' groups are all characterized by particularly problematic and stressful lifestyles, for example male homosexuals and intravenous drug abusers, while pregnancy, with its hormonal changes, inevitably precipitates AIDS in females carrying the virus.

In Third World countries AIDS appears to be associated with different risk factors (Gong and Shindler, 1986). For example, the epidemiology of African AIDS offers striking contrasts to that of North American or European AIDS. Transmission of AIDS occurs both from male to female and from female to male, and most Africans with AIDS are promiscuous heterosexuals, and some of the women were prostitutes. Few, if any, of African AIDS cases admit to homosexuality, intravenous drug abuse or blood transfusions.

At least two possibilities exist. First, there are several different AIDS viruses with different associated risk groups and subject to different external influences. Second, the differences discussed above are not only associated with the virus but (also) with group differences in susceptibility to the virus, which may be sex dependent and again be differentially affected by other factors. It is impossible to speculate here on whether there is a disadvantage in stress associated with promiscuity in heterosexual males in African cultures, although it would be ridiculous to deny such stress in the case of prostitution.

SITUATIONAL AND BEHAVIOURAL CONTROL OF PITUITARY–ADRENAL CORTICAL ACTIVITY UNDER STRESS

If this developing model of stress and health is valid, then it is important to ask what situational and behavioural factors appear to control possibly critical changes in pituitary–adrenal cortical activity. Some answer is provided by Henry (Henry 1982; Henry and Stephens, 1977).

Henry's Model

Situations which involve loss of status or power appear to be associated with the increased secretion of corticosteroids in a variety of different species (see Henry,

1982). For example, adrenal cortical activity is increased in the rejected consort in rhesus monkeys (Sassenrath, 1970), in the lost infant monkey (Smotherman *et al.*, 1979), and in the immobilized rat (Mikulaj and Mitro, 1973). Furthermore, experimental situations which involve some degree of uncertainty or low predictability are also associated with increased corticosteroid secretion in rats (for example, Coover *et al.*, 1971). Mason (1968) has reported that small increases in corticosteroid levels occurred in rhesus monkeys that had learned an avoidance response to electric shock, but these contrast markedly with the elevations in hormone levels which occurred in monkeys that had learned the avoidance response but that were then presented with unavoidable shocks. The withdrawal of the avoidance response was more effective in raising corticosteroid levels than the shock itself. Likewise, Levine and his colleagues (Weinberg and Levine, 1980) have somewhat similarly demonstrated that corticosteroid levels in monkeys exposed to high noise or shock, but with some means of control over the aversive stimulus, are equivalent to those levels found in control animals. However, they are significantly lower than levels found in animals experiencing the same stimuli with no effective control. There is good evidence for the sensitivity of this type of response (Hennessy *et al.*, 1979).

Clinical studies have associated changes in corticosteroid secretion with depression. The reliability with which depressed persons fail to suppress plasma cortisol after dexamethasone administration (for example, Carroll *et al.*, 1976) is so high that a positive test has been accepted as evidence that a depressive state exists (Schlesser *et al.*, 1980). The changes in corticosteroid activity which occur include increased secretion with increased episodes of secretion, increased periods of active secretion, and disruption of normal circadian patterns (Sachar, 1980).

There is other, clinical, evidence that corticosteroid activity is associated with the cognitive processes involved with coping with stress. Wolffe *et al.* (1964), in a prospective study of parents of leukemic children, demonstrated that the most meaningful differences in urinary 17-OHCS excretion were those between individuals. Consistently lower levels of urinary 17-OHCS were excreted by parents who had adopted successful methods of coping with their children's fatal illness (and re-established some control over their stressful situation—author). Although the evidence is correlational, it seems that while denial is a successful cognitive defence and maintains low corticosteroid activity, personality traits such as denial and repression seem to be associated with high levels of corticosteroids (Fox, 1978).

Henry (1982) has suggested that the common element in all cited examples is exposure to stressful situations in which the subject experiences either a low degree of control or a loss of control and possibly helplessness (Seligman, 1968; 1975; Garber and Seligman, 1980). Feedback providing information on the success of 'controlling' behaviour (coping) also seems to be important (Weinberg and Levine, 1980), and perhaps has a role not only in decision making and problem solving in stressful situations (Cox, 1987) but also in learning how to cope (see later).

Situations which thus involve mastery or the otherwise gaining of control, or where events become predictable, should be associated with decreased cortico-steroid secretion. Mandell (1980), for example, has recently discussed the circumstances surrounding 'elation', and has linked the experience of this pleasure to activity in the septal-hippocampal system (and thus possibly to pituitary–adrenal cortical function) under the control of situations involving status enhancement, with their implications for increased security and control.

Learning, Mastery and Coping

The pituitary–adrenal cortical system appears to be partially under the control of the hippocampus (Henry and Stephens, 1977; Henry and Meehan, 1981), and thus its function may possibly be associated with the cognitive processes involved in general and social learning and memory (O'Keefe and Dostrovsky, 1971; Sinnamon et al., 1978; Ely et al., 1977). Direct evidence of a role for the pituitary–adrenal cortical system in learning comes from psychopharmacological studies on the behavioural effects of cortisol, for example, and ACTH. Brain and Poole (1974) have shown that increasing the activity of the cortisol–ACTH system can enhance the acquisition of conditioned learning behaviour in albino mice. However, such effects on learning behaviour may be largely due to ACTH, and, in this situation, the action of this endocrine may be extra-adrenal. However, it is possible that the 'loser' in situations involving conflict and loss of status or control may show increased pituitary–adrenal cortical activity and, in a wider evolutionary sense, this may be adaptive in two very different ways. First, if the loser is injured, then the immunosuppression which may accompany increased corticosteroid levels may increase the likelihood that the animal will perish, thus enhancing the principle of 'survival of the fittest'. However, if the animal is not injured, then it may be freed by ACTH to learn new patterns of behaviour (coping) and to learn them more rapidly. There is now evidence for this latter effect, as Krieger and Martin (1981) point out in their review of brain peptides. The 'winner', however, may show a relative inflexibility in their behaviour, thus maintaining their successful pattern of coping with conflict etc.

It can be concluded from this research that the concepts of perceived control and power are important for the relationship between stress and health. From what has been reviewed, this should seem obvious in relation to physical ill-health, such as cancer, but it is also relevant to psychological disorders, and in particular to post-traumatic stress disorder.

POST-TRAUMATIC STRESS DISORDER

There is an increasing literature on post-traumatic stress disorder which has been reviewed in the context of police work by Hillas and Cox (1987).

The first official American psychiatric classification of psychological malfunction, the *Diagnostic and statistical manual of mental disorders* (DSM-I), was published in 1952. The response to stress was included under the heading 'gross stress reactions'. In the subsequent revision of the manual (DSM-II: in operation from 1968 until January 1980), the developing diagnostic dilemma associated with

Table 33.3   The diagnosis of post-traumatic stress disorder (from Hillas and Cox, 1978)

1. Having experienced an exceptionally stressful event, which could be diagnosed as the basis of the problem

2. Re-experiencing that event; this might occur in a number of ways:
   - (2a) recurrent painful and intrusive recollections of the event
   - (2b) repeated dreams and nightmares
   - (3c) a dissociative state, fortunately very rare, lasting anything from a few minutes to several days. The victim acts as though reliving the original situation once more. This tends to be triggered by either something in the environment or by an intrusive thought

3. Numbing or responses to, or involvement with, the external world:
   - (3a) feeling detached from all things occurring around in the environment
   - (3b) being unable to enjoy things which were pleasurable before the incident
   - (3c) having an inability to feel close to others, to feel intimacy, or to feel tenderness or sexuality

4. A variety of other symptoms, of which at least two must not have been present before the trauma:
   - (4a) being hyperalert or having an exaggerated startle response
   - (4b) suffering initial, middle or terminal sleep disturbance
   - (4c) experiencing guilt at surviving when others perished or guilt over the actions needed in order to survive
   - (4d) having a memory impairment and/or trouble in concentrating
   - (4e) avoiding situations likely to lead to recall of the event
   - (4f) suffering an intensification of symptoms when exposed to events, situations or activities which resemble or symbolize the original trauma, for example, 'uniforms' could act as trigger to survivors of the death camps

the psychological reactions to stress (and trauma) was highlighted by the removal of that heading. Diagnoses such as 'traumatic neurosis' or 'neurosis precipitated by trauma' were classified as 'anxiety neurosis' or 'transient situational disturbance'. However, in the most recent edition of the manual (DSM-III), there is once more provision for the diagnosis of a stress or trauma response syndrome—post-traumatic stress disorder (PTSD).

Diagnosis of PTSD is partly dependent on the identification of the severely stressful event or trauma which precipitated the disorder, and partly dependent on the recognition of a cluster of symptoms. DSM-III describes the various symptoms which together constitute PTSD. The essential features and effects which must be expressed by the patient include re-experiencing the event in some way (from nightmares through to flashbacks), becoming numb or insensitive and unresponsive to people and events, and probably suffering sleep and memory disturbances. A more detailed list of the symptoms is presented in Table 33.3.

There may also be anxiety or depression, occasionally in an extreme form, and the victim may become irritable and show aggressive outbursts with little or no provocation. For example, Helweg-Larson et al., (1952) reported that 75% of a sample of ex-prisoners that they examined showed neutotic symptoms, the most common of which were restlessness, fatigue and irritability.

The extent to which any of these symptoms are exhibited may vary from causing mild impairment of behaviour to the disruption of almost every aspect of daily life. Stratton (1983) reports that about 6 out of every 10 US police officers involved in shooting incidents suffer untoward psychological reactions (63%). About half of these are severely affected. Burgess and Holmstrom (1978) report that 25% of rape victims still do not regard themselves as fully recovered from their ordeal as long as 4 to 6 years after the event. Sleep disturbances and a general preoccupation with the event are the symptoms which tend to persist the longest. Marris (1958), for example, discovered that in 72 clinically normal widows, 80% suffered insomnia, and Glick *et al.* (1974) have reported that widows continually rework the events leading up to their husbands' deaths, compulsively reviewing the course of the illness or accident. Bornstein and Clayton (1972) have reported that up to 67% of people experience a mild to severe reaction on the anniversary of the death of a spouse.

Time Course

Several accounts of the time course of PTSD exist (Ross, 1968; Figley, 1985; Green *et al.*, 1985). These have been reviewed elsewhere (Hillas and Cox, 1987), but several points can be usefully made here.

The time course for PTSD varies from victim to victim. Although the diminished responsiveness usually begins soon after the event, it is not rare for there to be a latency period of a few months, or occasionally a few years, before the psychological reaction becomes apparent. This presents a major problem for the diagnosis of PTSD and the management of the post-trauma situation.

Overall, two types or patterns of PTSD appear to exist: (a) acute and (b) chronic or delayed. Acute PTSD begins within 6 months of the trauma and the symptoms tend not to last for more than a further 6 months. The prognosis for such victims is generally good. By contrast, chronic or delayed PTSD is diagnosed if the symptoms are delayed for at least 6 months and then persist for more than 6 months. It has been suggested that the delay may be caused by the trauma being internalized in an attempt to avoid immediate pain; the prognosis for such victims is not good.

Nature of the Trauma

Leopold and Dillon (1963) made an important point when they commented that most of the early literature on PTSD regarded the traumas experienced as being more or less homogeneous in their characteristics. It is now obvious that this is not so. Incidents vary both in real terms, but, more importantly, in the way they are perceived by the victim. Several possible dimensions are discernible in the nature of these traumas.

(1) The victim is alone (rape) or in a group (military combat).
(2) The trauma may have a man-made basis but be purely accidental (air crash) or be man-made and deliberate (terrorist bomb attack).
(3) It may be entirely natural and beyond human control (earthquake).

The victim need not be the simple recipient of the trauma. He or she may even be an 'initiator' of the incident, as with the shooting incidents experienced by the police or during combat. Whatever is the case, the available evidence suggests that PTSD may be more severe and longer lasting if the source is of human design, and involves loss of control, power or status.

The loss of power and control over an important aversive situation, and any associated loss of status (humiliation), may determine two possibly related outcomes: (a) increased glucocorticoid activity (see above), and (b) conditioned helplessness, and hence depression (see Seligman, 1968; 1975). Thus the pyschological trauma might have implications, not only for psychological illness, but also for physical disorder. There are data to suggest, for example, that there is an excess appearance of disease after bereavement, at least within the first 6 to 12 months, but possibly little excess after that (Jacobs and Ostfeld, 1977).

SUMMARY AND CONCLUSIONS

It is safe to conclude from the available evidence that there is some effect of the experience of stress on the person's health, both physical and psychological. However, more specific and focused research is required to describe the detail of this relationship and to deal with the issue of causality. Such research should necessarily address the description of the underlying psychological and physio-pathological mechanisms.

On balance, this evidence suggests that the experience of stress is a factor in the determination of:

(1) general psychological and social well-being, although this is almost implicit in most contemporary definitions of stress;
(2) some chronic degenerative diseases, in particular coronary heart disease and some forms of cancer; and
(3) psychological disorders, especially that now recognized as post-traumatic stress disorder.

The evidence suggests that aspects of the endocrine response to stress may be of importance in the developing pathology of some chronic degenerative diseases. Although much effort has been expended in understanding the link between activity in the sympathetic–adrenal medullary system and coronary heart disease, interest has now been expressed in the role of the pituitary–adrenal cortical mechanism and the glucocorticoids in producing a depression of immune system activity. Immuno-suppression may have implications for the control of cancer development, and some animal experiments and clinical observation have linked the experience of stress to the accelerated development of some forms of cancer.

One psychological notion that has recurred throughout the evidence reviewed in this chapter is that of control. It has been pointed up as an important factor determining the experience of stress and in coping. It has also been implicated as a factor in determining pituitary–adrenal cortical function, and in post-traumatic stress disorder. Further research on its possibly critical role in health is therefore indicated.

The final comment must concern the importance of work-related factors and their study. Many of the events and processes cited in the available literature as relevant to health are to do with the nature or experience of work or the work/home interface. Not surprisingly, therefore, much of the research has been set within an occupational health context. While there is not scope within the present chapter to develop this discussion, it would be foolish, on the weight of current evidence, to deny the importance of work and its study in connection with the stress–health relationship.

REFERENCES

Ader, R., & Friedman, S.B. (1965). Differential early experiences and susceptibilities to transplanted tumours in the rat. *Journal of Comparative and Physiological Psychology, 59*, 361–364.

Appley, M.H., & Trumbull, R. (1967). *Psychological stress*. New York: Appleton-Century-Crofts.

Bartrop, R.W., Luckhurst, E., Lazarus, L., Kiloh, L.G., & Penny, R. (1977). Depressed lymphocyte function after bereavement, *Lancet, i*, 834–836.

Beehr, T.A., & O'Hara, K. (1987). Methodological designs for the evaluation of occupational stress interventions. In S. Kasl & C. Cooper (eds), *Stress and health: Issues in research methodology*. Chichester: Wiley.

Bornstein, P.E. & Clayton, P.J. (1972). The anniversary reaction. *Diseases of the Nervous System, 33*, 470–472.

Brain, P.F., & Poole, A.E. (1974). The role of endocrines in isolation-induced intermale fighting in albino laboratory mice. I Pituitary–adrenocortical influences. *Aggression and Behaviour, 1*, 39–69.

Brown, G.M., & Heninger, G. (1976). Stress induced growth hormone release: psychologic and physiologic correlates. *Psychosomatic Research, 38*, 145–147.

Brown, G.M., & Reichlin, S. (1972). Psychologic and neural regulation of growth hormone secretion. *Psychosomatic Research, 34*, 45–61.

Burgess, A.W., & Holmstrom, L.L. (1978). Recovery from rape and prior life stress, *Research in Nursing and Health, 1*, 165–174.

Cannon, W.B. (1929). *Bodily changes in pain, hunger, fear and rage: An account of recent researches in the function of emotional excitement*. New York: Appleton-Century-Crofts.

Carroll, B.J., Curtis, G.C., & Mendels, J. (1976). Neuroendocrine regulation in depression. II Discrimination of depressed from non depressed patients. *Archives of General Psychiatry, 33*, 1039–1051.

Charters, C.A., Odell, W.D., & Thompson, C. (1969). Anterior pituitary function during surgical stress and convalescence. Radioimmunoassay measurement of blood TSH, LH, FSH and growth hormone. *Journal of Clinical Endocrinology and Metabolism, 29*, 63–71.

Contrada, R.J., & Krantz, D.S. (1987). Measurement bias in health psychology research designs. In S. Kasl & C. Cooper (eds), *Stress and health: Issues in research methodology*. Chichester: Wiley.

Coover, G.D., Ursin, H., & Levine, S. (1971). Plasma corticosterone levels during active avoidance learning in rats. *Journal of Comparative and Physiological Psychology, 82*, 170–176.

Cox, S., Cox, T., Thirlaway, M., & Mackay, C.J. (1982). Effects of simulated repetitive work on urinary catecholamine excretion. *Ergonomics, 25*, 1129–1141.

Cox, T. (1978). *Stress*. London: Macmillan.

Cox, T. (1984). Stress: a psychophysiological approach to cancer. In C.L. Cooper (ed.), *Psychosocial stress and cancer*. Chichester: Wiley.

Cox, T. (1985a). The nature and measurement of stress. *Ergonomics, 28*, 1155–1163.

Cox, T. (1985b). Repetitive work: occupational stress and health. In C.L. Cooper & M. Smith (eds), *Job stress and blue collar work*. Chichester: Wiley.

Cox, T. (1987). Stress, coping and problem solving. *Work and Stress, 1*, 5–14.

Cox, T., & Cox, S. (1985). The role of the adrenals in the psychophysiology of stress. In E. Karas (ed.), *Current issues in clinical psychology*, Vol. 2. New York: Plenum.

Cox, T., Cox, S., & Thirlaway, M. (1983). The psychological and physiological response to stress. In A. Gale & J.A. Edwards (eds), *Physiological correlates of human behaviour*. London: Academic Press.

Cox, T., & Mackay, C.J. (1981). A transactional approach to occupational stress. In N. Corlett & P. Richardson (eds), *Stress, work design and productivity*. Chichester: Wiley.

Cox, T., & Mackay, C.J. (1982). Psychosocial factors and psychophysiological mechanisms in the aetiology and development of cancers. *Social Science and Medicine, 16*, 381–396.

Cox, T., & Mackay, C.J. (1985). The measurement of self reported stress and arousal. *British Journal of Psychology, 76*, 183–186.

Cox, T., Thirlaway, M., & Cox, S. (1984). Occupational well being: sex differences at work. *Ergonomics, 27*, 499–510.

Cox, T., Thirlaway, M., Gotts, G., & Cox, S. (1983). The nature and assessment of general well being. *Journal of Psychosomaic Research, 27*, 353–359. (Paper based on presentation to the 26th Annual Conference of the Society for Psychosomatic Research, Royal College of Physicians, London, December.)

Crown, S., & Crisp, A.H. (1966). A short clinical diagnostic self rating scale for psychoneurotic patients. The Middlesex Hosptial Questionnaire (MHQ). *British Journal of Psychiatry, 112*, 917–923.

Denckla, W.D. (1978). Interactions between age and neuroendocrine and immune systems. *Federation Proceedings, 37*, 1263–1266.

Derogatis, L.R., Lipman, R.S., Rickels, K., Uhlenhuth, E.H., & Convi, L. (1974). The Hopkins Symptom Checklist (HSCL). In P Pichot (ed.), *Modern problems in pharmacopsychiatry*, Vol 7, Basel: Karger.

Diamant, J., & Byers, S.O. (1975). A precise catecholamine assay for small samples. *Journal of Laboratory and Clinical Medicine, 85*, 679–693.

Dimsdale, J.E., & Moss, J. (1980a). Plasma catecholamines in stress and exercise. *Journal of the American Medical Association, 243*, 340–342.

Dimsdale, J.E., & Moss, J. (1980b). Short term catecholamine response to psychological stress. *Psychosomatic Medicine, 42*, 493–497.

Ebbesen, P., & Rask-Nielsen, R. (1967). Influence of sex segregated groupings and of inoculation with subcellular leukemic material on development on non leukemic lesions in DBA/2, BALB/C and CBA mice. *Journal of the National Cancer Institute, 39*, 917–932.

Elmadjian, F., Hope, J.M., & Lamson, E.T. (1958). Excretion of epinephrine and norepinephrine under stress. In G. Incus (ed.), *Recent progress in hormone research*. New York: Academic Press.

Ely, D.L., Greene, E.G., & Henry, J.P. (1977). Effect of hippocampal lesion on cardiovascular, adrenocortical and behaviour response patterns in mice. *Physiology and Behaviour, 18*, 1075–1083.

Fabris, N., Pierpaoli, W., & Sorkin, E. (1971). Hormones and the immunological capacity III. The immunodeficiency disease of the hypopituitary Snell–Bagg dwarf mouse. *Clinical and Experimental Immunology, 9*, 209–225.

Figley, C.R. (1985). *Trauma and its wake. The study of treatment of post traumatic stress disorder*. New York: Brunner/Mazel.

Fisher, S. (1986). *Stress and strategy*. London: Lawrence Erlbaum.

Folch, H., & Waksman, B.H. (1974). The splenic suppressor cell. *Journal of Immunology, 113*, 127–139.

Fox, B.H. (1978). Premorbid psychological factors as related to cancer incidence. *Journal of Behavioural Medicine, 1*, 45–133.

Fox, B.H. (1981). Psychosocial factors and the immune system in human cancer. In R. Ader (ed.), *Psychoneuroimmunology*. New York: Academic Press.

Frankenhaeuser, M., & Gardell, B. (1976). Underload and overload in working life: outline of a multidisciplinary approach. *Journal of Human Stress, 2*, 35–46.

Friedman, M., & Rosenman, R. (1971). Type A behaviour pattern: its association with coronary heart disease. *Annals of Clinical Research, 3*, 300–312.

Funkenstein, D.H. (1956). Norepinephrine like and epinephrine like substances in relation to human behaviour. *Journal of Nervous and Mental Diseases, 124*, 58–68.

Garber, J., & Seligman, M.E.P. (1980). *Human helplessnesss*. New York: Academic Press.

Gisler, R.H. (1974). Stress and the hormonal regulation of the immune response in mice. *Psychotherapy and Psychosomatics, 23*, 197–208.

Glick, I.O., Weiss, R.S., & Parkes, C.M. (1974). *The first year of bereavement*. New York: Wiley.

Goldberg, D.P. (1972). *The detection of psychiatric illness by questionnaire*. Maudsely Monograph No. 21. London: Oxford University Press.

Gong, V., & Shindler, D. (1986). Questions and answers about AIDS. In V. Gong & N. Rudnick (eds), *AIDS: Facts and issues*. New Brunswick: Rutgers University Press.

Green, B.L., Wilson, J.P., & Lindy, J.D. (1985). Conceptualising post traumatic stress disorder: a psychosocial framework. In C.R. Figley (ed.), *Trauma and its wake*. New York: Brunner/Mazel.

Greene, W.A. (1970). Psychologic correlates of growth hormone and adrenal secretory responses of patients undergoing cardiac catheterisation. *Psychosomatic Medicine, 32*, 599–614.

Grierson, H.L. (1986). The immunology of AIDS. In V. Gong & N. Rudnick (eds), *AIDS: Facts and issues*. New Brunswick: Rutgers University Press.

Gurin, G., Veroff, J., & Feld, S. (1960). *Americans view of their mental health*. New York: Edinburgh.

Helweg-Larson, P., Hoffmeyer, H., Kieler, J., Thaysen, E.H., Thaysen, J.H., Thygensen, P., & Dwulff, M.H. (1952). Famine disease in German concentration camps: complications and sequels with special reference to tuberculosis, mental disorders and social consequences. *Acta Medica Scandinavica, 144*, 3.

Hennessy, M.B., Heybach, J.P., Vernikos, J., & Levine, S. (1979). Plasma corticosterone concentrations sensitivity reflect levels of stimulus intensity in the rat. *Physiology and Behaviour, 22*, 821–825.

Henry, J.P. (1982). The relation of social to biological processes in disease. *Social Science and Medicine, 16*, 369–380.

Henry, J.P., & Meehan, J.P. (1981). Psychosocial stimuli, physiological specificity and cardiovascular disease. In H. Weiner, M.A. Hofer & A.J. Stunkard (eds), *Brain behaviour and bodily disease*. New York: Raven Press.

Henry, J.P., & Stephens, P.M. (1977). *Stress, health and the social environment*. New York: Springer-Verlag.

Hillas, S., & Cox, T. (1987). *Post traumatic stress disorder in the police*, occasional paper. London: Police Scientific Research and Development Branch, Home Office.

Holroyd, K.A., & Lazarus, R.S. (1982). Stress, coping and somatic adaptation. In L. Goldberger & S. Breznitz (eds), *Handbook of stress*. New York: Free Press.

Irwin, J., & Anisman, H. (1984). Stress and pathology: immunological and central nervous system interactions. In C.L. Cooper (ed.), *Psychosocial stress and cancer*. Chichester: Wiley.

Jacobs, S., & Ostfeld, A. (1977). An epidemiological review of bereavement. *Psychosomatic Medicine, 39*, 344–357.

Jamasbi, R.J., & Nettesheim, P. (1977). Non immunological enhancement of tumour transplantability in x irradiated host animals. *British Journal of Cancer, 36*, 723–729.

Kasl, S.V. (1987). Methodologies in stress and health: past difficulties, present dilemmas and future directions. In S. Kasl & C. Cooper (eds), *Stress and health: Issues in research methodology*. Chichester: Wiley.

Komaki, J.L., & Jensen, M. (1986). Within group designs: an alternative to traditional control groups. In M.F. Cataldo & T.J. Coates (eds), *Health and industry*. New York: Wiley.

Kort, W.J., & Weijma, J.M. (1982). Effect of chronic light–dark shift stress on the immune response of the rat. *Physiology and Behaviour, 29*, 88–92.

Krieger, D.T., & Martin, J.B. (1981). Brain peptides. *New England Journal of Medicine, 304*, 944–951.

Kurokawa, N., Suematsu, H., Tamai, H., Esakai, M., Aoki, H., & Ikemi, Y. (1977). Effect of emotional stress on human growth hormone. *Journal of Psychosomatic Research, 21*, 231–235.

Laudenslager, M.L., Ryan, S.M., Drugan, R.C., Hyson, R.L., & Maier, S.F. (1983). Coping and immunosuppression: inescapable but not escapable shock suppresses lymphocyte proliferation. *Science, 221*, 568–570.

Laux, L., & Vossel, G. (1980). Theoretical and methodological issues in achievement related stress and anxiety research. In H.W. Krohen & L. Laux (eds), *Achievement, stress and anxiety*. New York: Hemisphere.

Lazarus, R.S. (1966). *Psychological stress and the coping process*. New York: McGraw-Hill.

Leopold, R., & Dillon, H. (1963). Psycho-anatomy of a disaster. *American Journal of Psychiatry, 119*, 913.

Leventhal, H., & Tomarken, A. (1987). Stress and illness: perspectives from health psychology. In S. Kasl & C. Cooper (eds), *Stress and health: Issues in research methodology*. Chichester: Wiley.

Levine, S., & Cohen, C. (1959). Differential survivial to leukemia as a function of infantile stimulation in DBA/2 mice. *Proceedings of the Society for Experimental and Biological Medicine, 104*, 180–183.

McGrath, J.E. (1970). *Social and psychological factors in stress*. New York: Holt.

Mackay, C.J. Cox, T., Burrows, G.C., & Lazzerini, A.J. (1978). An inventory for the measurement of self reported stress and arousal. *British Journal of Social and Clinical Psychology, 17*, 283–284.

Mandell, A.J. (1980). Towards a psychobiology of transcendence: God in the brain. In J.M. Davidson & R.J. Davidson (eds), *The psychobiology of consciousness*. New York: Plenum Press.

Marchant, J. (1967). The effects of different social conditions on breast cancer induction in three genetic types of mice by dibenz (a,h) anthracene and a comparison with breast carcinogenesis by 3 methylcholanthrene. *British Journal of Cancer, 21*, 750–754.

Marris, P. (1958). *Widows and their families*. London: Routledge & Kegan Paul.

Mason, J.W. (1968). A review of psychoendocrine research on the pituitary–adrenal cortical system. *Psychosomatic Medicine, 30*, 576–607.

Mikulaj, L., & Mitro, A. (1973). Endocrine functions during adaptations to stress. *Advances in Experimental Medicine and Biology, 33*, 631–638.

Miyabo, S., Hisada, T., Asato, T., Mizushima, N., & Ueno, K. (1976). Growth hormone and cortisol responses to psychological stress: comparison of normal and neurotic subjects. *Journal of Clinical Endocrinology and Metabolism, 42*, 1158–1162.

Monjan, A., & Collector, M.I. (1977). Stress induced modulation of the immune response. *Science, 196*, 207–208.

Noel, G., Suh, H.K., Stone, J.G., & Frantz, A.G. (1972). Human prolactin and growth hormone release during surgery and other conditions of stress. *Journal of Clinical Endocrinology and Metabolism, 36*, 840–841.

O'Keefe, J., & Dostrovsky, J. (1971). The hippocampus as a spatial map. Preliminary evidence from unit activity in the freely moving rat. *Brain Research, 34*, 171–175.

O'Riordan, J.H.L., Malan, P.G., & Gould, R.P. (1982). *Essentials of endocrinology*. London: Blackwell Scientific.

Peters, L.J., & Kelly, H. (1977). The influence of stress and stress hormones on the transplantability of a non immunogenic syngeneic murine tumour. *Cancer, 39*, 1482–1488.

Pierpaoli, W., Baroni, C., Fabris, N., & Sorkin, E. (1969). Hormones and immunologica capacity II. Reconstitution of antibody production in hormonally deficient mice by somatotrophic hormone, thyrotropic hormone and thyroxin. *Immunology, 16*, 217–230.

Rasmussen, A.F. (1969).Emotions and immunity. *Annals of the New York Academy of Science, 164*, 458–461.

Riley, V. (1979). Stress–cancer contradictions: a continuing puzzlement. *Cancer Detection and Prevention, 2*, 159–162.

Riley, V. (1981). Psychoneuroendocrine influences on immunocompetence and neoplasia. *Science, 212*, 1100–1109.

Riley, V., Fitzmaurice, M.A., & Spackman, D.H. (1981). Psychoneuroimmunologic factors in neoplasia: studies in animals. In R. Ader (ed.), *Psychoneuroimmunology*. New York: Academic Press.

Riley, V., & Spackman, D. (1977). Cage crowding stress: absence of effect on melanoma within protective facilities. *Proceedings of the American Association for Cancer Research, 18*, 173.

Riley, V., Spackman, D., McClanahan, H. & Santisteban, G.A. (1979). The role of stress in malignancy. *Cancer Detection and Prevention, 2*, 235–255.

Rogers, E.H. (1960). *The ecology of health*. New York: Macmillan.

Ross, H. (1968). Cited in Carson, S. (1982). Post shooting reaction. *The Police Journal, 64*, 30–32.

Sachar, E.J. (1980). Hormonal changes in stress and mental illness. In D.T. Krieger & J.C. Hughes (eds), *The interrelationship of the body's two major integrative systems*. Sunderland, Mass.: Sinauer Associates.

Sassenrath, E.N. (1970). Increased adrenal responsiveness related to social stress in rhesus monkeys. *Hormones and Behaviour, 1*, 238–298.

Schlesser, M.A., Winokur, G., & Sherman, B. (1980). Hypothalamic–pituitary–adrenal axis activity in depressive illness. *Archives of General Psychiatry, 35*, 737–743.

Seligman, M.E.P. (1968). Chronic fear produced by unpredictable electric shock. *Journal of Comparative and Physiological Psychology, 66*, 402–411.

Seligman, M.E.P. (1975). *Helplessness: On depression, development and death*. San Francisco: Freeman.

Selye, H. (1950). *Stress*. Montreal: Acta.

Sinnamon, H.M. Freniere, S., & Kootz, J. (1978). Rat hippocampus and memory for places for changing significance. *Journal of Comparative and Physiological Psychology, 92*, 142–155.

Smotherman, W.P., Hunt, L.E., McGinnis, L.M., & Levine, S. (1979). Mother–infant relations. *Developmental Psychobiology, 12*, 211–217.

Stratton, J.G. (1983). Traumatic incidents and the police. *Police Stress, 6*, 4–7.

Surwit, R.S., Williams, R.B., & Shapiro, D. (1982). *Behavioural approaches to cardiovascular disease*. New York: Academic Press.

Teshima, H., Kubo, C., Kihara, H., Imada, Y., Nagata, S., Ago, Y., & Ikemi, I. (1982). Psychosomatic aspects of skin diseases from the standpoint of immunology. *Psychotherapy and Psychosomatics, 37*, 165–175.

Wayner, E., Cox, T., & Mackay, C.J. (1979). Stress, immunity and cancer. In D.J. Oborne, M.M. Gruneberg & J.R. Eiser (eds), *Research in psychology and medicine*. London: Academic Press.

Weinberg, J., & Levine, S. (1980). Psychobiology of coping in animals: the effects of predictability. In S. Levine & H. Ursin (eds), *Coping and health*. New York: Plenum.

Wolffe, C.T., Friedman, S.B., Hofer, M.A., & Mason, J.W. (1964). Relationship between psychological defences and mean urinary 17-hydroxycorticosteroid excretion rates. *Psychosomatic Medicine, 26*, 576–591.

World Health Organisation (1946). *Constitution of the World Health Organisation (3)*. Geneva: WHO.

Yalow, R.S., Varsano-Aharon, N., Echmendia, E., & Berson, S. (1969). HGH and ACTH secretory responses to stress. *Hormone Metabolism Research, 1*, 3–8.

KEY WORDS

Stress, suboptimum health, well-being, demand, ability, constraint, support, control, adrenals, adrenal cortex, adrenal medulla, catecholamines, glucocorticoids, corticosteroids, immune system, immunocompetence, cancers, post-traumatic stress disorder.

Handbook of Life Stress, Cognition and Health
Edited by S. Fisher and J. Reason
© 1988 John Wiley & Sons Ltd.

34

Allostasis: A New Paradigm to Explain Arousal Pathology

Peter Sterling
and
Joseph Eyer
University of Pennsylvania School of Medicine, Philadelphia

INTRODUCTION

This chapter summarizes our joint effort as epidemiologist (J.E.) and neuro-biologist (P.S.) to understand the physiological basis for certain broad patterns of human morbidity and mortality. Age-specific death rates rise when intimate social relations are disrupted. This is observed in contemporary statistics, for example the mortality associated with bereavement, divorce, migration and overwork. It is also observed historically in the increased mortality of urban versus rural popula-tions and in the rise of age-specific death rates that accompanies modern eco-nomic development. The increases in all these examples are large (two- to ten-fold) and are observed for essentially all causes, so they cannot be explained by any single environmental factor such as air pollution or nutrition (Berkson, 1962; Eyer and Sterling, 1977).

Disruptions to intimate social relations, including war, migration, and eco-nomic development, affect most strongly youth entering the labor market. The size of a particular birth cohort is especially important because this affects the competitive experience of that cohort throughout its lifecycle. A small cohort entering the labor market during an economic expansion experiences relatively mild competition and has lower death rates from all causes. A large cohort entering the labor market during an economic contraction experiences greater competition and social disruption and has correspondingly higher mortality (Eyer and Sterling, 1977).

The major causes of death shift as a cohort ages, but high mortality in youth from one set of causes presages high mortality later from another set. The large cohort born after World War II ('baby boom') entered the labor market in the 1960s at the end of a long cycle of economic expansion. It experienced elevated mortality at ages 15–24 from accidents, homicide, and suicide, and at ages 30–34 from liver cirrhosis (due to alcoholism). This cohort is now reaching the age at which the important causes of death become renal, cerebral, and cardiovascular disease (see Figure 10 in Sterling and Eyer, 1981), causes for which hypertension is the largest single contributor. Cancer, too, becomes an important cause of death, though its main impact comes somewhat later. Our historical studies predict for this cohort an increase in mortality from these causes (Eyer and Sterling, 1977).

Having discovered these patterns, we could find no explanation for them in textbooks of physiology. No text explains, for example, why in modern society blood pressure rises with age (Eyer, 1975). Nor do they explain why this rise starts at the age when children enter the environment of school (Figure 34.1; Blumenthal *et al.* 1977). Texts do not explain why blood pressure is highest and hypertension most prevalent where social disruption is greatest, e.g. among the unemployed and (in the US) among blacks. The most common form of hypertension is called in textbooks 'essential', meaning of unknown cause. In certain

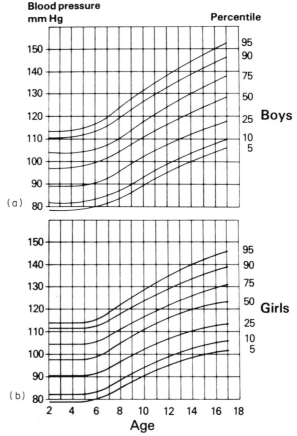

FIG. 34.1 Percentiles of diastolic blood pressure measurement (right arm, seated). (Reprinted from Blumenthal *et al.*, 1977.)

instances the epidemiological observations that we cite are acknowledged, but are given biological explanations that are unrelated to the social and psychological patterns. Thus, a standard explanation for elevated blood pressure in modern society is that salt consumption is excessive and beyond the kidney's capacity to excrete it. This is supposed to cause retention of excess salt water in the vascular system which causes the high blood pressure. Hypertension among blacks is commonly attributed to a genetic predisposition.

These explanations beg the questions *why* we eat so much salt and *why* the kidney fails to excrete it. Similarly, one needs to explain why the blood pressures of American and Caribbean blacks rise so much higher than those of the West Africans whose genes they share (Waldron, 1979). The only possible link between sociopsychological and physiological phenomena is the brain. Textbooks do not describe this link because the dominant conceptual model in physiology for a century has viewed the body as operating almost independently of the brain. Neurobiological studies of the 1960s and 1970s revealed many links between brain and soma, and appreciation of the richness of these links has accelerated in the 1980s. By now the evidence warrants abandoning the old conceptual model and adopting a new one in which the central nervous system is the pre-eminent regulatory influence on somatic physiology (Sterling and Eyer, 1981). Here, we review briefly the old model and present the new one, which accounts quite easily for the epidemiological findings.

HOMEOSTASIS VERSUS ALLOSTASIS

The principle of homeostasis is that to maintain stability an organism must hold all the parameters of its internal milieu constant (Bernard, 1865; Cannon, 1932). Deviations from normal are corrected automatically by local, 'negative feedback' mechanisms. Thus, normal blood sugar is about 80 mg/ml. A rise above this level can trigger release of insulin from the pancreas which leads to uptake of glucose by liver and muscle and restores blood glucose to normal. Similarly, normal blood pressure is about 110/70 mmHg. A rise above this level can trigger slowing of the heart, dilatation of the vessels, and excretion of salt and water by the kidneys. Those three factors—reduced cardiac output, enlarged vascular reservoir, and reduced blood volume—all contribute to restoring normal pressure.

The major thrust in physiological research for the last century has been to study isolated organs and tissues. It turns out that most organs function remarkably well when they are disconnected from the rest of the body and brain and placed in a dish. The pancreas releases insulin when glucose is added, and a slice of kidney pumps salt water. Consequently there has been great success in identifying the cellular and subcellular bases for local feedback control, and this has bolstered the idea that in the body the organs function autonomously.

On the other hand, when measurements of the internal milieu are made in an intact, unanesthetized organism, the results fit the homeostatic model very poorly. Consider Figure 34.2a, which is a continuous record of arterial blood pressure made from a normal adult human over a period of 24 hours (Bevan *et al.*, 1969). The pressure is by no means constant. Instead, there are many peaks and

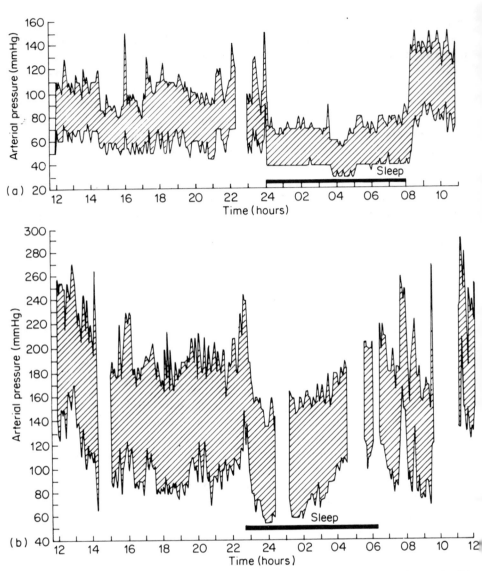

FIG. 34.2   (a) Arterial pressure from a normal subject plotted at 5-minute intervals. (b) Arterial pressure from a hypertensive subject. (Redrawn from Bevan *et al.*, 1969.)

troughs of varying size and duration. Some peaks are identified with specific behavioral states and environmental events. For example, the pressure fell between hours 15 and 16 when the subject was dozing in a lecture, and rose sharply at hour 16 when he awakened (briefly) to a jab from a pin. The pressure rose at hour 24 (midnight) when the subject engaged in sexual intercourse, and fell profoundly (as low as 50/30 mmHg) during sleep. At hour 08, when the subject was preparing to meet his work day, the pressure rose to the preorgasmic level of the previous night and remained there for hours.

It is obvious from this record that the idea of a 'normal' value toward which automatic mechanisms drive the blood pressure is a fiction. In one behavioral state the pressure is maintained low for a long period without restoration, and in another state it is held high for long periods, also without restoration. It makes no more sense to average the pressures from these different periods than it does to 'average' the states of sleep and wakefulness or the states of sexual arousal and satiety. Clearly, to achieve stability an organism must occupy each one of these different states and move flexibly between them. At each behavioral transition, the blood pressure must be reset to match the new state (see also Pickering et al., 1986).

An aroused behavioral state in which an organism is preparing to respond with some form of 'coping' behavior to an environmental challenge generally requires a rise in blood pressure. The early studies by Cannon emphasized acute, intense arousal engendered by pain, fear, and rage (Cannon, 1929). Later studies by Selye emphasized aroused behavioral states of somewhat longer duration and milder conditions (Selye, 1956). Whereas Cannon had studied animals prepared for immediate 'fight or flight', Selye studied animals under conditions of chronic frustration, for example a rat with its legs tied together for 24 hours. A still milder paradigm was introduced by Mason and colleagues in which an animal could avoid an electrical shock by watching for a signal and then pressing a lever (Mason, 1968). An aroused state can also be engendered in animals by disrupting a socially stable community, for example among mice by introducing a strange male into an established colony (Henry et al., 1967).

In all such animal models, when the acute or semichronic arousing stimulus is removed, the blood pressure falls. However, when the arousing stimulus is made chronic and removed only after a rather long period, the pressure may remain elevated. Thus, after many months of elevation in response to an avoidance conditioning paradigm, the high pressure in monkeys becomes sustained (Forsyth, 1969). Similarly, the elevated pressures evoked in rats as part of a 'defense response' by chronic brain stimulation also become sustained, even when the stimulation ceases (Folkow and Rubinstein, 1966). The elevated pressures in a mouse colony fall when the stranger is removed, but only if less then 6 months has elapsed; thereafter the pressure remains high even when the stranger is gone (Henry et al., 1967).

The question arises as to what other physiological parameters besides blood pressure covary with behavioral state. The answer is, essentially all of them (Table 34.1; Mason 1968, 1971, 1972). As blood pressure rises during arousal, there is a dramatic shift in the pattern of blood flow: more to muscle, less to the gut, kidney, and skin. Correspondingly, there is a metabolic mobilization to increase energy production. Glucose, amino acids, and fatty acids are released from their macro-molecular storage forms (glycogen, protein, and fat) and their blood levels rise. Synthesis of the storage forms is halted. Red blood cells and oxidative enzymes in the liver increase because these facilitate the energy mobilization. Other processes that use energy but that do not contribute to the metabolic mobilization are suppressed: the immune response declines as circulating white blood cells decrease and the thymus shrinks (Selye, 1956). Wound healing, bone growth and

Table 34.1   Catabolic state (arousal)

Increase
Blood pressure
Cardiac output
Retention of salt and water (to support blood pressure)
Blood to muscle
Breakdown of carbohydrate, fat, protein
Blood levels of glucose, fatty acids, amino acids
Circulating red cells
Production of red cells
Synthesis of oxidative enzymes (liver)

Decrease
Blood to kidney, skin, gut
Synthesis of glycogen, fat, protein
Repair, replacement, growth of bone
Replacement of cells with high turnover (gut, skin, etc.)
Production of cells for immune system (thymus, lymph nodes, bone marrow)
Sexual processes (endocrine, cellular, psychological, behavioural)

The *anabolic state* (relaxation) is accompanied by a reversal of the above pattern.

repair, replacement of the cellular lining of the gut, etc. all slow markedly. Thus, corresponding to the behavioral/psychological state of arousal there is a biochemical state of 'catabolism', that is, breakdown of metabolic compounds to produce energy. Corresponding to states of relaxation is a biochemical state of 'anabolism', that is, a rebuilding of energy stores, repair, and growth (Mason, 1972).

The catabolic mobilization accompanying arousal is accomplished by shifts in essentially all the known hormones. Catabolic hormones (those that promote energy production), e.g. epinephrine, norepinephrine, cortisol (glucocorticoids), growth hormone, glucagon, and thyroxine, increase. Anabolic hormones (those that promote growth and repair), e.g. insulin, estrogen, and testosterone, decrease. The timing of these changes is complex because certain hormones, such as epinephrine, cortisol, and growth hormone, serve the acute mobilization and rise almost instantaneously (seconds to minutes), while others, such as thyroxine and the sex hormones, have slower, modulatory roles and rise or fall over longer periods (hours to weeks). Other hormones that indirectly support energy production also change (Mason, 1968). For example, vasopressin (antidiuretic hormone), renin, angiotensin II, and aldosterone all increase (see Sterling and Eyer, 1981) and atripopeptin decreases (Eskay *et al.*, 1986). This pattern serves the aroused state by increasing the rate of circulation through the cardiovascular system (Fig. 34.3).

A list of some hormones associated with the catabolic and anabolic states is given in Table 34.2. It is notable that quite a few of them have been discovered only recently, e.g. the opiate hormones (enkephalin, dynorphin, and endorphin: Akil *et al.*, 1984), the cardiac hormone (atriopeptin: Manning *et al.*, 1985; Eskay *et al.*, 1986; Dillingham and Anderson,1986), and the immune system hormones (interleukins and thymosins: Goetzl, 1985). The discovery rate of new, physio-

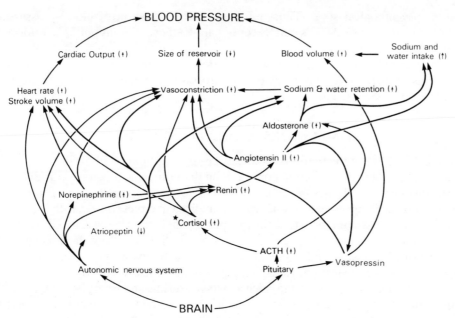

FIG. 34.3 Multiple, mutually reinforcing mechanisms to raise blood pressure during arousal. Negative feedbacks reset or overridden. (*Indicates that cortisol acts indirectly by enhancing receptor binding of norepinephrine.)

logically active peptides increases as techniques in molecular biology advance. *All physiologically active substances and processes discovered so far are regulated and therefore fluctuate with shifts in demand corresponding to shifts in behavioral

Table 34.2 Hormonal pattern during arousal

Catabolic hormones increase	Anabolic hormones decrease
Cortisol (glucocorticoids)	Insulin
Epinephrine	Calcitonin
Norepinephrine	Testosterone
Glucagon	Estrogen
Growth hormone	Prolactin
Antidiuretic hormone (vasopressin)	Luteininzing hormone
Renin	Follicle-stimulating hormone
Angiotensin	Gonadotrophin-releasing hormone (GnRH)
Aldosterone (mineralocorticoids)	Prolactin-releasing hormone (PRH)
Erythropoietin	Atriopeptin
Thyroxin	Thymosins
Parathormone	Lymphokines
Melatonin	Cytokines
Thyroid-releasing hormone (TRH)	
Adrenocorticotrophic hormone (ACTH)	
Enkephalin ⎫	
Dynorphin ⎬ opiates	
Endorphin ⎭	

and/or psychological state. Thus the contextual fluctuation of blood pressure illustrated in Figure 34.2 is not exceptional. Rather, it exemplifies a critical principle of physiology: to maintain stability an organism must *vary* all the parameters of its internal milieu and match them appropriately to environmental demands. We refer to this principle as allostasis, meaning 'stability through change'.

MECHANISMS OF ALLOSTASIS

To create allostatic fluctuations, connections are required from brain to soma. Such connections, elucidated in considerable detail by new methods introduced over the last few decades, are now known to be extremely rich. Electron microscopy permits nerve terminals to be visualized in direct contact with specific types of cell, and immunocytochemistry permits nerves to be visualized by the application of antibodies to specific neurochemicals. Such methods show that cells in most of the classical endocrine glands are contacted by nerves. Thus, cells in pancreas that secrete insulin, glucagon, and somatostatin are directly innervated; so are cells in thyroid that secrete calcitonin (see Sterling and Eyer, 1981). Organs not formerly considered to be endocrine are now recognized to contain special endocrine cells and these too are under neural control, for example cells in kidney that secrete renin (see Sterling and Eyer, 1981) and in heart that secrete atriopeptin (Eskay *et al.*, 1986). Tissues previously thought to be free of nerves, for example the metabolically active surfaces of bone (Hohmann *et al.*, 1986) and cells in tissues of the immune system such as spleen, thymus, and lymph nodes, are now known to be innervated (Felten *et al.*, 1985). All blood vessels, including those in the brain itself, are richly innervated. Thus, the brain has direct access through nerves to every tissue and especially to all the internal signalling systems such as the endocrines, blood vessels, and immune system.

The brain also synthesizes its own hormones which it releases into the blood; dozens are now identified, with the certainty that more are still to come. Each brain hormone acts at several levels, affecting (1) peripheral tissues and organs, (2) peripheral endocrine secretions that in turn affect tissues, and (3) pituitary secretion of hormones that alter both tissues and peripheral endocrines. For example, vasopressin released by the brain causes blood vessels to constrict, the kidney to decrease urine output, and the heart to increase blood output. It also stimulates aldosterone release from the adrenal, and ACTH release from pituitary. All these actions of vasopressin tend to increase blood pressure. Thus, neural control is multileveled, with the general form of a cascade (see Figure 34.3).

All the elements in the cascade tend to be mutually reinforcing and this provides the brain with powerful means to override local negative feedback mechanisms that would tend to oppose its commands. This can be appreciated in Figure 34.3, which summarizes the multiple mechanism for raising blood pressure. Clearly, if the brain raised pressure only be increasing cardiac output, pressure would tend to be reduced automatically by local mechanisms for vascular dilatation and renal excretion of salt and water. Similarly, if the brain raised pressure by suppressing salt-water excretion, cardiac output would be reduced automatically by local mechanisms. By controlling all the mechanisms simultaneously, the brain can enforce its command. Furthermore, it can effect the changes rapidly. The existence of these multiple, mutually reinforcing mechanisms is of great therapeutic significance, as we shall see.

The hormones and metabolites whose levels in allostasis are set by the brain also feed *back* to the brain, where they reinforce the original command. These feedbacks, like the feedforward mechanisms, also have the general form of a cascade. For example, the hormones angiotensin II and aldosterone, whose peripheral roles in raising blood pressure are shown in Figure 34.3, affect multiple regions in the brain. Angiotensin stimulates the area postrema in the medulla to cause further neural drive on the heart, vessels and kidney. Angiotensin also acts on the hypothalamus to increase release of vasopressin (Miselis, 1986). Most remarkably, angiotensin and aldosterone, the hormones that cause the kidney to save salt, act on the brain to increase the *appetite* for salt (Zhang *et al.*, 1983). This makes perfect sense since the same allostatic purpose is served by both mechanisms: increase the available salt in order to support the elevation of blood pressure. The newly discovered salt/water regulatory hormone, atriopeptin, is also found in the brain (Standaert *et al.*, 1986).

Allostasis, because it involves the whole brain and body rather than simply local feedbacks, is a far more complex form of regulation than homeostasis. Yet it offers definite advantages. One is that it permits a fine matching of resources to needs. In homeostasis, negative feedback mechanisms, uninformed as to need, force a parameter to a specific 'setpoint'. If blood pressure were actually determined in this way, that is, set to an average, 'normal' value, it would almost invariably be too high or too low for whatever was going on at the moment. Allostasis provides for continuous re-evaluation of need and for continuous readjustment of all parameters toward new setpoints. This makes the most effective use of the organism's resources.

Another advantage of allostasis is its design for *anticipating* altered need and achieving the necessary adjustments in advance. In homeostasis, when increased need creates an 'error' signal, negative feedback mechanisms may try to correct the error, but by then the required resources may be unavailable and the time needed for correction may be too long. Errors corrected by negative feedback can get dangerously large. For example, if one is called upon to leap into action from a sitting position, blood pressure to the head tends to fall as blood drains to the lower body by gravity. Homeostatic mechanisms would correct this, of course, but the error signal (fall in blood pressure to the head) would be associated with momentary dizziness. The most advantageous time for resetting is *before* one leaves the chair.

Similarly, if blood pressure is to be elevated, the time to save salt and water to support the rise is at the moment of elevation and not after much salt and water has been lost to urine so that new supplies are required. Further, if the elevation is to be sustained, new supplies will be needed eventually and the time to seek them is before the body's supply is exhausted. Finally, there is no way for a homeostatic regulatory system to benefit from experience. One learns to get up from the chair slowly if dizziness is a problem and to bring supplies of water and salt to a dry environment. All of these anticipatory regulations are achieved by allostatic mechanisms.

The insight provided by the allostatic model, that specific appetites serve anticipatory mechanisms for physiological regulation, is crucial. It makes comprehensible the relation between physiological need, diet, and pathology. An individual's tendency to eat salt and his kidney's tendency to save salt are driven in concert by the same hormones (aldosterone and angiotensin II; Figure 34.3) as part of an allostatic response to arousing stimuli. Because salt consumption and salt excretion are matched to the level of arousal by means of neuroendocrine mechanisms, they cannot logically be considered 'excessive'. If anything is to be considered 'excessive' in the sense that it leads to pathology, it must be the level of arousal itself.

ALLOSTATIC REGULATION OF THE IMMUNE RESPONSE

The organism's response to an infectious agent involves an extraordinary web of centrally organized, mutually reinforcing connections between the brain, endocrine, and immune systems. To fight a virus optimally requires: (1) recognizing it as foreign, (2) selectively producing white blood cells (leucocytes) to attack it specifically and not the body's own cells, (3) suppressing viral replication by raising body temperature, (4) redirecting metabolic energy to promote these activities, and (5) suppressing activities (and the hormones that promote them) that would compete with these needs. Thus, even though the immune system can initiate a response to the virus through local homeostatic mechanisms, the brain is required to develop full response. The brain needs information regarding the intensity of the infectious challenge so that it may weigh the seriousness of these demands. The brain also needs mechanisms to suppress the immune response in case other demands are more pressing (Kanigel, 1986; Goetzl, 1985).

It has been discovered recently that cells of the immune system secrete a host of chemical factors, called lymphokines and cytokines, that affect the brain (Figure 34.4; Hall et al., 1985; Felten et al., 1985). These include many peptide hormones that are also secreted by endocrine glands such as the adrenal and pituitary (Blalock et al., 1985). For example, leucocytes can release ACTH (Smith et al., 1986), endorphins (Smith et al., 1985), enkephalin (Zurawski et al., 1986), and thyroid-stimulating hormone (TSH; Geenan et al., 1986). The amount of ACTH released is substantial—enough to evoke from the adrenal a rise in cortisol comparable to that produced by moderate arousal (Besedovsky et al., 1986). There are additional factors secreted by leucocytes such as thymosins, interleukins, and interferons (Figure 34.4; Goetzl, 1985). All of these secreted factors, as in the case of hormones that control blood pressure, have local effects and also reinforcing effects on the brain. The details are far from completely clear, but the following examples may give some feeling for the broad organization.

The glucocorticoid hormones, whose secretions are evoked by leucocyte ACTH, suppress production of leucocytes except for those that specifically bind the infectious agent. Thus, these hormones play a key role in the development of selectivity in the immune response (Besedovsky et al., 1985). ACTH, cortisol, and

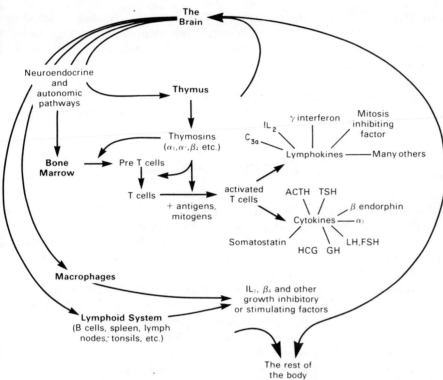

FIG. 34.4   Multiple pathways for the brain's influence on the immune system and for signals from the immune system to the brain. (See Goetzl (1985) for details.)

the opiate hormones also act on the brain to promote euphoria (Barnes, 1986; Shavit *et al.*, 1985). Interleukin IL1 binds to thermoregulatory neurons in the hypothalamus that promote a rise in metabolic rate (e.g. by promoting TSH secretion and thus activation of the thyroid) (Besedovsky *et al.*, 1986). IL1 also promotes sleep. Interferon acts peripherally to block viral replication and on the brain to cause lethargy. Thymosin B_4 promotes the development of the cellular immune response in the thymus and also binds in the hypothalamus to promote secretion of luteinizing hormone (LH). LH promotes elevation of sex hormones that in turn promote anabolic chemistry, mood, and behavior (Hall *et al.*, 1985). Thus, if the response to the virus were the only coping demand, the organism would tend to develop fever and go to sleep, accompanied by dreams of nurturance and pleasure that promote the endocrine state optimal for supporting its developing immune response.

On the other hand, if for some reason the level of arousal is very high, the brain will evoke secretion of much higher levels of ACTH, cortisol, and the other catabolic hormones (Bourne *et al.*, 1974). The immune system and the inflammatory response will be suppressed until the arousal resolves (Laudenslager *et al.*, 1983; Keller *et al.*, 1983; Schleiffer *et al.*, 1985). Then the body and brain can turn their attention once again to internal affairs and fight the infection. This general scheme may help explain why one often falls ill immediately after a period of intense arousal. The internal challenge has already been present for some time but the symptoms have been suppressed. When the level of catabolism called forth by the brain falls to a certain level, the processes engaged by the system of lymphokines and cytokines are then asserted. Thus, as for the cardiovascular system, the critical reason for having feedforward connections from the immune system to the brain is to permit allostasis, enabling the brain to weigh the internal versus external demands and to allocate resources accordingly.

REGULATION OF AROUSAL

Weiss (1972) documented four factors that regulate arousal. He measured the extent of gastric ulceration in pairs of rats 24 hours following their exposure to the identical series of tail shocks. When the shocks were administered at random intervals, ulceration in both rats was severe. However, when one rat was provided with a warning signal before each shock, its ulcers were greatly reduced compared to the control rat which received the identical shocks. Similarly, when a rat could prevent some shocks by pressing a lever, its ulcers were fewer than in the control rat which received the identical number of shocks but for which all the shocks were inescapable. When, following a lever press, a signal was provided to indicate a correct response, ulcers declined still further. Thus, *predictability*, a sense of *control*, and *feedback* all permit the organism to reduce its level of arousal. However, when *demand*, that is, the rate of required response, is made very high, these factors are overridden and the ulcers increase.

These experiments have been repeated in rats using several measures of immune response with the same result. The random, inescapable shocks cause immune suppression. When there is predictability, control, and feedback with regard to the shocks, the immune suppression declines, but when the demand for bar pressing to prevent shocks is elevated, the immune system is once more suppressed (Schleiffer et al., 1985; Keller et al., 1983; Laudenslager et al., 1983).

The Weiss experiments do not identify every factor controlling arousal in humans—for example, they omit the role of psychological defense mechanisms (see Wolff et al., 1964)—but they make much intuitive sense. The biological purpose of the aroused state is to allow an organism to 'cope' physiologically, behaviorally, and emotionally with specific environmental demands. When the environmental demands are identified, predicted, and demonstrably met, that is, when coping has been successful, arousal must be followed by a period of relaxation. This allows anabolic hormones to flow, restoring blood pressure, energy stores, the immune system, gut lining, and so on. It also allows restoration of a relaxed subjective state so that intimate social relations and spiritual ties can be restored that tend to be disrupted by the agonistic moods and behavior accompanying arousal. (In this context, it must be appreciated that essentially all the catabolic hormones, including epinephrine, cortisol, ACTH, thyroxine, TRH, and the opiates, in addition to their metabolic effects, tend to elevate mood, suppress fatigue and pain, and promote agonistic behavior (see Nemeroff and Dunn, 1984).) From this point of view one might consider the Sabbath as a cultural adaptation to ensure regular periods of physiological, interpersonal, and spiritual anabolism. Its progressive corruption in modern society reflects the continued unrestricted expansion of arousing activities and the loss of a potentially important source of anabolic time.

When demand and thus arousal become chronic, the brain–body system adapts at essentially all levels of organization. The muscle in blood vessel walls thickens and so becomes more effective in raising blood pressure. On the other hand, when the muscle is maximally relaxed, it no longer lowers the pressure quite as much. Furthermore, since the vessels are now always more constricted, they require a higher blood pressure than formerly to maintain the same resting blood flow (Folkow and Neill, 1971; Lund-Johanson, 1984). The vascular system becomes in a sense 'addicted' to higher pressure.

Similarly, the body becomes addicted to its own catabolic hormones. Many hormones act by binding to specific protein 'receptors' on the surfaces of and inside cells. It is now appreciated that a hormone's potency depends on the number of its receptor molecules available for binding as well as on the quantity of the hormone. Chronic elevation of a hormone generally leads to downward regulation of its receptors (see Friedhoff and Miller, 1983). Therefore, to obtain a given effect eventually requires a larger dose of the hormone. To the extent that subjective states such as appetite and mood are regulated by hormones binding to receptors in the brain, there will tend to be addiction of subjective state to arousal. That is, the higher the chronic levels of one's own opiates, cortisol, ACTH, angiotensin, and so on, the more dependent one's mood may become on keeping them high. When the level of arousal has been high for a long period due to high demand, entry into a relaxed condition may create an unpleasant state of withdrawal from one's own catabolic hormones. This could provide a physiological basis for an individual's continuing to seek conditions of high demand ('workaholism', Type A behavior).

Another neurophysiological mechanism for adaptation to chronic arousal is that the brain tends to create fixed automatisms out of previously flexible anticipatory responses. Just as a bell that has come to presage food causes salivation and a rise in insulin, so do hosts of signals, previously neutral, come to presage arousing events and automatically reinforce the aroused endocrine and subjective states. One potential consequence of all the mechanisms mentioned is that specific genes whose activities are associated with arousal may be switched irreversibly into the active state (Reisine et al., 1986; Yamamoto, 1985). If this were so for the genes controlling synthesis of any of the catabolic hormones or their receptors, the chronically aroused state could persist even in the absence of objectively arousing situations. Thus there are pathways at all levels from that of the genes, receptors, tissues, neural systems, subjective states, and the social system that tend through natural adaptive mechanisms to become addicted to chronic arousal and thereby make it permanent.

The tendency for the physiological consequences of chronic arousal to become self-maintaining is evident in the studies already cited. This includes the failure of blood pressure in monkeys, cats, and mice to return to normal when the chronically arousing stimuli are removed. It probably also explains, at least in part, why blood pressure in humans that is first labile in response to arousal can become permanently regulated at much higher than normal levels long after the chronically arousing stimuli are gone. Figure 34.2b, a 24-hour recording from a hypertensive individual, gives some feeling for this point. It can be seen that the pressure is not fixed at a specific level, but is modulated over a considerable range, falling in sleep and rising by day, just as the normal individual whose record was shown in Figure 34.2a. There continues to be allostatic regulation, but the average setpoint is much higher than normal.

PATHOLOGY FROM CHRONIC AROUSAL

One may expect, because arousal alters the level of virtually every regulatory chemical in the body and affects the metabolism and function of every system, that chronic arousal would lead to a variety of pathologies. Figure 34.5 indicates some of the main pathologies of the renal–cerebral–cardiovascular system and how they arise in a cooperative manner from multiple mechanisms all driven by arousal. The main problems are that chronic hypertension damages blood vessels in every organ and that elevated cholesterol and other blood lipids cause atherosclerosis in damaged vessels. Add to that increased viscosity and clotting tendency of the blood, and the potential for rupture or occlusion of vessels in kidney, brain, and heart becomes significant. Chronic stimulation of the now compromised heart by continuing signals of arousal, as well as by drugs whose consumption tends to accompany arousal (e.g. nicotine and caffeine), increase the chances of sudden coronary death (see Sterling and Eyer, 1981).

Diabetes, the fifth leading cause of death in the US, is a condition in which regulation of carbohydrate, fat, and protein metabolism is abnormal. Its sequelae are accelerated atherosclerosis and other forms of cardiovascular deterioration, increased protein breakdown, reduced immunity, and usually hypertension. The hormonal pattern in childhood-onset diabetes, lowered insulin and elevated glucagon, resembles the hormonal pattern of arousal. This is not to say that arousal causes the disease, but it certainly exacerbates the symptoms. This has been shown clearly for diabetic children in families in which interparental conflict is discharged through the child (Minuchin et al., 1978). In adult-onset diabetes, the timing of insulin secretion is abnormal so that the hormone is relatively ineffective and ultimately causes down regulation of its own receptors (Jacobs and Cuatrecasas, 1977). Chronic arousal would tend to exacerbate this conditon since the arousal hormones tend to antagonize insulin. Chronic arousal, because it tends to suppress insulin secretion, may also be one of the initiators of adult-onset diabetes. This disorder is especially prevalent among the obese. The prevalence of obesity is greatest in the most disrupted segments of the population, leading one to wonder whether the appetite for food, like salt, may be strongly driven by the catabolic hormones of chronic arousal.

Cancer, another leading cause of death at older ages, is connected in several ways to arousal level. There are external factors such as drug consumption and diet. Thus smoking contributes to lung cancer and alcohol consumption to cancers of the liver and pancreas, while excess animal fat and deficiency of fiber apparent-

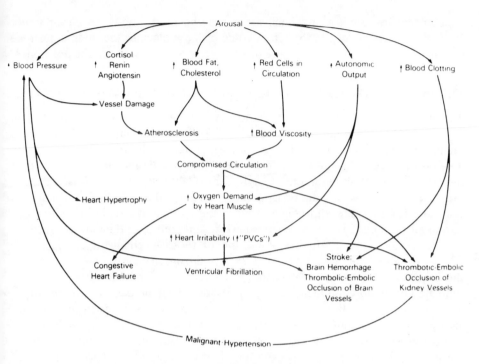

FIG. 34.5   Multiple mechanisms for renal, cerebral and cardiovascular pathology from chronic arousal. (Reprinted from Sterling and Eyer, 1981.)

ly contribute to colon cancer. The allostatic model suggests connections between appetite and physiological state; therefore, the modern craving for nicotine, alcohol, fat, and fiberless food may all be related to appetites driven by chronic arousal. The progressive contamination of our environment by asbestos, radiation, and organic chemicals is widely recognized to contribute to cancer. This is not linked to chronic arousal in any single individual; nevertheless, like the lapsing of the Sabbath already noted, it reflects a change of values that arises from and helps to reinforce chronic arousal as a societal pattern.

Cancers are also regulated by the body's immune and endocrine systems. Immunosuppressed humans and animals develop cancer at up to one hundred times the normal rate (Harris and Sinkovics, 1970). Female mice chronically aroused by handling and exposure to strangers show hypersecretion of cortisol, suppressed immune organs such as the thymus, and die at higher rates and earlier ages of virally evoked mammary tumors (Riley, 1975). In this case it appears that replication of the oncogenic virus is also directly stimulated by cortisol (Yamamoto, 1985). Rats subjected in the Weiss paradigm to inescapable and unpredictable shock develop tumors at higher rates than animals who can prevent or predict the shocks (Schleiffer et al., 1985). Recently, specific genes have been discovered whose activities are related to the development of cancer. It has been learned that the proteins coded by at least two of these so-called oncogenes are identical in structure to the receptor molecules for thyroid hormone and cortisol (Sap *et al.*, 1986; Weinberger *et al.*, 1986). Thus, some of the molecules that help determine whether cells become cancerous are direct targets for certain catabolic hormones.

DEFINITIONS OF HEALTH AND APPROACHES TO THERAPEUTICS

The homeostatic model defines health as a state in which all physiological parameters have 'normal' values. A value outside the normal range is said to be 'inappropriate', and thus a candidate for 'treatment'. The main treatment is to administer drugs that stimulate or suppress the somatic mechanisms that most directly control that parameter (Taylor and Caldwell, 1986). Thus, if blood pressure is above 140/90 mmHg, drugs are directed at the three basic mechanisms that raise the pressure: diuretics to reduce the volume of circulating salt water; vasodilators to increase the size of reservoir; antagonists of the beta-receptor to reduce the heart's output. To block one of these mechanisms is sometimes adequate, but frequently, as would be expected from the diagram in Figure 34.3, the brain uses the other mechanisms to compensate. Thus, a diuretic-induced reduction of blood volume may be compensated by an increase in cardiac output and by vasoconstriction; drug-induced vasodilatation is compensated by increased cardiac output, and so on (see Sterling and Eyer, 1981). When such compensations occur, additional drugs can be administered until all three mechanisms have been blocked. Another pharmacotherapy in the same spirit is to block the enzymatic conversion of angiotensin to its active form or to block the binding of this hormone to its receptors. These are potent treatments because angiotensin has many actions that affect all three of the somatic mechanisms for increasing pressure and many sites in the brain as well (see Figure 34.3). Further, in animals, blocking the central action of angiotensin is shown to reduce salt appetite (Weiss *et al.*, 1986; Moe *et al.*, 1984).

The pharmacological approach, despite its impressive ingenuity, contains an inherent tendency toward iatrogenesis. Because each hormone has multiple effects and each receptor type (alpha, beta, angiotensin, etc.) is widely distributed, every drug directed at restoring one parameter to normal necessarily causes other parameters to become 'inappropriately' high or low. For example, the diuretic treatment causes potassium to become inappropriately low and glucose, cholesterol and uric acid to become inappropriately high (Gifford, 1974). Consequently, the pharmacological reduction of blood pressure reduces the chances of a stroke, but the other effects *increase* the chances of a heart attack (Grimm, 1986; Leren and Helgeland, 1986). Additional drugs are commonly administered to restore these other parameters to normal (see Sterling and Eyer, 1981). Thus the therapeutic approach associated with the homeostatic model is inevitably associated with polypharmacy and iatrogenesis.

The other serious drawback is that the responsiveness of the organism is reduced. Pharmacological treatment that tries to clamp some parameter at its 'normal' value naturally prevents it from responding to increased demand at moments when that would be desirable. With blood pressure clamped low, the tolerance of a drug-treated hypertensive person for exercise is diminished, even though exercise might be therapeutic (Lund-Johanson, 1984). Further, the reduction of responsiveness is not limited (for reasons already noted) to the therapeutically targeted parameter. The drug treatments that reduce the tolerance of a hypertensive person for exercise may also render him lethargic and impotent (see Sterling and Eyer 1981).

The allostatic model defines health as a state of responsiveness. A parameter with values outside the normal range is not considered 'inappropriate' because every parameter is controlled by a multitude of mutually reinforcing signals. If a parameter has a value above or below normal, most likely there are multiple mechanisms forcing it there, and most likely the ultimate source of these signals is the brain. In this model, the elevated blood pressure of the hypertensive is considered to be entirely appropriate, and the question for exploration becomes 'appropriate to what?'.

The elevation of blood pressure may be appropriate to the arousing conditions of modern life. The chain of evidence linking the conditions of life to this disorder is now fairly complete. First, there is the epidemiological and behavioral evidence: (1) hypertension is greatest among human populations subjected to disruption of intimate social relations, (2) the pressure rise in the population to begins essentially at the moment children leave the family bosom and enter the uncertain and demanding environment of school, (3) hypertension can be produced experimentally in populations of animals by social disruption and in individual animals by arousing behavioral paradigms. Next, there is broad physiological evidence: (1) many neural and neuroendocrine mechanisms are available to elevate blood pressure and thus potentially to cause hypertension (see Figure 34.3), (2) chronic hypertension can be produced in animal models by stimulating the brain regions that activate these neural and neuroendocrine mechanisms, (3) these mechanisms are demonstrated to be active in the natural state under the arousing behavioral conditions associated with the development of hypertension, (4) pharmacological suppression of one mechanism for raising pressure is compensated by the other mechanisms, and this suggests that the target pressure is set by the brain.

Chronically elevated blood pressure is 'appropriate' in the allostatic model but it is certainly not healthy. When pressure is at high levels, there is no margin for responding to additional challenges or to opportunities for relaxation. Furthermore, high pressure leads inevitably to serious organic pathology (see Figure 34.5). Thus the allostatic model provides a scientific framework for recognizing the obvious, that health requires a decent balance between catabolism and anabolism.

The therapy suggested by the allostatic model is to reduce arousal. A prime objective, following the Weiss paradigm, would be to reduce demand by encouraging people to rest and play in proportion to their work and striving and to increase predictability, control, and feedback in their lives. Such steps would reduce *all* the neural and neuroendocrine drives on the multiple mechanisms for raising blood pressure. In contrast to pharmacotherapy, where blocking one mechanism evokes compensatory increases in others, reducing arousal would reduce pressure by the concerted action of multiple mechanisms.

Prevention and treatment of hypertension directed at the social and psychological levels are widely considered impractical compared to pharmocotherapy.

Yet, the experience of several decades with mass drug treatment for hypertension has raised doubts regarding its true practicality. Long-term drug treatment for mild and moderate hypertension reduces mortality from stroke but increases mortality from heart disease (Grimm, 1986; Leren, 1986; Freis, 1986a). Furthermore, the various unpleasant and iatrogenic effects of drug treatment cause enough patient non-compliance that pressure in the population remains uncontrolled. In fact, blood pressures in the large (baby boom) cohort that has experienced increased competition and chronic arousal since youth are higher than they were in the preceding small cohort at the corresponding age despite the wide availability of antihypertensive drugs (Eyer, 1980). Physicians enthusiastic about drug treatment for 20 years have sharply moderated their claims and are now recommending for mild hypertension simple follow-up visits and possibly relaxation training, diet and exercise (Chesney et al., 1986; Freis, 1986a; 1986b).

The highly technological treatments for the end-stages of disease related to chronic arousal are also proving to be of dubious practicality. Coronary artery bypass grafts (CABG) successfully reduce pain from angina but contribute hardly at all to longevity (see Sterling and Eyer, 1981; Chaitman et al., 1986; Cameron et al., 1986). Kidney dialysis and transplantation prolong life but at great psychological cost to the patient (Abrams et al., 1972). Treatments for the major cancers have been largely unsuccessful (Kolata, 1986). The technological approach is also very expensive. There are now about 250 000 CABGs per year in the US, at a cost of nearly $8 billion (Rimm et al., 1986). When the large cohort comes of age for this surgery, these figures might easily double. The cost of medical care now absorbs about 12% of the US GNP, and still grows. To continue on this path of highly technological treatment will progressively limit the possibilities for other uses of the social product. What proves practical in the long run may not be technology but rather investment in social structures and activities that rebuild and enrich communal life, that reduce demand and enhance predictability, control and feedback.

SUMMARY AND CONCLUSIONS

'Homeostasis', the central model in physiology and therapeutics for 100 years, is superseded by a new model, 'allostasis', that emerges from recent studies in neurobiology. Homeostasis emphasized that the body's internal environment is held constant by the self-correcting (negative feedback) actions of its constituent organs. Allostasis emphasizes that the internal milieu varies to meet perceived and anticipated demand. This variation is achieved by multiple, mutually reinforcing neural and neuroendocrine mechanisms that override the homeostatic mechanisms. The allostatic model, in emphasizing the subordination of local feedbacks to control by the brain, provides a strong conceptual framework to explain social and psychological modulation of physiology and pathology.

Acknowledgements

We thank Professor Charles Kahn for suggesting the term 'allostasis', Dr Noga Vardi for reading the manuscript, and Ms Judy Jackson for typing.

REFERENCES

Abrams, H. *et al.* (1972). Suicidal behavior in chronic dialysis patients. *American Journal of Psychiatry, 127,* 1199.

Akil, H., Watson, S.J., Young, E., Lewis, M.E., Katchaturian, H., & Walker, M.J. (1984). Endogenous opioids: biology and function. *Annual Review of Neuroscience, 7,* 223–255.

Barnes, D. (1986). Steroids may influence changes in mood. *Science, 232,* 1344.

Berkson, J. (1962). Mortality and marital status. *American Journal of Public Health, 52,* 1318.

Bernard, C. (1865). *An introduction to the study of experimental medicine.* New York: Dover Publications. (Published 1957.)

Besedovsky, H. *et al.* (1985). Immune-neuro-endocrine interactions. *Journal of immunology, 135(2),* Suppl., 750–754.

Besedovsky, H. *et al.* (1986). Immunoregulatory feedback between interleukin-1 and glucocorticoid hormones. *Science, 233,* 652–654.

Bevan, A.T. *et al.* (1969). Direct arterial pressure recording in unrestricted man. *Clinical Science, 369,* 329.

Blalock, J. *et al.* (1985). Peptide hormones shared by the neuroendocrine and immunologic systems. *Journal of Immunology, 135(2),* Suppl., 858–861.

Blumenthal, S. *et al.* (1977). Report on the task force on blood pressure control in children. *Pediatrics, 59,* Suppl., 797.

Bourne, H.R. *et al.* (1974). Modulation of inflammation and immunity by cyclic AMP. *Science, 184,* 19.

Cameron, A. *et al.* (1986). Bypass surgery with the internal mammary artery graft: 15-year followup. *Circulation, 74* (Suppl. III), III-17.

Cannon, W.B. (1929). *Bodily changes in pain, hunger, fear and rage: An account of recent researchers into the function of emotional excitement,* 2nd edn. New York: Appleton.

Cannon, W.B. (1932). *The wisdom of the body.* New York: W.W. Norton.

Chaitman, B.R. *et al.* (1986). The role of coronary bypass surgery for 'left main equivalent' coronary disease: the CASS registry. *Circulation, 74,* (Suppl. III). III-30.

Chesney, M.A. *et al.* (1986). Behavioral treatment of borderline hypertension. *Cardiovascular Journal of Pharmacology, 8,* (Suppl. 5), 557–563.

Dillingham, M.A., & Anderson, R.J. (1986). Inhibition of vasopressin action by atrial natiuretic factor. *Science, 231,* 1572–1573.

Eskay, R., Zukowska-Grojec, Z., Haass, M., Dave, J.R., & Zamir, N. (1986). Circulating atrial natiuretic peptides in conscious rats: regulation of release by multiple factors. *Science, 2321,* 636–638.

Eyer, J. (1975). Hypertension as a disease of modern society. *International Journal of Health Services, 5,* 539.

Eyer, J. (1980). Social causes of coronary heart disease. *Psychotherapy and Psychosomatics, 34,* 75–87.

Eyer, J., & Sterling, P. (1977). Stress-related mortality and social organization. *Review of Radical Political Economics, 9,* 1–16.

Felten, D. *et al.* (1985). Noradrenergic and peptidergic innervation of lymphoid tissue. *Journal of Immunology, 135(2),* Suppl., 755–765.

Folkow, B., & Neill, E. (1971). *Circulation.* London: Oxford University Press.

Folkow, B., & Rubinstein, E.H. (1966). Cardiovascular effects of acute and chronic stimulation of the hypothalamic defense area in the rat. *Acta Physiologica Scandinavica, 68,* 48.

Forsyth, R.P. (1969). Blood pressure responses to long-term avoidance schedules in the unrestrained rhesus monkey. *Psychosomatic Medicine, 31,* 300.

Freis, E.D. (1986a). Borderline mild systemic hypertension: should it be treated? *American Journal of Cardiology, 58,(7),* 642–645.

Freis, E.D. (ed.) (1986b). Symposium on borderline hypertension. *Journal of Cardiovascular Pharmacology 8,* Suppl. 5.

Friedhoff, A.J., & Miller, J.C. (1983). Clinical implications of receptor sensitivity modification. *Annual Review of Neuroscience, 6*, 121–148.

Geenan, V. *et al.* (1986). The neuroendocrine thymus: coexistence of oxytocin and neurophysin in the human thymus. *Science, 232*, 508.

Gifford, R.W. (1974). A practical guide to management. In *The hypertension handbook* (p. 83). West Point: Merck, Sharpe and Dohme.

Goetzl, E.J. (ed.) (1985). Proceedings of the conference on neuromodulation of immunity and hypersentivity. *Journal of Immunology, 135*(2), Suppl.

Grimm, R.H. (1986). The drug treatment of mild hypertension in the multiple risk factor intervention trial: a review. Proceedings of a symposium on treatment of hypertension and primary prevention of coronary heart disease. *Drugs, 31*, Suppl. 1, 13–21.

Hall, N.R. *et al.* (1985). Evidence that thymosins and other biologic response modifiers can function as neuroactive immunotransmitters. *Journal of Immunology, 135*(2), Suppl., 806–811.

Harris, J., & Sinkovics, J. (1970). *The immunology of malignant disease.* St Louis, Miss.: Mosby.

Henry, J.P., Meehan, J.P., & Stephens, P.M. (1967). The use of psychosocial stimuli to induce prolonged systolic hypertension in mice. *Psychosomatic Medicine, 29*, 408.

Hohmann, E.L., Elde, R.P., Rysavy, J.A., Einzig, S., & Gebhard, R.L. (1986). Innervation of periosteum and bone by sympathetic vasoactive intestinal peptide-containing nerve fibers. *Science, 232*, 868–871.

Jacobs, S. & Cuatrecasas, P. (1977). Cell receptors in disease. *New England of Medicine, 297*, 1383.

Kanigel, R. (1986). Where mind and body meet. *Mosaic, 17*, 52–60.

Keller, S.E., Weiss, J.M., Miller, N.E. & Stein, M. (1983). Stress-induced suppression of immunity in adrenalectomized rats. *Science, 221*, 1301–1304.

Kolata, G. (1986). Cancer progression data challenged. *Science, 232*, 932–933.

Laudenslager, M.L., Ryan, S.M., Drugan, R.C., Hyson, R.L., & Maier, S.E. (1983). Coping and immunosuppression: inescapable but not escapable shock suppresses lymphocyte proliferation. *Science, 221*, 568–570.

Leren, P., & Helgeland, A. (1986). The Oslo Hypertension Study. Proceedings of a symposium on treatment of hypertension and primary prevention of coronary heart disease. *Drugs, 31*, Suppl. 1, 40–49.

Lund-Johanson, P. (1984). Hemodynamic concepts in essential hypertension. *Triangle, 23*, No. 1. 13–24 (Sandoz).

Manning, P.T., Schwartz, D., Katsuvbe, N.C., Holmberg, S.W., & Needleman, P. (1985). Vasopressin-stimulated release of atriopeptin: endocrine antagonists in fluid homeostatis. *Science, 229*, 395–397.

Mason, J.W. (1968). Organization of endocrine mechanisms. *Psychosomatic Medicine, 30*, 565.

Mason, J.W. (1971). A reevaluation of the concept of 'nonspecificity' in stress theory. *Journal of Psychiatric Research, 8*, 323.

Mason, J.W. (1972). Organization of psychoendocrine mechanisms. In N.S. Greenfield & R.A. Sternbach (eds), *Handbook of psychophysiology.* New York: Holt, Rhinehart and Winston.

Minuchin, S., Rosman, B., & Baker, L. (1978). *Psychosomatic families. Anorexia nervosa in context.* Cambridge, Mass.: Harvard University Press.

Miselis, R. (1986). The visceral neuraxis in thirst and renal function. In G. de Caro, A.N. Epstein & M. Massi (eds), *The physiology of thirst and sodium appetite.* Plenum.

Moe, K.E., Weiss, M.L., & Epstein, A.N. (1984). Sodium appetite during captopril blockage of endogenous angiotensin II formation. *American Journal of Physiology, 247*, 356–R365.

Nemeroff, C.B., & Dunn, A.J. (eds) (1984). *Peptides, hormones, and behavior.* Spectrum.

Pickering, T.G. *et al.* (1986). Behavioral determinants of 24-hour blood pressure patterns in borderline hypertension. *Journal of Cardiovascular Pharmacology, 8*. Suppl. 5, 589–592.

Reisine, T., Affolter, H.-A., Rougon, G., & Barbet, J. (1986). New insights into the molecular mechanisms of stress. *Trends in Neuro Science, 9*, 574–579.

Riley, V. (1975). Mouse mammary tumors: alteration of incidence as apparent function of stress. *Science, 189*, 465.

Rimm, A.A. *et al.* (1986). Trends in coronary surgery. *Journal of the American Medical Association, 255*, 229–233.

Sap, J. *et al.* (1986). The c-erb-A protein is a high-affinity receptor for thyroid hormone. *Nature 324*, 635–640.

Schleiffer, S. *et al.* (1985). Stress and immunomodulation: the role of depression and neuroendocrine function. *Journal of Immunology, 135*(2), Suppl., 827.

Selye, H. (1956). *The stress of life.* New York: McGraw-Hill.

Shavit, Y. et al. (1985). Stress, opioid peptides, the immune system and cancer. *Journal of Immunology, 135*, Suppl., 834.

Smith, E. *et al.* (1985). Lymphocyte production of endorphins and endorphin-mediated immunoregulatory activity. *Journal of Immunology, 135*(2), Suppl., 779–782.

Smith, E. *et al.* (1986). Cortiocotropin releasing factor induction of leukocyte-derived immunoreactive ACTH and endorphins. *Nature, 321*, 881–882.

Standaert, D.G., Needleman, P., & Saper, C.B. (1986). Organization of atrio-peptin-like immunoreactive neurons in the central nervous system of the rat. *Journal of Comparative Neurology, 253*, 315–341.

Sterling, P., & Eyer, J. (1981). Biological basis of stress-related mortality. *Social Science and Medicine, 15E*, 3–42.

Taylor, S., & Calwell, A. (eds) (1986). Proceedings of a symposium on treatment of hypertension and primary prevention of coronary heart disease. *Drugs, 31*, Suppl., 1.

Waldron, I. (1979). A quantitative analysis of cross-cultural variation in blood pressure and serum cholesterol. *Psychosomatic Medicine, 41*, 582.

Weinberger, C. *et al.* (1986). The *c-erb-A* gene encodes a thyroid hormone receptor. *Nature, 324*, 641–646.

Weiss, M.L., Moe, K.E., & Epstein, A.N. (1986). Interference with central actions of angiotensin II suppresses sodium appetite. *American Journal of Physiology, 250*, R250–R259.

Weiss, J.M. (1972). Psychological factors in stress and disease. *Scientific American, 226*, 104.

Wolff, C.T., Friedman, S.B., Hofer, M.A., & Mason, J.W. (1964). Relationship between psychological defenses and mean urinary 17-hydroxycorticosteroid excretion rates. I. A predictive study of parents of fatally ill children. *Psychosomatic Medicine, 26*, 574–591.

Yamamoto, K.R. (1985). Steroid receptor regulated transcription of specific genes and gene networks. *Annual Review of Genetics, 19*, 209–252.

Zhang, D.-M., Stellar, E., & Epstein, A.N. (1983). Together intracranial angiotensin and systemic mineralocorticoid produce avidity for salt in the rat. *Physiology and Behaviour, 32*, 677–681.

Zurawski, G. *et al.* (1986). Activation of mouse T-helper cells induces abundant pre-proenkephalin mRNA synthesis. *Science, 232*, 772–775.

KEY WORDS

Stress, allostasis, homeostasis, hypertension, arousal, psychoneuriommunology, iatrogenesis, health.

Section V: Cognitive Developments With Implications for Coping and Health

Handbook of Life Stress, Cognition and Health
Edited by S. Fisher and J. Reason
© 1988 John Wiley & Sons Ltd.

35

Helping People Cope with the Long-Term Effects of Stress

IAN HOWARTH
The University of Nottingham
and
INEZ DOOTJES DUSSUYER
Community Services Victoria, Melbourne, Australia

INTRODUCTION

The effect of stress on mental and physical health has been amply documented in earlier chapters. So too have the factors which affect people's resistance to these adverse effects. Here we shall survey what is known about the effectiveness of psychological methods used to help people overcome the debilitating effects of stress on their long-term mental and physical health, and then consider ways in which these methods may be improved.

Psychological treatments in the past have been of two main types, the psychodynamic and the behavioural. Both are moderately but almost equally effective (e.g. Parloff *et al.*, 1986). Since they are based on irreconcilable theories and use totally different procedures, we must conclude that there is little support for either type of theory. In the absence of the understanding which derives from good theory, it is difficult to see how either psychodynamic or behavioural approaches may be improved.

Fortunately, there are several studies outside the behavioural and psychodynamic traditions which suggest where we should look for more effective helping strategies. For example, we know that stress affects different people in different ways and that people of low self-esteem are particularly susceptible to the adverse effects of stress (e.g. Kobasa, 1982). We also know that the effects of help depend critically on the self-esteem of the person being helped. Those of low self-esteem are difficult to help. So much so that help may further damage their self-esteem and make them even more vulnerable to the effects of stress. Since people of low self-esteem are more likely to seek help, those who provide help are in a difficult situation, which has been called the 'helping paradox' (Nadler and Fisher, 1986).

Competence and cognitive strategies are related to self-esteem, and it seems likely that more effective helping will concentrate on them rather than on self-esteem directly. One might hope that the new cognitive therapies will become more effective by doing just that, but at the moment there is no strong evidence that they are any better than the behavioural or psychodynamic therapies.

However, there are examples of highly effective interventions which suggest that really powerful forms of help or treatment are not impossible. Rodin and Langer (1977) halved the death rate in an old people's home by giving inmates a very small amount of extra responsibility. This may have had the effect of raising their self-esteem and hence inoculating them against the manifold stresses of growing old.

Ways of preserving or increasing people's control over their own lives have been suggested in other contexts, such as education and work. They are usually evaluated in terms of their effect on competence, but they are also likely to reduce the effects of stress provided they do not, at the same time, encourage people to attempt even more difficult and stressful tasks.

EVALUATIONS OF PROFESSIONAL HELP

People suffering from the effects of stress seek many types of help, from their workmates, from their families and friends, from general practitioners, from social workers, counsellors or psychotherapists, clinical psychologists or psychiatrists. Here we shall consider the type of help which they are likely to be given if it is believed that the problem is within themselves, rather than in their environment. This is always a simplification, as earlier chapters have shown. Stress reactions are best understood as a degree of incompetence or unhappiness, induced by the interaction between a particular individual and a particular environment. People could theoretically be helped by changing the environment, or the person, or the relationship (practical and conceptual) between the person and the environment. Many forms of help take the environment as given, or assume that changing the environment is a different sort of problem, e.g. political or managerial. They therefore address themselves to the task of changing the person or changing that person's conception of the environment or competence in dealing with it.

Professional practice is dominated by two contrasting approaches to the task of making the person more able to cope with the emotional consequences of stress. The older is the psychodynamic approach, which owes a great deal to Freud, but has, over the years, taken many different forms such as the client-centred approach of Carl Rogers. Different though they may be, all psychodynamic therapy and counselling assumes that people cannot cope because they are not thinking straight about their emotions. The basic method is to talk about the client's feelings and emotional responses until the client feels better and can face life with renewed hope.

The main alternative approach is behaviourist. This owes a great deal to the founders of behaviourism, J.B. Watson and B.F. Skinner, but moved into the clinical field following the pioneering work of Wolpe on the treatment of phobias.

The behaviourist assumption is that emotions are an epiphenomenon which cannot be directly treated. The essence of the problem is assumed to be the existence of inappropriate habits which interfere with the ability to cope adaptively. Treatment consists of extinguishing these bad habits by refusing to reward them, and training new ones by more appropriate reinforcement schedules. More recently, an attempt has been made to combine these two approaches. For example, cognitive behaviour modification tries to induce more appropriate thoughts about emotional problems by explicitly rewarding them.

There are now about 500 reasonably good studies of the effectiveness of the different forms of psychotherapy. These have been reviewed many times, most recently by obtaining average estimates of effectiveness in a meta analysis (e.g. Smith *et al.*, 1980). The best of the recent reviews have concluded that the psychodynamic and behavioural approaches are equally effective for most problems, although behavioural treatments may be marginally more effective for phobias and obsessions (e.g. Parloff *et al.*, 1986). There are also some well-controlled experimental comparisons, such as that of Sloane *et al.* (1975). These authors report the results of separating the people seeking help from a large outpatients facility into three groups by an entirely random process. One group was told that treatment would be delayed, another was sent to behaviourally orientated therapists and the last to psychodynamic therapy. After treatment the two treated groups were judged by independent observers to be in better shape than the waiting group, but there were no significant differences between the two treated groups. Follow-up several weeks later left this conclusion unchanged.

The most recent reviews (e.g. Parloff *et al.*, 1986; Stiles *et al.*, 1986) have tried to make sense of the apparent equivalence of different forms of treatment. It has been suggested that despite their surface differences, the therapeutic effect may be due to some similar features of the therapeutic encounter. This is the most likely explanation, but we have no good evidence concerning the nature of this common element, only speculations.

Various placebo treatments have also been tried in an attempt to isolate the essential feature of therapy. Unfortunately most of these are almost as good as formal treatment (Prioleau *et al.*, 1983), so that they also must share whatever is common to psychodynamic and behavioural therapies. The impression that psychotherapists do not know what they are doing is confirmed by the evidence that the extent of training received by the therapist has no more effect than the type of training. About 20 studies have compared the effectiveness of highly trained (professional) therapists and counsellors with that of untrained or very briefly trained therapists (paraprofessionals). Two meta analyses have been done to estimate the average difference in the effectiveness of professionals and paraprofessionals. Hattie *et al.* (1984) concluded, paradoxically, that the relatively untrained paraprofessionals were more effective than the professionals. Berman and Norton (1985) criticized Hattie *et al.* for including some poorly designed studies in the meta analysis. Restricting their analysis to the 15 best conducted studies, they concluded that there was no evidence of any difference in the effectiveness of therapists as a function of training. Equally, there is little evidence that therapists become more effective with experience (e.g. Brehmer, 1980).

Social case work is a form of counselling combined with practical help which is designed to help people in social difficulties to overcome them and to learn to cope better in future. Evaluations of the efforts of social workers show that the practical help they provide, e.g. with cash and housing, is appreciated by their clients but that the counselling element is not appreciated. When outcome measures are used there is very little evidence that the clients' autonomy is increased; if anything, they tend to become rather dependent on the social worker (Brewer and Lait, 1980).

Drug addiction and crime are sometimes thought to be effects of deprivation and to that extent may also be regarded as long-term effects of stress (Howarth, 1976). Professionally organized rehabilitation is dramatically unsuccessful with these groups; much less successful than with the emotionally disabled. This may be because there are well-established subcultures which support drug addicts and criminals in a way which reinforces rather than extinguishes their behaviour. It may also be because the success of rehabilitation programmes in these fields is judged by more objective criteria. A very important study by McCord (1978) suggests that objective evaluations may always present a more dismal picture than subjective evaluations. She traced, 30 years later, almost all the 500 boys who had taken part in a well-controlled study—a counselling programme for potentially delinquent boys. Those in the treated group remembered the programme well and only 13% thought it had not helped them. Two-thirds thought it had helped them, and some believed that without it they might have taken to a life of crime. However, the objective data, obtained from health, criminal and employment records, told a different story. The group which had received approximately 5 years counselling were less healthy, more criminal and less successful in their jobs. If we had both objective and subjective evidence for the effectiveness of all professional help, it would be easier to make confident judgements about its effectiveness.

This is a very depressing literature. It is now clear that there is not enough empirical evidence to sustain the interminable theoretical writing which characterizes this subject. At the moment, only one strong theoretical statement is possible, i.e. that the subject does not make sense.

If we are to derive new understanding and insight we must look elsewhere. In particular, we will now look at factors which affect resistance to stress and at experimental studies of helping.

FACTORS AFFECTING RESISTANCE TO STRESS

If we are to help people cope with the effects of stress, we must also hope that what we do will make them more resistant to stress in future. To make this more likely, we should be aware of the factors which are associated with resistance to stress. The main ones are physical health, personality, social support and previous experience. We shall deal with each of these in turn.

Physical Health

Physical health, in the sense of good health, is commonly assumed to improve our resistance to stress, while poor health reduces our resistance. This has never been scientifically documented, perhaps because it never occurs to anyone to question it. However, there are several studies which have shown that activities which promote physical health also improve mental health and resistance to stress (Orwin, 1973; Shephard, 1983). Whether the resistance is a consequence of the activities themselves, which require self-discipline, or of the improved health which follows, we do not know.

Personality

Personality, in contrast, has frequently been shown to be related to resistance to stress. Kobasa (1982) has shown that 'hardy' personalities seem comparatively resistant to stress. Measures of the 'hardy' personality used seven different types of questions. Those which indicated 'alienation from self', nihilism, external locus of control, powerlessness and lack of vigour were most effective in picking out the type of non-hardiness which correlated with adverse effects of stress. Many of the questions in the test battery resemble those found in measures of self-esteem.

Several similar studies have picked out personality factors which may affect people's susceptibility to stress. These include 'learned resourcefulness' (the opposite of learned helplessness), neuroticism, dispositional optimism, cognitive flexibility, effective problem-solving strategies, social skills, financial assets and social support (see Kessler *et al.* (1985) for a review and further references).

This is a formidable list, but it does suggest a certain coherence, rather like Kobasa's 'hardy' personality. Kobasa developed her concepts within an 'existential theory of personality'; but the above list suggests a more cognitive approach. We therefore suggest that resistance to the adverse effects of stress is greatest when the person has the social, intellectual and physical resources to deal with the stressful problems and the confidence and determination to make use of them.

No test battery has yet been developed to measure exactly this constellation of personal characteristics, so we do not know whether it would have a more powerful relationship to stress resistance than the 'hardiness' scale of Kobasa. But it does have the advantage of suggesting intervention strategies which might be used to improve people's ability to cope. These will be considered again when we look at the experimental studies of helping.

Social Support

Social support is the one element in our list which has been extensively studied. There is very general agreement that social support can mitigate the effects of stress. The evidence for this view comes from studies of specific groups who have experienced a particular form of stress or distress and also from studies of the general population.

Brown *et al.* (1962) suggested that when schizophrenics returned to their families, the relapse rate depended upon the kind of support they received. In particular it was found, and has been independently confirmed (e.g. Vaughan and Leff, 1976; Goldstein, 1983), that the greater the amount of 'expressed emotion' the convalescent schizophrenic encountered, the greater the likelihood of relapse.

In this context, 'repression' appears to be desirable rather than undesirable.

Brown and Harris (1978) found that among women who experienced life stress, 40% of those who did not have a close confidant were depressed, while only 4% of those who did have a close confidant, such as a boyfriend or husband, were depressed. This sort of result has been replicated several times (e.g. Miller and Ingham, 1976; Slater and Deprie, 1981).

There are still methodological difficulties with these studies since they are correlational. Hence we do not know if social support prevents stress breakdown or if those who are likely to breakdown under stress are also less likely to have good social relationships with the sort of people who could help them. Intervention studies could distinguish between these two possibilities, but only in the special case of the convalescent schizophrenics has this been tried (Boyd et al., 1981). Fortunately, in this case the intervention was successful, but we can draw no conclusions from this about other populations.

Even within the correlational design, there is some indication that different sorts of people need different sorts of handling by their family and friends. Kobasa (1982) found that a supportive family was associated with less illness in stressed executives only if they were 'hardy' personalities. For the non-hardy, the association went the other way, with greater illness being associated with more, rather than less, family support. A very similar interaction with personality is found in the experimental study of help which will be discussed in the next section. The adverse effects of social support may be limited to family support since, in a later paper, Kobasa and Puccetti (1983) failed to find the same curious interaction in relation to support from the boss at work. However, they did report a correlation between hardiness and the likelihood of support from the boss, suggesting that it is easier to offer help to hardy personalities or that hardy personalities may seek help more effectively.

There has been much controversy about the interaction of social support and stress. Some authors propose a 'buffering hypothesis' (e.g. Cobb, 1976) whereby social support is associated with better health only in the case of people who are highly stressed (as in the study by Brown and Harris, 1978). Others, on the other hand, have found that social support is associated with better health even in those who are not particularly stressed. For example, 2334 people enrolled in a health insurance programme were sent the usual questionnaires twice with 1 year in between. Associations were found between both life events and social support and health measured 1 year later. But there was no interaction between the two and hence no support for the 'buffering hypothesis'.

However, the most recent review, by Kessler and McLeod (1984), has concluded that the most methodologically adequate studies support the 'buffering hypothesis' and suggest that emotional support is more effective than more social involvement or social activity. (They do not comment on the involvement of the supporters in problem-solving activities.)

Learned Helplessness

In 1975, Seligman proposed a major new theory of the effects of experience on resistance to stress. He proposed, essentially, that failure to control one's environment leads to a reduction in competence, associated in humans with depression. Stated in this way, it can be regarded as the obverse of the phenomenon of 'learning to learn' observed 30 years earlier by Harlow (1949). While the theory has had some success, the past 10 years have revealed anomalies which have required several revisions of the theory (e.g. Abramson *et al.*, 1978; Alloy and Abramson, 1982; Baumeister, 1982; Baumgardner *et al.*, 1986; Garber and Hollen, 1980).

The main additions to helplessness theory have been the recognition that depression is associated with learned helplessness only if the uncontrollable events are unpleasant; that we can distinguish between events which no-one can control (universal helplessness) and those which only we fail to control (personal helplessness); that we can distinguish between events which will always be uncontrollable and those which are only temporarily so; and, finally, various authors have distinguished the effects of private feelings of helplessness and public presentations of ourselves and our competence.

The essence of these reformulations is the realization that our reactions to failure depend crucially on the way we explain it, on how we respond to that explanation and how public or private the failure is. Brockner (1979), for example, showed that people of low self-esteem were more prone to feelings of personal helplessness and were more affected in their performance on a second task by their success or failure in an earlier task. They were even more affected if they were naturally self-conscious or made more so by the presence of a mirror. Strong personalities, however, may respond reactively (Brehm, 1966; Baum and Gatchel, 1981), i.e. by trying harder on future tasks when weaker people may give up. Even strong personalities may give up in the face of an impossible task. The effect this has on future tasks is at the moment difficult to predict, although we now have enough (rather common sense) explanatory concepts to be able to explain almost any result after the event.

EXPERIMENTAL STUDIES OF HELPING

There are at least three comparatively unrelated literatures on helping. The first concerns the giving of help and why people do not always give it when it is needed (Darley and Latané, 1968; Smithson *et al.*, 1983). We shall not discuss this, except to say that the adverse effects of help may explain some of the reluctance to give help, which is seen at its most extreme in the 'unresponsive bystander'. The second deals with the effects of different styles of help on the task in hand. This is an enormous literature on learning, instruction, teaching and intellectual development. The third concerns longer term reactions to help, for example on self-esteem and on future competence. We shall deal briefly with each of these in turn.

There are many different approaches to teaching and instruction, but the most important can be fitted into three broad categories. The first is the behaviourist, or 'bottom-up', approach which assumes the task of the instructor is to provide the elements of knowledge in a logical order and allows the general principles to emerge later. The second is the cognitive, or 'top-down', approach which assumes that learning will be more effective if the instructor starts with the broad principles of what must be learned and then allows the student to have more or less control of the order in which he or she acquires the elements. The third is interactive and assumes that both bottom-up and top-down approaches have their place and that that place must be determined by an interaction between the pupil and teacher. We shall concentrate on the last-mentioned, drawing heavily on the ideas of Piaget, Vygotsky and Bruner (see, for example, Wertsch, 1985; Bruner, 1966).

Piaget believed that the role of the instructor, or helper, was to present the learning child with experiences which were slightly discrepant from current understanding. In this way the child would develop more powerful understanding. Vygotsky characterized the tolerable degree of discrepancy as the 'zone of proximal development', which is the gap between what a child can do unaided and what it can do with help. Bruner went further than either Vygotsky or Piaget in requiring the teacher to have a clearly structured idea of what it is the child needs to learn. All three theorists conceive instruction as an interactive process in which the chief elements are what the child knows already, the goal which the instructor sets, the child's conception of the speed with which learning can take place and the direction in which it should go, and the instructor's conception of the appropriate direction and speed of learning. Particularly from Bruner and Vygotsky, we get a view of learning as a negotiation between teacher and pupil, who have to agree about what is possible and desirable.

These descriptions of the process of instruction have not been rigorously tested but have been extremely influential. They can be regarded as descriptions of what happens during the most effective period of childhood learning—when the child is learning to be physically skillful, to talk and to be otherwise socialized.

These conceptions of teaching seem to apply best to individual tuition; but the relative success of education can be understood if we assume that the negotiation of what is possible has occurred culturally over a long period of time. However, there is a documented weakness in the educational systems of most advanced countries, whose less able students over the age of 11 seem to have very great difficulty acquiring important linguistic and mathematical concepts which the brighter pupils mastered releatively easily at a younger age (Husen, 1977; Hart, 1981). One possible explanation of this follows from the discovery that over the age of 11, children begin to make the distinction between effort and ability (Nicholls and Miller, 1983), and that before that age children do not show the performance impairments after failure which are one of the chief indicators of learned helplessness (Miller, 1985). Miller set out to compare 'egotism' (Frankel and Snyder, 1978) as an alternative to learned helplessness as an explanation of the cognitive effects of failure. It is suggested that the 'egotist' is concerned to avoid threats to his self-esteem, such as appearing to be of low ability, and hence avoids, or does not try to succeed in, tasks in which he is not sure of success. This is contrasted with the learned helplessness theory of Abramson et al. (1978) which, according to Miller, regards loss of competence as a more automatic consequence of a perceived inability to control events. Miller found that failure in a figure-matching task lowered performance on a subsequent anagram task for sixth grade children (aged 12+) but not for second grade children (aged 8+). He explained the difference in terms of Nicholls' finding that, under the age of 11, children do not distinguish between failure due to lack of ability and failure due to lack of effort, and claimed that his finding supported the 'egotism' hypothesis. The logic of this argument is highly questionable, since one could equally well argue that the distinction between effort and ability is central to many of the reformulations of the learned helplessness theory.

Whatever the preferred explanation, all recent work and reformulations of the learned helplessness theory suggest that it can be fitted comfortably within an evolutionary framework and that the reduction of ambition and competence, which has been demonstrated many times to follow failure, can improve our biological 'fitness'. Learned helplessness, together with learning to learn, provides a form of negative feedback which will crudely ensure that we try to learn or to perform what is within our capacity but do not exceed it. It may be that failure shrinks our conception of our own 'zone of proximal development.'. If this is correct, then learned helplessness is only handicapping when our conception of what we are capable of learning or doing is unnecessarily or unrealistically timid. This may be one of the consequences of failure at school and is a major problem in all systems of universal education. It may also be one of the handicapping effects of stress.

The factors which affect our own conception of our competence are perhaps most clearly indicated in experimental studies of the longer term effects of help.

The most impressive of the studies of the effects of help is that by de Paulo *et al.* (1981), who asked female students to do two tasks, one after the other. The first was a pattern completion task, the second an anagram task. When the first task was completed the subjects passed their papers to another female who was also supposed to be a subject but who was, in fact, a confederate of the experimenters. She marked it and returned it with a mark of 35% for the subject. The subjects also marked the confederate's paper, which always merited a mark of 95%. The confederate also added various remarks on the bottom of the subjects' answer sheets. These remarks were of different types for different subjects. Some were helpful comments on how to do the pattern task, some socially supportive ('good luck on the next task'), some threatening ('I guess this is hard for you'). The subjects then moved on to the second task, performance on which provided the dependent variable.

The pattern of results was different for subjects of high and low self-esteem. Those of high self-esteem did better on the second task if they had received a helpful hint about the first task. This improvement was greater if it was accompanied by a threatening remark than if it was accompanied by a supportive remark. In contrast, low self-esteem subjects did less well on the second task if they had received help on the first, and this deterioration was also greater if accompanied by a threatening rather than a supportive remark. This pattern of results suggests that high self-esteem subjects try harder when paired with someone who is apparently more competent than they are and who emphasizes this by trying to help and by making a disparaging remark. It contrast, low self-esteem subjects suffer from a loss of competence under the same conditions.

It is interesting that the greatest improvement in competence in those of high self-esteem, and the greatest deterioration in competence in those of low self-esteem, are produced by the same task-oriented and challenging kind of help. Socially supportive, non-task-oriented help is less helpful to those of high self-esteem and less damaging to those of low self-esteem.

This is unfortunately the only study of the effects of help in one task on competence in an unrelated task. But the effect may be related to the greater sensitivity of those of low self-esteem to the effects of failure (e.g. Brockner, 1979), and the pattern of results is very similar to that obtained by Kobasa (1982) for the effects of social support on executives under stress. There is a real possibility that these effects are at least reasonably common. If this is so, then the comparative ineffectiveness of professional help, and the lack of any theory about it which makes sense, may be partly a result of a failure to treat different personalities differently when trying to help them overcome the effects of stress, and partly a result of the likelihood that any kind of help may be damaging to people of low self-esteem (Nadler and Fisher, 1986).

There is a reasonably extensive literature on the effects of help on people's self-concepts and how this depends on the personality of the one being helped, on the similarity of helper and helpee, on the possibility of returning the help, on the presence or absence of a mirror, and on many other factors (Nadler and Fisher, 1984; Coates et al., 1983).

One of the puzzling features of these studies is the finding that people of low self-esteem do not mind seeking help (Tessler and Schwartz, 1972), and that their self-esteem does not suffer as a result (Nadler et al., 1976). In contrast, in experimental studies, people of high self-esteem are likely to suffer a lowering of self-esteem if they accept help from a similar person but not from a dissimilar person (Nadler et al., 1976). This result seems inconsistent with the finding that it is the performance of people of low self-esteem which is damaged by help rather than that of the high self-esteem subjects in the study of de Paulo et al. (1981). This apparent conflict of evidence remains to be resolved, but it does not prevent us speculating about the relative effectiveness of different sorts of help for different sorts of people. Those of high self-esteem can be challenged, while those of low self-esteem need to be encouraged. At the same time we must be alert to the possibility that high self-esteem can be threatened by insensitive help, perhaps even more than by failure.

IS A SYNTHESIS POSSIBLE?

Ideas encountered in the literature on learned helplessness, instruction and the experimental studies of helping show an interesting convergence and make up for the disappointing state of older theories of helping.

We are left with a picture of individuals coping with the demands life makes of them and, at the same time, trying to discover which sort of problems they can solve and which they should leave to someone else. In other words, we are all trying to discover what sort of person we are, and a very important aspect of our personality is our competence at different tasks, both old and new. The most important strategy we use is, very sensibly, to follow up on the things we do best and to give up on those we do badly. But this strategy can go horribly wrong if it is poorly tuned. If we respond only to success and ignore failure, we are likely to become more and more ambitious and to attempt to do things beyond our scope. If we respond only to failure, we are likely to become less and less enterprising and fail to make use of what competence we possess. This analysis has obvious similarities to Gray's (1971) description of aggression and anxiety as being due to differential sensitivities to positive and negative reinforcement. Sensitivity to failure has been blamed for some aspects of depression. Insensitivity to failure may be an important aspect of mania.

The greater sensitivity of people of low self-esteem to the effects of failure (Brockner, 1979) and the possibly greater sensitivity of the non-hardy to the effects of stress (Kobasa, 1982) suggest that it may not be too difficult to pick out those people who are likely to be most affected by stress. What is more difficult is to devise optimal helping strategies for different people in different circumstances.

There are fortunately some very encouraging examples of successful interventions whose effects are much greater than the usual 50% better than nothing which is the commonest finding in evaluations of psychological help. Perhaps the most cheering of these is that of Rodin and Langer (1977), referred to earlier. They gave pots of flowers to all the inmates of a large old people's home. Half of them were given responsibility for looking after the flowers. The other half were told that the nurses would look after the flowers. There were some other small differences, largely concerned with exhorting the first group to take control of other small features of their lives. There was an immediate difference in morale and activity in the two groups. Eighteen months later, 30% of the group with less responsibility, but only 15% of the group with greater responsibility, had died. One is reminded of the apparent life-extending qualities of political power. It may be that we shorten the lives of our old people when we do too much for them, and particularly when we take away from them responsibility for their own environment.

Schultz (1976) produced a very similar improvement in morale by allowing old people more control of the times and duration of visits from students. But when he returned 18 months latr, the death rate was greater in the group given greater responsibility (Schultz and Hanusa, 1978). This seems like a contradictory result, but it is not. Rodin and Langer left their pots of flowers behind during the 18 months' interval before the follow-up study so that the differences in control remained. Schultz' students stopped visiting immediately after the initial study, so that the group given greater control lost it rather suddenly.

These results are in stark contrast to the comparative ineffectiveness of counselling, psychotherapy and social case work. In these studies, the main problem is the ethical dilemmas posed by doing research on variables which have such a dramatic effect (Rodin et al., 1982). One would like to know if giving the old people even more responsibility would have prolonged their lives still further. It seems likely that too much responsibility could have had just as bad an effect as too little, since with too much responsibility and too many things to do, the old people may have again lost their sense of their own competence.

The evidence is not yet strong, but it does suggest a totally different approach to helping people cope with stress. It suggests that in all aspects of our lives we are competent, but within limits. If too many demands are made of us, we lose control. If too few, there is no control to be exercised. We know that there is an optimum rate at which children can be taught and at which adults can be persuaded to adopt new attitudes. All of these phenomena may be consequences of our attempts to understand ourselves and our relationship to our environment. If this analysis is correct, the best way to help people cope with stress should be by a cooperative problem-solving approach which gives optimum responsibility to the stressed persons but which also protects them from the most adverse effects of their long- or short-term incompetence.

This theory has some similarity with Karasek's (1979) model of job strain. He regards demand and control as independent variables and believes that stress is greatest when demand is high but control is low. This model has face validity in employment contexts where control is more a feature of the place of the individual in the organization and of the organizational style in the workplace, rather than of the particular job which is being done. But, in less constrained situations, control and demand are highly correlated because it is more difficult to succeed with more demanding tasks. Under these circumstances, perception of control or ability may be more determined by experience, ability and personality, than by external constraints.

SUMMARY AND CONCLUSIONS

The commonest theories of helping, derived from either psychodynamic or behaviourist theories, are clearly inadequate since they lead to no observable relationship between practice and outcome. This does not mean that help is ineffective, merely that we do not know why.

In contrast, theories of instruction which suggest that help must be closely related to the students' existing knowledge and to the students' expectations of their own abilities, provide a more powerful framework for understanding the effects of stress and of our more or less successful attempts to help people overcome the adverse effects of failure.

REFERENCES

Abramson, L.Y., Seligman, M.E.P., & Teasdale, J.D. (1978). Learned helplessness in humans: Critique and reformulation. *Journal of Abnormal Psychology, 87(1)*, 49–74.

Alloy, L.B., & Abramson, L.Y. (1982). Learned helplessness, depression, and the illusion of control. *Journal of Personality and Social Psychology, 42(6)*, 1114–1126.

Baum, A., & Gatchel, R.J. (1981). Cognitive determinants of reaction to uncontrollable events: Development of reactance and learned helplessness. *Journal of Personality and Social Psychology, 40(6)*, 1078–1089.

Baumeister, R.F. (1982). A self-presentational view of social phenomena. *Psychological Bulletin, 91(1)*, 3–26.

Baumgardner, A.H., Heppner, P.P., & Arkin, R.M. (1986). Role of causal attribution in personal problem solving. *Journal of Personality and Social Psychology, 50(3)*, 636–643.

Berman, J.S., & Norton, N.C. (1985). Does professional training make a therapist more effective? *Psychological Bulletin, 98(2)*, 401–407.

Boyd, J.L., McGill, C.W., & Falloon, I.R.H. (1981). Family participation in the community rehabilitation of schizophrenics. *Hospital Community Psychiatry, 32(9)*, 629–632.

Brehm, J.W. (1966). *A theory of psychological reactance*. New York: Academic Press.

Brehmer, B. (1980). In one word: Not from experience. *Acta Psychologica, 45*, 223–241.

Brewer, C., & Lait, J. (1980). *Can social work survive?* London: Temple Smith.

Brockner, J. (1979). The effects of self esteem, success–failure and self-consciousness on task performance. *Journal of Personality and Social Psychology, 37*, 1732–1741.

Brown, G.W., & Harris, T.O. (1978). *Social origins of depression: A study of psychiatric disorder in women*. London: Tavistock.

Brown, G.W., Monck, E.M., Carstairs, G.M., & Wing, J.K. (1962). The influence of family life on the course of schizophrenia illness. *British Journal of Preventative and Social Medicine, 16*, 55–68.

Bruner, J.S. (1966). *Toward a theory of instruction*. Cambridge, Mass.: Harvard University Press.

Coates, D., Renzaglia, G.J., & Embree, M.C. (1983). When helping backfires: Help and helplessness. In *New Directions in Helping, I*. London: Academic Press.

Cobb, S. (1976). Social support as a moderator of life stress. *Psychosomatic Medicine, 38(5)*, 300–314.

Darley, J.M., & Latané, B. (1968). Bystander intervention in emergencies: Diffusion of responsibility. *Journal of Personality and Social Psychology, 10*, 202–214.

de Paulo, B.M., Brown, P.L., Ishii, S., & Fisher, J.D. (1981). Help that works: The effects of aid on subsequent task performance. *Journal of Personality and Social Psychology, 41*, 478–487.

Frankel, A., & Snyder, M.L. (1978). Poor performance following unsolvable problems: learned helplessness or egotism? *Journal of Personality and Social Psychology, 36*, 1415–1423.

Garber, J., & Hollen, S.D. (1980). Universal versus personal helplessness in depression: belief in incontrollability or incompetence. *Journal of Abnormal Psychology, 89*, 56–66.

Goldstein, M.J. (1983). Family interaction: Patterns predictive of the onset and course of schizophrenia. In H. Stierlin, L.C. Wynne, & M. Wirsching (eds), *Psychosocial interventions in schizophrenia* (pp. 5–19). New York: Springer-Verlag.

Gray, J. (1971). *The psychology of fear and stress*. London: Weidenfeld & Nicolson.

Harlow, H.F. (1949). The formulation of learning sets. *Psychological Review, 51*, 51–65.

Hart, K.M. (ed.) (1981). *Children's understanding of mathematics: 11–16*. London: John Murray.

Hattie, J.A., Sharpley, C.F., & Rogers, H.J. (1984). Comparative effectiveness of professional and paraprofessional helpers. *Psychological Bulletin, 95*, 534–541.

Howarth, C.I. (1976). The psychology of urban life. In G.A. Harrison & J.B. Gibson (eds), *Man in urban environments*. London: Oxford University Press.

Husen, T. (ed.) (1977). *International study of achievement in mathematics, Vols. I and II*. Chichester: Wiley.

Karasek R. (1979). Job demands, job decision latitude, and mental strain; implications for job design. *Administrative Science Quarterly, 24*, 285–308.

Kessler, R.C., & McLeod, J. (1984). Social support and psychological distress in community surveys. In S. Cohen & L. Syme (eds), *Social support and health*. New York: Academic Press.

Kessler, R.C., Price, R.H., & Wortman, C.B. (1985). Social factors in psychopathology: Stress, social support, and coping processes. *Annual Review of Psychology, 36*, 531–572.

Kobasa, S.C. (1982). The hardy personality: Toward a social psychology of stress and health. In G.S. Sanders & J. Suls (eds), *Social psychology of health and illness*. New Jersey: Lawrence Erlbaum.

Kobasa, S.C., & Puccetti, M.C. (1983). Personality and social resources in stress resistance. *Journal of Personality and Social Psychology, 45*, 839–850.

McCord, J. (1978). A thirty-year follow-up of treatment effects. *American Psychologist, March*, 284–289.

Miller, A. (1985). A developmental study of the cognitive basis of performance impairment after failure. *Journal of Personality and Social Psychology, 49(2)*, 529–538.

Miller, P., & Ingham, J.G. (1976). Friends, confidants and symptoms. *Social Psychiatry, II*, 51–58.

Nadler, A., & Fisher, J.D. (1984). Effects of donor–recipient relationships on recipients' reactions to aid. In E. Staub *et al.* (eds), *Development and maintenance of prosocial behavior. International perspectives on positive morality*. New York: Plenum.

Nadler, A., & Fisher, J.D. (1986). The role of threat to self-esteem and perceived control in recipient reactions to help: Theory development and empirical validation. *Advances in Experimental Social Psychology, 19*, 81–122.

Nadler, A., Fisher, J.D., & Streufert, S. (1976). When helping hurts: The effects of donor–recipient similarity on recipient self esteem on reactions to aid. *Journal of Personality and Social Psychology, 44*, 392–409.

Nicholls, J.G., & Miller, A. (1983). The differentiation of the concepts of difficulty and ability. *Child Development, 54*, 951–959.

Orwin, A. (1973). The 'running treatment': A preliminary communication on a new use for old therapy (physical activity) in the agoraphobic syndrome. *British Journal of Psychiatry, 122*, 175–179.

Parloff, M.B., London, P., & Wolfe, B. (1986). Individual psychotherapy and behavior change. *Annual Review of Psychology, 37*, 321–349.

Prioleau, L., Murdock, M., & Brody, N. (1983). An analysis of psychotherapy versus placebo studies. *The Behavioral and Brain Sciences, 6*, 275–310.

Rodin, J., Bohm, L., & Wack, J.T. (1982). Control, coping and aging: Models for research and intervention. In L. Bickman (ed.), *Applied social psychology annual, Vol. 3* (pp. 153–180). Beverly Hills: Sage.

Rodin, J., & Langer, E.J. (1977). Long-term effects of a control-relevant intervention with the institutionalized aged. *Journal of Personality and Social Psychology, 35(12)*, 897–902.

Schultz, R. (1976). Effects of control and predictability in the physical and psychological well-being of the institutionalised aged. *Journal of Personality and Social Psychology, 33*, 563–573.

Schultz, R., & Hanusa, B.H. (1978). Long term effects of control and predictability enhancing interventions: Findings and ethical issues. *Journal of Personality and Social Psychology, 36*, 1194–1201.

Seligman, M.E.P. (1975). *Helplessness: On depression, development and death*. San Francisco: W.H. Freeman.

Shephard, R.J. (1983). Employee health and fitness: The state of the art. *Preventative Medicine, 12*, 644–653.

Slater, J., & Deprie, R.A. (1981). The contributions of environmental events and social support to serious suicide attempts in primary depressive disorder. *Journal of Abnormal Psychology, 90*, 275–285.

Sloane, R.B., Staples, F.R., Cristol, A.H., Yorkston, N.J., & Whipple, K. (1975). *Psychotherapy versus behavior therapy*. Cambridge, Mass.: Harvard University Press.

Smith, M.L., Glass, G.V., & Miller, T.I. (1980). *The benefits of psychotherapy*. Baltimore: Johns Hopkins.

Smithson, M., Amato, P.R., & Pierce, P. (1983). *Dimensions of helping behaviour*. Oxford: Pergamon.

Stiles, W.B., Shapiro, D.A., & Elliott, R. (1986). Are all psychotherapies equivalent? *American Psychologist, 41*, 165–180.

Tessler, R.C., & Schwartz, S.H. (1972). Help seeking, self-esteem, and achievement motivation: An attributional analysis. *Journal of Personality and Social Psychology, 21*, 318–326.

Vaughan, C.E., & Leff, J.P. (1976). The influence of family and social factors on the course of psychiatric illness: A comparison of schizophrenic and depressed neurotic patients. *British Journal of Psychiatry, 129*, 125–137.
Wertsch, J.V. (1985). *Vygotsky and the social formation of mind*. Cambridge, Mass.: Harvard University Press.

KEY WORDS

Stress, help, helping, coping, learned helplessness, learning to learn, control, responsibility, zone of proximal development, instruction, ability, effort, self-esteem, locus of control, task, social support, demand, help seeking, effects of help, strain, psychotherapy, counselling, psychodynamic, behaviourist, competence, incompetence, depression, resistance to stress, hardiness.

Handbook of Life Stress, Cognition and Health
Edited by S. Fisher and J. Reason
© 1988 John Wiley & Sons Ltd.

36

Confiding Traumatic Experiences and Health

JAMES W. PENNEBAKER
Southern Methodist University, Dallas

INTRODUCTION

Major life events are associated with subsequent psychological and physiological problems. Over the last two decades, an increasing number of studies indicate that the deleterious effects of major life events can be buffered by strong social support networks (Cohen and Syme, 1982; Wallston *et al.*, 1983). Unfortunately, very little attention has been devoted to the meaning of the events for the individual. For example, many upheavals, such as death of a spouse, being laid off from work, etc., are 'socially acceptable'. That is, when they occur, the victims can discuss the events with their social support network. Other experiences are less acceptable and thus are not discussed to the same degree. For example, when individuals are raped or molested, have served as soldiers in an unpopular war such as in Vietnam, or are involved in illicit relationships, they may not be able to discuss the event with anyone—even though they may still maintain a large and stable network of friends. In cases such as these, the act of *not* discussing or confiding the event with another may be more damaging than having experienced the event per se.

Since the early 1980s, we have been examining the health and physiological consequences of confiding versus not confiding in others about a traumatic event. Our work indicates that the failure to confide represents a special case of the larger construct of inhibition. Traumatic events associated with inhibition are more likely to be the focus of obsessive thoughts for several years or decades. Further, such events are ultimately associated with a number of major and minor diseases (for more detailed discussion, see Pennebaker, 1985; Pennebaker and Susman, in press).

At present, our theory can be summarized by three general propositions.

Preparation of this manuscript was made possible by grants from the National Science Foundation (BNS 86–06764) and the National Heart, Lung, and Blood Institute (HL32547).

1. To actively inhibit ongoing behavior, feelings, or thoughts requires physiological work. Short-term inhibition is reflected in phasic autonomic changes (e.g. skin conductance, heart rate, and blood pressure increases). Long-term inhibition is associated with stress-related diseases such as infections, ulcers, etc.

2. The more that individuals inhibit thoughts, emotions, and behavior, the more they think about the behaviors that are being inhibited (i.e. obsessive thinking) or, in some cases, actively work to avoid thinking about them. Obsessive thinking and the resultant anxiety are associated with increased physiological activity.

3. Confiding or consciously confronting the perceptions and feelings associated with a traumatic event allows for the integration or cognitive reorganization of the event. The confiding act, then, allows individuals to 'forget' or to otherwise put the event behind them—thus reducing physiological activity by negating the need for further obsessing and inhibiting.

Certain events are more likely to be associated with inhibition than others. When individuals do not or cannot discuss significant personal experiences for fear of punishment, guilt, or hurting others, they often must hold back from conveying their conscious thoughts and feelings to others. As we discuss in greater detail below, certain highly charged emotional events such as sexual traumas, divorce, and other events associated with humiliation are particularly likely to be inhibited.

If inhibition is related to short-term physiological changes, a number of possible links to long-term disease processes can be made. An implication of this work is that we know that social support is a vague construct that, nonetheless, is related to health. Hopefully, we can identify one of the mediating variables that may work independently of number of close friends. That we are linking our research to traumatic events not typically examined in the traditional life events literature will give us a better understanding of the long-term health implications of such traumas as concentration camp experience, incest, child abuse, etc. Indeed, the health consequences of traumas such as these may last the entire lifespan.

In the remainder of this chapter, the research that we have conducted related to confiding and inhibition will be summarized. We conclude the chapter with speculations about the processes underlying the benefits of confronting a trauma.

INHIBITION OF THOUGHTS, FEELINGS AND BEHAVIORS REQUIRES PHYSIOLOGICAL WORK

Short-Term Inhibition

Freud (e.g. 1915/1963) posited that not only was the act of initially repressing a thought effortful, but that continuous energy was needed to keep a thought suppressed. He did not focus, however, on the physiological mechanisms related to effort or energy expenditure. In some of the earliest experiments with human inhibition, Alexander Luria (1932) provided compelling evidence that when individuals were told to try to inhibit their expression of specific thoughts via hypnosis, they demonstrated increases in several autonomic channels. Particularly intriguing, Luria found that manipulated attempts to inhibit thoughts, feelings, or behaviors resulted in increased physiological activity and gross cognitive impairments (e.g. longer reaction times in response to simple and complex stimuli).

In recent years, Jeffrey Gray (1975) has argued that specific regions in the central nervous system are variously related to behavioral inhibition and to behavioral activation. In reviewing a large number of animal studies, Gray indicates that blocking the action of the behavioral inhibition system (which is associated with neural pathways in the septum and hippocampus) by drugs or lesions results in the animal's inability to inhibit activity that may result in punishment (i.e. passive avoidance paradigm).

In an extension of Gray's work, Fowles (1980) provides evidence indicating that behavioral inhibition is specifically linked to skin conductance activity in humans, whereas behavioral activation is associated with increased cardiovascular action. When individuals must restrain naturally occurring behavior, electrodermal activity increases whereas other autonomic nervous system activity is not directly affected. In a recent test of this idea, individuals who were induced to deceive an experimenter inhibited overt behaviors such as eye movements and facial expressions while, at the same time, their immediate skin conductance levels (SCLs) increased markedly (Pennebaker and Chew, 1985). Other work implicates cardiovascular activity as a reflection of bodily movement or other somatic activity (Obrist, 1981). Interestingly, a large number of studies point to the fact that blood pressure and heart rate changes can also reflect increased cognitive work (Lacey, 1956).

Long-Term Inhibition

Whereas brief instances of behavioral inhibition covary with increases in SCL, recent clinical and personality research suggests that individuals classified as chronic inhibitors yield higher overall autonomic levels and are at higher risk for a number of diseases. For example, Buck (1984) reports that individuals who tend to be low in overt emotional expressiveness have higher overall SCLs than those who are expressive. Similarly, individuals rated as high in repressive coping styles (Weinberger et al., 1979) or highly or overly socialized (e.g. Waid and Orne, 1982) have higher SCLs than non-repressors or those classified as poorly socialized. Finally, several studies suggest that individuals rated as inhibited or repressed are more prone to such problems as hypertension (McClelland, 1979), physical illness in general (Blackburn, 1965), and higher mortality rates following diagnosis of breast cancer (Derogatis et al., 1979).

DISCLOSURE OF TRAUMATIC EVENTS IS PHYSICALLY AND COGNITIVELY BENEFICIAL

If the failure to discuss traumatic or stressful events is physiologically harmful, it would follow that disclosing these events should be beneficial. Three recent studies suggest that talking or writing about major upheavals may ultimately reduce health problems as well as unwanted thoughts about the events. These studies also point to some of the underlying processes that may explain the long-term benefits of confession.

Immediate Autonomic Changes

Recall that the inhibition of behavior has been shown to relate to skin conductance levels. In two related experiments, Pennebaker et al. (1987) demonstrated that when individuals disclosed extremely personal and stressful life events, their skin conductance levels dropped. In the two studies, subjects were divided into high disclosers and low disclosers, based on what they disclosed into a tape recorder (experiment 1) or to an anonymous 'confessor' (experiment 2). All subjects talked about a traumatic event in their life and a trivial topic—what they planned to do in the hours following the experiment.

In line with inhibition predictions, talking about traumatic events was associated with lower skin conductance among the high disclosers than talking about trivial issues. Low disclosers, on the other hand, showed an opposite pattern of results. The cardiovascular measures (systolic and diastolic blood pressure, heart rate) dramatically increased *while* talking about traumatic events and, to a lesser degree, trivial events. Nevertheless, following the traumatic disclosures, blood pressure and heart rate dropped to levels at or below baseline.

Cognitive Benefits

Common responses to a traumatic event involve intrusive, unwanted thoughts and the denial or blocking of thoughts about the event (Lang, 1977; Zilberg et al., 1982). When individiuals discuss an upsetting experience, several processes contribute to help the victim. Confiding in others often allows for social comparison feedback, coping information, and various forms of positive reinforcement (e.g. Lazarus and Folkman, 1984). In addition, the mere act of talking about a personal trauma makes an individual feel closer to the one who is being confided to—thus increasing the powers of social support (Jourard, 1971). Of particular significance is that confiding in others or even writing about the event helps the person to organize cognitively or work through (Horowitz, 1976), reframe (Meichenbaum, 1977), and find meaning to the experience (Silver et al., 1983). If these cognitive effects are accomplished, the individual should be better able to put the trauma behind him.

Although it is commonly assumed that talking about an event helps the person to cope, very little empirical evidence is available to support such a contention. Recently, Pennebaker and O'Heeron (1984) surveyed a stratified sample of individuals whose spouses had died the previous year by suicide or automobile accident. Although the sample size was small (19 cases, representing a return rate of 61%), three important effects emerged. First, the more that respondents talked with others about their spouse's deaths, the fewer health problems they reported during the following year. Second, the more that subjects ruminated or thought about their spouses' deaths, the more the health problems the following year. Third, the more that individuals talked with others about the death, the *less* they ruminated about the deaths.

The results from the Pennebaker and O'Heeron study suggest a possible inverse causal relationship between talking about an event and ruminating about it.

Indeed, recent laboratory studies by Wegner and his colleagues indicate that individuals required to suppress a thought are more likely to ruminate about it at a later time if given the opportunity (see Wegner, Chapter 37 in this volume; also, Wegner *et al.*, 1987). These patterns of findings are particularly important given that long-term ruminating or obsession about a traumatic upheaval is undoubtedly stressful and deleterious to health over time (cf. Rachman and Hodgson, 1980).

Long-Term Physical Benefits

In their development of the cathartic method, Breuer and Freud (1895/1966) emphasized the importance of 'the talking cure' in the relief of hysterical symptoms by encouraging the patient to discuss all major aspects of earlier traumatic experiences. Alexander (1950) noted that in some cases physiological problems such as asthma, ulcer, or high blood pressure could be relieved by allowing the patient to confess repressed desires. Jourard (1971), a pioneer of self-disclosure research, noted that either talking with others or even writing about one's problems could ultimately reduce and/or prevent health problems.

In a recent attempt to learn what aspects of disclosing traumatic events could influence long-term health, Pennebaker and Beall (1986) required 46 healthy undergraduates to write about either the most traumatic and stressful experience of their lives or about trivial assigned topics for four consecutive days. Of those assigned to write about traumatic events, one experimental group wrote about the facts surrounding the traumas but not their feelings about the traumas (trauma-factual condition), another about their feelings concerning the traumas but not the facts (trauma-emotion), and a third about both their feelings and the facts concerning the traumas (trauma-combination group). Across the four experimental sessions, subjects in the trauma-emotion and the trauma-combination conditions reported feeling the most upset after writing and demonstrated increases in systolic blood pressure compared to the control and trauma-factual subjects.

Most important, however, was that subjects in the trauma-combination cell visited the student health center for illness in the 6 months following the experiment significantly less than those in the other conditions (Figure 36.1). Six-month follow-up questionnaires also showed a consistent pattern indicating that trauma-combination and trauma-emotion subjects felt healthier, reported fewer illnesses, and fewer days restricted activity due to illness.

Although the Pennebaker and Beall study suffers from some weaknesses, it nevertheless suggests that written—and anonymous—disclosure of traumatic experiences, while initially unpleasant for the individual, may ultimately reduce physician visits and improve health perceptions. Further, for long-term benefits to accrue, it appears to be important for the person to disclose not only the event but also the emotions aroused by the event.

In a recent extension of these findings, Pennebaker *et al.* (in press) sought to learn if writing about traumatic experiences had a direct impact on immune function. Over four consecutive days, 50 healthy undergraduates were randomly assigned to write about either the most upsetting events of their lives or about

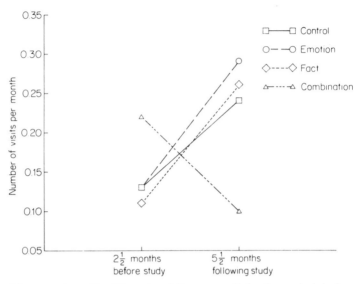

FIG. 36.1   Mean number of health center visits per month for the periods before and after the experiment (from Pennebaker and Beall, 1986).

superficial topics. Blood samples were drawn from the participants before the first day of writing, the last day of writing, and a third time 6 weeks later. Using a blastogenic procedure, two related immune assays (relying on the mitogens Con A and PHA) were performed on the blood samples that measured the action of T-lymphocytes. In addition to the immune assays, we were also able to collect autonomic, physician visit, and self-report data from all of the subjects over the course of the study.

Two particularly exciting results emerged from the immune study. First, compared to controls, individuals who wrote about traumas exhibited improved immune function from the final day of the experiment through the 6-week follow-up. As in the earlier study, trauma subjects also evidenced a significant drop in health center visits for illness after participating in the experiment relative to controls. Second, subjects in the trauma group were asked each day: 'To what degree did you write about something which you have previously held back telling others?' Those who reported confronting previously inhibited topics were labeled high disclosers and those below the median in the response to the item were called low disclosers. As would be predicted, high disclosers showed significantly greater immune improvements than low disclosers from before to after the writing portion of the study (Figure 36.2).

Summary

Taken together, the results indicate that confronting extremely traumatic experiences is associated with immediate reductions in skin conductance, and with long-term positive changes in obsessional thinking, immune function, and illness behavior. Individuals who benefit most from our experimental paradigm appear

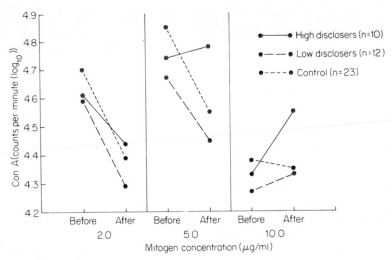

FIG. 36.2   Lymphocyte response to three levels of ConA stimulation before and after the writing sessions (from Pennebaker *et al.*; in press).

to be those who are currently living with the trauma and who focus on the thoughts and feelings associated with the experience. In the following section, we will explore some possible explanations for these effects.

POSSIBLE EXPLANATIONS FOR THE VALUE OF CONFRONTING TRAUMAS

Although the various studies indicate that writing or talking about upsetting experiences is physically beneficial, we have not satisfactorily addressed why the link exists. This is an issue that we are far from understanding. Nevertheless, our work points to both cognitive and social factors that may contribute to the value of talking about one's problems. Although we briefly discuss each one, it is important to acknowledge that these domains are incomplete and not mutually exclusive.

Cognitive Correlates of Disclosure

The act of confronting traumas forces the individual to think about them in different ways. Several processes are at work in helping the person to overcome their long-term effects. In addition to helping the person to understand and assimilate the events, confronting a trauma forces the individual to translate the event into language, to externalize the event, and to allow a form of self-expression.

Meaning and Assimilation

A number of therapists and researchers point to the value of talking with others about traumatic experiences in helping to bring about a new understanding of the experiences. Cognitive therapists, for example, stress the importance of seeing an event from a different perspective. By talking or writing about an event, the individual reframes it, which results in a deeper understanding of it (Meichenbaum, 1977). Along similar lines, a group of social psychologists have stressed the importance of finding meaning to an event (cf. Wortman and Silver, 1980; Silver *et al.*, 1983). Across several studies, these researchers have verified that individuals who find meaning in tragic events (e.g. paralysis following a swimming accident, sudden death of an infant) cope much better than those who do not find meaning.

The primary value of reframing or finding meaning in a trauma is that it helps the individual to organize and assimilate the experience. According to Horowitz (1976), traumas are unique in impinging on all aspects of life. Although most daily experiences are easily assimilated and stored in memory, the emotional content, magnitude, and uniqueness of traumas impede this process. The act of talking or writing about overwhelming traumas helps to bring about assimilation for several reasons. First, the act of communicating the event forces some degree of organization or structure. Second, by talking about the event several times, the individual gradually levels and sharpens different parts of the experience. As portions are understood, they become assimilated. This process may continue until the entire experience is assimilated and cognitively 'filed away'. Third, repeated writing or talking about the trauma helps to bring about the habituation of the emotional response to the event (Rachman, 1980). Fourth, talking or writing about an event forces the individual publicly to acknowledge its existence and impact. The person can no longer work to deny the nature of it.

The Role of Language

Disclosing a traumatic experience is beneficial, in part, because it converts the experience from images to language. The process of coding information linguistically accomplishes several goals. First, because images are psychologically large, diffuse, and changing over time, converting them to language forces some degree of temporal organization. Further, writing and, to a somewhat lesser degree, talking are relatively slow processes that require the sequencing of thoughts and feelings. Otherwhelming images are reduced to a surprisingly small number of words. In our experience, we have found that most people who have suffered unimaginably horrible experiences run out of things to write about them in a few hours over several days.

A second goal of converting traumas into language was discussed by Freud (1915/1963) and Breuer and Freud (1895/1966). In Freud's view, the ability to use language to describe an event was the prime marker of the event's presence in consciousness. Freud noted that one of the dangers of traumas was that individuals suppressed or repressed the thoughts of the events while their associated emotions of anxiety remained in consciousness. One goal of therapy was to bring these thoughts, or ideation, into consciousness and to link them with their appropriate feelings. The birth of the cathartic method came about as Breuer and Freud discovered that their patients benefitted from talking in detail about the thoughts and feelings they harbored about their upsetting experiences. Talking—

even in a stream of consciousness mode—crystallized forgotten and important thoughts, thus simplifying the process of connecting traumatic ideation and emotion.

A third factor associated with the translation into language concerns the possible changes that occur in the central nervous system. Although a traumatic experience may be coded in different forms throughout the cortex, an individual who actively avoids confronting the trauma may experience trauma-relevant feelings associated with negative affective areas in the right cortical hemisphere (cf. Davidson, 1980). However, these experiences may be consciously kept from the language-production regions of the brain in the left hemisphere. The individual who is actively inhibiting thoughts and feelings associated with trauma, then, should exhibit more general cortical activity than one who has not experienced a trauma. Further, this activity should be asynchronous from one brain region to another. That is, one part of the cortex may be 'reliving' a portion of the trauma, whereas another may be actively avoiding it by engaging in obsessions or compulsions. Once a trauma is translated into language, however, the trauma-relevant information would be stored and processed in similar ways in more brain regions. In short, this would reduce the overall independent processing of the same information within separate cortical areas. These ideas, which are quite speculative, are currently being examined in our laboratory.

Externalizing the Event

I am not the kind of person that routinely makes lists. However, whenever I am about to move or go on vacation, I am forced to make lengthy lists of last-minute tasks to perform. Before making the list, I actively juggle the tasks in my mind for several days. Once the list is completed, however, I have transferred my memory from within my head to a piece of paper. Other researchers have noted how we can view memory as external to our brains. Wegner (1986; Wegner *et al.*, 1985), for example, has provided fascinating examples of how partners in a marriage or intimate relationship gradually become repositories of specific types of information. One spouse may remember restaurants, the other may keep track of movies. (One can readily see how divorce can make people stupid.)

As with list-making or marriage, we can also construe the act of writing about a trauma as a method of externalizing a traumatic experience. Once it has been written down or told to another, the memory and value of it have been preserved. There is now less of a reason to rehearse the event actively. Individual interviews indicate that people often view what they have written as part of themselves. Indeed, they are often reticent to give their essays away—not so much because of the anonymity, but rather they want to be able to refer back to their thoughts and feelings in the future.

The Drive Toward Self-Expression

When under great conflict, individuals have been known to produce major literary works. Eugene O'Neill's *Long day's journey into night*, Sylvia Plath's *The bell jar*, Alexandre Solzhenitsyn's *Cancer ward*, and hundreds of other masterpieces express the fundamental psychological fears and traumas of the authors. A parallel phenomenon occurs within the visual arts, music composition, and dance. The stark photography of Diane Arbus, the twisted visions of Van Gogh, the conflicted musical themes of Antonin Dvorak or Hank Williams Jr, or the haunting choreography of Alvin Ailey or Robert Fosse attest to the expression of core conflicts across a variety of media.

As has been suggested by other psychologists (cf. Maslow, 1970), individuals may have a basic drive towards self-expression. When this drive is blocked, tension results. One reason that our experiments may be successful in promoting health is that they encourage a fundamental form of self-expression. If needs concerning self-expression are being fulfilled, we would expect comparable autonomic and immune system changes when people use alternative methods to express themselves. Individual case studies in our laboratory indicate that artistically talented individuals show a greater drop in skin conductance when drawing pictures in expressing earlier traumas than when asked to write about the traumas. In short, the method of self-expression that people are most familiar with may result in the greatest benefits. Interestingly, we would predict that long-term benefits would depend on the person's expressing their basic thoughts and feelings surrounding significant traumas or conflicts.

Social Factors Associated with Disclosure

On the surface, our studies indicate that the benefits of confronting deeply personal experiences can accrue without the presence of other people. Careful inspection of our findings, however, indicates that presumably private disclosure is, in part, a social act. In this section, we first point to the act of disclosing to a symbolic other. We then speculate how confronting traumas allows for closer human relationships and, in some cases, greater allegiance to political and religious institutions.

Private Disclosure as a Symbolic Social Interaction

Most forms of psychotherapy emphasize the ongoing interaction between therapist and client. Presumably, the more supportive and accepting the therapist, the greater potential gains for the client (cf. Rogers, 1961). In addition to offering unconditional positive regard, the therapist provides important feedback to the client concerning the coping strategies and objective evaluation of threats (cf. Lazarus and Folkman, 1984). Even though discussing a trauma with others clearly can be advantageous, our studies indicate that the benefits of confronting traumas can occur in the absence of any social feedback.

Although individuals in our studies express their traumas in writing or into a microphone, assuming anonymity and confidentiality, many have noted that they hoped that someone would read or hear what they would say. Indeed, following the immune study where 25 of the 50 subjects wrote about traumas for four consecutive days, we included several questionnaire items that assessed the importance of anonymity and the degree to which they would like others to read their essays. Not surprisingly, most trauma subjects (over 70%) claimed that it was extremely important that their essays were anonymous. Ironically, of those who felt anonymity was important, 60% reported that they would either not mind (27%) or would very much like (33%) people they did not know to read their essays. In response to a third question, only 16% of the trauma subjects claimed that they would very much like to have their essays thrown away without anyone ever reading them.

These findings suggest that people write or talk about traumas to an imaginary or symbolic other (cf. Mead, 1934). Future studies must examine the nature of the symbolic other in far greater detail. For example, addressing an earlier trauma with the imagined audience being one's parents, therapist, minister, friend, political leader, or God, would undoubtedly result in different interpretations of the same event. Indeed, writing or talking about a personal experience within a certain context helps to integrate one's self-view with the context itself.

Disclosure in Human Interactions

To disclose a significant traumatic experience is a highly personal and intimate action. In revealing core aspects of themselves, individuals risk fundamental assaults on their egos. Ideally, when a person discloses personal traumas to another, a significant bond either exists or is strengthened between the two. Indeed, researchers in the area of self-disclosure have documented how the sharing of personal secrets is associated with increased liking between the two (e.g. Derlega, 1984) and overall reduced feelings of isolation or loneliness (Davis and Franzoi, 1986; Derlega and Berg, in press).

Based on earlier experience, individuals learn to associate safe self-disclosure with positive feelings of warmth and acceptance. Through this conditioning, subjects in our studies may have more readily disclosed intimate secrets than they otherwise would have. A key to this approach is a past history of instances of safe and positively reinforced self-disclosure. Those who have revealed their deepest secrets and have been met with punishment, denial, or other negative experience would be less likely to disclose in the future (as with our low disclosers) and, perhaps, to exhibit overall higher repressive coping styles and poor health.

The clinical literature is replete with case studies wherein individuals have been punished after disclosing traumatic events. For example, when women victims of incest tell their mothers of their experience, a surprisingly high percentage of the mothers either blame the daughter or deny the event occurred (Silver et al., 1983). From all indications, the punishment of disclosure is particularly damning from both a social and clinical perspective. First, of course, punishment of intimate disclosures represents a basic rejection of self and one's self-view. Second, the social balance between the discloser and disclosee is often permanently affected, resulting in gross inequity in the relationship (e.g. Hatfield, 1982).

Implications for Thought Reform and Religious Conversion

While intimate forms of self-disclosure can be self-defining, denigrating, or exhilarating, it is little wonder that there are potential dangers of using the paradigm we have presented in this chapter. The integration of the self-view with the social context, along with the corresponding affective elements, are evident within several institutions that attempt to influence basic thoughts and values.

Most thought-reform techniques rely heavily on various forms of public acknowledgement of private personal experience. In China, Vietnam, and other countries, the political regimes in power encourage individuals publically to confess their weaknesses, past traumas, and ideological shortcomings in self-criticism groups. In our own culture, self-help groups, such as the popular training or T-groups of the 1960s or the more recent commercial ventures such as EST, place a premium on the public sharing of traumatic experiences and personal weaknesses. Similarly, most contemporary religious groups, including traditional Catholics, fundamentalist Christians and followers of Reverend Moon (the Moonies), encourage the confessing of personal trauma and sin to either the priest or fellow members of the church. Groups as diverse as the Mormons and Quakers proscribe that their members maintain detailed personal journals of their thoughts and feelings. Finally, virtually all Western religions strongly urge the admission of traumatic and personal experience to their gods in the form of prayer.

Most institutions promote intimate disclosure while, at the same time, making the values of the institutions salient. Many religions, for example, expect individuals to talk about deeply personal experiences within the context of the particular religious doctrines. As we have discussed, the disclosure of basic elements of one's self aids in assimilating these elements into memory. If, at the same time, new or alien values are explicitly or implicitly present, these values should have a higher probability of being integrated with other aspects of the self. Are similar processes occuring in our experiments? If so, are particular values being conveyed within the laboratory setting? Although we would like to delude ourselves into believing that our studies are value free, a number of implicit values may well impinge on our subjects' self-definitions. Given that all of our students are enrolled in psychology courses and are participating in order to satisfy course requirements, we may unwittingly be 'converting' many of these students to some of the fundamental precepts of current psychological thinking. Future research demands that we explore the role that confronting traumatic experience may have on the shaping of value systems in general.

SUMMARY AND CONCLUSIONS

The act of inhibiting thoughts, emotions, and behaviors is physiologically and cognitively taxing. Across several studies, individuals who are required to confront previously inhibited life experiences show reductions in autonomic activity and improvements in immune function and physical health. The disclosure of traumas is cognitively beneficial because it promotes the assimilation of the events, it translates the images of the events into language, and provides a sense of detachment from the experiences. Socially, the actual or symbolic disclosure of personal experiences to others usually strengthens human relationships and assimilates peoples' self-definitions with those individuals or institutions in whom they confide.

REFERENCES

Alexander, F. (1950). *Psychosomatic medicine*. New York: Norton.

Blackburn, R. (1965). Emotionality, repression-sensitization, and maladjustment. *British Journal of Psychiatry, III*, 399–400.

Breuer, J., & Freud, S. (1895/1966). *Studies on hysteria*. New York: Avon.

Buck, R. (1984). *Communication of emotion*. New York: Guilford.

Cohen, S., & Syme, S. (eds) (1982). *Social support and health*. Orlando: Academic Press.

Davidson, R.J. (1980). Consciousness and information processing: A biocognitive perspective. In J.M. Davidson & R.J. Davidson (eds), *The psychobiology of consciousness*. (pp. 11–46). New York: Plenum Press.

Davis, M., & Franzoi, S. (1986). Adolescent loneliness, self-disclosure, and private self-consciousness: A longitudinal investigation. *Journal of Personality and Social Psychology, 51*, 595–608.

Derlega, V.J. (1984). Self-disclosure and intimate relationships. In V.J. Derlega (ed.), *Communication, intimacy, and close relationships* (pp. 1–9). Orlando: Academic Press.

Derlega, V.J., & Berg, J. (eds) (In press). *Self-disclosure: Theory, research and therapy*.

Derogatis, L.R., Abeloff, M.D., & Melisaratos, N. (1979). Psychological coping mechanisms and survival time in metastatic breast cancer. *Journal of the American Medical Association, 242*, 1504–1508.

Fowles, D.C. (1980). The three arousal model: Implications of Gray's two-factor theory for heart rate, electrodermal activity, and psychopathy. *Psychophysiology, 17*, 87–104.

Freud, S. (1963). Repression. In *General psychological theory* (pp. 104–115). New York: Collier. (Original work published 1915.)

Gray, J. (1975). *Elements of a two-process theory of learning*. New York: Academic Press.

Hatfield, E. (1982). Passionate love, compassionate love, and intimacy. In M. Fisher & G. Stricker (eds), *Intimacy*. New York: Plenum Press.

Horowitz, M.J. (1976). *Stress response syndromes*. New York: Jacob Aronson.

Jourard, S.M. (1971). *Self-disclosure: An experimental analysis of the transparent self*. New York: Wiley.

Lacey, J.I. (1956). The evaluation of autonomic responses: Toward a general solution. *Annals of the New York Academy of Science, 67*, 123–164.

Lang, P. (1977). Imagery and therapy. *Behavior Therapy, 8*, 862–886.

Lazarus, R., & Folkman, S. (1984). *Stress, appraisal, and coping*. New York: Springer-Verlag.

Luria, A. (1932). *The nature of human conflicts*. New York: Liveright.

Maslow, A.H. (1970). *Motivation and personality*, 2nd end. New York: Harper & Row.

McClelland, D.C. (1979). Inhibited power motivation and high blood pressure in men. *Journal of Abnormal Psychology, 88*, 182–190.

Mead, G.H. (1934). *Mind, self, and society*. Chicago: University of Chicago Press.

Meichenbaum, D. (1977). *Cognitive-behavior modification: An integrative approach*. New York: Plenum Press.

Obrist, P.A. (1981). *Cardiovascular psychophysiology: A perspective*. New York: Plenum Press.

Pennebaker, J.W. (1982). *The psychology of physical symptoms*. New York: Springer-Verlag.

Pennebaker, J.W. (1985). Traumatic experience and psychosomatic disease: Exploring the roles of behavioral inhibition, obsession, and confiding. *Canadian Psychology, 26*, 82–95.

Pennebaker, J.W., & Beall, S. (1986). Confronting a traumatic event: Toward an understanding of inhibition and disease. *Journal of Abnormal Psychology, 95*, 274–281.

Pennebaker, J.W., & Chew, C.H. (1985). Deception, electrodermal activity, and the inhibition of behavior. *Journal of Personality and Social Psychology, 49*, 1427–1433.

Pennebaker, J.W., Hughes, C., & O'Heeron, R.C. (1987). The psychophysiology of confession: Linking inhibitory and psychosomatic processes. *Journal of Personality and Social Psychology, 52*, 781–793.

Pennebaker, J.W., Kiecolt-Glaser, J.K., & Glaser, R. (in press). Disclosure of traumas and immune function: Health implications for psychotherapy. *Journal of Consulting and Clinical Psychology.*

Pennebaker, J.W., & O'Heeron, R.C. (1984). Confiding in others and illness rate among spouses of suicide and accidental death victims. *Journal of Abnormal Psychology, 93,* 473–476.

Pennebaker, J.W., & Susman, J.R. (in press). Disclosure of traumas and psychosomatic processes. *Social Science and Medicine.*

Rachman, S.J. (1980). Emotional processing. *Behavior Research and Therapy, 18,* 51–60.

Rachman, S.J., & Hodgson, R.J. (1980). *Obsessions and compulsions.* Englewood Cliffs, NJ: Prentice-Hall.

Rogers, C. (1961). *On becoming a person: A therapist's view of psychotherapy.* Boston: Houghton-Mifflin.

Silver, R.L., Boon, C., & Stones, M.H. (1983). Searching for meaning in misfortune: Making sense of incest. *Journal of Social Issues, 39,* 81–102.

Waid, W.M., & Orne, M.T. (1982). Reduced electrodermal response to conflict, failure to inhibit dominant behaviors, and delinquent proneness. *Journal of Personality and Social Psychology, 43,* 769–774.

Wallston, B.S., Alagna, S.W., DeVallis, B.M., & DeVallis, R.F. (1983). Social support and physical health. *Health Psychology, 2,* 367–391.

Wegner, D.M. (1986). Transactive memory: A contemporary analysis of the group mind. In B. Mullen & G.R. Goethals (eds), *Theories of group behavior* (pp. 185–208). New York: Springer-Verlag.

Wegner, D.M., Guiliano, T., & Hertel, P.T. (1985). Cognitive interdependence in close relationships. In W.J. Ickes (ed.), *Compatible and incompatible relationships* (pp. 253–276). New York: Springer-Verlag.

Wegner, D.M., Schneider, D.J., Carter, S.R., & White, T.L. (1987). Paradoxical effects of thought suppression. *Journal of Personality and Social Psychology, 53,* 5–13.

Weinberger, D.A., Schwartz, G.E., & Davidson, R.J. (1979). Low-anxious, high-anxious, and repressive coping styles: Psychometric patterns and behavioral and physiological responses to stress. *Journal of Abnormal Psychology, 88,* 369–380.

Wortman, C.B., & Silver, R.L. (1980). Coping with undesirable life events. In J. Garber and M. Seligman (eds), *Human helplessness* (pp. 279–375). New York: Academic Press.

Zilberg, N.J., Weiss, D.S., & Horowitz, M.J. (1982). Impact of event scale: A cross validation study and some empirical evidence supporting a conceptual model of stress response syndromes. *Journal of Consulting and Clinical Psychology, 50,* 407–414.

KEY WORDS

Psychosomatics, inhibition, confession, obsessions, consciousness, post-traumatic stress disorder, religion, self-disclosure, self-expression, stress, emotion, trauma.

Handbook of Life Stress, Cognition and Health
Edited by S. Fisher and J. Reason
© 1988 John Wiley & Sons Ltd.

37

Stress and Mental Control

DANIEL M. WEGNER
Trinity University, San Antonio, Texas

INTRODUCTION

Normally, we seem to have a measure of control over our thinking. We often attend to things just by wanting to do so, and attend away as well when it suits us. The luxury of mental control is frequently lost, however, when we encounter everyday stresses. Small stresses occupy our minds with worry and distract us from the things we would like to think about; large stresses wrest our attention away repeatedly, sometimes chronically, and leave us wondering if we can control our minds at all. This chapter is concerned with the nature of mental control, the effect of stress upon it, and the tactics that may be useful in regaining mental control in the face of stress.

FORMS OF MENTAL CONTROL

If we have any mental control, it seems to start with our ability to influence our focus of attention. William James held that 'effort of attention' is the 'essential phenomenon of will' (1890, p. 562), meaning by this that one can willfully perform an action by means of directing one's attention toward the idea of the action. Mental control in this kind of analysis is viewed as the first step toward 'will power', and so stands as a key to any other kind of control we might claim to have. To control our movements, our emotions, our addictions, our desires, our diets, or anything else, we must first control our attention.

Attention Control

James' analysis of the 'effort of attention' was limited to one aspect of attention control, *concentration*. He noted only that we had the occasional capacity to attend toward things at will. A more complete analysis would also include the complementary attentional enterprise often emphasized by Freud (e.g. 1915/ 1957)—*suppression*, or the capacity to attend away from things at will.

These two processes are interdependent. An act of concentration seems to entail a simultaneous suppression, in that concentrating on item A depends on suppressed attention to items that are not A. This is the classic problem addressed by filter theories of attention (e.g. Broadbent, 1958). As a rule, theorists have claimed that we must somehow process, at least minimally, the information that we do not consciously heed, if only to filter that information out of awareness. By the same token, suppressing typically entails concentration as well. The suppression of an item usually will require concentrating on some other items—unless we manage somehow to become completely unconscious.

Despite these links of concentration and suppression, when we exert mental control we normally seem to energize only one of the processes. We can explicitly attempt to concentrate (and implicitly suppress), or explicitly try to suppress (and implicitly concentrate). In either case, we appear then to overcome willfully the background processes that usually guide our attention when we are not exerting control. These processes, like the ones that control breathing when we are not taking a breath 'on purpose', seem to work quite automatically. There are automated processes that parallel concentration, drawing our attention toward items that have salient stimulus properties and away from items that are non-salient (Kahneman, 1973). There are automated processes that parallel suppression, drawing our attention away from items that have extreme stimulus properties and toward items that are less extreme (Berlyne, 1960).

The basic processes of concentration and suppression could be responsible for starting and stopping a wide array of mental processes. This activity makes mental control a major aspect of metacognition. In the case of metamemory (Flavell and Wellman, 1977), for example, it appears that people who concentrate on certain features of the task of remembering may gain in mental control, in that they increase their ability to use their memory systems more effectively. Judgment processes might also be brought under control by attention deployment or withdrawal (Wegner and Vallacher, 1981). Any mental processes or contents that are open to awareness are the potential target of control attempts, each a possible target of the will.

Control Failure

Our capacities for concentration and suppression seem only partially effective. For example, on three different occasions I asked a group of 33 undergraduate subjects to spend 30 seconds thinking of a coffee cup. They were also asked to make a mark on a piece of paper each time their attention drifted off the topic in the time period, if it did so. The mean number of marks was 3.3 in a 30-second period, indicating that attention drifts away frequently even when people are willing it to stay on a certain item. At the same three points, I also asked this group to spend a 30-second period *not* thinking of a coffee cup. They were asked to make a mark each time they thought about the item, if they did. The mean number of marks was 3.7, showing that suppression is an imperfect mental control process as well. People do not seem able to control their attention for longer than about 10 seconds under these conditions.

It is difficult to discern just what one should have expected from a study of this kind. Given that the subjects were constrained to perform a behavior upon each control failure (making the mark), one might argue that the response contingency itself could remind subjects of the potential of failure and lead them to fail. Nonetheless, similar processes might normally accompany natural mental control, in that *internal* responses to concentration or suppression failure would usually occur to serve the same function as the external marks. The failure to concentrate should prompt an internal response to return to the focus, whereas a failure to suppress should prompt an internal response to begin suppression anew. In other words, because any control failure would tend to elicit subsequent reactions, the failure rate observed in this, admittedly contrived, demonstration might not be very far removed from that people could experience in daily life.

It does seem, however, that failures associated with concentration are less conspicuous than those associated with suppression. A failure to concentrate, because it leaves the person attending to *anything* other than the initial focus, is likely to be difficult to notice. It is not heralded by the arrival of any particular item in consciousness (rather by a disappearance), and unless one is specifically anticipating a disappearance, the new entry to awareness will signal little at all. A failure to suppress a thought, in turn, is signalled clearly by the presence of the unwanted thought. The thought once driven away is easy to recognize on its return, and the failure is duly noted.

This analysis suggests that, by and large, cognitive failures that come from concentration lapses will be non-salient whereas those that arise from suppression lapses will be noticed by the person. In essence, one only notices concentration failures some time later, whereas suppression failures are immediately evident. Perhaps this is why there is no unitary label for concentration lapses in diagnostic categories for psychopathology. We could speak of attention deficits, perhaps, or dementias of some kind. Suppression lapses, however, are well known in terms of a familiar category: obsessional thinking. Indeed, a wide array of psychopathologies involve failures in suppression, the occurrence of unwanted thoughts, or unusual preoccupations. Janet (1925) even held that all mental disorder could be traced to the occurrence of 'fixed ideas'. It is not too surprising that normal individuals experience profound lapses of this kind as well (Berry, 1916–1917; Rachman and de Silva, 1978).

Obsession recommends itself, then, as a prototypical failure of mental control. For this reason, it is worthwhile to examine in some detail the relationship between stress and obsession; we may learn from this analysis how stress impinges on mental control generally. So, although stress has been identified as a critical precursor of yet other lapses of mental control, especially those related to concentration (see, for example, Fisher, 1984; Reason, Chapter 22 in this volume), our concern here is an understanding of what stress may do to affect suppression and obsession.

ORIGINS OF OBSESSION

Obsession and suppression can be difficult concepts to separate at a simple definitional level. This is because they both pertain to unwanted thoughts. When a thought is 'unwanted', it often qualifies as a worry or obsession, and at the same time appears to be a candidate for suppression. It is only when we consider the frequency, intrusiveness, or vividness of the thought that we can begin to see obsessive thoughts as more than merely 'unwanted' (see, for example, Rachman and Hodgson, 1980; Reed, 1985).

This ambiguity in the definition of obsession, however, suggests a useful way of distinguishing between two quite different sources of obsessional thinking. On the one hand, obsessions may originate because the thoughts themselves are truly abhorrent and become unwanted. Such obsessions stem from traumatic origins, and have been documented repeatedly in several literatures. On the other hand, though, it may be that certain obsessions originate from nearly arbitrary origins, becoming problematic only because of the development of excessive desires for suppression. The 'unwanting' itself promotes the problem. This second category of obsession development has not been fully documented in the empirical literature, and thus must be examined in detail. In this section, each source of obsessional thought is considered in turn.

Traumatic Obsession

People acquire obsessive thoughts as the direct result of exposure to traumatic, stressful events. This fact was recognized by Freud (e.g. 1959) in a theory of traumatic neuroses, and has been demonstrated in many studies. When one loses a spouse or child in a motor vehicle accident, for instance, it is likely that one will continue to ruminate about the loss for years (Lehman et al., 1987). Being the victim of incest is likewise a trauma of major proportions, one that commonly engenders disturbing, obsessive thoughts that may in some cases last a lifetime (Silver et al., 1983). Witnessing a terrorist attack can produce distressing thoughts that reappear over a prolonged period, both in wakefulness and in dreams (Ayalon, 1983). Obsession in response to traumatic events like these is widely recognized as a natural occurrence.

Phenomena that echo this relationship have been found in circumstances that are much less extreme. Horowitz (1975) demonstrated in a series of experiments, for example, that exposure to filmed traumatic events leads people to report intrusive, repetitive thoughts afterwards. These thoughts typically center on the traumatic event. At a more global level, related results were obtained in a study I conducted with a group of subjects who were asked to rate their daily level of overall stress, and their daily level of unwanted thoughts, for a period of 42 consecutive days. The correlation between these daily ratings was reliably greater than zero for 21 of the 33 subjects, with a median value of 0.31. It may be that even some relatively minor daily stresses give rise to rumination, but because the causal direction of the correlation is not yet known, this conclusion is uncertain.

Although there is considerable unanimity in the literature regarding the existence of traumatic obsession, there is much less agreement on why it is so persistent. One argument is that affective processes are primary in the development of memory (cf. Zajonc, 1980), and that the obsessive retrieval of a memory is produced when the memory has strong affective content. Laboratory research has indicated that affective or evaluative judgments of neutral stimuli enhance memory for those stimuli (Hyde and Jenkins, 1969); soliciting affective reactions to pictures of faces makes subjects more inclined to remember those faces as well (Patterson and Baddeley, 1977). Traumatic experience may induce obsession because sufficient affect is marshalled to create an extraordinarily strong memory trace, a cognitive representation that holds the trauma in a central position in the overall memory organization. One might not even be able to recall specifics of the incident, but still associate severe affective reactions with stimuli linked with the incident (Jacobs and Nadel, 1985). In this view, suppression might follow an obsessive thought—but it would remain an afterthought, a weak response to an otherwise overpowering mental event.

A second explanation of the persistence of ruminations following traumatic stress is that the ruminations are coping strategies. Epstein (1983) has argued that reliving a trauma can have palliative effects over time, producing an eventual habituation to the stressful stimulus. In this view, the normal response to any disturbing event is a brief obsession, a tendency to think about the event in an effort to understand it. This is effective in many cases, but becomes troublesome when the trauma is particularly severe. Habituation may be complicated in these instances because of the person's tendency to avoid thinking about the trauma whenever the rumination occurs. This line of theorizing implicates suppression in the continued momentum of obsession, in that pre-emptive suppression may prevent the person from achieving complete habituation.

A third interpretation of chronic rumination following trauma is the idea that the emotional reaction to the trauma must be expressed. Freud held that such expression, or *abreaction*, was necessary (e.g. Breuer and Freud, 1895), and his idea has been reiterated in many forms since. Lindemann (1944) believed that full expression of grief at the time of bereavement was necessary to avoid subsequent rumination, but that later grief expression could serve this purpose as well. Rachman (1980) developed the theory of emotional expression more fully to represent this process in other domains. And, most recently, Pennebaker (1985) has shown in a number of investigations that significant health problems occur in individuals who fail to confide their traumatic experiences to others. This perspective also might hold suppression responsible for continued rumination, in that the impulse to suppress could interfere with full expression of emotion.

A decision on the relative validity of these approaches to the longevity of traumatic obsessions will require extensive inquiry. We seem in this case to know quite clearly what can cause an obsession, and the major concern is with the efficacy of competing theories regarding its cure. All of these various formulations do hold in common, however, an underlying assumption. In each case, it is regarded as fairly obvious that a desire for mental peace makes suppression a standard reaction to obsessive, unwanted thoughts. This notion that suppression must only *follow* obsession can be challenged by a different view of obsessive thought origins.

Synthetic Obsession

It is conceivable that obsessions can arise from suppression, without stemming from any particular traumatic experience. Such an origin might account for the variety of obsessions people develop that seem to center on relatively mundane matters, concerns that are not obviously linked with any specific stressor. The obsessions people develop about weight gain, cleanliness, lost loves, jealousies, health, orderliness, the safety of loved ones, sexual inadequacies, feared victimization, personal improprieties, and on and on, are often difficult to trace to traumas. Now, as Freud (1901/1953) suggested, potentially traumatic origins for many pedestrian obsessions might be masked by childhood amnesia (cf. Wetzler and Sweeney, 1986). Yet certain obsessions seem to be constructed right before our eyes in adulthood. It might be more straightforward to start fresh with these cases and to consider the possible beginnings of obsession in the process of thought suppression.

All it takes to start is a desire to suppress a thought. The desire is difficult to satisfy at first, because the task of thought suppression is not easy. We fret over the suppression for a bit, wondering why we have trouble getting rid of this particular thought. Eventually we seem to succeed, however, as we become drawn to the other thoughts of daily life. For one or another reason, though, we are then reminded somehow of the suppressed thought, and at this point it looms slightly larger in mind. Something has happened to make it more noticeable, and we attend to it, perhaps again with the hope of wishing it away. It is more difficult to dispel this time, and we wonder why almost everything seems to remind us of the unwanted idea. We suppress it again, and again it returns with even greater insistence, eventually to visit our minds emphatically and frequently, beyond our now feeble attempts at control. And, in the turmoil, we may become highly anxious about our mental state as the result of yet other stresses that are wholly unrelated. This is the typical course of development of a synthetic obsession.

How might this sequence of events occur? The initial wish to avoid a thought could arise from several sources, none particularly unusual or traumatic. The motivation to avoid thoughts of food and eating, for instance, could arise from the simple desire to lose weight. *Self-control* strategies usually depend on individuals exercising their wills to suppress certain thoughts related to the actions being controlled. So, we try to avoid thoughts of tobacco, alcohol, heroin, or the like, in a period of abstinence, and extend this rule to all addictive substances. Similarly, it could be important to suppress thoughts of socially or personally disapproved actions as well, especially if these are problems of self-control. People who are trying to stop gambling, committing crimes, or seeing a cruel partner may view their problems as addictions and engage thought suppression as an aid.

One might also pursue thought suppression in a variety of other social circumstances. A need for *secrecy*, or, more generally, for deception in the service of positive self-presentation, could incline individuals to suppress thoughts. It is dangerous to rehearse the revelation of a lie while in the presence of the person being deceived, for example. And it is particularly distressing that the presence of the person from whom we must keep the awful truth of some fact almost inevitably brings the fact to our minds. The need to keep a secret creates considerable mental turmoil when we face the people we deceive, for we have multiple incompatible actions in mind. To tell or not to tell? Mental disturbances related to this conflict are likely to get us into trouble. This will prompt us either to avoid people who do not know our secrets, or to suppress the secret thoughts at least for the duration of the encounter.

And, finally, there may be some thoughts we suppress at first simply in the pursuit of *mental peace*. An idea may be replaying itself in our minds for no apparent reason, but we think it is happening too often. Although it does not interfere with particular behaviors (as in the case of ideas suppressed during self-control or secrecy), this idea may concern us merely in that it is a preoccupation. We note that we have a 'worry', and we wish it would go away. We have a little bump and we think of cancer, for instance, but we have not seen a physician. We sense it soon after we wake in the morning, and it intrudes occasionally all day. Rather than control the situation that the worry is about, though, we become concerned that we are worrying and treat it as a problem of mental control. We decide we are silly for worrying, so we try to set the thought of the bump aside.

None of these sources of suppression appears particularly strong or persistent. The pressures for self-control, secrecy, or mental peace may come and go, producing in their moments only the briefest interest in maintaining a suppression of thought. For this reason, we could easily question their efficacy in the production of an obsession. It is only because of additional processes that occur following initial suppressions that these first attempts to block a thought might serve as the seeds of obsessive rumination. The processes that energize the synthesis of an obsession can be categorized in terms of (1) rebound effects, (2) positive feedback processes, and (3) arousal-transfer processes.

Rebound effects occur when the person stops suppressing and gives license to the rumination. Unwanted thoughts can become more frequent and intrusive following an attempt at suppression than they were before it. After a diet, for example, a person might become quite preoccupied with the very thoughts of food that he or she was attempting to suppress. There is evidence that a history of dietary restraint can cause obesity (Polivy and Herman, 1985). It is also well established that the breakdown of abstinence from any addictive substance typically yields more than a 'sampling' of the substance, rather a complete relapse of addiction (Marlatt and Parks, 1982). The abstaining alcoholic falls 'off the wagon' not with one drink but with many.

Likewise, in other spheres, the person who has tried to suppress thoughts of, say, a child dying, a lover leaving, or an accident happening, may find many related thoughts crowding into consciousness when just a first image is allowed. The legacy of Freudian theory has tended to obscure this possibility because Freud (e.g. 1915/1957) popularized the idea that people are regularly capable of repression, the complete expulsion of unwanted thoughts from memory. Research has revealed this eventuality to be rare and perhaps non-existent in the form in which Freud envisioned (e.g. Erdelyi and Goldberg, 1979; Geiselman *et al.*, 1983; Holmes, 1974). Suppressed thoughts are not necessarily erased from memory—only from attention—and thus are always available for activation and even possible preoccupation. The developmental patterns of such rebound phenomena are not yet well established in the experimental literature, and this problem is the focus of much of the remainder of this chapter. If such rebound effects reliably occur, they provide the substance for yet further amplification through positive feedback and arousal-transfer processes.

Positive feedback processes would be likely to occur as the immediate result of suppression-induced rebound. A positive feedback mechanism is one that produces adjustments in a behavior or thought process *away* from some set level each time it cycles (von Bertalanffy, 1968). When the individual suppresses a thought and experiences a subsequent rebound of preoccupation with that thought, renewed suppression attempts would often be produced. Failure to suppress a desire for food after a diet, for example, could lead to an eating binge; this, in turn, might motivate a return to the diet and its associated attempts to suppress thoughts of food. This second occurrence of suppression, however, might be somewhat more difficult than the first, if only because the intervening rebound has strengthened the obsession. Over time, repeated cycles of suppression and obsession would occur, perhaps escalating in intensity with repeated suppression failures. This positive feedback process could turn a mere whim to suppress into a disturbing synthetic obsession.

Ruminations established in this way could be susceptible to further amplification through arousal-transfer processes. These processes, of course, have been identified in many inquiries inspired by the Schachter and Singer (1962) model of emotion. This work indicates that people are often mistaken about their emotional states. Non-specific arousal that arises from various stressors can make the person seek out possible causes, misattribute the arousal to them, and thus experience an emotional state that was not truly the cause of the arousal. There is enough research in this area to indicate that the translation of one emotional state to another could be a fairly common occurrence (e.g. Zillman, 1983). Worry about a newly synthesized obsession, after all, would be a handy factor to blame in the arousal misattribution process. The minor stresses of everyday life at work and at home might be forgotten as sources of emotion, and the arousal coming from them could be transferred to a synthetic obsession (cf. Borkovec *et al.*, 1983). Worry about the development of the obsession, in turn, could fuel more suppression and perhaps further rebound effects.

Relations Between Obsession Processes

The distinction between traumatic and synthetic obsessions seems to be a natural one, as it can account for the very different topics that obsessions may embrace. The distinction also allows an understanding of the different roles that stress may play in the development of mental control difficulties. Major stresses may engender obsessions directly, leading to problems in mental control that are focused primarily on the themes of the original trauma. Minor stresses, in turn, or even the anxieties that come from unresolved responses to major stresses, can serve to fuel a sequence of events that produces odd, idiosyncratic, and sometimes arbitrary obsessions. These mental control problems are synthetic, in that they are built from a suppression process gone awry. In trying to avoid a thought, however briefly, we find the thought repeating itself, kindled by insidious processes that usually lie outside our scope of awareness. It is transformed, given promotive circumstances, into a synthetic obsession that seems every bit real.

It is through translations such as these, then, that obsessions can seem to generate one another, overtake one another, or spring into existence in groups. The person who is one day a hypochondriac may the next be ruminating about a household insect problem or entertaining obsessive jealous thoughts of a spouse. The trauma that causes one obsession can provide the arousal to inflame others that seem, on the surface, to be wholly unrelated to the first. These interrelations make individual case histories confusing and complex, full of ambiguities only to be resolved when we recognize that obsessions can be traumatic or synthetic.

THOUGHT SUPPRESSION AND OBSESSION

The evidence for the development of synthetic obsession is fairly recent and still largely suggestive. Although it is clear that obsessions with food and other addictive substances can arise from suppression in natural settings (cf. Polivy and Herman, 1985), the evidence linking suppression to obsession more generally comes principally from laboratory studies. These studies do provide, however, a set of findings that appear to correspond well with processes and outcomes observed in realistic cases of obsession and preoccupation.

The White Bear Study

Experimental participants were asked by Wegner *et al.* (1987, Experiment 1) to spend a period of 5 minutes verbalizing the stream of their consciousness for a tape recorder. They were asked merely to think aloud, verbalizing every thought, feeling, or image that came to mind, and were assured that the recordings would be completely confidential. This period served to accustom subjects to the reporting technique to be used for the experiment.

Some research participants were then asked to continue their reporting, but now to follow an additional instruction: 'In the next 5 minutes, please verbalize your thoughts as you did before, with one exception. This time, try not to think of a white bear. Every time you say white bear or have white bear come to mind, though, please ring the bell on the table before you.' This suppression instruction typically led participants to ring the bell repeatedly (a mean of 6.07 times in 5 minutes) and mention 'white bear' from time to time as well (1.59 mentions). This level of thought is interesting in light of the instruction, but it is far lower than the level observed when a separate group of participants was asked to follow expression instructions—attempting to think of a white bear. Their bell rings averaged 11.82 and mentions occurred a mean of 11.52 times in 5 minutes. Nonetheless, it is noteworthy that complete suppression was initially difficult to manage.

These suppression and expression subjects were then asked to perform the complementary tasks. Those who had suppressed were now asked to think about white bear, whereas those who had expressed were now asked to stop thinking about white bear. This manipulation produced an increased level of expression in the group that had initially suppressed the thought. These subjects rang the bell an average of 15.71 times and mentioned white bear an average of 14.35 times, a level significantly greater than that shown by the subjects in the expression period in the group that performed no initial suppression. The mere act of avoiding a thought for 5 minutes, it seems, made subjects oddly inclined to signal a relative outpouring of thought occurrences when they were subsequently allowed to express the thought.

The observed pattern resembles quite strikingly the hypothesized rebound effect, an incipient obsession produced by suppression. A number of other features of the data in the study lend further credence to such an interpretation. For instance, it was found that responding in the 'rebound' period (expression following suppression) increased reliably over the time interval—whereas it decreased reliably over the same interval in each of the other experimental periods. Moreover, those subjects who were the better suppressors at first were found to be more expressive later on when given license in the expression period. This correlational relationship did not hold among subjects who expressed first; here, the more expressive subjects also showed more thought tokens in the suppression period. In short, the better a subject was at following an initial instruction to suppress, the more likely the subject was to show the rebound of thought expression.

Why does this rebound effect occur? A possible answer to this question is suggested by the think-aloud protocols we collected as people were trying to suppress the thought. Almost invariably, people would say 'Okay, if I can't think of white bear, I'll think of something else.' They then would turn their attention toward items in the room, toward plans for the day, or toward yet other things, in an attempt to distract themselves from the white bear. This process of self-distraction may be responsible for producing the rebound effect. To understand how, it is necessary to consider the nature of self-distraction in some detail.

Self-Distraction Processes

When psychologists study distraction, they usually provide subjects with distracting stimuli. So, for example, in learning that distraction may be an effective technique of pain control, researchers have standardly provided subjects with instructions to focus internally on a particular stimulus, or have provided subjects with an external stimulus to consider (McCaul and Malott, 1984). When people try to distract *themselves*, however, a quite different process seems to occur. The person rummages briefly through memory, or through what is presently in view, and selects a distracting stimulus. This could be a lightbulb, for instance, or the thought of a friend's wedding, but in any case it is selected arbitrarily by the person at the time. The person searches for anything that is 'not a white bear', using the unwanted thought as a *negative cue* for further thinking.

This feature of natural self-distraction usually accompanies the suppression process to produce the rebound effect. In essence, the person attempts to suppress the thought of white bear, say, by looking at a lightbulb and thinking about it instead of the white bear. This is not very intriguing, and attention eventually wanders back to white bear. Then, the person might think of something else, maybe the friend's wedding, to use it in the self-distraction attempt. This, too, is not very interesting for long, and perhaps fails to lead the person's thoughts far enough away from the white bear task, so attention returns again to the to-be-suppressed stimulus. In these repeated attempts at self-distraction, all the person has succeeded in doing is creating associations in memory between white bear and the failed distracters—the lightbulb and the wedding.

Such associations would not normally arise if the person were merely trying to think about a white bear. An expression task of this kind would only lead the person to investigate ideas that are already associated with white bear—perhaps to include thoughts of the North Pole, eskimos, or the zoo. Therefore, thought suppression introduces a unique propensity to create new associations with the unwanted thought. As the result of a poorly focused, wide-ranging self-distraction procedure, the person comes to attach the unwanted thought to every distracter that has come to mind. The person's environment, in consequence, now contains a number of new reminders of white bear, and any other thoughts that were current on the person's mind may similarly now be attached to white bear as well. This seems to be the usual effect of unfocused self-distraction.

It is easy to see that unfocused self-distraction could supply the cognitive underpinnings for a well-developed preoccupation. Once the person had suppressed a thought with sufficient frequency in a particular setting, many of the features of that setting would be imbued with cues for the retrieval of the unwanted thought. The lightbulb, for example, is not a white bear, nor is the friend's wedding. As long as the individual remains in the setting that contains all these distracters from the unwanted thought, the thought itself should be especially available for retrieval.

This explanation was tested by Wegner *et al.* (1987, Experiment 2). In this study, some subjects replicated the conditions of the original white bear research, whereas others undertook to suppress the white bear thought with the aid of a *focused distraction* instruction. These subjects were encouraged not to think of white bear in a suppression period, and were instructed that whenever white bear came to mind, they were to think of a red Volkswagen instead. This single focus was planned to cut short the tendency to think of anything at all whenever white bear was to be avoided, and so to eliminate the associative linking of white bear to these various ongoing thoughts. The results revealed that the intervention was effective, in that the rebound effect was wholly undermined. (It should be noted, though, that the rebound effect remained alive and well in those subjects who participated in expression following suppression, but without the aid of the focused distraction instruction.)

In a related experiment conducted by Wegner *et al.* (1988), the unfocused self-distraction hypothesis was subjected to a different sort of test. Here, the participants were presented with specific contexts for thought in the first and second experimental periods. Some subjects were exposed to conditions designed to replicate the general arrangements of the original study. Because subjects in the original study spent both the suppression and expression periods in the same room with little change, subjects in this condition of the present experiment were shown a relatively unchanging context—a slide show featuring a sequence of photos of related items (either classroom scenes or household appliances).

Other subjects, in contrast, were presented with different contexts for their suppression and expression tasks. They were shown either the slides of classrooms in one period and the appliances in the other, or vice versa. This variation was designed to reduce the degree to which the attachment of the unwanted thought to thoughts of the present context during suppression could transfer to the (new) context in the subsequent expression period. Although subjects would still be in an experiment (with all its contextual trappings), at least one key feature of their environment would change between periods, perhaps enough to supply fewer cues for retrieval of white bear during expression.

The results supported this analysis. Subjects whose context was changed from suppression to expression showed little evidence of a rebound effect even though the effect was again observed among those whose context was left unchanged. A constant context appears necessary for the elevation of expression scores following suppression above those observed in subjects without such initial suppression. These findings substantiate the idea that a natural strategy of *unfocused self-distraction* underlies the development of preoccupations following suppression.

Alleviating Synthetic Obsession

People trying not to think of white bears in the laboratory can, apparently, get into the very trouble that seems to foster the development of synthetic obsessions in everyday life. They engage in a cognitive strategy that, at face value, appears to improve their condition. They think of anything other than their unwanted thought. This strategy brings only passing relief, though, because it infects their every distracting idea with the germ of the rumination they wish to dispel. These distracters, when again encountered, are reminders of the thought that has been suppressed.

One measure to be taken to weaken synthetic obsessions would be the adoption of a limited array of distracters. Like the red Volkswagen in the focused distraction study, this special set of distracting thoughts might not aid in suppression at once. But over time, they could keep the rebound from happening. The suppressed thought would only be cued by the limited set of ideas that had been used for self-distraction—certain items around the house, perhaps, or religious icons, or the people one looks to under stress. This limitation would keep the remaining universe of thoughts generally free of contamination with the unwanted thought.

Another strategy suggested by this research would be a change of context. Like subjects who have changed from watching slides of classrooms and are now watching those wonderful household appliances instead, people who change contexts leave unwanted thoughts behind. The old context contains all the things one turned to for solace or distraction in the throes of the unwanted thought, and these now have become tarnished themselves. The new context is free of reminders about what one did not want to think, and for this reason will serve to stimulate fewer memories of the unwanted thought. A vacation, a new home, a change of outfits or friends, might be particularly useful to promote a change of mind.

Beyond the recommendations that flow from these studies, there are some further possibilities suggested by the more general developmental conditions of synthetic obsession. Even though the rebound effect can be seen as an early contributor to synthetic obsession, it seems unlikely that a fully bothersome obsessional state would be achieved by this means alone. It may more often be the case that rebounding preoccupations are given impetus by repeated, escalating occurrence in the presence of physiologically arousing stimulation of some kind. Prolonged arousal, then, could have extreme effects on obsession development. This realization points toward relaxation as a general treatment for synthetic obsession as well. As this technique is already well established as a useful therapy (Rachman and Hodgson, 1980), the present analysis has only an additional vote to add.

Ultimately, the most general advice suggested by these findings is to stop stopping. Thought suppression is, after all, a form of mental control, and thus it should be to some extent voluntary. Therapies that depend on a paradoxical tactic of 'flooding' people with the unwanted thought appear to be much more effective than thought-stopping techniques or other suppression-promoting interventions (e.g. Reed, 1985). So, although not suppressing might sometimes be the very last thing a person would want to do, it could be the best. Telling a trusted friend, writing about the problem, or even making a public scene could be healthy steps (cf. Pennebaker, 1985), as these activities would be incompatible with suppression. Finding conditions under which the person could feel comfortable, or at least able, to stop suppressing for a time, could be the key to overcoming synthetic obsessions.

SUMMARY AND CONCLUSIONS

The inquiries examined in this chapter range over a variety of problems in the relationship between stress and mental control. The analysis has centered on the notion that the relationship between these factors may be reciprocal in an important sense. Stress may induce lapses in mental control. In particular, traumatic stess can often cause obsessional thinking. But it appears that mental control may also be a precursor of self-induced stress. There is evidence that certain attempts to suppress thoughts may have the unfortunate effect of stimulating preoccupation with those very thoughts, sometimes to the point of a synthetic obsession. And, because people often can be alarmed by their own cognitive processes (Mandler, 1979), they enter into periods of stress that are largely traceable to mental control.

There is a broad program of research required on the problem of synthetic obsession, as it is only vaguely understood at this point. We know that certain phenomena in laboratory studies of thought suppression and field studies of self-control point to such an effect, but few investigators to date have seriously entertained the possibility that *many* obsessions, addictions, preoccupations, or sharply focused mental states might be manufactured by this process. Synthetic obsessions are certainly more than laboratory curiosities, but their role in the general scheme of cognitive failures is only now becoming evident. At the minimum, synthetic obsessions might be little more than the worries we have when we are failing at thought suppression. At the extreme, however, synthetic obsessions could be major flaws in the fabric of mental peace, frailties that endanger us to the stresses of everyday life.

Acknowledgements

Several ideas presented here arose in talks with James Pennebaker, David Schneider and Richard Wenzlaff, and I am grateful for this help. Thanks are also due to Anne Blake, Mary Dozier, and Toni Giuliano for their comments on an earlier draft.

REFERENCES

Ayalon, O. (1983). Coping with terrorism: The Israeli case. In D.J. Meichenbaum & M.E. Jaremko (eds), *Stress reduction and prevention* (pp. 293–339). New York: Plenum Press.

Berlyne, D.E. (1960). *Conflict, arousal, and curiosity*. New York: McGraw-Hill.

Berry, C.S. (1916–1917). Obsessions of normal minds. *Journal of Abnormal Psychology, 11*, 19–22.

Bertalanffy, L. von (1968). *General system theory*. New York: Braziller.

Borkovec, T.D., Robinson, E., Pruzinsky, T., & DePree, J.A. (1983). Preliminary exploration of worry: Some characteristics and processes. *Behavioral Research and Therapy, 21*, 9–16.

Breuer, J., & Freud, S. (1895/1955). *Studies on hysteria*. In J. Strachey (ed.), *The standard edition of the complete psychological works of Sigmund Freud*, Vol. 2. London: Hogarth.

Broadbent, D. (1958). *Perception and communication*. London: Pergamon.

Epstein, S. (1983). Natural healing processes of the mind: Graded stress inoculation as an inherent coping mechanism. In D. Meichenbaum & M.E. Jaremko (eds), *Stress reduction and prevention* (pp. 39–66). New York: Plenum Press.

Erdelyi, M.H., & Goldberg, B. (1979). Let's not sweep repression under the rug: Toward a cognitive psychology of repression. In J.F. Kihlstrom & F.J. Evans (eds), *Functional disorders of memory* (pp. 355–402). Hillsdale, NJ: Erlbaum.

Fisher, S. (1984). *Stress and the perception of control*. London: Lawrence Erlbaum Associates.

Flavell, J.H., & Wellman, H.M. (1977). Metamemory. In R.V. Kail, Jr & J.W. Hagen (eds), *Perspectives on the development of memory and cognition*. Hillsdale, NJ: Erlbaum.

Freud, S. (1901/1953). The psychopathology of everyday life. In J. Strachey (ed.), *The standard edition of the complete pyschological works of Sigmund Freud*, Vol. 6. London: Hogarth.

Freud, S. (1915/1957). Repression. In J. Strachey (Ed.), *The standard edition of the complete psychological works of Sigmund Freud*, Vol. 14 (pp. 146–158). London: Hogarth.

Freud, S. (1959). *Beyond the pleasure principle*. New York: Bantam.

Geiselman, R.E., Bjork, R.A., & Fishman, D.L. (1983). Disrupted retrieval in directed forgetting: A link with posthypnotic amnesia. *Journal of Experimental Psychology: General, 112*, 58–72.

Holmes, D.S. (1974). Investigation of repression: Differential recall of material experimentally or naturally associated with ego threat. *Psychological Bulletin, 81*, 632–653.

Horowitz, M. (1975). Intrusive and repetitive thoughts after experimental stress. *Archives of General Psychiatry, 32*, 1457–1463.

Hyde, T.W., & Jenkins, J.J. (1969). The differential effects of incidental tasks on the organization of recall of a list of highly associated words. *Journal of Experimental Psychology, 82*, 472–481.

Jacobs, W.J., & Nadel, L. (1985). Stress-induced recovery of fears and phobias. *Psychological Review, 92*, 512–531.

James, W. (1890). *Principles of psychology*. New York: Holt.

Janet, P. (1925). *Principles of psychotherapy*. London: Allen and Unwin.

Kahneman, D. (1973). *Attention and effort*. Englewood Cliffs, NJ: Prentice Hall.

Lehman, D.R., Wortman, C.B., & Williams, A.F. (1987). Long-term effects of losing a spouse or child in a motor vehicle crash. *Journal of Personality and Social Psychology, 52*, 218–231.

Lindemann, E. (1944). Symptomatology and management of acute grief. *American Journal of Psychiatry, 101*, 141–148.

Mandler, G. (1979). Thought processes, consciousness, and stress. In V. Hamilton & D.M. Warburton (eds), *Human stress and cognition* (pp. 179–201). Chichester: Wiley.

Marlatt, G.P., & Parks, G.A. (1982). Self-management of addictive behaviors. In P. Karoly & F.H. Kanfer (eds), *Self-management and behavior change* (pp. 443–488). New York: Pergamon.

McCaul, K.D., & Malott, J.M. (1984). Distraction and coping with pain. *Psychological Bulletin, 95*, 516–533.

Patterson, K.E., & Baddeley, A.D. (1977). When face recognition fails. *Journal of Experimental Psychology: Human Learning and Memory, 3*, 406–417.

Pennebaker, J.W. (1985). Inhibition and cognition: Toward an understanding of trauma and disease. *Canadian Psychology, 26*, 82–95.

Polivy, J., & Herman, C.P. (1985). Dieting and binging: A causal analysis. *American Psychologist, 40*, 193–201.

Rachman, S. (1980). Emotional processing. *Behavior research and therapy, 18*, 51–60.

Rachman, S., & de Silva, P. (1978). Abnormal and normal obsessions. *Behavior Research and Therapy, 16*, 233–248.

Rachman, S., & Hodgson, R.J. (1980). *Obsessions and compulsions*. Englewood Cliffs, NJ: Prentice-Hall.

Reed, G.F. (1985). *Obsessional experience and compulsive behavior*. Orlando: Academic Press.

Schachter, S., & Singer, J. (1962). Cognitive, social, and physiological determinants of emotional state. *Psychobiological Review, 69*, 379–399.

Silver, R.L., Boon, C., & Stones, M.H. (1983). Searching for meaning in misfortune: Making sense of incest. *Journal of Social Issues, 39*, 81–102.

Wegner, D.M., Schneider, D.J., Carter, S., & White, T. (1987). Paradoxical effects of thought suppression. *Journal of Personality and Social Psychology, 53*, 1–9.

Wegner, D.M., Schneider, D.J., McMahon, S., & Mitchell, M. (1988). Taking obsessions out of context. Unpublished research data.

Wegner, D.M., & Vallacher, R.R. (1981). Commonsense psychology. In J. Forgas (ed.), *Social cognition: Perspectives on everyday understanding* (pp. 225–246). London: Academic Press.

Wetzler, S.E., & Sweeney, J.A. (1986). Childhood amnesia: An empirical demonstration. In D.C. Rubin (ed.), *Autobiographical memory* (pp. 191–201). Cambridge: Cambridge University Press.

Zajonc, R.B. (1980). Feeling and thinking: Preferences need no inferences. *American Psychologist, 35*, 151–175.

Zillman, D. (1983). Transfer of excitation in emotional behavior. In J.T. Caccioppo & R.E. Petty (eds), *Social psychophysiology*. New York: Guilford Press.

KEY WORDS

Concentration, suppression, metacognition, metamemory, fixed ideas, obsession, traumatic obsession, abreaction, synthetic obsession, self-control, secrecy, mental peace, rebound effect, repression, arousal-transfer, white bear, self-distraction, negative cue.

Handbook of Life Stress, Cognition and Health
Edited by S. Fisher and J. Reason
© 1988 John Wiley & Sons Ltd.

38

The Costs and Benefits of Coping

Wolfgang Schönpflug and Wolfgang Battmann
Freie Universität, Berlin

INTRODUCTION

Theories of coping have predominantly dealt with the benefits of coping. Taxonomies of coping styles were constructed, the individual consistency of coping styles was assessed, and the match between stressors and coping styles was evaluated (cf. Lazarus and Folkman, 1984; Moos and Billings, 1982). This research is based on the optimistic presupposition that coping is a problem-solving procedure, and there may be optimal ways of coping for each combination of stressors and individuals suffering from these stressors. However, other studies have also tried to elaborate some negative aspects of coping. Favoring a more pessimistic perspective, they have analyzed coping attempts as problem-generating procedures (cf. Cohen *et al.*, 1986; Schönpflug, 1985; 1986a). Evidently, theories of stress and coping could gain more sophistication and ecological validity if positive and negative aspects could be combined within the same theoretical model. Such a model should support an analysis of the costs and benefits ensuing from a stressing situation. The model should be action oriented, and should describe costs and benefits as originating from the coping attempts initiated for mastery of stressing situations.

RESOURCES

There are several ways of classifying resources (Schönpflug, 1986b). Distinctions can be made between (a) structural and energetic resources, (b) internal and external resources, and within the external resources, and (c) the natural, technical and social aids (including metaphysical agents in the mind of the believers). Structural resources are instrumental for attaining specific goals. Examples from the internal domain are personal skills, or muscles, or working memory, whereas machines and friends are examples for structural resources from the environment. Energetic resources are needed to activate the structural ones. Examples from the internal domain are biochemical excretions which tune the organism for physical and mental acts; an example from the environment is gasoline which if combusted drives an engine. Typically, energetic resources are consumed fast, whereas structural resources serve their purpose for longer time intervals. Thus, the supply of biochemical agents stimulating the contraction of muscles may easily be exhausted by extended or intense secretion, whereas the working memory structure may be filled to its limits repeatedly without suffering from a substantial loss.

In the context of stress and coping, resources serve a double function. On the one hand, they are functional in coping: personal skills, friends and technical aids help in the mastery of stressors. On the other hand, the need for resources is also the origin of stress. In the cognitive theory, three specifications of stress are distinguished: challenge, loss, and threat (cf. Lazarus and Folkman, 1984). These concepts clearly relate to resources. Challenge can only be conceived of as relating to resources such as skills, friends or tools to be acquired; threat and loss relate to the same resources being jeopardized or already gone.

That stress derives from the need for resources which are functional in resolving stress constitutes a circular reasoning. This circular reasoning, however, can serve as a background for evaluating stressful transactions.

BENEFITS: SAVINGS OF AND GAINS IN RESOURCES

If stressors are defined as problems, successful coping can be treated as a process of problem solving. Taking the three above-mentioned specifications of stress— namely challenge, loss, and threat—as points of departure, it is easy to determine what has to be accomplished by successful coping. In the case of challenge, coping will comprise the identification and the overcoming of barriers, until control or possession of new resources is achieved. In the case of threat, coping is successful if a reduction of available resources is prevented. Similarly, coping with loss will be regarded as successful if compensating for the deprivation of resources.

These three redefinitions of coping refer to an active coping mode, a mode which is directed to actual changes in the state of resources. However, there are also other modes of coping such as subjective reappraisal. Subjective reappraisal will, in general, alter the evaluation of resources; a universal tactic is the cynical attitude of lowering esteem, i.e. derogation of a challenging, threatened or lost object (cf. Ellis, 1978). If an individual succeeds in lowering the esteem of resources at stake, the experience of challenge, loss or threat related to these resources will decrease. Therefore, cognitive coping with a stressor may serve the same purpose as active coping.

Evidently, there are two economical principles which determine benefits of coping: conservation and growth. The former calls for saving of available resources, the latter for enlarging one's resources. How benefits of coping are assessed is a matter of methodological orientation. On the behavioral level, the effects of active coping have to be considered. Then, benefits can be assessed in terms of the savings or expansion of objective resources. On the cognitive level, the analysis of perceived resources provides the evidence for mental representations of resource utilization.

The principles of conservation and growth may be universally valid or may be limited in their scope. At the first glance, they seem not to account for 'paratelic' phenomena (Apter, 1982) such as mountain climbing or sky diving (Zuckerman *et al.*, 1980). Some individuals, or all individuals in some situations, seem to enjoy spending their resources. They seem to look for stress rather than avoiding it. Possibly the joys of spending are typical for situations and individuals with rich supply or low demand of resources (Scitovsky, 1976). A more refined analysis may succeed in explaining how 'paratelic' phenomena could follow the principles of conservation and growth, but this is beyond the scope of the present chapter.

FAILURE: ABSENCE OF BENEFITS DESPITE COPING ATTEMPTS

There are many reasons why coping attempts may fail. In general, two classes of failing actions can be distinguished: action slips and erroneous actions (Norman, 1981; Reason, 1979). Action slips are behaviors which do not follow original intentions, as in the case of mistakes in spelling or motor response. Some planned actions are correctly executed, but are not functional. An example of an erroneous action is a letter to a high-ranking politician concerning a local noise complaint; the letter, though correctly written, might not serve its purpose if the case does not fall into the recipient's perview.

The origins of failures may stem from any component of the action chain: from faulty cognitive representations of individuals and their environment (e.g. invalid estimation of personal skills, failure to detect obstacles), from inappropriate goal setting (e.g. unrealistic level of aspiration), from inefficient action strategies, from interference in the execution of actions, and from inappropriate sampling and evaluation of feedback (Schönpflug, 1985).

Failures will, in general, not produce benefits. They will not contribute to conservation and growth of resources. Therefore, the experience of failure is likely to become a stressing factor itself. If repeatedly encountered, it may successively induce feelings of challenge, threat, and loss (Schwarzer *et al.*, 1984).

Although the failure to produce benefits per se does not constitute a cost factor, the incidence of failures may become the starting point for additional costly activities. A general strategy is repetition of the activity which has been failing (e.g. repeating a class after failing the finals). In addition, failures call for orienting and modifying activities such as searching for the reasons for former failures and improvement of both the former activity and its situational conditions. These additional activities may become highly demanding and complex (e.g. participation in state committees investigating the educational system). Possibly, it is the need for active correction which contributes heavily to the dissatisfaction and incompleteness reported after failure (Mahler, 1933).

PROBLEM GENERATION: NEW SOURCES OF COSTS AS RESULTS OF COPING ATTEMPTS

As with all kinds of human behavior, coping attempts may yield both side- and after-effects. These effects may be positive or negative. An example of a positive side-effect of coping is finding a true friend while fighting a flood emergency. A negative effect is overrunning a pedestrian while driving to the hospital. Both positive and negative effects may be anticipated or unexpected. Whether anticipated or unforeseen, negative effects vary in the degree to which they are instrumental for the purpose of coping. For instance, breaking a wall may or may not be judged as helpful while extinguishing the fire in a house. Effects can also be rated as evitable or inevitable. If foreseen and judged either as instrumental or inevitable, negative effects of coping behavior may explicitly be taken into account at the planning stage.

Thus, in contrast to the more optimistic traditional approach to the notion of coping, the above analysis underlines the need to consider the negative consequences. Problems may arise because of the use of coping strategies and these may cause further stress. It is often argued that stress is not always imposed on an individual—it may be self-created. A particular source of stress which could seem self-imposed could be the consequence of coping strategies. It may be the coping process itself which makes things worse rather than better (Lumsden, 1975; Schönpflug, 1982).

New problems generated during the course of coping attempts may deplete or destroy resources. Coping can lead to loss of structural resources from the environment (e.g. death of a partner in a rescue action, breaking of tools during repair work) as well as to loss of personal structural resources (e.g. severance of a limb). The same is true for energetic resources (see next section).

Predictable loss of resources due to coping will induce feelings of threat, as is the case with predictable loss of resources due to external factors. Therefore, individuals may develop a specific fear of coping (Fuchs, 1976).

New problems arising from coping attempts may also augment the demands on an individual. At least in some cultural settings, they create conditions which require specific actions. Typical actions after causing new problems are eliminative in nature (e.g. cleaning polluted soil around a factory), substitutive (e.g. replacing spoiled material), or compensatory (e.g. giving a formal excuse) (Schönpflug, 1985).

OPERATIONAL COSTS OF COPING

Among the resources lost in the course of coping are the personal energetic resources invested in coping. After coping with a stressor, individuals suffer from performance decrements in subsequent tests: they show less tolerance to others, as expressed in increased aggression and decreased helping (Cohen, 1980); they report fatigue and exhaustion after prolonged, strenuous work, and such complaints have been validated in biochemical studies on catecholamine excretion (Frankenhaeuser, 1986). It should be noted that it was the observation of performance decrements after coping with noise which prompted Glass *et al.* in 1969 to introduce the concept of 'psychic costs of adaptation' into the theory of stress. The term 'psychic costs of adaptation' may be used as a metaphor for any behavioral handicap which follows the confrontation with a stressor. However, the meaning of the phrase also implies the cause of such behavioral handicaps.

One cause can be specified as the loss of personal energetic resources in the process of coping. For the purpose of better discrimination between loss of personal energetic resources and loss of structural or external resources, the former will be called 'operational costs'.

The nature of operational costs is not sufficiently clear as the issue of human energetics, in general, needs further clarification. However, it can be stated that energetics and operational costs are reflected in measures of arousal, attention, emotionality, and effort, and that all these phenomena seem to have a biological basis (Hockey *et al.*, 1986; Posner and Rothbart, 1986). It will be argued later in this chapter that operational costs in stressful situations derive from two different types of behavior: orientation to the nature and the origins of stressors, and the control of features of the stress. This argument rests on the assumption that both orientation and control may constitute highly complex behavior patterns comprising sensory, mental, emotional and motor components. An example of such a complex orienting activity is seeing a doctor for a radiographic inspection. A matching example for complex control activity is cooking a diet for healing gastroenteritis.

Operational costs are mostly transient; they accumulate during the period of activity, but individuals recover from energy expenditure during periods of rest or relaxation. However, there are suggestions that the balance between expenditure and recovery may be disturbed. If this should be the case, the state of exhaustion becomes chronic and pathogenic symptoms result. One of the suggestions is that significant involvement in challenging situations may not only induce transient elevations of blood pressure and pulse rate, but in the long run may also increase the risk of cardiovascular diseases (e.g. Pittner *et al.*, 1983). In the same way, proneness to other physical and mental disorders can be attributed to chronic stress (Levine and Ursin, 1980; Cohen *et al.*, 1986).

To a certain extent, there should be no active response without operational costs. However, there is also a reasonable possibility that some individuals operate at a higher level of costs than is justified by the demands of the situation. This issue has been brought up by Strelau (1983) on the basis of Tomaszewski's (1967) theory of the functional structure of activity. Tomaszewski distinguishes between productive and auxiliary goals and activities. A productive activity is directly devoted to an outcome which primarily motivates the pattern of behavior (e.g. driving a tourist to the airport). Auxiliary activities do not directly contribute to productivity, but rather monitor, prepare and protect it (e.g. checking the pressure of car tyres, filling an extra tank of gasoline). Strelau points out that there are considerable interindividual differences in the involvement in auxiliary acts; he relates this involvement to a temperamental dimension of reactivity.

Individuals exhibit consistent preferences for a specific style of coping with their problems. But as long as they can follow their preferred style, their achievement seems not to be affected by it. More specifically, low reactives seem to perform as well with few auxiliary acts as high reactives do with many (e.g. Klonowicz, 1986). In consequence, high reactives can be described as putting in more effort for the same result, or as investing more operational costs. Similar ideas have been developed concerning individuals differing in their anxiety score. High-anxious subjects were found to report more effort and fatigue, to spend longer time on mental tasks, and to execute a larger number of operations while working on mental tasks; however, in the pertinent studies, the high-anxious subjects produced as many correct solutions as the low-anxious subjects (Eysenck, 1983; Schönpflug, 1984; Wieland-Eckelmann, 1986).

Further investigations are needed into the origins and functions of costly coping styles. Possibly they are generalizations from behavior which has proved to be adjustive in tricky task situations, among them situations offering highly salient risks with low probability of occurrence (e.g. accidents in nuclear power plants). Another possibility is that acts beyond the minimal productive behavior yield information which is required for self-regulation (e.g. providing safety cues).

BENEFITS AND COSTS OF SUPPORTS

Stress originates from a discrepancy between demands and available resources. This proposition has become a pivot in cognitive stress theories (e.g. Lazarus and Folkman, 1984). The proposition can be extended to read: operational costs, as discussed above, increase with demands and decrease with resources (e.g. Schönpflug, 1983). Since resources contribute to savings of operational costs, they are beneficial.

On the other hand, the utilization of resources may also raise costs. Unless operating automatically or driven by external agents, they have to be monitored and controlled by the user. Thus, specific operational costs arise on the side of the user. More specifically, in order to initiate and maintain support from partners and tools, the investment of effort, attention or energy, in general, is required.

EFFECTIVE COPING AS A RESOURCE MANAGEMENT PROCESS

During stressful transactions, costs and benefits from several sources may combine. For a more systematic account, some prototypical stress situations should be analyzed.

One prototype is a situation offering one potential stressor or a set of such stressors. The first response to situational stressors is internal or external orientation (e.g. observation of own bodily pains, seeing a doctor for a medical diagnosis). As elaborated above, the sensory, mental, emotional and motor involvement in orienting behavior is associated with operational costs. These operational costs, contingent on specific tasks or problems, can be assumed to determine the initial stressing impact of these tasks and problems. Unless these tasks and problems vanish for external reasons, they may permanently stimulate orienting behavior and hence cause a continuous drain of personal energetic resources. One way of stopping this drain is directly to terminate the process of orientation. This can be accomplished by perceptual defence, reappraisal and palliation of emotions (e.g. Lazarus, 1983; Lazarus and Folkman, 1984).

Another way is to eliminate the tasks and problems at hand which have become the objects of costly orientation. This can often be accomplished by active coping, i.e. by exerting control. As has also been mentioned above, the sensory, mental, emotional and motor involvement in the control process raises the same kinds of operational costs as does orientation. This creates a trade-off problem. Operational costs from control have to be compared with operational costs from continued orientation, and a decision in favour of control is only warranted if the latter costs are outbalanced by the former (Schönpflug, 1983). It should be remembered that (as described above) in the determination of operational costs invested, the available supports play an important role.

There are at least two features complicating the balancing procedure. First, in the process of active coping, orientation and control mostly overlap; this means that costs of control increase while costs of orientation are not yet saved. Second, within the period of control, the costs may well exceed the costs of orientation. In consequence, within the period of active control, operational costs will accumulate, and the pay-off of active coping may seem poor. However, this judgement may only be valid in short perspective. Within a sufficiently long time perspective, accumulated costs arising during a limited period of efficient control may well be outweighed by savings thereafter.

A second protoypical case is failure. Operational costs of coping attempts, particularly of attempted control, arise, but the initial tasks and problems persist and call for resumed orientation and control. Thus, in face of continued costs, failing actions can never be evaluated as paying off.

The third prototypical case is problem generation. New problems necessitate the investment of more resources. Of course, some of the prototypical cases can go together: both successful efforts and failure in solving an old problem may result in the creation of a new problem. Then the costs from the prototypical cases combine (Cohen et al., 1986; Schönpflug, 1986a).

In conclusion, coping can be interpreted as a resource management process. This process aims at optimizing the network of resources available to a person according to the above-mentioned principles of conservation and growth and in a long-time perspective. During coping, the individual repeatedly makes decisions on the allocation and the consumption of resources. Allocation of resources is a primary decision; resources once allocated require capacity and are not available for another purpose at the same time (e.g. allocation of attention to a signal, allocation of a computer unit to a calculation task). Some of the resources allocated will not undergo substantial changes during the period of allocation; as stated above, this is a feature of the structural resources. Other resources—typically the energetic ones—will be diminished while being allocated (e.g. suffering from fatigue after prolonged work, burning of coal).

Resource management will encompass tasks such as matching of energetic and structural resources (e.g. providing electricity for an engine) and matching different structural resources (e.g. supplying a tractor for a farmhand). Typically, it will call for matching of personal resources to external ones (e.g. gaining physical strength to handle a power saw, acquiring skills for instructing collaborators). As a main feature, resource management will balance the benefits and costs as defined above, and the efficiency of coping will be evaluated by the trade-off between benefits gained and costs invested.

Resource management will be most dramatic when there are scarce resources and urgent needs. It may happen that a whole network of resources collapses if one single element is missing (e.g. lack of air for an individual, breakdown of electricity in a workshop). The occurrence of an element falling below a limit which is critical for the maintenance of a larger network characterizes specific emergency situations. In these situations, an excessive investment of resources may occur to avert an extended collapse. High stress situations seem to reflect such a state of affairs.

WHEN COSTS EXCEED THE BENEFITS: DELIBERATE DISENGAGEMENT

With the experience or the prospect of costs outweighing the benefits of coping, deliberate disengagement becomes an economic option. Schönpflug (1985) distinguishes between disengagement as giving up and disengagement as an instrumental act.

Disengagement as giving up is a transition to passivity in face of a stressor (Cohen et al., 1986). In the literature, passivity has been interpreted as adjustive if the stressor is uncontrollable or a task situation taxes a person's resources too heavily. As an example of an uncontrollable stressor, Baum et al. (1983) present the case of the Three Mile Island nuclear power plant. Inhabitants from the neighborhood of the plant are described as resigned, but not distressed, as the decline of property prices does not permit them to move away. Schönpflug (1983) reports experiments in which task difficulty and intellectual capacity were varied systematically. If performance level deteriorated as a function of increasing discrepancy between task difficulty level and personal skills, subjects first reacted with an increased effort, but switched to a guessing strategy thereafter. When the correct solution had to be selected from a set of alternatives, and despite effort expenditure the performance approached the chance level, use of a guessing strategy did not influence performance but reduced the effort and emotional strain involved. In the context of everyday life, giving up in face of experienced or anticipated loss of structural and external resources (mainly damage of objects, bodily violations) is a well known phenomenon.

Within groups sharing common solidarity standards, disengagement may also become instrumental for transferring a task to somebody else. Delegation of tasks may be a matter of mutual exchange when one service is traded in for another. The central argument for receiving or expecting help is inferiority of own resources relative to the resources of another person or a group (Fisher et al., 1983). Communications on high need but low availability of resources serve as persuasions for stipulating help.

Handicaps or lack of resources may be subjectively conceived of and verbally stated in the process of communication; this is what Snyder and Smith (1982) have designated as self-handicapping strategies in impression formation. Handicaps or lack of resources may also be objectively produced. An example from experimental research is the choice of a presumably inhibitory drug in anticipation of failure (Berglas and Jones, 1978). Examples from real-life situations include destruction of internal resources (e.g. self-mutilation of soldiers before combat) and external resources (e.g. sabotage in industry). In such cases statements or generation of problems are motivated by the intention of deliberate disengagement; in the process of resource management, they are sophisticated strategies to create the conditions for delegation of tasks or for giving up.

SOME APPLICATIONS: COSTS AND BENEFITS OF COOPERATION, PLANNING AND FEEDBACK

The utilization of personal and external resources has frequently been discussed in the psychological literature; cost–benefit analyses served the purpose of explaining decisions between and evaluations of multidimensional objects. Studies from our own laboratory are presented because they were explicitly designed and conducted to demonstrate and test some aspects of our behavior economics approach to stress and coping. We selected three examples to represent a variety of psychological domains to which the stress paradigm can be applied.

Cooperation

The first example belongs to the domain of social cooperation (Battmann, in preparation). Subjects worked in dyadic units on administrative tasks. They were assigned 42 tasks requiring division of labor and 14 tasks not permitting division of labor. The tasks requiring division of labor consisted of two subtasks to be solved in succession. For example, one class of shared tasks required the calculation of expenses for a new employee in a business firm. The first stage in this task was to establish a proper classification of the new employee according to his age, qualifications, etc. Once the employee was placed in a category, the total expenses could be calculated according to family status, company regulations, etc. The tasks were solved in a dialogue with a data-base computer system. Each partner could only take over one of the subtasks, and credit was given to both partners, but only for a complete solution. If one partner failed, the other partner lost his credit. Extra tasks were introduced as 'complaints' to be solved by one partner individually; the extra tasks were also problems from public and business administration and were solved in a dialogue with the data-base system. The system provided information on the performance of the person and the partner, in the same way. A task, once started, was terminated when a solution was entered. There was a premium payment for correct solutions, but this payment was equally split between the partners involved.

The subjects were classified as high or low in intelligence in accordance with scores on intelligence tests. Information concerning the partner was fabricated and described in terms of 'efficiency'. Half of both the high and low intelligent subjects were made to believe that they cooperated with a highly 'efficient' partner, whereas it was suggested to the other half that the partner was low in efficiency.

The most relevant effects observed were as follows. (a) Both low and high intelligent subjects reached more correct solutions, and therefore more credits, if they cooperated with a highly 'efficient' partner. (b) Subjects who were low or high in intelligence both spent more time on their tasks, if cooperating with a high 'efficient' partner. (c) Subjects of low intelligence took over the highest number of extra tasks if cooperating with an 'efficient' partner, but the lowest number if the performance of their partner was low. (d) Calls for feedback were more frequent if the partner is more 'efficient'. (e) Low intelligence subjects expressed increased satisfaction if cooperating with a high 'efficient' partner; but within this group the proportion of persons expressing the wish to change the partner for any further sessions was highest.

Obviously, this is a task system which permits social support, but also induces a social–emotional and mental load. A high efficient partner helps to gain material and emotional rewards from work, and this can be regarded as beneficial. But there is also a considerable price for these rewards in terms of prolonged working time, monitoring of both the personal interactions and the outcome of coopera-tion, together with a need to satisfy efficient partners. Thus the paradoxical finding is that, in terms of extra tasks taken over, weak partners give more support to strong partners than vice versa. In consequence, there were more emotional conflicts for the weaker member of a heterogeneous dyad.

Thus, our findings augment the growing body of data on the benefits of social resources (Cohen and Syme, 1985, Sarason and Sarason, 1985). But, simul-taneously, they corroborate the notion, only recently discussed (Hobfoll, 1985), that there are costs attached to the utilization of social resources.

Planning

Another example is anticipatory planning. In a laboratory experiment (Batt-mann, 1984), subjects had to play the role of the supervisor of a chain of department stores. Within an experimental day, the supervisor had to visit twelve stores which were scattered over the whole city. In each store, two problems from a pool of office tasks (accounting, marketing, hiring personnel) waited for the supervisor's decision. The plan of the city and the location of stores were simulated on a computer display, and so was the route which the subject actually took through his fictitious environment.

The subjects received credits for the tasks solved correctly. By saving time, they could earn an extra premium. The shops were not open all day, so time could be lost by arriving too early or too late. An opportunity for effective planning was thus part of the task. Subjects were free to arrange their route in advance and to fix appointments at different shops. In addition, they could revise their plans; but changes had to be made well in advance and became effective only after a delay of half an hour in system time.

The subjects were split into two groups according to their scores in an intelligence test. One half of each group received explicit planning instructions and was instructed to plan ahead; the other half of the group was not explicitly instructed and motivated to do so.

The following findings are of interest. (a) In terms of performance, groups with planning instructions were superior: they used shorter routes, spent less time in driving, and were more efficient in avoiding delays after arriving at the shops. Lower intelligence led to impaired performance. (b) Planning creates demand

and is accompanied by more mental involvement. Subjects with planning instructions consulted the city map more often and checked and changed their appointments more frequently. Subjects of either high or low intelligence did not show conspicuous differences in organizing the route when given planning instructions. Subjects of low intelligence were significantly less active than those of high intelligence when no explicit planning instructions were given. (c) Subjective reports and physiological measures of involvement showed that for low intelligent subjects scores were raised if planning instructions were given; but for high intelligent subjects the scores were higher, if planning instructions were lacking.

Obviously, the subjects who follow the planning instructions enjoy benefits which have already been discussed in the literature: by constructing and backing up a realistic cognitive model of their actions they avoid disorganization and, hence, effort and frustration during execution (Hacker, 1985). However, the costs of planning come into the picture, as well. The construction and backing up of plans put demands on individuals. They call for monitoring of actual states, comparisons between plans and actual states, and adaptation of plans to cope with deviation in actual states; such processes impose a mental load on individuals. In addition, the construction of plans may provoke worries concerning external difficulties, internal shortcomings and their adverse consequences, some of which may never be encountered while actually performing the task. In consequence, also an emotional load is associated with planning. Therefore, the question arises whether and when planning pays off. Under the conditions of the described experiment, the payoff appears to be high for more intelligent subjects but lower for the less intelligent ones. The more intelligent subjects do better in carrying the load of planning than the less intelligent subjects; but the intelligent subjects also report more irritation from the disorganization of unplanned work. Thus, avoiding disorganization by active planning yields a better trade-off for the high than for the low intelligent subjects.

Feedback

A third example is feedback. Positive feedback may be described as 'the heart of learning' (Anzai and Simon, 1979). It indicates the appropriateness of coping strategies, confirms that future events of a similar category can be mastered (Raynor, 1982), and, finally, gives the individual a 'warm glow of success' (Isen, 1970). However, the reverse is true for negative feedback turning it into a potent stressor. Therefore, in general, individuals expecting a negative outcome avoid feedback (Meyer and Starke, 1982; Sachs, 1982).

The difficulty of balancing the costs and benefits of feedback seeking is demonstrated in a series of laboratory studies with administrative tasks similar to the office work described above (Battmann, 1988). Using a data-base system, subjects had to calculate wages, decide about promotions and placements of employees. The data-base system offered, in addition, performance feedback indicating the correctness of the results, the quality of work, as well as a comparison with the performance of a control group. Subjects had to solve up to 120 tasks distributed over four sessions. Anxiety, intelligence, and the costs of obtaining feedback were used as independent variables. Anxiety was hypothesized to be associated with the need to reduce uncertainty and worries; intelligence was hypothesized to be associated with the need to improve performance. In one study, a delay between the request and the exposition of feedback information was introduced in order to vary the costs of obtaining the information.

The four most relevant results are as follows. (a) As for most realistic tasks, the informational value of feedback was limited: it explained only about 10% of the variance of performance. Such feedback can be a help in reducing uncertainty, but supports learning only marginally. (b) High-anxious individuals requested more performance feedback and rated it as more important than did low-anxious subjects. In addition, they reduced the request rate less strongly when feedback followed higher cost. (c) Feedback requests helped high-anxious subjects to attenuate their affective state. Uncertainty and emotional load decreased when feedback was available without cost, and increased when high cost constrained the use of the information. (d) Low-intelligent subjects solved considerably fewer tasks than high-intelligent ones, and, in general, requested less feedback. However, within the low-intelligent subjects, two groups can be differentiated: those giving up and those trying to gain control. The latter group showed a strong interest in learning and requested feedback primarily to improve the working strategy. However, since feedback supported learning only marginally, these subjects showed no improved performance but, instead, a considerable increase in emotional load due to the high rate of negative feedback received.

The results demonstrate both benefits and costs of feedback seeking as factors in coping and, in addition, allow a tentative evaluation of the balance between costs and benefits. For high-anxious subjects, feedback proved to be a powerful means for the regulation of the affective state; it helped to reduce uncertainty and worries. The need for feedback is most evident in the high-cost condition. Despite increased operational costs, anxious subjects tried to establish a satisfying feedback rate. As the growing uncertainty in this group reveals, this attempt was not a complete success. However, these subjects rated the feedback as particularly helpful. Therefore, the payoff may be regarded as positive.

However, as argued previously, due to adverse side-effects, the costs can outweigh the benefits of feedback. This is demonstrated by the low-intelligent subjects who sought feedback for its informational value. The strong need for feedback felt by these subjects is expressed in the readiness to tolerate frequent negative feedback. But this strategy did not pay off; instead of being rewarded by increasing performance, subjects began to feel the cumulative effects of emotional load.

A Short Outlook

In the future, more task situations can be studied which will yield more measures of psychological benefits and costs. However, what is needed more than an accumulation of measures is a rationale which provides a basis for comparison of different measures by construction of precise equivalence statements. Then, a dynamic balance of the economic features of coping in various task situations could be set up, and both trade-off and payoff functions in behaviour could be determined.

SUMMARY AND CONCLUSIONS

This chapter contrasts the benefits of efficient coping with the costs of coping attempts. Benefits and costs are defined as concepts related to personal, natural, technical and social resources. Benefits result from conservation and growth of resources, whereas costs originate from the loss of resources. The main sources of costs identified in this chapter are the operational costs of coping and the generation of new problems in the course of coping. In this context, coping is defined as a resource management process, and cost–benefit analyses are advocated for stressful situations.

Three examples of potentially stressful situations, to which a cost–benefit analysis has been applied, are presented: social cooperation, planning a days work, and requests for feedback. The examples demonstrate some benefits of coping; but they also give evidence that there are no benefits without costs, although there may be costs which are not balanced by benefits.

REFERENCES

Anzai, Y., & Simon, H.A. (1979). The theory of learning by doing. *Psychological Review*, 86, 124–140.

Apter, M.J. (1982). *The experience of motivation. The theory of psychological reversals*. London: Academic Press.

Battmann, W. (1984). Regulation und Fehlregulation im Verhalten. IX. Entlastung und Belastung durch Planung. *Psychologische Beiträge*, 26, 672–691.

Battmann, W. (1988). Requests of feedback as a means of self-assessment and affect optimization. *Motivation and Emotion*, 12, 57–74.

Battmann, W. (in preparation). Regulation und Fehlregulation im Verhalten. XIII. Entlastung und Belastung durch Kooperation. *Psychologische Beiträge*.

Baum, A., Fleming, R., & Singer, J.E. (1983). Coping with victimization by technological disaster. *Journal of Social Issues*, 39, 117–138.

Berglas, S., & Jones, E.E. (1978). Drug choice as a self-handicapping strategy in response to noncontingent success. *Journal of Personality and Social Psychology*, 36, 405–417.

Cohen, S. (1980). After effects of stress in human performance and social behavior: A review of research and theory. *Psychological Bulletin*, 88, 82–108.

Cohen, S., & Syme, S.L. (eds) (1985). *Social support and health*. New York: Academic Press.

Cohen, S., Evans, G.W., Stokols, D., & Krantz, D.S. (1986). *Behaviour, health, and environmental stress*. New York: Plenum.

Ellis, A. (1978). What people can do for themselves to cope with stress. In C.L. Cooper & R. Payne (eds), *Stress at work* (pp. 209–222). New York: Wiley.

Eysenck, M. (1983). Anxiety and individual differences. In G.R.J. Hockey (ed.), *Stress and fatigue in human performance* (pp. 273–298). Chichester: Wiley.

Fisher, J.P., Nadler, A., & DePaulo, D.M. (1983). *New directions in helping* (3 volumes). New York: Academic Press.

Frankenhaeuser, M. (1986). A psychobiological framework for research on human stress and coping. In M.H. Appley & R. Trumbull (eds), *Dynamics of stress* (pp. 101–116). New York: Plenum.

Fuchs, R. (1976). Furchtregulation und Furchthemmung des Zweckhandelns. In A. Thomas (ed.), *Psychologie der Handlung und Bewegung* (pp. 97–162). Meisenheim: Hain.

Glass, D.C., Singer, J.E., & Friedman, L.N. (1969). Psychic costs of adaptation to an environmental stressor. *Journal of Personality and Social Psychology, 12,* 200–210.

Hacker, W. (1985). Activity: A fruitful concept in industrial psychology. In M. Frese & J. Sabini (eds), *Goal directed behavior: The concept of action in psychology* (pp. 262–283). Hillsdale, NJ: Erlbaum.

Hobfoll, S.E. (1985). Limitations of social support in the stress process. In I.G. Sarason & B.R. Sarason (eds), *Social support: Theory, research and applications* (pp. 391–414). Dordrecht: Nijhoff

Hockey, G.R.J., Coles, M.G.H., & Gaillard, A.W.K. (1986). Energetical issues in research on human information processing. In G.R.J. Hockey, A.W.K. Gaillard & M.G.H. Coles (eds), *Energetics and human information processing* (pp. 3–21). Dordrecht: Nijhoff.

Isen, A.M. (1970). Success, failure, attention, and relation to others: The warm glow of success. *Journal of Personality and Social Psychology, 15,* 265–273.

Klonowicz, T. (1986). Reactivity and performance: The third side of the coin. In J. Strelau, F.H. Farley & A. Gale (eds), *The biological bases of personality and behaviour* Vol. 2 (pp. 119–126). Washington: Hemisphere.

Lazarus, R.S. (1983). Costs and benefits of denial. In S. Breznitz (ed.), *Denial of stress* (pp. 1–30). New York: International Universities Press.

Lazarus, R.S., & Folkman, S. (1984). *Stress, appraisal, and coping.* New York: Springer.

Levine, S., & Ursin, H. (eds) (1980). *Coping and health.* New York: Plenum.

Lumsden, D.P. (1975). Towards a systems model of stress: feedback from an anthropological study of the impact of Ghana's Volta River project. In I.G. Sarason & C.D. Spielberger (eds), *Stress and anxiety* Vol. 2 (pp. 191–228). New York: Wiley.

Mahler, W. (1933). Ersatzhandlungen verschiedenen Realitätsgrades. *Psychologische Forschung, 18,* 27–89.

Meyer, W.-U., & Starke, E. (1982). Seeking information about one's ability in relation to self-concept of ability: a field study. *Personality and Social Psychology Bulletin, 8,* 501–507.

Moos, R.H., & Billings, A.G. (1982). Conceptualizing and measuring coping resources and processes. In L. Goldberger & S. Breznitz (eds), *Handbook of stress* (pp. 212–230). New York: Free Press.

Norman, D.A. (1981). Categorization of action slips. *Psychological Review, 88,* 1–15.

Pittner, M.S., Houston, B.K., & Spiridigliozzi, G. (1983). Control over stress, Type A behavior pattern, and response to stress. *Journal of Personality and Social Psychology, 44,* 627–637.

Posner, M.I., & Rothbart, M.K. (1986). The concept of energy in psychological theory. In G.R.J. Hockey, A.W.K. Gaillard & M.G.H. Coles (eds), *Energetics and human information processing* (pp. 23–40). Dordrecht: Nijhoff.

Raynor, J.O. (1982). Future orientation, self-evaluation, and achievement motivation: Use of an expectancy × value theory of personality functioning and change. In N.T. Feather (ed.), *Expectations and actions* (pp. 97–124). Hillsdale, NJ: Erlbaum.

Reason, J. (1979). Actions not as planned: The price of automatization. In G. Underwood & R. Stevens (eds), *Aspects of consciousness* Vol. 1 (pp. 67–89). London: Academic Press.

Sachs, P.R. (1982). Avoidance of diagnostic information in self-evaluation of ability. *Personality and Social Psychology Bulletin, 8,* 242–246.

Sarason, I.G., & Sarason, B.R. (eds) (1985). *Social support: Theory, research and applications.* Dordrecht: Nijhoff.

Schwarzer, R., Jerusalem, M., & Stiksrud, H.A. (1984). The developmental relationship between test anxiety and helplessness. In H.M. van der Ploeg, R. Schwarzer & C.D. Spielberger (eds), *Advances in test anxiety research* Vol. 3 (pp. 73–79). Lisse: Swets & Zeitlinger.

Schönpflug, W. (1982). Coping and the generation of stress. In W. Bachmann & I. Udris (eds), *Mental load and stress in activity* (pp. 18–23). Amsterdam: North-Holland.

Schönpflug, W. (1983). Coping efficiency and situational demands. In G.R.J. Hockey (ed.), *Stress and fatigue in human performance* (pp. 299–330). Chichester: Wiley.

Schönpflug, W. (1984). Activity style of anxious individuals. In H.M. van de Ploeg, R. Schwarzer & C.D. Spielberger (eds), *Advances in test anxiety research* Vol. 3 (pp. 163–172). Hillsdale, NJ: Erlbaum.

Schönpflug, W. (1985). Goal directed behavior as a source of stress: Psychological origins and consequences of inefficiency. In M. Frese & J. Sabini (eds), *Goal directed behavior: The concept of action in psychology* (pp. 172–188). Hillsdale, NJ: Erlbaum.

Schönpflug, W. (1986a). Behavior economics as an approach to stress theory. In M.H. Appley & R. Trumbull (eds), *Dynamics of stress* (pp. 81–98). New York: Plenum.

Schönpflug, W. (1986b). Effort regulation and individual diferences in effort expenditure. In G.R.J. Hockey, A.W.K. Gaillard & M.G.H. Coles (eds), *Energetics and human information processing* (pp. 271–284). Dordrecht: Nijhoff.

Scitovsky, T. (1976). *The joyless society*. New York: Oxford University Press.

Snyder, C.R., & Smith, I.W. (1982). Symptoms as self-handicapping strategies: The virtues of old wine in a new bottle. In G. Weary & H.I. Mirels (eds), *Integration of clinical and social psychology* (pp. 104–127). New York: Oxford University Press.

Strelau, J. (1983). *Temperament, acitivity, personality*. New York: Academic Press.

Tomaszewski, T. (1967). Aktywnosz czowieka. In M. Maruszewski, J. Reykowski & T. Tomaszewski (eds), *Psychologia jako nauka c czlowieku* (pp. 53–84). Warszawa: Kalaszka i Wiedza.

Wieland-Eckelmann, R. (1986). Regulation und Fehlregulation im Verhalten. XI. Zur Makro- und Mikrostruktur des Leistungshandelns. *Psychologische Beiträge, 28*, 457–487.

Zuckerman, M., Buchsbaum, M.T., & Murphy, L. (1980). Sensation seeking and its biological correlates. *Psychological Bulletin, 38*, 187–214.

KEY WORDS

Adaptation, anxiety, appraisal, catecholamines, challenge, cooperation, coping, cost–benefit analysis, disengagement, efficiency, effort, failure, feedback, loss, planning, problem generation, psychic benefits, psychic costs, reactivity, resource conservation, resource enlargement, resourced management, resources, self-handicapping, social support, stress, technical support, threat.

Author Index

715

Subject Index